Essentials of Consultation-Liaison Psychiatry

Based on
The American Psychiatric Press
Textbook of
Consultation-Liaison Psychiatry

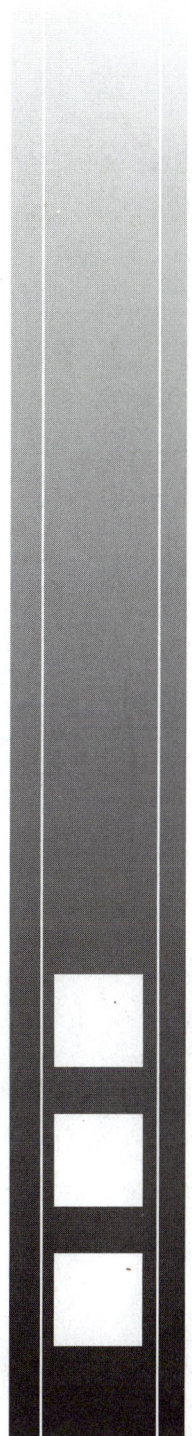

Essentials of Consultation-Liaison Psychiatry

Based on
The American Psychiatric Press
Textbook of
Consultation-Liaison Psychiatry

Edited by
James R. Rundell, M.D.
Michael G. Wise, M.D.

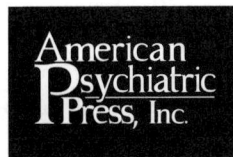

American
Psychiatric
Press, Inc.

Washington, DC
London, England

Copyright © 1999 American Psychiatric Press, Inc.
ALL RIGHTS RESERVED
Manufactured in the United States of America on acid-free paper
02 01 00 99   4 3 2 1
First Edition

American Psychiatric Press, Inc.
1400 K Street, N.W., Washington, DC   20005

Library of Congress Cataloging-in-Publication Data
Essentials of consultation-liaison psychiatry : based on the American
    Psychiatric Press textbook of consultation-liaison psychiatry /
    edited by James R. Rundell, Michael G. Wise. — 1st ed.
        p.   cm.
    Includes bibliographical references and index.
    ISBN 0-88048-801-8 (alk. paper)
    1. Consultation-liaison psychiatry.   I. Rundell, James R., 1957–   .
II. Wise, Michael G., 1944–   .   III. American Psychiatric Press.
IV. American Psychiatric Press textbook of consultation-liaison
psychiatry.
    [DNLM: 1. Mental Disorders—diagnosis.   2. Mental Disorders—
therapy.   3. Psychiatry.   4. Referral and Consultation.   WM 140
E78 1999]
RC455.2.C65E87   1999
616.89—dc21
DNLM/DLC
for Library of Congress   98-54234
                                                                         CIP

British Library Cataloguing in Publication Data
A CIP record is available from the British Library.

Contents

Section I
General Principles

Section II
Psychiatric Disorders in General Hospital Patients

Section III
Clinical Consultation-Liaison Settings

Section IV
Treatment

Contributors

Susan E. Abbey, M.D., F.R.C.P.C.
Assistant Professor, Department of Psychiatry, University of Toronto; and Director, Psychosomatic Medicine Program, The Toronto Hospital, Toronto, Ontario, Canada

Mark D. Beale, M.D.
Assistant Professor, Department of Psychiatry and Behavioral Sciences, Medical University of South Carolina, Charleston, South Carolina

Duane S. Bishop, M.D.
Associate Professor, Department of Psychiatry and Human Behavior, Brown University, Providence, Rhode Island

John Michael Bostwick, M.D.
Chief, Consultation-Liaison Psychiatry, Wilford Hall Medical Center, Lackland Air Force Base, Texas

Anthony J. Bouckoms, M.D.
Director, Consultation-Liaison Psychiatry, Hartford Hospital; Associate Professor of Psychiatry, University of Connecticut; and Assistant Medical Director, Institute of Living, Hartford, Connecticut

William Breitbart, M.D.
Associate Professor of Clinical Psychiatry, Cornell University Medical College; and Associate Attending Psychiatrist, Memorial Sloan-Kettering Cancer Center, New York City

Lewis M. Cohen, M.D.
Director, Psychiatric Consultation Service, Baystate Medical Center, Springfield, Massachusetts; and Clinical Assistant Professor of Psychiatry, Tufts Medical School, Boston, Massachusetts

Eduardo A. Colón, M.D.
Director, Consultation Psychiatry Service, Hennepin County Medical Center, Minneapolis, Minnesota; and Associate Professor of Psychiatry, University of Minnesota Medical School, Minneapolis, Minnesota

Jeffrey L. Cummings, M.D.
Director, UCLA Alzheimer's Disease Center, Professor of Neurology and Psychiatry & Biobehavioral Sciences, UCLA School of Medicine; and Chief, Behavioral Neuroscience Section, Psychiatry Service, West Los Angeles Veterans Affairs Medical Center, Los Angeles, California

Richard S. Epstein, M.D.
Clinical Professor, Department of Psychiatry, Uniformed Services University of the Health Sciences, F. Edward Hebert School of Medicine, Bethesda, Maryland

Fawzy I. Fawzy, M.D.
Professor, Department of Psychiatry and Biobehavioral Sciences, School of Medicine, University of California, Los Angeles, California

Marc D. Feldman, M.D.
Associate Professor of Psychiatry; Vice Chairman for Clinical Services; Medical Director, Center for Psychiatric Medicine, Department of Psychiatry and Behavioral Neurobiology, University of Alabama at Birmingham, Birmingham, Alabama

Charles V. Ford, M.D.
Professor of Psychiatry; Director, Neuropsychiatry Clinic; Director, Division of Adult Services, Department of Psychiatry and Behavioral Neurobiology, University of Alabama at Birmingham, Birmingham, Alabama; and President (1995–1996), Academy of Psychosomatic Medicine

Richard J. Frances, M.D.
Director, Department of Psychiatry, Institute for Psychotherapy and Counseling of Hackensack Medical Center, Hackensack, New Jersey; and Professor of Clinical Psychiatry, University of Medicine and Dentistry of New Jersey, New Jersey Medical School, Newark, New Jersey

John E. Franklin, Jr., M.D.
Associate Professor of Psychiatry and Behavioral Sciences, Northwestern University Medical School, Chicago, Illinois

Gregory Fricchione, M.D.
Associate Professor of Psychiatry, Harvard Medical School, Brigham and Women's Hospital, Boston, Massachusetts

Alan J. Gelenberg, M.D.
Professor and Head, Department of Psychiatry, University of Arizona, Arizona Health Sciences Center, Tucson, Arizona

Kevin F. Gray, M.D.
Director, Memory Disorders Clinic, Dallas Veterans Affairs Medical Center; and Assistant Professor of Psychiatry and Neurology, University of Texas Southwestern Medical School, Dallas, Texas

Donna B. Greenberg, M.D.
Assistant Professor of Psychiatry, Harvard Medical School; and Psychiatrist and Director of Medical Student Teaching, Massachusetts General Hospital, Boston, Massachusetts

Ibrahim Gunay, M.D.
Geriatric Psychiatrist, Department of Psychiatry and Biobehavioral Sciences, University of California, Los Angeles School of Medicine, Neuropsychiatric Institute and Hospital; and the Geriatric Psychiatry Program of the West Los Angeles Veterans Affairs Medical Center, Los Angeles, California

Robert E. Hales, M.D.
Professor and Vice Chairman, Department of Psychiatry, University of California, Davis; and Medical Director, Sacramento County Mental Health Division and Treatment Center

Richard C. W. Hall, M.D.
Medical Director, Psychiatric Programs, Florida Hospital, Center for Psychiatry, Orlando, Florida; Clinical Professor of Psychiatry, University of Florida, Gainesville, Florida

Mark H. Halman, M.D., F.R.C.P.C.
Director, HIV Psychiatry Program, The Wellesley/St. Michaels Mental Health Service; and Lecturer in Psychiatry, University of Toronto, Toronto, Ontario, Canada

Peter Halperin, M.D.
Physician-in-Chief, Marino Center for Progressive Health, Cambridge, Massachusetts; and Instructor in Psychiatry, Harvard Medical School, Tufts Medical School, Boston, Massachusetts

Alisa K. Hoffman, Ph.D.
Staff Psychologist, Department of Psychiatry, University of California School of Medicine, Los Angeles, California

Jimmie Holland, M.D.
Vice Chairman, Department of Psychiatry, Cornell University Medical College; and Chief, Psychiatry Service, Wayne E. Chapman Chair of Psychiatric Oncology, New York City

John S. Jachna, M.D.
Assistant Professor, University of Arizona College of Medicine; and Acting Chief of Psychiatry; Director, Consultation-Liaison Psychiatry, Tucson, Arizona

Karen M. Johnson, M.D.
Assistant Professor of Psychiatry and Behavioral Sciences, Emory University School of Medicine; and Chief, Consultation-Liaison Service, Grady Memorial Hospital, Atlanta, Georgia

Roger Kathol, M.D.
Professor of Internal Medicine and Psychiatry; Director, Medical Psychiatry, University of Iowa, Iowa City, Iowa

Charles H. Kellner, M.D.
Professor and Deputy Chair, Department of Psychiatry and Behavioral Sciences, Department of Neurology, Medical University of South Carolina, Charleston, South Carolina

Mark W. Ketterer, Ph.D.
Senior Bioscientific Staff, Henry Ford Health Sciences Center, Case Western Reserve University School of Medicine, Detroit, Michigan

Richard L. Kradin, M.D.
Associate Pathologist, Assistant Physician, Department of Medicine; Consultant Psychoimmunologist, Department of Psychiatry; Massachusetts General Hospital; and Associate Professor of Pathology, Harvard Medical School, Boston, Massachusetts

Richard D. Lane, M.D.
Associate Professor, Department of Psychiatry, Arizona Health Sciences Center, Tucson, Arizona

Susan G. Lazar, M.D.
Clinical Professor of Psychiatry and Behavioral Sciences, George Washington University Medical School, Washington, D.C.; Clinical Professor of Psychiatry, Uniformed Services University of the Health Sciences, F. Edward Hebert School of Medicine, Bethesda, Maryland; and Teaching Analyst, Washington Psychoanalytic Institute, Washington, D.C.

Don R. Lipsitt, M.D.
Clinical Professor, Department of Psychiatry, Harvard Medical School, Boston, Massachusetts

Andrew B. Littman, M.D.
Director, Behavioral Medicine, Division of Preventive Cardiology, and Department of Psychiatry, Massachusetts General Hospital; and Associate Professor, Harvard Medical School, Boston, Massachusetts

R. Bruce Lydiard, M.D., Ph.D.
Department of Psychiatry and Behavioral Sciences, Medical University of South Carolina, Charleston, South Carolina

J. Stephen McDaniel, M.D.
Assistant Professor of Psychiatry, Department of Psychiatry and Behavioral Sciences, Emory University School of Medicine; and Medical Director, Mental Health Services, Grady Infectious Disease Program, Atlanta, Georgia

George B. Murray, M.D.
Associate Professor of Psychiatry, Harvard Medical School, Massachusetts General Hospital, Boston, Massachusetts

Kevin W. Olden, M.D., F.A.C.P.
Assistant Clinical Professor of Medicine (Gastroenterology) and Psychiatry, University of California, San Francisco, California

Robert O. Pasnau, M.D.
Professor, Department of Psychiatry and Biobehavioral Sciences; and Assistant Dean, University of California School of Medicine, Los Angeles, California

L. Russell Pet, M.D.
Senior Psychiatry Resident, Department of Psychiatry and Human Behavior, Brown University, Providence, Rhode Island

Michael K. Popkin, M.D., F.A.P.M.
Chief of Psychiatry, Hennepin County Medical Center, Minneapolis, Minnesota; and Professor of Psychiatry and Medicine, University of Minnesota Medical School, Minneapolis, Minnesota

Richard Pounds, M.D.
Assistant Professor, University of Kentucky Medical School; Director, Consultation-Liaison Psychiatry; and Co-Director, Child and Adult Forensic Psychiatry Clinic, Lexington, Kentucky

Alvin M. Rouchell, M.D.
Head, Consultation-Liaison Service, Department of Psychiatry, Ochsner Clinic; and Clinical Professor of Psychiatry, Tulane University School of Medicine, New Orleans, Louisiana

James R. Rundell, M.D.
Professor of Psychiatry, Uniformed Services University of the Health Sciences, Bethesda, Maryland; and Chief of Medical Staff, 86th Medical Group, Ramstein Air Base, Germany

John L. Shuster, Jr., M.D.
Director, Division of Medical/Surgical Psychiatry; Director, Psychiatric Consultation Service; Assistant Professor of Psychiatry, University of Alabama School of Medicine at Birmingham, Birmingham, Alabama

Jonathan M. Silver, M.D.
Associate Professor of Clinical Psychiatry, Columbia University College of Physicians & Surgeons; and Director, Columbia Presbyterian Psychiatric Associates, New York City

Gregory E. Simon, M.D., M.P.H.
Staff Psychiatrist, Mental Health Service, Group Health Cooperative of Puget Sound; and Research Assistant Professor, Department of Psychiatry and Behavioral Sciences, University of Washington, Seattle, Washington

Robert I. Simon, M.D.
Clinical Professor of Psychiatry and Director, Program in Psychiatry and Law, Georgetown University School of Medicine, Washington, D.C.

Christine E. Skotzko, M.D.
Assistant Professor of Psychiatry, University of Maryland at Baltimore School of Medicine; and Medical Director, Substance Abuse Treatment Unit, Baltimore Veterans Administration Medical Center, Baltimore, Maryland

Gary W. Small, M.D.
Associate Professor, Department of Psychiatry and Biobehavioral Sciences, University of California, Los Angeles School of Medicine; and Director, Geriatric Psychiatry Consultation Service, West Los Angeles Veterans Affairs Medical Center, Los Angeles, California

Theodore A. Stern, M.D.
Chief, The Avery D. Weisman, M.D., Psychiatry Consultation Service, Massachusetts General Hospital; and Associate Professor of Psychiatry, Harvard Medical School, Boston, Massachusetts

Nada L. Stotland, M.D.
Associate Professor, Departments of Psychiatry and Obstetrics/Gynecology, University of Chicago, Chicago, Illinois

James J. Strain, M.D.
Professor of Consultation-Liaison Psychiatry and Behavioral Medicine, Mount Sinai School of Medicine; and Director, Division of Behavioral Medicine, Mt. Sinai Medical Center, New York City

Thomas B. Strouse, M.D.
Assistant Clinical Professor of Psychiatry, UCLA School of Medicine; and Director, Psychosocial Services, Cedars-Sinai Comprehensive Cancer Center, Los Angeles, California

Richard L. Strub, M.D.
Chairman, Department of Neurology, Ochsner Clinic; and Clinical Professor of Neurology, Tulane University School of Medicine, New Orleans, Louisiana

George E. Tesar, M.D.
Chairman, Department of Psychiatry and Psychology, Cleveland Clinic Foundation, Cleveland, Ohio

John G. Tierney, M.D.
Clinical Assistant Professor of Psychiatry, Emory University Medical School, Atlanta, Georgia

Paula T. Trzepacz, M.D.
Associate Professor of Psychiatry, University of Pittsburgh School of Medicine, Western Psychiatric Institute and Clinic, University of Pittsburgh Medical Center, Pittsburgh, Pennsylvania

Robert J. Ursano, M.D.
Professor of Psychiatry and Neuroscience; Chairman, Department of Psychiatry, Uniformed Services University of the Health Sciences, F. Edward Hebert School of Medicine, Bethesda, Maryland

Edward A. Walker, M.D.
Assistant Professor, Department of Psychiatry and Behavioral Sciences, University of Washington, Seattle, Washington

Jeffrey B. Weilburg, M.D.
Assistant Professor of Psychiatry, Harvard Medical School; and Instructor in Psychiatry, Massachusetts General Hospital, Boston, Massachusetts

David K. Wellisch, Ph.D.
Professor-in-Residence, Department of Psychiatry, University of California School of Medicine, Los Angeles, California

Ilona Wiener, M.D.
Assistant Clinical Professor of Psychiatry, Columbia University College of Physicians & Surgeons; and Assistant Attendng Psychiatrist, Columbia Presbyterian Medical Center, New York City

John W. Winkelman, M.D., Ph.D.
Instructor in Psychiatry, Harvard Medical School; and Medical Director, Sleep Disorders Center, McLean Hospital, Boston, Massachusetts

Michael G. Wise, M.D.
Clinical Professor of Psychiatry, Louisiana State University School of Medicine and Tulane School of Medicine, New Orleans, Louisiana; and Clinical Professor of Psychiatry, Uniformed Services University of the Health Sciences, F. Edward Hebert School of Medicine, Bethesda, Maryland

Deane L. Wolcott, M.D.
Director, Psychological Services, Comprehensive Cancer Centers, Inc., and Pain Management Services, Salick Health Care, Inc., Los Angeles, California

Jonathan L. Worth, M.D.
Instructor in Psychiatry, Harvard Medical School; and Associate Psychiatrist, Massachusetts General Hospital, Boston, Massachusetts

Stuart C. Yudofsky, M.D.
D.C. and Irene Ellwood Professor and Chairman, Department of Psychiatry and Behavioral Sciences, Baylor College of Medicine; and Psychiatrist-in-Chief, The Methodist Hospital, Houston, Texas

Preface

In 1987, we wrote the *Concise Guide to Consultation Psychiatry*. We endeavored to make that book practical and clinically focused. It became one of the most popular books of the Concise Guide series and found its way into the laboratory coat pockets of many psychiatrists, psychiatric fellows and residents, nonpsychiatric physician colleagues, and medical students. The American Psychiatric Press subsequently agreed to publish a comprehensive textbook of consultation-liaison psychiatry, employing the same successful approach used for the *Concise Guide*.

Consultation-liaison psychiatrists often refer to textbooks from disciplines related to the consultation-liaison/medical-surgical psychiatry field, such as behavioral medicine, behavioral neurology, and neuropsychiatry. Indeed, these textbooks are referenced frequently throughout this textbook. However, clinicians who evaluate and treat medically ill patients with psychiatric syndromes need a unifying, comprehensive, and practical textbook. The demand for such a comprehensive textbook has increased with efforts to attain "added qualifications" status for consultation-liaison psychiatry. That effort requires a textbook that consolidates the body of knowledge important to the field.

For the first time, *The American Psychiatric Press Textbook of Consultation-Liaison Psychiatry* brought together clinical leaders in the consultation-liaison field to share their knowledge, experience, and research. An impressive group of almost 100 authors described their clinical experience in the evaluation and treatment of psychiatric disorders in patients with concomitant medical or surgical illness.

The purpose of *Essentials of Consultation-Liaison Psychiatry* is to present the body of knowledge of consultation-liaison psychiatry in a clinically concise manner. This book is a primary resource for psychiatrists who perform consultation and liaison work, treat patients with concurrent psychiatric and medical-surgical conditions, or use a medical model in their general psychiatry practice. It is also designed for psychiatry residents rotating on consultation-liaison services; physicians and health care professionals in related fields such as internal medicine, neurology, family practice, neuropsychology, and behavioral health psychology; as well as medical and mental health colleagues who have a strong interest in neurobehavioral syndromes that occur in medical and surgical patients.

Psychiatrists who consult with medical-surgical patients with psychiatric symptoms must understand unique aspects of evaluation and treatment in a variety of clinical settings. To aid in this process, the textbook is organized into four sections: General Principles, Psychiatric Disorders in General Hospital Patients (e.g., depressive syndromes, anxiety syndromes), Clinical Consultation-Liaison Settings (e.g., neurology, rehabilitation medicine, primary care), and Treatment. Although this occasionally results in overlap among chapters, we believe that this is the best approach for learning about consultation and liaison work. Knowledge about the diagnosis and differential diagnosis of psychiatric syndromes, as well as the context of care delivery, improves the psychiatrist's ability to render effective recommendations in a language and manner relevant to the clinical setting. For example, we foresee that a clinician who consults on a disoriented posttransplant patient may refer to chapters on mental status examination, delirium, and transplantation. In addition, readers will discover that the text is applicable to both outpatient and inpatient medical-surgical populations. Psychiatrists who are working in primary care settings will find this textbook as useful as psychiatrists who are consulting or treating patients in tertiary care subspecialty settings.

The emerging consensus among psychiatrists is that long-established principles of consultation-liaison psychiatry hold the key to psychiatry's future. These principles view the psychiatrist as someone who is 1) an expert in the mental status examination, 2) knowledgeable about medical conditions and treatments, 3) able to communicate with other physicians using the vocabulary and metaphors of medicine, 4) skilled at forming a comprehensive biopsychosocial differential diagnosis, 5) comfortable working with medical-surgical colleagues, 6) skilled in both psychopharmacology and psychotherapy, 7) cost-effective, and 8) able to work in a variety of unique medical and surgical settings.

This textbook would not have been published without the support and efforts of many people. First, we thank the chapter authors for their outstanding work and scholarly manuscripts. We also thank them for their patience; we often asked authors to write and rewrite several drafts before their work was finished. We asked authors to add tables where appropriate. Useful tables are not easy to construct. We hope that the reader will appreciate the authors' efforts to produce tables with clinically relevant material that are amenable to copying, putting on notecards, and carrying in laboratory coat pockets. Chapter authors universally responded

to our litany of perfectionistic requests with grace and good humor—we thank them.

We also want to express our gratitude to the textbook's editorial board. Each member peer reviewed several chapters and provided vision, guidance, and focus as we endeavored to create a textbook to unify the body of knowledge contained in consultation-liaison psychiatry. We also want to thank the chapter reviewers who were not part of the editorial board: Drs. Andrea DiMartini, Steven Dubovsky, Frank Fernandez, Ken Hoffman, Valerie Holmes, Michael Jellinek, James Levenson, John Lion, Steven McDaniel, Mary Moskowitz, Quentin Regestein, Judith Roheim, Kathy Sanders, and Gary Small. The outstanding staff at American Psychiatric Press deserves praise for publishing this textbook and for their hard work on it.

A special thanks goes to Cheryl Balot, who has kept us organized and on track with tight timelines. It is a logistical nightmare to keep track of the efforts, not to mention the locations, of almost 100 authors. At any point in time, the 44 chapters contained in this textbook were at different stages of review, rewriting, and editing. Cheryl has been a lighthearted, patient, and persistent organizer of this entire effort. This textbook would not exist without her.

Finally, we thank our families for their patience and forbearance during the years of hard work this textbook required. Only they know the night and weekend hours that this project required. They never asked us to stop, slow down, quit, or let someone else do it. Somehow they understood that this textbook was a critical effort for all of those medical-surgical patients who experience stigma, undiagnosed psychiatric conditions, and untreated psychiatric illnesses.

James R. Rundell, M.D.
Michael G. Wise, M.D.

Dedication

This textbook is dedicated to several important people. I dedicate the book first to my father, who died in 1993 of complications of multiple sclerosis. We experienced firsthand the devastating effects of brain disease on every aspect of life.

I also dedicate this textbook to two psychoanalysts—M. Richard Fragala, M.D., and Robert Ursano, M.D.—giants of medicine in the military. They taught me the importance of seeing consultation-liaison patients in the context of their life trajectories rather than as mere cross-sectional collections of signs and symptoms.

Finally, I dedicate this book to Ned Cassem, M.D., and George Murray, M.D., mentors in the truest sense of the word. These pages are heavily influenced by their collective wisdom and experience.

—James R. Rundell, M.D.

I dedicate this textbook to several important people. The first and foremost is Buffy, my wife. Without her tolerance and consistent encouragement, this textbook would not exist.

I also dedicate this textbook to three of my mentors—Thomas Hackett, M.D., Ned Cassem, M.D., and George Murray, M.D. Each taught me valuable lessons that helped to shape this book and my career.

To Tom Hackett, who was an unassumingly brilliant, indefatigable, always curious, and kind man. It is regrettable that future consultation-liaison psychiatrists will not know him.

To Ned Cassem, who is the consummate, erudite clinician. His uncompromising drive for excellence in teaching and clinical treatment is unparalleled.

To George Murray, who is the ultimate observer and interpreter of behavior. His unrelenting questions about the patient's behavior, or my emotional response to the patient, during a consultation were eye-opening and always instructive.

—Michael G. Wise, M.D.

We also dedicate this book to Cheryl Balot, who for the last 8 years has nurtured this textbook from birth to adulthood. We thank her for her selfless contribution to this book.

—James R. Rundell, M.D., and Michael G. Wise, M.D.

Introduction

George Henry's paper published by the *American Journal of Psychiatry* in 1929 marks the beginning of consultation-liaison psychiatry as we know it today (Lipowski 1992). From these origins, now almost 3,000 American psychiatrists devote at least 25% of their professional time to consultation-liaison activities (Noyes et al. 1992). These past 65-plus years were fertile soil for the intellectual growth of psychosomatic medicine, somatopsychic medicine, the roles of stress in the etiology of disease states, and the beneficial effects of social support systems. These important ideas have found wide support among medical professionals and the general public (Lipowski 1987). As a result, and because of the pioneering work by persons such as Eugene Meyer, George Henry, Helen Flanders Dunbar, and Edward Billings, consultation-liaison psychiatrists have been at the forefront of the progressive incorporation of psychiatry into the mainstream of modern medicine.

Consultation-liaison psychiatry is increasingly accepted as an important part of psychiatric education. The American Council on Graduate Medical Education requires clinical experience in consultation-liaison psychiatry for all general psychiatry residents. Standards for consultation-liaison fellowship training have been established; standards for consultation-liaison training in general psychiatry residency programs are forthcoming (Ford et al. 1994). This growing body of systematically collected medical-scientific knowledge, as well as the efforts of a number of national leaders, led to the recommendation by the American Psychiatric Association that consultation-liaison psychiatry be formally recognized as a subspecialty by the American Board of Psychiatry and Neurology. The evolution of consultation-liaison psychiatry as a defined and recognized subspecialty has driven an often vigorous debate as to the goals and limits of the field of psychiatry (Wise and Ford 1991). Irrespective of the ultimate outcome, there is little question that consultation-liaison psychiatry meets the criteria for a subspecialty as defined by the American Psychiatric Association (Lipowski 1992). The most clinically relevant of these subspecialty criteria form the four sections of this textbook: clinical skills, a knowledge base about specific medical and psychiatric disorders, defined patient-based clinical settings, and specific treatment modalities.

The specific skills required of the consultation-liaison psychiatrist include 1) the ability to conduct detailed mental status examinations and to interpret findings in conjunction with modern technological tests such as neuroimaging; 2) the capacity to assess the potential for suicidality, aggression, and agitation within a medical-surgical setting; 3) the capacity to apply medical, legal, and ethical principles in the psychiatric management of physically ill patients; and 4) the ability to work with and clearly communicate findings and recommendations to nonpsychiatric physicians, other health care workers, and families. The consultation-liaison psychiatrist must also be knowledgeable about psychiatric and medical comorbidity, the various psychiatric presentations of medical illnesses, and the use of medical symptoms or simulated physical disease to communicate psychosocial distress. In addition, expertise in the diagnosis and management of delirium, dementia, depression, anxiety, and the effects of toxic substances is essential in the medical setting.

The traditional setting for the practice of consultation-liaison psychiatry is the general hospital. Within this medical environment, especially in highly specialized areas such as transplantation, psychiatrists increasingly function as integral parts of medical care teams. As general medicine is less hospital-based and more outpatient-oriented, consultation-liaison psychiatrists have made this shift. Outpatient consultation-liaison services are increasingly common.

In the past, the liaison psychiatrist was at times stereotypically depicted as a pleasant, pipe-smoking gentleman wearing a tweed jacket who, with much time on his hands, proselytized for the psychosocial model. Assuming that was ever an accurate description, we can confidently say that this stereotype has changed. Present-day consultation-liaison psychiatrists, both men and women, must possess a fund of knowledge about the physiological/psychological responses to advanced technologies and high-stress medical settings, the interactions and psychotropic effects of a wide variety of medications, and the emotional responses to advanced therapies such as in vitro fertilization and organ transplantation. With effective integration of the consultation-liaison psychiatrist into the treatment team, the components of psychiatric liaison and consultation merge. The results include education of health care personnel about psychological issues, improvements in patient care, and attention to systemic issues that influence the quality of life for both patients and care providers. Each medical care setting has its own micro-ecological characteristics; the consultation-liaison psychiatrist must know how to best meet the needs of specific programs and providers. For example, the characteristics and psychi-

atric issues of an intensive care unit differ greatly from those of a physical medicine and rehabilitation center.

The value of a psychiatric consultation to the patient, to the physician seeking consultation, or to a system depends on the success of recommendations made. Philosophical formulations, regardless of how accurate, are useless unless they positively influence diagnosis, management, or treatment of the patient. In order to do this, the consultation-liaison psychiatrist must communicate clearly and know psychiatric medications and their interactions with those medications used for medical-surgical illness. This textbook contains a detailed discussion of psychopharmacology. Nonpharmacological interventions are also important. Behavioral techniques are invaluable in the treatment of patients with somatization syndromes including chronic pain. Psychotherapy, particularly that which is focused on acute problems, is an essential treatment for many medically ill patients. Early psychiatric consultation, with diagnosis and treatment of psychiatric comorbidity, not only improves the quality of life for the medical patient but, as research described in this textbook demonstrates, often results in shorter hospitalizations and reduced costs and resource utilization.

This textbook brings together the body of knowledge and skills that defines the subspecialty of consultation-liaison psychiatry. During the past 65 years, scientific knowledge about interrelations between psychological factors and medical illness has greatly advanced. Yet, past publications of consultation-liaison pioneers make it obvious that many issues remain remarkably unchanged. Among these issues are the personal motivations and enthusiasm of consultation-liaison psychiatrists, which are qualities possessed by all great clinicians. I believe that most consultation-liaison psychiatrists would endorse the words of orthopedic surgeon Lorin Stephens in an address he made to a graduating medical school class: " . . . to be a physician, to be permitted to be invited by another human being into his life in the circumstances of the crucible which is illness, to be a trusted participant in the highest of dramas, for these privileges I am grateful beyond my ability to express . . . " (Werner and Korsch 1976, p. 327).

Although the twenty-first century consultation-liaison psychiatrist will use knowledge and skills that we cannot envision, he or she must retain a commitment to medical excellence, a respect for patients, and a love of medicine. Consultation-liaison psychiatrists exemplify these qualities and will remain "real doctors" who are participants in the high dramas of birth, illness, and death.

Charles V. Ford, M.D.

REFERENCES

Ford CV, Fawzy FI, Frankel BL, et al: Fellowship training in consultation-liaison psychiatry. Psychosomatics 35:118–124, 1994

Lipowski ZJ: The interface of psychiatry and medicine: toward integrated health care. Can J Psychiatry 32:743–748, 1987

Lipowski ZJ: Consultation-liaison psychiatry at century's end. Psychosomatics 33:128–133, 1992

Noyes R, Wise TN, Hayes JR: Consultation-liaison psychiatrists; how many are there and how are they funded? Psychosomatics 33:123–127, 1992

Werner ER, Korsch BM: The vulnerability of the medical student: posthumous presentation of L.L. Stephens' ideas. Pediatrics 57:321–328, 1976

Wise TN, Ford CV: Subspecialization at the crossroads. Psychosomatics 32:121–123, 1991

Section I

General Principles

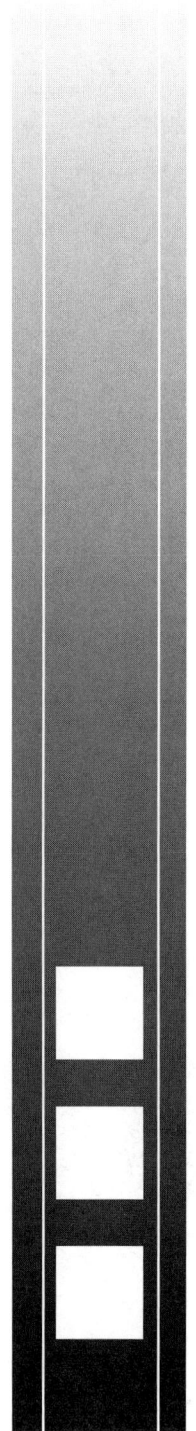

Chapter 1

Liaison Psychiatry

James J. Strain, M.D.

A distinction must be made between a consultation service and a consultation liaison service. A consultation service is a rescue squad. It responds to requests from other services for help with the diagnosis, treatment, or disposition of perplexing patients. At worst, consultation work is nothing more than a brief foray into the territory of another service, usually ending with a note written in the chart outlining a plan of action. The actual intervention is left to the consultee. Like a volunteer firefighter, a consultant puts out the blaze and then returns home. Like a volunteer fire brigade, a consultation service seldom has the time or manpower to set up fire prevention programs or to educate the citizenry about fireproofing. A consultation service is the most common type of psychiatric-medical interface found in the departments of psychiatry around the United States today.

A liaison service requires manpower, money, and motivation. Sufficient personnel are necessary to allow the psychiatric consultant time to perform services other than simply interviewing troublesome patients in the area assigned to him. He must be able to attend rounds, discuss patients individually with house officers, and hold teaching sessions for nurses. Liaison work is further distin-

guished from consultation activity in that patients are seen at the discretion of the psychiatric consultant as well as the referring physicians. Because the consultant attends social service rounds with the house officers, he is able to spot potential psychiatric problems. (Hackett and Cassem 1979, p. 5)

Liaison psychiatry is positioned at the interface of psychiatry and medicine. It includes not only the traditional psychiatric consultation on an individual patient, but going beyond this essential task to establish the psychiatrist as a bona fide member of the medical-surgical team. Establishing a liaison relationship means that the psychiatrist will be in contact with all the psychiatric and medical comorbidity on a unit or ward, and not only be consultant to those identified and referred. In epidemiological terms liaison psychiatry attempts to deal with the **denominator** of the prevalence of psychiatric morbidity in the medical setting, whereas consultation psychiatry, by the very nature of the referral process, is involved only with the **numerator.** (Strain and Strain 1988, p. 76)

Consultation is the method by which one medical discipline interacts with another. It requires that one discipline discern when the needs of another discipline are extant. Data demonstrate that at least with regard to psychiatry, the medical-surgical specialties recognize relatively few patients with psychiatric morbidity, and when they do, relatively few are referred (Fulop and Strain 1985; Strain et al. 1991; Wallen et al. 1987). The traditional consultation process imposes a sampling bias for establishing clinical needs; the process also hampers research to investigate prevalence, mind-body interactions, outcome of interventions, and cost-offset studies or mechanism issues (Strain et al. 1986).

The consultation methodology limits needed psychiatric, biopsychosocial, and behavioral assessments and interventions that have been demonstrated to affect not only mental health but also general health. Liaison psychiatry enters the system of the medical-surgical setting to access the denominator—the entire patient cohort—and is not restricted to the numerator, the limited referred patient population. Liaison psychiatry also interacts with the other disciplines (such as medical, nursing, social work) to expand the physician's ability to detect, treat, and/or refer those patients who have mental disorders (and to assist caregivers with their own emotional impediments in dealing with a patient); to affect systems of medical care; to involve the patient's support system; and to conduct research on the interaction of medical and psychiatric comorbidity.

PSYCHIATRIC AND MEDICAL COMORBIDITY IN THE GENERAL HOSPITAL

Saravay and Lavin (1994) reviewed 21 studies: 7 international, of which 1 was retrospective, 2 were cross-sectional, and 4 were prospective, and 14 in the United States, of which 7 were retrospective and 7 were prospective (with no control for severity of illness in 4 of the prospective studies). Of the 21 studies described,

16 (76%) found a significant association between psychiatric or psychological and medical comorbidity and increased length of stay (LOS). Of the studies with populations of greater than 110 (to avoid a type II error), 87% demonstrated statistically significant results. Twelve of the 21 studies examined geriatric patients.

Saravay and Lavin (1994) also reviewed three generations of United States studies. The retrospective studies all found significant correlations between psychiatric and psychological comorbidity and LOS (Ackerman et al. 1988; Billings 1941; Brezel et al. 1988; Cushman 1988; Dvoredsky and Cooley 1986; Fulop et al. 1987; Lyons et al. 1988). Of the three prospective studies that did control for severity of illness or other confounding variables (the second-generation studies), the two that failed to show significance had small samples (Levenson et al. 1986; Rogers et al. 1989).

Three of the four third-generation studies (prospective and controlled for severity of illness, degree of functional impairment, or other potentially confounding variables) had significant results. Narain et al. (1988) observed that cognitive impairment predicted nursing home placement within 6 months after discharge. Francis et al. (1990) found a significant positive association in geriatric patients between delirium and LOS. Levenson et al. (1990) observed significant positive associations between depression, anxiety, cognitive impairment, and pain on the one hand and LOS and expenses on the other. Saravay et al. (1991) also demonstrated an association between cognitive impairment, depression, and psychopathology on the Symptom Checklist—90 (SCL-90; Derogatis et al. 1974) and increased LOS, more frequent hospitalization, and more days spent hospitalized during a 4-year period. These studies are denominator based (i.e., included the entire patient cohort). Examining inpatients only, and not taking into account the severity of illness, impairs the value of research findings (i.e., using the consultation patient—a referred subset of the population—limits the conclusions that can be drawn).

PSYCHIATRIC INTERVENTIONS IN THE INPATIENT MEDICAL SETTING

Inpatient hospital care remains the most expensive health care service delivery component in our medical care system. Several variables other than the patient's medical condition contribute to the length of hospitalization. Zimmer (1974) observed in more than 2,500 patients that 11.8% of all hospital days could not be accounted for by physical needs. Glass et al. (1978) reported that for 363 hospitalized medical-surgical inpatients, 18% of the hospital days were secondary to social rather than physical factors. Mason et al. (1980) reported that social factors were critical in the decision to admit 21% of patients to a metropolitan hospital. Boaz (1979) described how the LOS for patients admitted on an emergency basis was strongly affected by social factors. Therefore, psychiatric and psychosocial factors affect every phase of hospitalization: 1) admission (the factors are reasons for admitting a patient or represent "pressures" to admit a patient), 2) the hospital stay itself, and 3) discharge and aftercare placement.

In the early 1970s, Berkman and Rehr (1972, 1973) reported that biopsychosocial needs were typically identified late in the hospitalization, if at all, by the referral method commonly employed by social services. Decreasing the lag time (i.e., shortening the time before psychosocial intervention during hospitalization) was hypothesized to enhance patient care and decrease LOS. Currently, social services are part of the medical-surgical team, do not await referral, and are involved with the entire ward population (the denominator); they have moved from the consultation to the liaison model.

Most studies of inpatient medical populations are flawed because of one or more confounding factors, including problems of measurement and instrumentation; lack of randomization of control and experimental samples; transfer effects from experimental to control environments (i.e., the effect of the intervention extending to the control setting); failure to consider the seriousness of the medical illness, the number of medical and psychiatric diagnoses, and the complexity of medical and surgical interventions; and poor statistical management of physiological and psychosocial data. Billings (1936) was the first investigator to demonstrate improved biopsychosocial status and earlier hospital discharge after a psychiatric intervention. Bonilla et al. (1961) found improved well-being and reduced complaints of pain on a surgical service after hypnosis. Boone et al. (1981) reported that early and comprehensive social intervention improved psychosocial well-being and reduced LOS by 1.25 days ($P = .001$, $F = 10.10$, df = 1,362) in an experimental group compared with a control cohort. However, the investigators did not control for transfer effect (the control group thereby mitigated the difference in the intervention). The intervention permitted early access to every patient (the liaison method) without awaiting referral (i.e., a consultation request) and resulted in a cost-offset effect.

Levitan and Kornfeld (1981) documented in orthopedic patients that a psychiatric liaison approach, in contrast to the traditional consultation approach, resulted in a cost offset—earlier discharge and more discharges to home than to a nursing home (LOS was 30 vs. 42 days, and discharge to home was 16 vs. 8 patients, respectively, for the experimental and control cohorts [$P < .05$]).

Ackerman et al. (1988) described the effect of coexisting depression and the timing of psychiatric consultation on medical inpatients' LOS. They found that 11% of the variance in LOS in the control and experimental populations was accounted for by the timing of the consultation. Psychiatric consultations that occurred earlier in the hospital stay were associated with an LOS closer to that expected from the diagnosis-related group (DRG) system.

Levenson et al. (1992) examined the psychiatric and economic outcomes of psychiatric consultation guided by screening in general medical patients. Although they found neither psychosocial improvement nor earlier discharge—hospital stays were quite short to begin with—these results may have been accounted for by studying heterogeneous medical populations, having only a one-time visit by the psychiatrist, utilizing "indirect" interventions implemented through the consultee with less than 50% concordance with the consultant's recommendations, working with an inner-city disadvantaged population, and examining patients whose preintervention LOS was already short.

Strain et al. (1991) studied liaison psychiatry interventions versus traditional consultation in elderly hip fracture patients at two different sites—Mount Sinai Hospital (MSH) in New York City and Northwestern Memorial Hospital (NMH) in Chicago—using identical assessment and intervention designs. All patients were assessed by the psychiatrist at admission and treated with psychological and/or pharmacotherapy after a review of all medications. Patients were discussed in weekly multidisciplinary ombudsman rounds (Strain and Hamerman 1978), and psychosocial/psychological issues were presented at discharge planning. Treatment was coordinated with the social worker, the patient's significant others, and the treatment team. In the comparison (traditional consultation) group, fewer than 10% (MSH) and 3% (NMH) were referred for consultation, whereas in the experimental (liaison) cohort, 70%–80% received assessment and intervention when indicated. (The remaining patients refused to sign informed consent and therefore had to be excluded.)

The liaison intervention, in contrast to the consultation approach, 1) detected significant DSM-III-R (American Psychiatric Association 1987) psychiatric morbidity (56%), 2) resulted in less depression and cognitive impairment at discharge, 3) decreased LOS by 2 days, 4) led to fewer rehabilitation days, and 5) resulted in no rehospitalizations within a 12-week follow-up period. The confounds of age, sex, severity of illness, number of psychiatric diagnoses, bone density, complexity of orthopedic procedures, stability of fracture, socioeconomic class, study site, and year of study were all taken into account in the regression analysis, which revealed that 11% of the variance in the difference in cost could be explained by assessment and intervention. There was no transfer of cost from the inpatient to the outpatient component in the episode of illness. In fact, not only were inpatient costs reduced, but postdischarge—12-week ambulatory—costs were diminished as well. The liaison approach resulted in increased psychiatric well-being and significant cost offset at both hospitals (e.g., MSH $20,000 cost of intervention resulted in a $167,000 savings, a 1:8 cost-offset ratio).

CONCEPTUAL FRAMEWORK OF LIAISON PSYCHIATRY

Although consultation remains the cornerstone of the liaison process, the emphasis of the latter differentiates these two models of psychiatric intervention. The pedagogical thrust of liaison psychiatry and the attempt to formalize patient care compared with the "catch-as-catch-can" format of the consultation model are underscored by the aims of liaison psychiatry (Strain and Grossman 1975) to

■ Practice primary, secondary, and tertiary prevention
■ Foster case detection and triage methodologies
■ Provide continuing education to the nonpsychiatric staff to promote assessment, treatment, and/or referral of mental disorders

■ Develop basic biopsychosocial knowledge

■ Promote structural or methodological changes in the medical setting to enhance detection and treatment of mental disorders

The practice of liaison psychiatry differs from consultation in yet another way: it cannot charge third-party payers for its efforts and, instead, depends on support from a host department, hospital administration, federal grants, or innovative funding procedures.

MODELS OF PSYCHIATRIC TRAINING FOR PRIMARY CARE PHYSICIANS

Another approach to describing liaison psychiatry is its role in teaching certain mental health concepts to primary care physicians, who see the majority of patients with mental health problems in the United States. Strain et al. (1985) and Pincus et al. (1983) reviewed the literature, examined National Institute of Mental Health (NIMH) grant proposals, interviewed funding agency personnel, and made 35 site visits to internal medicine, general primary care medicine, and family practice residency training programs supported by the NIMH and the Health Resources Services Administration (HRSA). Based on this survey, we described six models of mental health training for the nonpsychiatric physician (Figure 1–1) (Strain et al. 1987).

1. Consultation model. This is the standard medical consultation approach based on the case method (i.e., the consultee initiates the

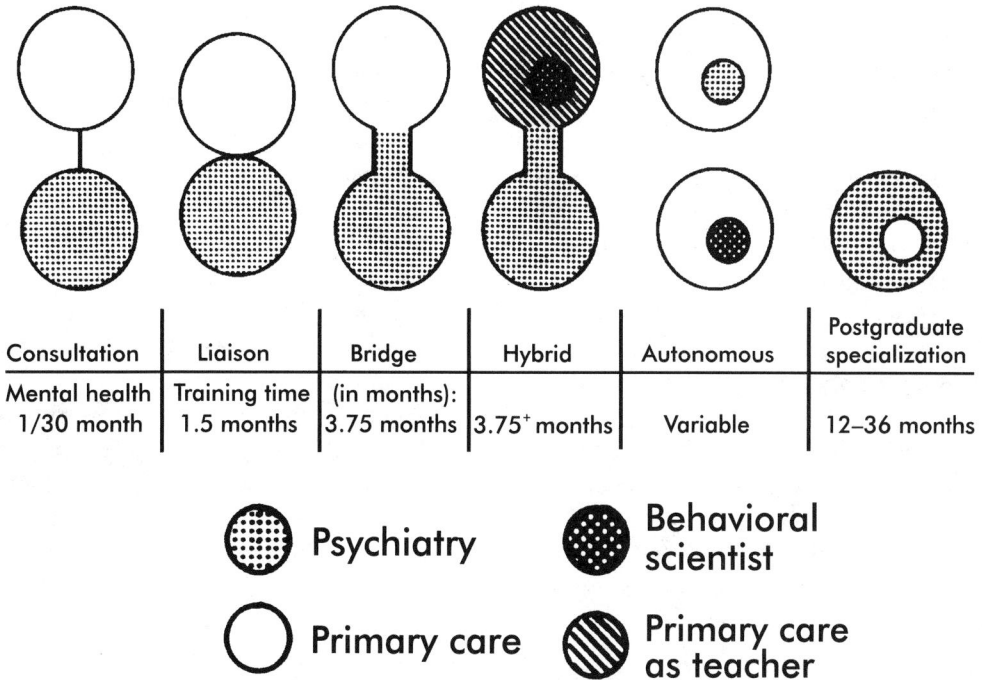

Consultation	Liaison	Bridge	Hybrid	Autonomous	Postgraduate specialization
Mental health 1/30 month	Training time 1.5 months	(in months): 3.75 months	3.75$^+$ months	Variable	12–36 months

Psychiatry   Behavioral scientist

Primary care   Primary care as teacher

Figure 1–1. Models of primary care training in mental health. (Bridge, hybrid, autonomous, and postgraduate are variants of the liaison model.) *Source.* Reprinted from Pincus HA, Strain JJ, Houpt JL, et al: "Models of Mental Health Training in Primary Care." *Journal of the American Medical Association* 249:3065–3068, 1983. Copyright 1983, American Medical Association. Used with permission.

consult and receives no formal, structured teaching such as didactic sessions, seminars, and precepting).

2. Liaison model. In addition to the elements of the consultation model, formal, structured, pedagogical exercises are employed to teach basic knowledge and skills. A psychiatrist-teacher often becomes part of a medical or surgical unit and team.

3. Bridge model. A psychiatrist-teacher, affiliated with a department of psychiatry, is assigned to one primary care teaching site (often an ambulatory training site) for a major portion of his or her time; teaching is structured.

4. Hybrid model. Teaching is provided by a psychiatrist, a behavioral scientist (i.e., psychologist, social worker, or sociologist) who is part of a multidisciplinary team, and the primary care faculty.

5. Autonomous model. The psychiatrist is hired by the primary care group and has no formal connection with a department of psychiatry, or psychosocial teaching is provided exclusively by a nonpsychiatrist behavioral scientist (i.e., psychologist, social worker, or sociologist) not affiliated with a department of psychiatry.

6. Postgraduate specialization model. The primary care physician is trained in a mental health setting for 1 or 2 years, gaining considerable expertise in detecting, diagnosing, and treating mental health disorders.

Internal medicine employed the formal psychiatric consultation model for 68% of its mental health training, compared with 30% and 22.5% for family practice training and general primary care training, respectively. Internal medicine rarely used a psychiatric rotation but relied on the medical inpatient setting for 80% of its mental health training. The modal internal medicine resident requested three or four psy-

chiatric consultations per year and spent an average of less than 15 minutes per case with the consultant. Consequently, the accumulated mental health teaching via the psychiatric consultation model resulted in 3–4 hours of instruction over the course of an internal medicine residency for those residents inclined to initiate a consultation.

The consultation method of relating with medicine was the weakest model that psychiatry offered. When the consultation model was used in primary care and family practice, it was relegated to a minor role because these specialties relied primarily on nonpsychiatric behavioral scientists for most of their teaching. They preferred a liaison relationship with the teacher rather than with an intermittent, itinerant consultant.

Another classification system was presented by Greenhill (1977), in which he described five variations of liaison psychiatry:

1. The *basic liaison model* typically involves a psychiatrist from a department of psychiatry who is assigned to a medical-surgical unit for the express purpose of teaching.
2. The *critical care model* provides for the assignment of mental health personnel to critical care units rather than to clinical departments.
3. The *biological model* is a more exacting variation of the critical care model that emphasizes neuroscience, psychopharmacology, and psychological management. The psychiatrist acts as a member of diagnosis-centered treatment units (e.g., dysphoria clinic, pain center, psychopharmacology clinic).
4. The *milieu model* emphasizes the group aspects of the patient care–group process, staff reactions and interactions, interpersonal theory, and creation of a therapeutic environment on the ward.
5. The *integral model* is emerging as a result of social pressure on medicine. It relies

more on hospital governance than on triage by physicians. The aforementioned models of liaison programs depend on consultation with patients and staff and on working relationships with physicians. This model is based, in addition, on the inclusion of psychological care as an integral factor available to function openly at the point of administrative and clinical need.

The integrated human services model of consultation-liaison psychiatry remedies the isolation among mental health disciplines in the medical setting and lack of integrated formal structure that characterize the traditional consultation mode.

CONCLUSION

Physicians in the medical specialties increasingly have been turning to mental health disciplines other than psychiatry for training and collaborative care of their patients. Many reasons have been postulated. Nonpsychiatric mental health care workers 1) charge less, 2) are easier to incorporate into the medical-surgical team (e.g., social worker's daily presence on the ward, making team rounds, knowledge about the majority of patients and multidisciplines, willingness to interact with families), 3) are comfortable employing the problem level of diagnosis rather than a formal psychiatric taxonomy, and 4) are willing to provide posthospital ambulatory care for patients identified during hospitalization (e.g., to follow patients through an episode of illness). Liaison psychiatry has attempted to address these mandates prescribed by the medical-surgical specialties.

As long as psychiatry's relation with the other specialties of medicine is formulated on the consultation model (and its reliance on the medical inpatient), the ability of primary care physicians to adequately meet the needs of the de facto mental health service (Regier et al.

1978) will become even more attenuated. With the current revolution in health care that mandates primary care as the "gatekeeper" for health care, primary care will be the locus for initial assessment and treatment of psychiatric disorders. One of the first guidelines is for depression in primary care (Depression Guideline Panel 1993a, 1993b). This guideline is promulgated in two volumes: *Detection and Diagnosis* and *Treatment of Major Depression*. It carefully details how to manage depression in primary care and when to refer to other mental health specialists. Primary care must have bridges to psychiatry that far exceed the bridge to psychiatry provided by the consultation model if it is to effectively treat depression in the United States. The limited training received by use of the consultation model will not provide the knowledge and skill for this goal. Even the liaison model commonly practiced in the inpatient setting will not be sufficient. Rather, psychiatry will have to liaison with primary care in the way that the "bridge" and the "hybrid" models propose: a sufficient pedagogic forum to transmit knowledge and skills so that primary care physicians can adequately assess, treat, and/or refer patients to ensure that they receive adequate care. Katon and Gonzales (1994) have shown the need for an extended relationship with primary care to share sufficient knowledge to affect the primary care physician's performance with depressive disorders. Liaison psychiatry defines the next generation of interaction with other medical disciplines and is positioned to move well beyond the traditional consultation mode.

REFERENCES

Ackerman AD, Lyons JS, Hammer JS, et al: The impact of coexisting depression and timing of psychiatric consultation on medical patients' length of stay. Hosp Community Psychiatry 39:173–176, 1988

American Psychiatric Association: Diagnostic and Statistical Manual of Mental Disorders, 3rd Edition, Revised. Washington, DC, American Psychiatric Association, 1987

Berkman BG, Rehr H: The sick role cycle and the timing of social work intervention. Social Service Review 46:567–580, 1972

Berkman BG, Rehr H: Early social service case finding for hospitalized patients: an experiment. Social Service Review 47:256–265, 1973

Billings EG: Teaching psychiatry in a general hospital. JAMA 107:635–639, 1936

Billings EG: Value of psychiatry to the general hospital. Hospitals 15:30–34, 1941

Boaz R: Utilization review and containment of hospital utilization. Med Care 17:315–330, 1979

Bonilla K, Quigley W, Bowers W: Experiences with hypnosis on a surgical service. Mil Med 126:364–370, 1961

Boone CR, Coulton CJ, Keller SM: The impact of early and comprehensive social work services on length of stay. Soc Work Health Care 7:1–9, 1981

Brezel BS, Kassenbrook JM, Stein JM: Burns in substance abusers and in neurologically and mentally impaired patients. J Burn Care Rehabil 9:169–171, 1988

Cushman LA: Secondary neuropsychiatric complications in stroke: implications for acute care. Arch Phys Med Rehabil 69:877–879, 1988

Depression Guideline Panel: Depression in Primary Care, Vol 1: Detection and Diagnosis. Clinical Practice Guideline, No 5. Rockville, MD, U.S. Department of Health and Human Services, Public Health Service, Agency for Health Care Policy Research, AHCPR Publ No 93-0050, 1993a

Depression Guideline Panel: Depression in Primary Care, Vol 2: Treatment of Major Depression. Clinical Practice Guideline, No 5. Rockville, MD, U.S. Department of Health and Human Services, Public Health Service, Agency for Health Care Policy Research, AHCPR Publ No 93-0051, 1993b

Derogatis LR, Lipman RS, Rickels K, et al: The Hopkins Symptom Checklist (HSCL): a self-report symptom inventory. Behavioral Science 19:1–15, 1974

Dvoredsky AE, Cooley HW: Comparative severity of illness in patients with combined medical and psychiatric diagnoses. Psychosomatics 27:625–630, 1986

Francis J, Martin D, Kapoor WN: A prospective study of delirium in hospitalized elderly. JAMA 263:1097–1101, 1990

Fulop G, Strain JJ: Patients who self-initiate a psychiatric consultation. Gen Hosp Psychiatry 7:267–271, 1985

Fulop G, Strain JJ, Vita J, et al: Impact of psychiatric comorbidity on length of hospital stay for medical/surgical patients: a preliminary report. Am J Psychiatry 144:878–882, 1987

Glass R, Mulvihill M, Smith H, et al: The 4-score: an index for predicting a patient's non-medical hospital days. Am J Public Health 8:751–755, 1978

Greenhill MH: The development of liaison programs, in Psychiatric Medicine. Edited by Usdin G. New York, Brunner/Mazel, 1977, pp 115–191

Hackett T, Cassem N: The Massachusetts General Hospital Handbook of Psychiatry. St Louis, MO, Mosby, 1979

Katon W, Gonzales J: A review of randomized trials of psychiatric consultation liaison studies in primary care. Psychosomatics 35:268–278, 1994

Levenson JL, Hamer R, Silverman JJ, et al: Psychopathology in medical inpatients and its relationship to length of hospital stay: a pilot study. Int J Psychiatry Med 16:231–236, 1986

Levenson JL, Colenda CC, Larson DB, et al: Methodology in consultation-liaison research: a classification of biases. Psychosomatics 31:367–376, 1990

Levenson JL, Hamer RM, Rossiter LF: A randomized controlled study of psychiatric consultation guided by screening in general medical inpatients. Am J Psychiatry 149:631–637, 1992

Levitan S, Kornfeld D: Clinical and cost benefits of liaison psychiatry. Am J Psychiatry 138:790–793, 1981

Lyons JS, Larson DB, Burns BJ, et al: Psychiatric comorbidities and patients with head and spinal cord trauma: effects on acute hospital care. Gen Hosp Psychiatry 10:292–297, 1988

Mason W, Bedwell C, Zwaag R, et al: Why people are hospitalized: a description of preventable factors leading to admission for medical illness. Med Care 18:147–163, 1980

Narain P, Rubenstein LZ, Wieland GD, et al: Predictors of immediate and 6-month outcomes in hospitalized elderly patients: the importance of functional status. J Am Geriatr Soc 36: 775–783, 1988

Pincus HA, Strain JJ, Houpt JL, et al: Models of mental health training in primary care. JAMA 249:3065–3068, 1983

Regier DA, Goldberg ID, Taube CA: The 'de-facto' US Mental Health Services System: a public perspective. Arch Gen Psychiatry 35:685–693, 1978

Rogers MP, Liang MH, Daltroy LH, et al: Delirium after elective orthopedic surgery: risk factors and natural history. Int J Psychiatry Med 19: 109–121, 1989

Saravay SM, Lavin M: Psychiatric comorbidity and length of stay in the general hospital: a review of outcome studies. Psychosomatics 35:233–252, 1994

Saravay SM, Steinberg MD, Weinschel B, et al: Psychological comorbidity and length of stay in the general hospital. Am J Psychiatry 148:324–329, 1991

Strain JJ, Grossman S: Psychological Care of the Medically Ill: A Primer in Liaison Psychiatry. New York, Appleton-Century-Crofts, 1975

Strain JJ, Hamerman D: Ombudsmen (medical psychiatric) rounds: an approach to meeting patient-staff needs. Ann Intern Med 88:550–555, 1978

Strain JJ, Strain JW: Liaison psychiatry, in Modern Perspectives in Clinical Psychiatry. Edited by Howells JG. New York, Brunner/Mazel, 1988, pp 76–101

Strain JJ, Gise LH, Houpt JL, et al: Models of mental health training in primary care. Psychosom Med 47:95–110, 1985

Strain JJ, Fulop G, Strain JW, et al: Use of the computer for teaching in the psychiatric residency. Journal of Psychiatric Education 10:178–186, 1986

Strain JJ, George LK, Pincus HA, et al: Models of mental health training for primary care. Psychosom Med 49:88–98, 1987

Strain JJ, Lyons JS, Hammers JS, et al: Cost offset from a psychiatric consultation-liaison intervention with elderly hip fracture patients. Am J Psychiatry 148:1044–1049, 1991

Wallen J, Pincus HA, Goldman HH, et al: Psychiatric consultations in short term hospitals. Arch Gen Psychiatry 44:163–168, 1987

Zimmer J: Length of stay and hospital bed misutilization. Med Care 14:453–462, 1974

Chapter 2

Mental Status Examination and Diagnosis

Michael G. Wise, M.D.
Richard L. Strub, M.D.

The mental status examination (MSE) is to the consultation-liaison psychiatrist what the cardiac examination is to the cardiologist or the neurological examination is to the neurologist. To perform effective psychiatric consultation, one must be able to perform a complete MSE and integrate the findings with historical and behavioral information, as well as psychological, neurological, physical, and laboratory information, to arrive at a final diagnosis. The components of the MSE include assessment of general appearance and behavior, affect and mood, thought processes and content, perceptions (delusions, hallucinations), judgment, and insight. In addition, assessment of cognitive function, such as level of consciousness or awareness, attention, speech, orientation and memory, and abstracting ability, is essential.

It is unfortunate that cognitive impairment is not always recognized by nonpsychiatric medical personnel. In a study of elderly patients referred for evaluation, substantial cognitive dysfunction went unrecognized by the referring physician in 73% of the patients; cognitive dysfunction was related to medications 75% of the time (Kallman and May 1989).

Psychiatrists often depend too heavily on verbal communication and testing to exclude a medical or substance-induced psychiatric disorder—referred to in this chapter as *secondary disorders*. For that reason, psychiatrists will miss nonverbal cognitive impairment if the patient's ability to communicate is reasonably good. Formal tests of right-hemisphere, or nondominant, brain function are as important as the more traditional tests of verbal function that are the domain of the left hemisphere. The psychiatrist who asks the patient to remember three verbal items but does not ask the patient to recall three shapes succumbs to this pitfall and essentially ignores testing a major part of the brain's function (Ovsiew 1992).

Finally, mental status testing in a general hospital environment is difficult. Hospital rooms are noisy, and there are many distractions, such as intravenous alarms, a roommate who is groaning or loudly conversing with visitors, or a harried nurse or phlebotomist who must have immediate access to the patient. In addition, the patient being examined is sick, often frightened, and sleep deprived. As a result, the consultation-liaison psychiatrist can identify gross deficits much more readily than subtle abnormalities. Before testing, the psychiatrist should always ensure that the patient has his or her usual sensory aids (e.g., hearing aid or glasses).

The mental status test is separated into two categories: noncognitive and cognitive (Table 2–1).

Table 2–1.   Components of a mental status examination

Noncognitive

  Appearance and behavior
  Affect and mood
  Thought process and content
  Perceptions
  Abstracting abilities
  Judgment
  Insight

Cognitive

  Level of consciousness and awareness
  Attention
  Speech and language
  Orientation
  Memory

Source.   Reprinted from Strub RL, Wise MG: "Differential Diagnosis in Neuropsychiatry," in *The American Psychiatric Press Textbook of Neuropsychiatry,* 2nd Edition. Edited by Yudofsky SC, Hales RE. Washington, DC, American Psychiatric Press, 1992, p. 231. Used with permission.

NONCOGNITIVE COMPONENTS OF THE MENTAL STATUS EXAMINATION

Evaluating a patient with changes in noncognitive abilities is often more difficult than evaluating a patient who has abnormalities in cognitive function. Noncognitive changes are more subjective and are often symptomatic of a primary psychiatric disorder. Certain features help the clinician identify such patients. First, the clinician must know the epidemiology of common psychiatric disorders (Figure 2–1). For example, a 60-year-old man with no prior psychiatric problems who is referred for evaluation of new-onset "schizophrenia" virtually never has schizophrenia. A medical condition or substance-induced etiology is typically responsible for this patient's mental status changes.

Appearance and Behavior

The MSE begins the instant the psychiatrist sees the patient. From that moment on, information is collected and hypotheses are formulated about the patient's diagnosis. The patient's physical appearance, attitude, and behavior should be described simply without using jargon. Judgmental terms that imply a diagnosis—for example, "She acted hysterically" or "He exhibited borderline characteristics"—should be avoided. Not only do these imply a diagnosis, but they are not helpful and are usually wrong. How the patient looks and behaves during the examination should be reported. Behavior such as increased or decreased body movements, posturing, pacing, tremor, and choreiform or dyskinetic movements should be described. For patients who appear ill, depressed, angry, distractible, anxious, or disheveled, the clinician should state specific aspects of the patients' appearance or behavior that led to these conclusions. An accurate, unbiased description of behavior and appearance aids diagnosis.

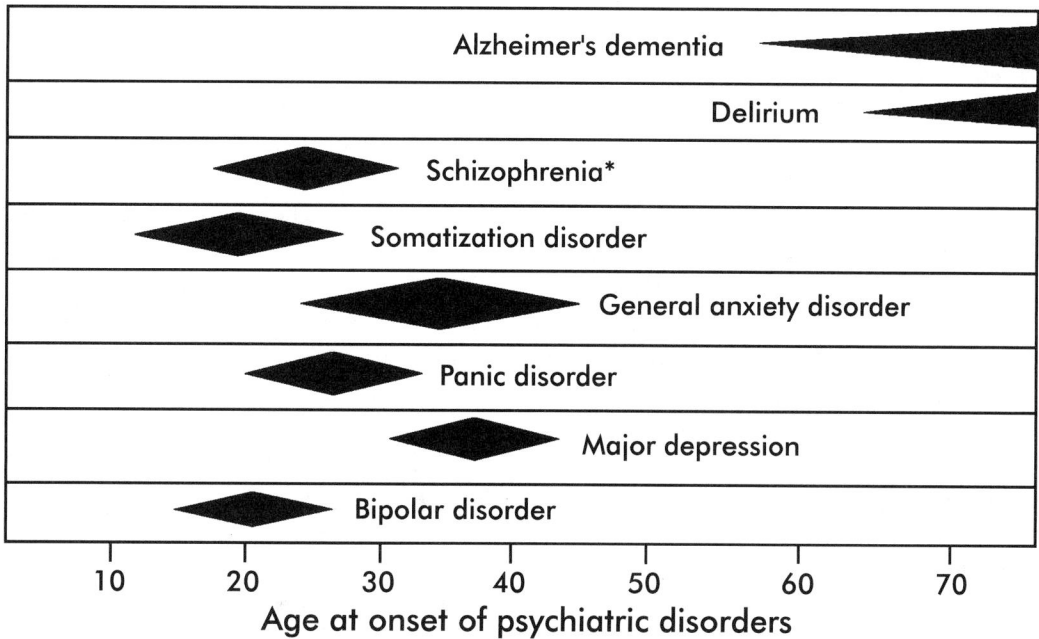

Figure 2–1. Epidemiology of common psychiatric disorders. *Earlier onset in males. *Source.* Reprinted from Strub RL, Wise MG: "Differential Diagnosis in Neuropsychiatry," in *The American Psychiatric Press Textbook of Neuropsychiatry,* 2nd Edition. Edited by Yudofsky SC, Hales RE. Washington, DC, American Psychiatric Press, 1992, p. 231. Used with permission.

Affect and Mood

Mood is the patient's pervasive and sustained emotional state. Terms used to describe mood are dysphoric, elevated, euthymic, expansive, and irritable. Affect refers to more rapid fluctuations in the patient's emotional state. If the patient's affect does not change during the interview (e.g., patient is constantly depressed, emotionless, or elated), that would, in all likelihood, represent the patient's mood. When reporting affect, the parameters used are range, intensity, lability, and appropriateness. Affective range may be full (e.g., the patient shows a wide range of emotional states during the interview), or affect may be restricted to a particular state (e.g., depressed). Affective intensity among patients can also vary greatly (e.g., from the extreme rage seen in a borderline patient to the flat or affectless expression typically observed in a patient with Parkinson's disease).

Affective lability denotes that the patient fluctuates rapidly from one affective state to another; this often indicates a toxic or medical etiology. Affect is also described as either appropriate or inappropriate to the topic being discussed. For example, a patient who describes the recent, traumatic death of a loved one appears sad (appropriate expression of affect); however, another patient during a similar discussion appears elated and laughs (inappropriate expression of affect).

Consultation-liaison psychiatrists frequently see medical and substance-induced mood disorders. In a study of 755 hospitalized patients consecutively seen in psychiatric consultation (Rundell and Wise 1989), 87% of patients with mania and 38% of patients with depression warranted a DSM-III-R (American Psychiatric Association 1987) diagnosis of organic mood disorder. Medical illnesses, such as thyroid disease, can markedly alter mood. A patient with hyperthyroidism can become manic (Lishman 1987) or depressed (Gold et al. 1981).

Medications are also implicated as causes for depression, and numerous medications are reported to cause mania (Krauthammer and Klerman 1978). Two classic examples of medications that cause depression are reserpine and α-methyldopa (Benson et al. 1983). On the other hand, corticosteroids, particularly when given in high doses such as after organ transplantation, commonly cause mood elevation and may cause a manic episode (Rundell and Wise 1989; Wise et al. 1988).

Thought Processes and Content

Thought processes and thought content are judged by the patient's quality and quantity of speech and behavior. How does the patient respond to a question? Is his or her answer responsive to the question asked (goal directed), or does he or she ramble purposelessly (tangential)? The pattern of thoughts is also an important measure of thought processes. The patient's thoughts may move extremely rapidly from one idea to another (flight of ideas), may not relate in an understandable way (loose associations), or may stop suddenly (thought blocking). The patient's thought content or major themes reflect the patient's concerns, including obsessional preoccupation, suicidal or homicidal ideation, or irrational beliefs.

Disordered thinking is seen in secondary disorders, such as delirium, dementia, and substance-induced disorders, and in primary thought disorders, such as schizophrenia, mania, and psychotic depression (D. W. Black et al. 1988). Patients with primary thought disorders are usually younger and have no related medical illness, clouding of consciousness, or disorientation, but they do have a psychiatric history and predominantly auditory hallucinations. Patients with secondary thought disorders usually have an older age at onset, associated medical illness(es) and medication(s), fluctuating consciousness, disorientation, non-

auditory hallucinations, and fleeting, poorly systematized delusional beliefs but no psychiatric history.

A patient's behavior may also reflect abnormal thought content. A patient who is reluctant to talk and leers suspiciously at the examiner is displaying paranoid behavior, even if he or she denies it. A patient who is oriented and alert during an examination but who was combative and urinated in the corner of his or her hospital room last night is, or at least was, delirious.

Perceptions

Disorders of perception include illusions (misinterpretation of a real sensory experience), hallucinations (a sensory perception in the absence of an external stimulus), delusions (a false belief), and ideas of reference (an incorrect interpretation that events have direct reference to oneself). In addition to directly questioning the patient about misperceptions, the physician should question nurses and family whether the patient attends to nonapparent stimuli, mentions hallucinations, makes bizarre comments, or behaves inappropriately. The patient who denies misperceptions but responds to hallucinations illustrates the importance of observing behavior during assessment.

Hallucinatory perception can be visual, auditory, tactile, olfactory, gustatory, or kinesthetic. Although cultural variations are important, hallucinations that occur in an awake individual are almost always symptomatic of a pathological process. Auditory hallucinations are more typical of primary psychiatric disorders, such as schizophrenia, mania, or psychotic depression; one notable exception is alcoholic hallucinosis, in which vivid auditory hallucinations occur in a fully oriented alcoholic patient (Victor and Hope 1958). Hallucinations that involve other sensory modalities are more typically associated with secondary disorders. (For a more detailed discussion, see Cummings 1985.)

Abstracting Abilities

Educational level is a strong determinant of one's ability to abstract. Bedside testing is usually done by asking the patient to interpret simple proverbs, such as "People who live in glass houses should not throw stones." If the patient replies "Because the glass will break," that is a concrete answer. Concrete interpretations are commonly found in three groups: 1) individuals with less than a high school education, 2) patients with schizophrenia, and 3) patients with dementia. Proverbs are also diagnostically helpful when the patient gives a bizarre and personalized reply such as "That's what they do to crack people like me." Bizarre proverb interpretation almost always signifies psychosis.

Judgment

Judgment is the ability to anticipate the consequences of one's behavior and to behave in a culturally acceptable way. Recent behavior is the best way to determine a patient's judgment. For example, the confused, paranoid patient with an acute myocardial infarction who believes he or she is about to be killed in the hospital, spits out his or her medications, and states, "I'm leaving here now!" has very poor judgment. Examiners will sometimes ask the same patient questions like "What would you do if you found a stamped, sealed, addressed envelope in the street?" to assess judgment. These types of questions are less adequate than the "common sense" standard of recent behavior.

Insight

Insight can have a wide range of meanings, including a simple awareness of one's own symptoms or a complex psychological awareness of conscious and unconscious determinants of one's behavior (Feher et al. 1989). In general,

insight is present if the patient realizes that a problem exists, that his or her thinking and behavior may contribute to that problem, and that he or she may need assistance.

◼ COGNITIVE COMPONENTS OF THE MENTAL STATUS EXAMINATION

Psychiatric residents and medical students who rotate on psychiatric consultation-liaison services and some experienced psychiatrists fall prey to two fallacies about testing cognitive function:

1. *Cognitive deficits are obvious during an interview or lengthy conversation.* This statement is true for patients with substantial cognitive dysfunction such as severe dementia or delirium; however, cognitive deficits are not obvious in most patients with mild to moderate global deficits or in many patients with focal neuropsychiatric deficits.
2. *Screening MSEs, such as those described later in this chapter, are sufficient to detect cognitive deficits.* Two frequently used examinations—the Mini-Mental State Exam (MMSE; Folstein et al. 1975) and the Cognitive Capacity Screening Examination (CCSE; Jacobs et al. 1977)—do not identify many patients who have cognitive deficits. In a neurosurgical population with known brain lesions, Schwamm et al. (1987) reported a false-negative rate of 43% with the MMSE and 53% with the CCSE.

Level of Consciousness

Psychiatric consultation is often requested for patients who experience a rapid or recent change in mental status. In most instances, the patient is either lethargic (not as alert as would be expected) or agitated and disruptive after surgery or some medical intervention. In addition to changes in arousal, such patients often exhibit altered thought content. This change in both alertness and thought content produces the clouded consciousness that is typical of the confusional behavior seen in delirium (Lipowski 1990).

Any patient who is difficult to arouse or who will not remain alert without constant stimulation is usually physically ill. However, other clinical situations may produce or mimic a decreased level of consciousness. For example, sleepiness, boredom, simple intoxication, or a primary sleep disorder may all produce lethargy. In addition, depressed patients with significant psychomotor retardation are sometimes withdrawn and very slow to respond. They are, however, rarely confused or lethargic in the sense used here. Also, a few patients will actually feign unconsciousness (i.e., so-called psychogenic unresponsiveness). One should consider this diagnosis only after a complete medical and neurological evaluation has not yielded a more plausible explanation. Such patients usually have a psychiatric history and/or significant current environmental chaos to explain their behavior.

Attention

The capacity to direct and maintain one's attention while screening out extraneous and irrelevant stimuli is a fundamental yet highly complex cognitive function (Berlucchi and Rizzolatti 1987; McGhie 1969). Inattention (the breakdown of selective attention) and distractibility are common and clinically significant neuropsychiatric symptoms. Inattention can also complicate the entire evaluation process (Mesulam 1985; Pribram and McGuinness 1975). For example, an inattentive patient will frequently fail tests of memory or calculation on the basis of inattention alone. Therefore, the clinician must use caution in the interpretation of cognitive failure in an inattentive patient.

Tests of attention include the Forward Digit Span and A Test for Vigilance (Strub and Black 1985). Digit span is a standard psycho-logical test for attention. The patient must immediately repeat a series of numbers that are read to him or her in a slow, clear fashion. Five digits forward is the minimum required for normal. Backward digit span may depend on visuospatial processing as well as attention (F. W. Black 1986). In the vigilance test, the patient is presented letters at a rate of one per second and is asked to signal each time the letter A is spoken. A single error is considered abnormal.

In addition to conditions in which patients display global inattention, there is a special type of inattention called hemiattention or hemineglect (Kinsbourne 1970). In this condition, patients are attentive to only half of their body and the extrapersonal space on the same side and neglect the other half. This syndrome is most frequently manifested as a left hemiattention in a patient who has had a right-hemisphere brain lesion (Weinstein and Friedland 1977).

Because it is nonspecific, inattention only indicates the presence of a problem. For the consultation-liaison psychiatrist, inattention is equivalent to the sedimentation rate for the internist. Its clinical significance is more fully appreciated when combined with more specific symptoms.

Speech and Language

Brain disease, particularly dominant-hemisphere insults, frequently disrupts a patient's speech and language. Speech defects include the slurred speech of the intoxicated patient, the soft trailing speech of the patient with Parkinson's disease, and the dysphonia and dysarthria of the patient with amyotrophic lateral sclerosis. Language disturbances, specifically aphasias, refer to defects in word choice, comprehension, and syntax seen when language areas of the brain are affected.

The consultation-liaison psychiatrist must develop a systematic way to screen for aphasia. A simple way to do this is a bedside test, such as the pocket-sized Aphasia Screening Battery

(Reitan 1984). Table 2–2 lists the clinical characteristics of aphasia syndromes.

First, the patient's spontaneous speech should be observed and its rate, rhythm, and fluency should be described. If speech is disorganized, absent, or bizarre, the clinician should suspect a psychotic process and must rule out an organic etiology. Next, comprehension must be tested. This is particularly important when the patient is on a respirator and normal speech is not possible. Yes-or-no questions should be asked. For example, "Do you put on your socks before your shoes?" "Is there a tree in the room?" and "Can an elephant ride a tricycle?" [The psychiatrist should also note whether the patient smiles when asked absurd questions.] If the patient misses the humorous aspect of these questions, it usually means significant cognitive impairment, severe fear (terror), or depression.

Other aspects of speech that are tested include repetition (e.g., the patient is asked to repeat "no ifs, ands, or buts"), naming (the patient is asked to name both common and less frequently used items), reading, and writing. Agraphia accompanies aphasia and is also very frequently seen in patients with delirium (Chedru and Geschwind 1972).

Orientation

Questions about orientation to self, time (year, month, day, and time of day), location, and circumstance, when answered correctly by the patient, are usually recorded in the medical chart as "oriented X 4." This phrase is used loosely by nonpsychiatric physicians, surgeons, and nurses. It typically means that the patient is not obviously confused. It does not mean that the patient was formally tested.

Memory

Memory loss is a common symptom seen by the consultation-liaison psychiatrist and has many different causes. Memory loss can be symptomatic of either a primary or a secondary psychiatric disorder. The patient's history is very useful in sorting through the differential diagnosis of memory dysfunction. In general, in patients younger than 40 years, especially those with a history of previous or concomitant emotional problems, a psychiatric disorder is the most likely explanation for their amnesia; however, elderly people with progressive memory loss more frequently have a type of dementia. More detailed discussions of memory testing are found in works by Strub and Black (1985, 1988), Squire and Butters (1984), and Victor et al. (1989).

Questions about orientation provide a basic test of recent memory. In addition, the patient should be asked to remember four unrelated objects, such as tulip, eyedropper, brown, and ball. The patient should immediately repeat them to ensure that he or she has properly heard and understood the words. After conversing with the patient about other things for about 3 minutes, the patient is asked to repeat the words. If the patient cannot recall the words, the psychiatrist should check whether the words were not encoded into memory or were encoded but cannot be retrieved. Such differentiation can be made by giving the patient clues. Patients who did not learn the words are not aided by prompting, whereas patients who learned the words but cannot access them quickly will recall with prompting. Testing memory for designs is also easy. The patient should be asked to replicate designs used to test constructional praxis. The examiner can use a three-word/three-shape test, such as that described by Weintraub and Mesulam (1985).

It is more difficult to test remote memory because the examiner must know whether the information given by the patient is correct or confabulated. The clinician can ask the patient to name the last five presidents or, better yet, about important world events that almost everyone knows.

Table 2–2. Clinical characteristics of aphasia

Type	Characteristic						Associated deficits	Emotional reaction
	Speech	Comprehension	Repetition	Naming	Writing	Reading		
Broca's	Nonfluent	Intact	Impaired	Impaired	Impaired	Impaired	Right hemiparesis	Despair
(Patient cannot articulate and is frustrated; speech is sparse [or absent] and telegraphic.)								
Wernicke's	Fluent	Impaired	Impaired	Impaired	Impaired	Impaired	Hemianopsia ± hemisensory loss	Unaware
(Patient articulates well but speaks nonsense and does not understand.)								
Conduction	Fluent	Intact	Impaired	Impaired	± Impaired	Intact	±Hemisensory loss	Frustration
(Like Wernicke's aphasia except patient can understand and is aware of deficits.)								
Anomic	Fluent	Intact	Intact	Impaired	± Impaired	Intact	Varies	± Aware
(Patient cannot name objects but describes their use; makes lame excuses for deficit.)								
Global	Nonfluent	Impaired	Impaired	Impaired	Impaired	Impaired	Right hemiparesis, hemisensory loss, hemianopsia	Unaware
(Very large lesion, marked impairment.)								

Source. Reprinted from Wise MG, Rundell JR: *Concise Guide to Consultation Psychiatry*, 2nd Edition. Washington, DC, American Psychiatric Press, 1994, p. 13. Used with permission.

SCREENING MENTAL STATUS EXAMINATIONS

A number of bedside examinations will screen patients for cognitive dysfunction (Folstein et al. 1975; Isaacs and Kennie 1973; Jacobs et al. 1977; Katzman et al. 1983; Kiernan et al. 1987; Reitan 1958; Taylor et al. 1987). Screening MSEs are very useful for physicians who do not normally perform an MSE as part of their examination. For the consultation psychiatrist, who is an expert in cognition and its measurement, screening MSEs are only one part of a more extensive cognitive examination. Sometimes the score on an MSE such as the MMSE will influence a physician who doubts a psychiatrist's opinion but who believes "hard" data. In addition, serial screening MSEs are useful when following the clinical course of a patient with delirium or dementia.

The MMSE is probably the most widely used and best-known screening MSE. The MMSE tests orientation, memory (registration and recall), attention, calculation, language (naming, repetition, ability to follow complicated commands, reading, and writing), and constructional ability. It takes about 5 minutes to administer, can be administered serially to follow a patient's clinical course, and is a reliable and valid test in medical patients (Anthony et al. 1982; Nelson et al. 1986; Strub and Black 1977).

Various MMSE cutoff scores are proposed to indicate delirium or dementia. A score of 20 or less may indicate impairment (Folstein et al. 1975); however, Mungas (1991) proposed that a score of 0–10 corresponds to severe cognitive impairment, 11–20 to moderate impairment, 20–25 to mild impairment, and 25–30 to questionable impairment or intact function. Delirium and dementia are not the only reasons for a low score on the MMSE. Other reasons include deafness, blindness, mutism, inability to understand English, aphasia, mental retardation, lack of cooperation, and an educational level less than eighth grade. The clinician must ensure that the patient has his or her usual sensory aids before testing, such as a hearing aid or glasses. Regardless of the reason for a low score on the MMSE, the information has clinical relevance.

Other Useful Tests of Cognitive Function

The consultation-liaison psychiatrist must have expertise on how to administer several tests, even when the patient is bedridden or on a respirator. In this section, we describe a few tests that we have found to be clinically useful. Lishman's classic text *Organic Psychiatry* (Lishman 1987) has an excellent detailed discussion of cognitive function and psychometric tests.

The Bender-Gestalt Test (Bender 1938) examines the patient's ability to copy designs. Nine designs are presented to the patient, one at a time, and he or she is asked to copy them. Errors suggest brain dysfunction, and error-free performance strongly supports the absence of brain disease. Memory can be tested for designs by asking the patient to reproduce the figures after a brief period has elapsed.

The Blessed Dementia Scale consists of two parts, which can be used separately or together (Blessed et al. 1968). One part measures the patient's ability to perform everyday activities, and the other measures the patient's ability to perform on information-memory-concentration tests. Information about daily activities is provided by a knowledgeable family member or close friend.

Draw a Clock Face is another useful bedside test that should be part of the core MSE (Lishman 1987). (See Chapter 7, Figure 7–1, in this volume, for a further explanation of this test.)

The Marie Three-Paper Test provides a quick assessment for comprehension problems and receptive aphasia (Lishman 1987). Three different-sized pieces of paper are placed in front of the patient. He or she is told to take the biggest piece and hand it to the examiner, take the smallest piece and throw it to the ground, and take the middle-sized one and place it in his or her pocket.

The Reitan-Indiana Aphasia Screening Test is a pocket-sized, easily administered, brief aphasia screen (Reitan 1984). This test gives a reasonable survey of aphasic symptoms, including ability to copy, name, spell, write, read, calculate, and demonstrate use of an object (ideomotor praxis).

The Set Test is a test of verbal fluency designed to screen elderly patients for dementia (Isaacs and Kennie 1973). The patient is asked to name 10 items from each of 4 categories. A useful mnemonic to recall the categories is F-A-C-T—fruits-animals-colors-towns. The patient is asked to name 10 fruits, then to name 10 animals, and so on. The score is the total number of items named, with a maximum score of 40. In patients age 65 or older, scores below 15 are clearly abnormal and indicate impairment.

The Trail Making Test (Trail Part A and B) consists of several circles distributed on a sheet of paper (Reitan 1958). In Part A, the circles contain numbers, and the patient is asked to connect the numbers in sequence by drawing a line as quickly as possible from one circle to the next. In Part B, each circle contains either a number or a letter. The patient is asked to alternate between numbers and letters (1, then A, then 2, then B, and so on). Both Trail Part A and B are timed tests, and age-corrected norms are available. More than one error on either test is usually significant.

A Test for Vigilance measures the ability to sustain attention. For example, a series of letters is read at a rate of one per second, and the patient is asked to raise his or her hand each time the letter *A* is read.

THE CONSULTATION-LIAISON PSYCHIATRIST AS NEUROPSYCHIATRIST

The consultation-liaison psychiatrist who can administer a variety of cognitive tests and a brief neurological examination will be able to identify cognitive and neurological deficits. If the psychiatrist also has a knowledge of neuropsychiatry, he or she can organize and understand symptoms within the context of brain-behavior relationships and identify specific clinical syndromes, such as dementia, left-hemisphere lesions, and delirium.

Neurological Examination

The consultation-liaison psychiatrist, during a consultation, will often need to perform a basic neurological examination. A neurological examination is essential in any patient with cognitive dysfunction, suspected somatoform or conversion disorder with neurological complaints, or malingering. The examination does not have to be time-consuming. The patient's history frequently will suggest deficits.

A basic bedside neurological examination consists of the following:

1. Check deep tendon reflexes for symmetry. Check for the presence of a Babinski reflex. Some clinicians also check for primitive reflexes (snout, grasp, glabellar, and palmomental), although the usefulness of frontal release signs has been challenged (Fogel and Eslinger 1991; Ovsiew 1992). The presence of two or three primitive reflexes may be more useful in the diagnosis of dementia (Ovsiew 1992).
2. Check muscle strength for asymmetry, weakness, tone, or embellishment.
3. Observe the gait and associated arm movements.
4. Examine cranial nerve function.
5. Check the distribution of any sensory complaints.
6. Check for signs of meningeal irritation, such as neck stiffness, headache, or Kernig and Brudzinski signs.

Knowledge of brain-behavior relationships is important for psychiatrists to function well as consultants in the hospital setting. The consultation psychiatrist must understand neurological terminology. The following list contains a few commonly used neurological terms. The prefix *a* means complete loss of ability (e.g., aphasia is the loss of ability to comprehend or express speech), and the prefix *dys* means an impaired ability (e.g., dysphasia means an impairment in the ability to comprehend or express speech).

- *Abulia*—loss of willpower
- *Acalculia*—loss of the ability to do mathematical calculations
- *Agnosia*—loss or diminution of the ability to recognize familiar objects
- *Agraphia*—loss of the ability to express thought in writing
- *Alexia*—loss of the ability to read (acquired)
- *Apraxia*—loss or impairment of the ability to use objects correctly
- *Ataxia*—impaired motor coordination
- *Dysarthria*—disturbance of articulation of speech caused by muscle dysfunction
- *Dyslexia*—disturbance of the ability to read
- *Dysphasia*—impaired ability to comprehend, elaborate, or express speech
- *Dysprosody*—speech that is not of the normal pitch, rhythm, and variation

SUMMARY

Effective psychiatric consultation in patients who are medically ill requires many clinical skills and the ability to integrate diverse pieces of information into a diagnosis. Essential skills for the consultation-liaison psychiatrist are the ability to perform a comprehensive MSE, especially the ability to test cognitive functions at the patient's bedside, and to perform a brief neurological and focused physical examina-

tion. These data are combined with historical information (e.g., patient's medical and psychiatric history, medications, laboratory results) and the clinician's knowledge of medicine, psychiatric disorders, defense mechanisms, characterology, and brain-behavior relationships to formulate a diagnosis. This sophisticated process is essential to the proper diagnosis and treatment of medically ill patients who develop psychiatric symptoms.

REFERENCES

American Psychiatric Association: Diagnostic and Statistical Manual of Mental Disorders, 3rd Edition, Revised. Washington, DC, American Psychiatric Association, 1987

Anthony JC, LeResche L, Niaz U, et al: Limits of the 'Mini-Mental State' as a screening test for dementia and delirium among hospital patients. Psychol Med 12:397–408, 1982

Bender L: A Visual Motor Gestalt Test and its Clinical Use. New York, American Orthopsychiatric Association, 1938

Benson D, Peterson LG, Bartay J: Neuropsychiatric manifestations of antihypertensive medications. Psychiatr Med 1:205–214, 1983

Berlucchi G, Rizzolatti G: Special issue: selective visual attention. Neuropsychologia 25 (no 1A): 1–145, 1987

Black DW, Yates WR, Andreasen NC: Schizophrenia, schizophreniform disorder, and delusional (paranoid) disorders, in The American Psychiatric Press Textbook of Psychiatry. Edited by Talbott JA, Hales RE, Yudofsky SC. Washington, DC, American Psychiatric Press, 1988, pp 357–402

Black FW: Digit repetition in brain-damaged adults: clinical and theoretical implications. J Clin Psychol 42:770–782, 1986

Blessed G, Tomlinson BE, Roth M: The association between quantitative measures of dementia and of senile changes in the cerebral gray matter of elderly subjects. Br J Psychiatry 114:797–811, 1968

Chedru F, Geschwind N: Writing disturbances in acute confusional states. Neuropsychologia 10:343–353, 1972

Cummings JL: Clinical Neuropsychiatry. Orlando, FL, Grune & Stratton, 1985, pp 5–16

Feher EP, Doody R, Pirozzolo FJ, et al: Mental status assessment of insight and judgment. Clin Geriatr Med 5:477–498, 1989

Fogel BS, Eslinger PJ: Diagnosis and management of patients with frontal lobe syndromes, in Medical-Psychiatric Practice, Vol 1. Edited by Stoudemire A, Fogel BS. Washington, DC, American Psychiatric Press, 1991, pp 349–392

Folstein MF, Folstein SE, McHugh PR: Mini-Mental State: a practical method for grading the cognitive state of patients for the clinician. J Psychiatr Res 12:189–198, 1975

Gold MS, Pottash ALC, Extein I: Hypothyroidism and depression: evidence from complete thyroid function evaluation. JAMA 245:1919–1922, 1981

Hales RE, Yudofsky SC: The American Psychiatric Press Textbook of Neuropsychiatry. Washington, DC, American Psychiatric Press, 1987

Isaacs B, Kennie AT: The Set Test as an aid to the detection of dementia in old people. Br J Psychiatry 123:467–470, 1973

Jacobs JW, Bernhard MR, Delgado A, et al: Screening for organic mental syndromes in the medically ill. Ann Intern Med 86:40–46, 1977

Kallman H, May HJ: Mental status assessment in the elderly. Prim Care 16:329–347, 1989

Katzman R, Brown T, Fuld P: Validation of a short orientation-memory-concentration test of cognitive impairment. Am J Psychiatry 140:734–739, 1983

Kiernan RJ, Mueller J, Langston JW, et al: The neurobehavioral cognitive status examination: a brief but differentiated approach to cognitive assessment. Ann Intern Med 107:481–485, 1987

Kinsbourne M: The cerebral basis of lateral asymmetries in attention. Acta Psychol (Amst) 33:193–201, 1970

Krauthammer C, Klerman GL: Secondary mania. Arch Gen Psychiatry 35:1333–1339, 1978

Lipowski ZJ: Delirium: Acute Confusional States. New York, Oxford University Press, 1990

Lishman WA: Organic Psychiatry, 2nd Edition. Oxford, UK, Blackwell Scientific, 1987, pp 78–125

McGhie A: Pathology of Attention. Middlesex, UK, Penguin Books, 1969

Mesulam M-M: Attention, confusional states, and neglect, in Principles of Behavioral Neurology. Edited by Mesulam M-M. Philadelphia, PA, FA Davis, 1985, pp 125–140

Mungas D: In-office mental status testing: a practical guide. Geriatrics 46:54–66, 1991

Nelson A, Fogel BS, Faust D: Bedside cognitive screening instruments: a critical assessment. J Nerv Ment Dis 174:73–83, 1986

Ovsiew F: Bedside neuropsychiatry: eliciting the clinical phenomena of neuropsychiatric illness, in The American Psychiatric Press Textbook of Neuropsychiatry, 2nd Edition. Edited by Yudofsky SC, Hales RE. Washington, DC, American Psychiatric Press, 1992, pp 89–126

Pribram KH, McGuinness P: Arousal, activation and effort in the control of attention. Psychol Rev 82:116–149, 1975

Reitan RM: Validity of the Trail Making Test as an indicator of organic brain damage. Percept Mot Skills 8:271–276, 1958

Reitan RM: Aphasia and Sensory-Perceptual Deficits in Adults. Tucson, AZ, Neuropsychology Press, 1984

Rundell JR, Wise MG: Causes of organic mood disorder. J Neuropsychiatry Clin Neurosci 1:398–400, 1989

Schwamm LH, Van Dyke C, Kiernan RJ, et al: The Neurobehavioral Cognitive Status Examination: comparison with the Cognitive Capacity Screening Examination and the Mini-Mental State Examination in a neurosurgical population. Ann Intern Med 107:486–491, 1987

Squire LR, Butters N (eds): Neuropsychology of Memory. New York, Guilford, 1984

Strub RL, Black FW: The Mental Status Examination in Neurology. Philadelphia, PA, FA Davis, 1977

Strub RL, Black FW: The Mental Status Examination in Neurology, 2nd Edition. Philadelphia, PA, FA Davis, 1985

Strub RL, Black FW: Neurobehavioral Disorders: A Clinical Approach. Philadelphia, PA, FA Davis, 1988

Strub RL, Wise MG: Differential diagnosis in neuropsychiatry, in The American Psychiatric Press Textbook of Neuropsychiatry, 2nd Edition. Edited by Yudofsky SC, Hales RE. Washington, DC, American Psychiatric Press, 1992, pp 227–243

Taylor MA, Sierles FS, Abrams R: The neuropsychiatric evaluation, in Textbook of Neuropsychiatry. Edited by Hales RE, Yudofsky SC. Washington, DC, American Psychiatric Press, 1987, pp 3–16

Victor M, Hope JM: The phenomenon of auditory hallucinations in chronic alcoholism: a critical evaluation of the status of alcoholic hallucinosis. J Nerv Ment Dis 126:451–481, 1958

Victor M, Adams RD, Collins GH: The Wernicke-Korsakoff Syndrome and Related Neurologic Disorders Due to Alcoholism and Malnutrition, 2nd Edition. Philadelphia, PA, FA Davis, 1989

Weinstein EA, Friedland RP (eds): Hemi-Inattention and Hemispheric Specialization (Advances in Neurology Series, Vol 18). New York, Raven, 1977

Weintraub S, Mesulam M-M: Mental state assessment of young and elderly adults in behavioral neurology, in Principles of Behavioral Neurology. Edited by Mesulam M-M. Philadelphia, PA, FA Davis, 1985, pp 71–123

Wise MG, Rundell JR: Concise Guide to Consultation Psychiatry, 2nd Edition. Washington, DC, American Psychiatric Press, 1994, pp 11–30

Wise MG, Brannan SK, Shanfield SB, et al: Psychiatry aspects of organ transplantation (letter). JAMA 260:3437, 1988

Chapter 3

Behavioral Responses to Illness: Personality and Personality Disorders

Robert J. Ursano, M.D.
Richard S. Epstein, M.D.
Susan G. Lazar, M.D.

What is personality? How is it related to medical illness? These challenging questions are stimuli to much science and to much ancient and modern intellectual thought. A great deal of the activities of the consultation-liaison psychiatrist involve understanding the interaction between personality and disease.

Personality may be understood as a cluster of behavioral responses that depend on a person's past experiences, biological propensities, social context, and view of the future. The patient's past experiences form the lenses through which the patient looks at the present world and, in this way, directs the pattern of future behaviors. Although we are still only beginning to understand the contributions of bi-ology to behavior, we know that biology is the underpinning of basic human feelings such as anxiety and excitement and therefore, from infancy, directs individuals' needs for security, novelty, and avoidance. Social context is measured in gross form by questions such as "Living alone or with family?" But, more important, we measure our social context by the complex web of interpersonal relationships that make up our world and influence our behavior.

The patient's view of the future is often overlooked as a major organizer of behavior. Perhaps it is most noticed with the dying patient; too often, physicians and other providers assume the patient has "no future." The patient's behavior, however, may become organized by his or her own notion of the future.

For example, the future may be the issue of who will come to visit today or whether remaining tasks can be accomplished—including saying good-bye (Ursano and Fullerton 1991).

Personality is not static. It changes throughout the life cycle, from childhood to adulthood to old age (Colarusso and Nemiroff 1981). The patient's personality interacts with and is reactive to the individuals on the treatment team. These interactions may be realistic or influenced by past interpersonal relationships (e.g., transference and countertransference). One of the consultation-liaison psychiatrist's goals is to understand how the patient's personality contributes to the patient's illness, treatment, and adaptation. With this understanding, the consultation-liaison psychiatrist can recommend interventions that will maximize good medical treatment, healthy behaviors, and the patient's sense of hope and realistic expectations for the future.

■ PATIENT'S RESPONSE TO ILLNESS

Most individuals are highly resilient and cope well with an illness or injury. The consultation-liaison psychiatrist is usually consulted when personality issues complicate the treatment of an illness or hinder the patient's cooperation with the medical or nursing staff. Anxiety, agitation, depression, hostility, uncooperativeness, or even psychosis may reflect an adverse interaction between the patient's personality and the illness, which requires psychiatric consultation.

Defense Mechanisms

Understanding the patient's defense mechanisms is one way to identify the patient's behavioral tendencies both during times of acute stress and throughout the life cycle. DSM-IV (American Psychiatric Association 1994, pp. 751–757) contains a proposed axis for further study that assesses defense mechanisms and

coping styles—the Defensive Functioning Scale. Characteristic defense mechanisms are identified from the present and past history of the patient, the mental status examination, and observations of how the patient relates to others. The Defensive Functioning Scale organizes these defense mechanisms into defense levels: high adaptive level, mental inhibitions (compromise formation) level, minor image-distorting level, disavowal level, major image-distorting level, action level, and level of defensive dysregulation. Denial is a disavowal-level defense mechanism sometimes seen in consultation-liaison patients. Denial may be identified in the patient who avoids any expression of fear or depression about a serious prognosis. A patient in denial who avoids painful conflicts or illness-related life issues may further complicate the course of a chronic medical illness. A patient who shortly after being told he or she has cancer talks of fears of his or her pet cat not being fed is likely to be using displacement, a mental inhibition (compromise formation)–level defense. Some degree of regression is commonly seen in frightened patients who may become extremely dependent on and demanding of the medical staff. These patients often give mixed and conflicting "calls" for help that are impossible to satisfy.

Patients with borderline, schizoid, paranoid, schizotypal, antisocial, and dependent personality disorders often display a spectrum of less mature defense mechanisms. These patients are especially vulnerable to more pronounced regression leading to poor cooperation with the medical team. Patients who try to pit the medical staff against one another and attribute blame and evil intent to their caregivers are exhibiting splitting. The consultation-liaison psychiatrist, called to intervene in such situations, must try to be empathic and accepting even in the face of a hostile, accusatory patient. Simultaneously, the psychiatrist may need to encourage an alienated, divided, and sometimes overtly hostile medical staff to present a united front to the patient and to correct any actual lapses in empathy. Reestablishing empathy, responsiveness, and respect toward the patient, regardless of how irrational the patient's complaints may have been, is one of the most difficult tasks of the consultant.

A patient's characteristic defense mechanisms can stir powerful feelings in his or her primary physician and treatment team. These feelings are often the focus of the psychiatric consultation. The consultation-liaison psychiatrist's feelings toward the patient are important data. If the patient stimulates dislike, hate, strong attraction, or sexual thoughts, the physician or others on the treatment team may want to ignore or disown these feelings. However, these feelings can profoundly influence the primary physician's responses to the patient.

Groves (1978) identified four types of patients who stir dislike and hate in physicians: 1) dependent clingers, 2) entitled demanders, 3) manipulative help rejectors, and 4) self-destructive deniers. All manifest an insatiable dependency that may evoke hate, avoidance, and distrust in caregivers. All of these patients may have an atypical, agitated depression or another underlying psychiatric disorder; thus, it is critical to consider such conditions and treat them if present.

Helplessness and Control

Patients with acute, life-threatening medical illnesses frequently experience fear and helplessness. Not knowing enough facts about their illness and treatment increases the sense of helplessness. A monitor- and machine-laden intensive care unit, critical care unit, or recovery room may heighten a patient's sense of isolation and fear. When a critical care patient is oriented and attentive, his or her anxiety usually decreases with information about the realities of his or her condition and what he or she can do to actively exert some control over his or her situation and recovery. At the same time, consultation-liaison psychiatrists can also help medically ill patients accept the inevitable demands of the hospital, their loss of autonomy, and their dependency on the treatment team (Perry and Viederman 1981a, 1981b). For type A cardiac patients, information that provides an opportunity for more control over their illness can greatly enhance the doctor-patient relationship and assuage fears and uncooperativeness. A sense of control over one's illness can also empower the cancer patient who experiences pessimism and depression (Lederberg et al. 1990).

Shame and Guilt

Patients often react with shame and guilt if their lifestyles have contributed to their illness. This may be especially true for illnesses that result from smoking, substance abuse, and risky sexual behaviors. A nonjudgmental, empathic, and supportive stance by the consultation-liaison psychiatrist is important with these patients. Encouraging ventilation of self-criticism and guilty ruminations can increase cooperativeness, improve the patient's mood, and strengthen the doctor-patient relationship.

■ DOCTOR-PATIENT RELATIONSHIP: WORKING ALLIANCE AND SUPPORTIVE INTERVENTIONS

As with all patients, clinicians doing a psychiatric consultation should avoid both the pseudo-analytic, unresponsive posture and the rigidly "biological" impersonal approach (Perry and Viederman 1981a, 1981b). On the other hand, an overly sympathetic stance, which over-identifies with the patient's problems, may leave the patient wondering, "Where is the doctor?" and diminish the patient's feelings of hope. Davis (1968) used tape-recorded evaluations of 154 new patients at a general medicine clinic to study how various combinations of patient and physician interactive styles affected treatment compliance. He found that compliance was significantly reduced if both patient and doctor had a formal relationship and rejected or withheld help from each other. Patients in this situation became antagonistic and withdrew. Patients who were very active and authoritative with a physician who passively acquiesced were even more noncompliant with the doctor's recommendation. Davis (1968) concluded that the physician, including the consultation-liaison psychiatrist, is best served by a style that can engage the patient with "a spontaneity tempered by rational control and intent" (p. 276).

One goal of most psychiatric consultations with medically ill patients is improved adaptation and mastery of the illness situation and its treatment. The patient is truly dependent on the physician, and the physician and other care providers must comfortably accept this burden and opportunity. In brief psychotherapy in hospitalized patients, the consultation-liaison psychiatrist usually will strengthen the patient's defenses rather than explore them (see Lipsitt, Chapter 33, this volume).

Obtaining a patient's Psychodynamic Life Narrative (Perry and Viederman 1981a, 1981b) may help the consultation-liaison psychiatrist to identify adaptive coping mechanisms. In this process, the psychiatrist does a careful psychiatric history and psychodynamic evaluation to help the patient develop a new understanding of his or her illness in the context of his or her unique history, character, life situation, and personal goals.

Transference and Countertransference

All patients have positive and negative reactions to their physician. Many patients have more dramatic transference reactions to their physician and other caregivers. Illness, hospitalization, pain, and fear increase the frequency and intensity of transference reactions. The physician may be seen as a reliable parent or authority figure from the past. Alternatively, the physician may be viewed with fear and suspicion as a disappointing figure from the past (Ursano et al. 1991). Manifestations of the transference to the physician and the medical staff often prompt the request for a psychiatric consultation. During the assessment, the patient may also have similar transference feelings toward the consultation-liaison psychiatrist. Often, however, the patient's transference feelings to the consultation-liaison psychiatrist are less intense because the consultant has had less contact with the patient. Therefore, these distortions of the patient–treatment team relationship can perhaps be worked out with the consultation-liaison psychiatrist's help. It is helpful for the consultation-liaison psychiatrist to remember that "there but for the grace of God go I." This reminder that the patient and the treating physician are caught in this web of the past helps the psychiatrist to see the situation more clearly.

Similarly, all patients elicit in their physicians—both their primary physician and the consultation-liaison psychiatrist—positive or negative reactions or full countertransference responses. Countertransference can be in either of two forms: a response to the patient or an identification with the patient's feelings and beliefs. In the first case, an older patient may remind the physician of a paternal figure. Such a patient who is hostile, suspicious, and demanding and subtly or overtly blames the physician might make the physician feel too defensive and rejecting. The consultant might find himself or herself forgetting to see the patient on rounds or making pointed and angry jokes about the patient. This overreaction is the physician's countertransference. The physician might then realize that his or her reaction was similar to the reaction he or she had to a past figure who was demeaning and belittling. Alternatively, the countertransference may show up as an identification: the physician might agree with the patient's views of the world without verifying them, perhaps assuming that the patient's treatment staff were really evil or not caring. In both countertransference situations, the consultation-liaison psychiatrist should do a thorough evaluation and obtain information from the treatment team. Using one's reactions to a patient as information to help understand what the treatment team experiences can help the consultation-liaison psychiatrist recommend effective interventions.

A major task for the consultation-liaison psychiatrist is to forge a therapeutic alliance with the patient and to help the patient form an alliance with the medical and surgical treatment team. To do this, the consultation-liaison psychiatrist may need to address the transference of the patient and/or the countertransference of the staff. The psychiatrist should empathize with the patient's specific fears and foster a sense of mastery and control. This may alleviate anxiety and regression and reinforce more mature cooperation. The psychiatrist often must help other physicians and staff avoid defensive postures that are stimulated by countertransference responses such as being too competitive, solicitous, or detached. When the consultation-liaison psychiatrist can convey to the house staff and the nurses an understanding of the patient's behaviors based on present and past events in the patient's life, the treatment team's reactions to the patient may change substantially. Helping physicians and staff understand what it is about a particular patient that makes them feel uncomfortable can help the staff better tolerate strong affect. Often, when the caregivers can see the patient's concerns, they can return to their usual role of wanting to alleviate the patient's suffering. The consultation-liaison psychiatrist facilitates this process by both modeling and explaining how best to react supportively in the face of the patient's regressive behavior and defenses (Perry and Viederman 1981a, 1981b).

■ PERSONALITY DISORDERS AND SOMATIC ILLNESS

Classification and Assessment

Personality traits—characteristic behavioral response patterns—are the typical ways that an individual thinks, feels, and relates to others. These traits are often called chronic or severe. When these patterns are fixed, inflexible, unresponsive to changes in the environment, and maladaptive, they can result in psychological and social dysfunction and may constitute a personality disorder.

The psychiatric diagnostic classification system (DSM-IV) causes some major problems for the study of the personality disorders because the clinically recognized dysfunctional personalities are not limited to the types listed in that system (see Table 3–1). The various taxonomic systems for classifying characterological features, including Hippocrates' four humors and Fourier's 810 character types, are thoroughly discussed by Frances and Widiger (1986). There is considerable overlap between the various systems, although different terms are often used for the same idea (McCrae and Costa 1990).

A five-factor model of personality (Dembrowski and Costa 1987; T. W. Smith and Williams 1992; Wise 1992) has been used to study the relation between individual traits and somatic diseases. This system of classifying personality traits was derived from a factor analysis of approximately 18,000 adjectives in the English language used to describe personality

Table 3–1. DSM-IV Axis II disorders

Cluster A: odd or eccentric characteristics

Paranoid personality disorder
Schizoid personality disorder
Schizotypal personality disorder

Cluster B: dramatic, emotional, or erratic characteristics

Antisocial personality disorder
Borderline personality disorder
Histrionic personality disorder
Narcissistic personality disorder

Cluster C: anxious or fearful characteristics

Avoidant personality disorder
Dependent personality disorder
Obsessive-compulsive personality disorder

characteristics (McCrae and Costa 1990). The five factors McCrae and Costa found included neuroticism, extroversion, openness, agreeableness, and conscientiousness (see Table 3–2).

The American Psychiatric Association's classification of personality disorders has evolved through an interesting series of revisions of the *Diagnostic and Statistical Manual of Mental Disorders* (Blashfield and McElroy 1989). The current version, DSM-IV, relies on a nontheoretical set of categories. Diagnosis is based on meeting a threshold number of symptoms. Because of considerable symptom overlap among the various Axis II conditions, personality disorders have been described as "fuzzy sets" (Livesley 1986). Although the personality disorders are divided into A, B, and C clusters in DSM-IV (see Table 3–1), this grouping has not received much support from a clinical or practical standpoint (Widiger and Rogers 1989).

Axis II diagnoses are defined by symptom "menus" that range from 7 to 10 items. Depending on the disorder, at least 4 or 5 symptoms are necessary before a specific Axis II diagnosis can be made. This results in a

Table 3–2.   Five-factor system of personality traits

Neuroticism

   Tendency toward negative affects (e.g., anxiety, depression, self-consciousness, poor impulse control, and angry or hostile thoughts)

Extroversion

   Tendency to be outgoing and talkative

Openness to experience

   Tendency to be curious, interested, and creative

Agreeableness

   Tendency to be good-natured and trusting; a negative score on this dimension consists of an antagonistic, rude, and behaviorally aggressive style

Conscientiousness

   Tendency to be ambitious and goal directed

numerical anomaly that can bias the prevalence of the different disorders in epidemiological studies. For example, there are 210 possible combinations of symptoms by which an individual can meet criteria for the diagnosis of antisocial personality disorder (4 symptoms out of 10) but only 35 ways that a person could receive a diagnosis of avoidant personality disorder (4 symptoms out of 7). Humorists might conclude from this situation that it is more difficult to be shy than to be psychopathic.

Some investigators have criticized the diagnostic reliance on behavioral checklists. Although diagnosis based on discrete behavior has relatively high reliability, it does not address personality traits detected by studying the patient's characteristic defense mechanisms (Grossman 1982), psychometric test results, or longitudinal clinical observations. Because of these shortcomings, many aspects of a patient's personality dysfunction are overlooked in the DSM-IV classification system.

Clinical observational studies have shown that other characterological disturbances exist in addition to the official list of Axis II conditions that qualify as personality disorders (see Table 3–3). Many of these conditions, such as alexithymia and type A behavior pattern, have been of great interest to consultation-liaison psychiatrists. Some conditions, such as dysthymia, cyclothymia, and multiple personality disorder, are categorized by the DSM classification committee as Axis I disorders, although they are more characteristic of the usual understanding of a personality disorder.

Alexithymia is an impaired ability to perceive or express emotions. In an extreme form, it might qualify as a personality disorder because the individual's characteristic way of dealing with feelings is maladaptive and inflexible. However, based on the operational definition, reliable measurement of alexithymia is difficult. In various studies, alexithymia was highly prevalent in patients with psychosomatic conditions, chronic psychogenic pain, and psychological conditions affecting a physi-

Table 3–3.   Personality disturbances not included in the official list of Axis II conditions

DSM-IV diagnosis provided for further study

Depressive personality disorder
Passive-aggressive personality disorder (negativistic personality disorder)

Listed as Axis I disorders

Dysthymia
Cyclothymia
Dissociative identity disorder (formerly multiple personality disorder)

Other personality disturbances

Type A behavior pattern
Alexithymia
Pain-prone disorder (Blumer and Heilbronn 1982)

ological disorder (Krystal 1988; Lesser and Lesser 1983; Taylor 1984; Taylor et al. 1990).

Diagnosis

Obtaining the comprehensive history necessary for diagnosing a personality disorder is time-consuming and difficult. This is particularly problematic for consultation-liaison psychiatrists, who often must propose practical recommendations to the referring physician after a relatively short evaluation. In addition, patients with somatic complaints often have physical pain and are fatigued, distractible, and sometimes not cooperative with extensive diagnostic evaluations. It is also difficult to differentiate a characteristic behavioral pattern from acute stress disorder or typical behavior during a significant illness or hospitalization. For patients who have several Axis II conditions, it may take several hours of interviewing, along with collateral information obtained from family members, to establish a reliable diagnosis. For these reasons, consultation-liaison psychiatrists initially tend to focus on the most prominent and remediable psychiatric symptomatology and defer Axis II assessment until the patient is discharged to his or her usual environment.

Some patients' chronic physical disorders or Axis I conditions (e.g., bipolar disorder, posttraumatic stress disorder) are sometimes misdiagnosed as personality disorders because the clinician incorrectly assesses the onset and chronicity of the symptoms. Consequently, it is important during the evaluation to determine whether the personality traits and behaviors observed during the mental status examination are long-standing, stable maladaptations that predate the present stressful clinical situation. Patients may behave much differently in the hospital than they do at home. Collateral information from family members is a critical part of this process.

The high comorbidity of Axis I and Axis II disorders (Dowson 1992; Goldsmith et al. 1989; Widiger and Rogers 1989) also creates diagnostic difficulties. The inflexible and maladaptive coping behaviors used by patients with personality disorders make them more likely to develop depression and anxiety syndromes (Widiger and Rogers 1989). The ideal assessment of personality disorders should combine the patient's self-report, the report of a close family member, the clinician's assessment of the presence or absence of specific behaviors, assessments over time as an outpatient, and a diagnostic evaluation of comorbid conditions.

Epidemiology

The epidemiology of personality disorders in medical-surgical patients has been limited by the nosological fuzziness of the personality disorders, the comorbidity of Axis II and Axis I disorders, the difficulty in making cross-sectional assessments at times of great duress, and the fact that epidemiological assessments of Axis II disorders are time-consuming and expensive. Therefore, it is not surprising that present estimates of the prevalence of personality disorders range widely from study to study, even in physically healthy populations. More efficacious and reliable instruments are needed to overcome these problems.

Merikangas and Weissman (1986) reviewed the epidemiological studies of the prevalence of personality disorders in the general population. Four studies conducted between 1951 and 1963, with a total of 5,471 individuals, suggested that the prevalence of personality disorders ranged from 6% to 9%.

In many patients with personality disorders in hospital settings who are referred to consultation-liaison psychiatrists, their conditions are not always recognized and written in the medical record. Personality disorder diagnoses are almost never included in hospitalization discharge summaries. Hales et al. (1986) found that only 4.5% of the patients in their series of 1,065 patients referred within a military hospital received an Axis II diagnosis, even though 16.5% of all referrals were made because of behavior difficulties (e.g., adjustment difficulties or conflict with physicians and staff). They suggested that military psychiatrists may have been reluctant to diagnose a condition that could lead to the patient's administrative discharge from the military. In contrast, in a prospective study of psychiatric consultations seen in a family practice clinic, Katon et al. (1981) found that 25% of the patients received a personality disorder diagnosis.

Mounting evidence suggests that somatization is associated with Axis II disorders. In a prospective study of 100 patients with somatizing illness (not somatization disorder) referred to a hospital-based consultation-liaison psychiatric service, Katon and colleagues (1984) made a definite personality disorder diagnosis in 37%. This rate was significantly higher than the level found in patients without somatizing illness (16%). Histrionic personality disorder was diagnosed in 12% of the patients with somatizing illness but in only 2% of those without somatizing illness.

Interaction of Personality Disorders and Somatic Illness

The relatively fixed behavioral response patterns found in patients with personality disor-

ders can affect somatic illness in many ways, and vice versa. For example, maladaptive behaviors, such as alcohol use, can directly increase the risk of diseases, such as liver disease, or not using a seat belt can increase the risk of traumatic injury. Alternatively, chronic medical conditions, such as chronic pain or life-threatening chronic illness, can lead to maladaptive chronic behavioral patterns (e.g., expectation of disappointment and rejection).

The patient's personality greatly influences his or her likelihood of seeking versus delaying appropriate treatment or adhering to versus interfering with needed treatment. This problem may reflect specific "hypertrophied" defenses of the personality disorder (e.g., denial) or may be a specific negative transference reaction. Frances and Widiger (1986) emphasized that character pathology is often at the core of negative transference manifestations that interfere with a patient's ability to seek out and cooperate with treatment. This problem is very important and difficult to manage in patients whose passive-aggressiveness leads them to act out marked resentment against their treating physicians or family members who are concerned about their health.

Personality disorders per se can be major etiological factors in somatic symptomatology. In most cases of factitious disorder, a personality disorder is at the core of the patient's inappropriate need to be in the patient role. Many of these patients exhibit borderline, self-defeating, and antisocial features. In a consecutive series of 1,288 patients referred to a consultation-liaison psychiatric service, Sutherland and Rodin (1990) found that 10 (0.8%) patients received a diagnosis of factitious disorder. One patient feigned psychiatric symptoms, and the other patients presented with a variety of somatic symptoms, such as self-inflicted trauma and infections. Elliott (1987) reviewed clinical observations of patients with Munchausen syndrome and suggested that masochistic personality features were prominent.

Personality disorders can also influence

use of medications, both prescribed and over-the-counter, particularly the use of hypnotic and psychotropic medications. Allgulander et al. (1990) studied a sample of 30,344 Swedish twins. They found that individuals with a diagnosis of neurosis or personality disorder, as defined by ICD-8 (World Health Organization 1968) criteria, were 11 times more likely to use sedative-hypnotic and other psychotropic drugs than were individuals without such a diagnosis.

Poor health care habits and improper attention to early symptoms of an impending medical condition can lead to the exacerbation or early onset of a disease. For example, Small et al. (1970) found that most of their sample of 100 patients with passive-aggressive personality disorder had frequent somatic complaints and neglected their personal hygiene. Failure to maintain good physical hygiene is a way that passive-aggressive patients act out their anger toward individuals they depend on in their lives.

A somatic presentation is also very common in dissociative identity disorder (DID), formerly called multiple personality disorder (Ross et al. 1990), and may be higher than that found in other psychiatric conditions. Ross et al. (1989) found that 35% of patients with DID also met criteria for somatization disorder.

Stoudemire and Thompson (1983) examined the ways that patients with certain personality disorders become noncompliant with medication. Denial was a characteristic defense mechanism that interfered with the patient's ability to either acknowledge the presence of somatic illness or realistically appraise the risks of refusing treatment. They also noted that patients with borderline personality disorder often experience considerable difficulty trusting their physicians and that their impulsiveness and self-destructive behavior hamper cooperation with medical recommendations. Patients with paranoid or schizoid personality disorders are often highly suspicious of authority figures such as physicians.

Laihinen (1991) reported that dermatological conditions often become chronic because of a personality disorder, emotional immaturity, untreated depression, and pleasure from scratching. Kellner (1983) found that patients with DSM-III (American Psychiatric Association 1980) hypochondriasis who had concurrent personality disorders were less likely to improve with psychotherapy than patients with hypochondriasis who did not have a personality disorder.

Patients with personality disorders probably constitute the group with the highest likelihood of stimulating countertransference reactions that lead to nontherapeutic staff and physician behaviors. The patient's personality disorder may interfere with the physician's or the medical staff's ability to function and respond as appropriate caregivers. This may lead to avoiding the patient, being unable to notice a change in symptom pattern, or assigning the patient's care to the least skilled member of the medical team. In this way, countertransference problems of caregivers elicited by the patient's personality disorder can influence the patient's clinical outcome.

Patients with borderline, self-defeating, paranoid, passive-aggressive, and antisocial personality disorders are particularly likely to engender anger, confusion, and frustration in their caregivers. When these feelings interfere with the care of the patient or are out of proportion to the events, a countertransference reaction is likely to be present and must be addressed. The excessive demandingness of masochistic patients with somatic illness can especially irritate the treatment team (Elliott 1987). Patients who "doctor shop" and become labeled as "crocks" frequently have a masochistic character (Lipsitt 1970). Their self-defeating method of seeking help results in physicians not taking their complaints seriously because their symptoms appear impervious to relief. These patients may unconsciously request caring rather than cure (Lipsitt 1970). They experience the physician's impatient therapeutic zeal as a rejection because they feel unworthy of care without their suffering. One way of avoiding a sadomasochistic struggle with such patients is to offer them conservative ongoing care that is not predicated on symptomatic results.

CONCLUSION

Assessment of the patient's personality is a necessary part of a comprehensive psychiatric consultation. The consultation-liaison psychiatrist observes the patient's present characteristic defense mechanisms and gathers information about previous response patterns. Patterns of relating to the treatment team and the consultation-liaison psychiatrist provide data on the patient's present defense mechanisms, level of psychological defensive functioning, and potential transference reactions. In addition, the consultation-liaison psychiatrist's feelings about the patient can provide valuable clinical information. Personality disorders per se are also common in medically ill patients. As with personality styles, personality disorders influence the medical illness and are influenced by it. The presentation of an illness and styles of relating to the caregivers can be influenced by a personality disorder. The consultation-liaison psychiatrist "translates" the description of the patient's "pain" from the language and behavior of a unique personality to the language of the treating physician and vice versa.

REFERENCES

Allgulander C, Nowak J, Rice JP: Psychopathology and treatment of 30,344 twins in Sweden, I: the appropriateness of psychoactive drug treatment. Acta Psychiatr Scand 82:420–426, 1990

American Psychiatric Association: Diagnostic and Statistical Manual of Mental Disorders, 3rd Edition. Washington, DC, American Psychiatric Association, 1980

American Psychiatric Association: Diagnostic and Statistical Manual of Mental Disorders, 4th Edition. Washington, DC, American Psychiatric Association, 1994

Blashfield RK, McElroy RA: Ontology of personality disorder categories. Psychiatric Annals 19: 126–131, 1989

Blumer D, Heilbronn M: Chronic pain as a variant of depressive disease: the pain-prone disorder. J Nerv Ment Dis 170:381–406, 1982

Colarusso CA, Nemiroff RA: Adult Development. New York, Plenum, 1981

Davis MS: Variations in patients' compliance with doctors' advice: an empirical analysis of patterns of communication. Am J Public Health 58:274–288, 1968

Dembrowski TM, Costa PT: Coronary prone behavior: components of the type A pattern and hostility. J Pers 55:211–235, 1987

Dowson JH: Assessment of DSM-III-R personality disorders by self-report questionnaire: the role of informants and a screening test for comorbid personality disorders (STCPD). Br J Psychiatry 161:344–352, 1992

Elliott RL: The masochistic patient in consultation-liaison psychiatry. Gen Hosp Psychiatry 9: 241–250, 1987

Frances AJ, Widiger T: The classification of personality disorders: an overview of problems and solutions, in Psychiatry Update: American Psychiatric Association Annual Review, Vol 5. Edited by Frances AJ, Hales RE. Washington, DC, American Psychiatric Press, 1986, pp 240–257

Goldsmith SJ, Jacobsberg LB, Bell R: Personality disorder assessment. Psychiatric Annals 19: 139–142, 1989

Grossman S: A psychoanalyst-liaison psychiatrist's overview of DSM III. Gen Hosp Psychiatry 4:291–295, 1982

Groves JE: Taking care of the hateful patient. N Engl J Med 298:883–887, 1978

Hales RE, Polly S, Bridenbaugh H, et al: Psychiatric consultations in a military general hospital. Gen Hosp Psychiatry 8:173–182, 1986

Katon W, Williamson P, Ries R: A prospective study of 60 consecutive psychiatric consultations in a family medicine clinic. J Fam Pract 13:47–55, 1981

Katon W, Ries RK, Kleinman A: Part II: a prospective study of 100 consecutive somatization patients. Compr Psychiatry 25:305–314, 1984

Kellner R: Prognosis of treated hypochondriasis. Acta Psychiatr Scand 67:69–79, 1983

Krystal H (ed): Integration and Self-Healing: Affect, Trauma, Alexithymia. Hillsdale, NJ, Analytic Press, 1988, pp 144–146

Laihinen A: Assessment of psychiatric and psychosocial factors disposing to chronic outcome of dematoses. Acta Derm Venereol Suppl (Stockh) 156:46–48, 1991

Lederberg M, Massie MJ, Holland JC: Psychiatric consultation to oncology, in American Psychiatric Press Review of Psychiatry, Vol 9. Edited by Tasman A, Goldfinger SM, Kaufmann CA. Washington, DC, American Psychiatric Press, 1990, pp 491–514

Lesser IM, Lesser BZ: Alexithymia: examining the development of a psychological concept. Am J Psychiatry 140:1305–1308, 1983

Lipsitt DR: Medical and psychological characteristics of "crocks." Psychiatry in Medicine 1:15–25, 1970

Livesley WJ: Trait and behavioral prototypes of personality disorder. Am J Psychiatry 143:728–732, 1986

McCrae RR, Costa PT: Personality in Adulthood. New York, Guilford, 1990

Merikangas KR, Weissman MM: Epidemiology of DSM-III Axis II personality disorders, in Psychiatry Update: American Psychiatric Association Annual Review, Vol 5. Edited by Frances AJ, Hales RE. Washington, DC, American Psychiatric Press, 1986, pp 258–278

Perry S, Viederman M: Adaptations of residents to consultation/liaison psychiatry, I: working with the physically ill. Gen Hosp Psychiatry 3:141–147, 1981a

Perry S, Viederman M: Adaptation of residents to consultation/liaison psychiatry, II: working with the "nonpsychiatric staff." Gen Hosp Psychiatry 3:149–156, 1981b

Ross CA, Heber S, Norton GR, et al: Somatic symptoms in multiple personality disorder. Psychosomatics 30:154–160, 1989

Ross CA, Miller SD, Reagor P, et al: Structured interview data on 102 cases of multiple personality disorder from four centers. Am J Psychiatry 147:596–601, 1990

Small IF, Small JG, Alig VB, et al: Passive-aggressive personality disorder: a search for a syndrome. Am J Psychiatry 126:973–983, 1970

Smith TW, Williams PG: Personality and health: advantages and limitations of the five-factor model. J Pers 60:395–423, 1992

Stoudemire A, Thompson TL II: Medication noncompliance: systematic approaches to evaluation and intervention. Gen Hosp Psychiatry 5:233–239, 1983

Sutherland AJ, Rodin GM: Factitious disorders in a general hospital setting. Psychosomatics 31:392–399, 1990

Taylor GJ: Alexithymia: concept, measurement, and implications for treatment. Am J Psychiatry 141:725–732, 1984

Taylor GJ, Bagby RM, Ryan DP, et al: Validation of the alexithymia construct: a measurement-based approach. Can J Psychiatry 35:290–297, 1990

Ursano RJ, Fullerton CS: Psychotherapy: medical intervention and the concept of normality, in The Diversity of Normal Behavior. Edited by Offer D, Sabshin M. New York, Basic Books, 1991, pp 39–59

Ursano RJ, Sonnenberg SM, Lazar SG: Concise Guide to Psychodynamic Psychotherapy. Washington, DC, American Psychiatric Press, 1991

Widiger TA, Rogers JH: Prevalence and comorbidity of personality disorders. Psychiatric Annals 19:132–136, 1989

Wise TN: Psychiatric management of functional gastrointestinal disorders. Psychiatric Annals 22:606–611, 1992

World Health Organization: International Classification of Diseases, 8th Revision. Geneva, World Health Organization, 1968

Chapter 4

Suicidality

John Michael Bostwick, M.D.
James R. Rundell, M.D.

Suicide, even in the psychiatric population, is a rare event, and the demographic risk factors alone will identify many more patients potentially at risk than imminently in danger of dying (Goldberg 1987). Unfortunately, no epidemiological factors represent an individual's suicidal intent—the essential variable in suicide prediction (Davidson 1993). Yet this absence of specific suicide attempt predictors is no cause for therapeutic nihilism. A suicide threat is a statement of ambivalent distress about something of meaning to the patient that must be understood if he or she is to be helped.

EPIDEMIOLOGY

General Population

Completed suicide. It is reported that more than 30,000 Americans kill themselves each year. The actual number is undoubtedly higher because many suicides are never identified as such or are reported as accidents or other causes of death. At 12 deaths per year per 100,000 Americans—0.5%–1% of all deaths in the United States—suicide is now the eighth leading cause of death (Roy 1989). The known suicide rate is nearly identical to what it was in 1900 (Monk 1987).

The suicide rate in men is three times higher than in women, and the rate for whites is almost twice that for blacks (Roy 1989). People who are socially isolated or who are widowed, divorced, or separated have higher rates of suicide than those who have ongoing, supporting relationships with friends and family (Monk 1987).

Suicide assessment begins with epidemiological analysis. With the first glance at the hospital card or consult request, the consultant already has many demographic clues to the patient's relative suicide risk. The consultation-liaison psychiatrist thus begins to build a formulation of suicide risk on an epidemiological foundation. Traditionally, epidemiological studies have shown that suicide attempters are more likely to be younger, female, and married and to use pills, whereas completers are more likely to be older, male, and single and to use violent means (Fawcett and Shaughnessy 1988). However, it must be remembered that anyone at any age may contemplate or execute suicide.

Over the course of the life cycle, men and women have different patterns of suicide. For men, suicide rates gradually rise during adolescence, increase sharply in early adulthood, and parallel advancing age up to the 75- to 84-year age bracket, at which time they reach a rate of 22.0 suicides per 100,000 (Shneidman 1989). Suicide rates for women peak in midlife and then decline, in contrast to the bimodal peaks for men. Suicide methods tend to be more violent and lethal for men, who are more likely to die by hanging, drowning, and shooting. Women are less likely to die in suicide attempts because they are more likely to choose the less lethal methods of wrist cutting and overdose (Kaplan and Klein 1989; Morgan 1989).

In the general population, psychiatric disorders—particularly depression and alcoholism—are associated with the vast majority of retrospectively studied completed suicides. Of 134 suicides in St. Louis County, MO, 94% had diagnosable psychiatric disorders and an additional 4% had terminal medical illness. Forty-seven percent of those who died had major depression, and 24% had alcoholism.

Attempted suicide. It is false security to regard attempted suicides as a discrete category from completed ones (Table 4–1). For some reason, many patients with a potentially lethal suicide attempt survive (Kellner et al. 1985). Some characteristics nonetheless distinguish surviving attempters from those who die. Although men die as a result of suicide at higher rates than women, women attempt at higher rates than men. Men tend to use more lethal, less reversible means (e.g., shooting, hanging), whereas women are more likely to attempt suicide by overdosing on medication. Patients who overdose are more likely to survive because they have time after the act to reconsider (or be found) and undergo medical treatment, an option not so frequently available after a jump or a gunshot wound.

Medically Ill Patients

Physical disease is an independent suicide risk factor present among a high proportion of people who commit suicide (Kontaxakis et al. 1988). Physical illness is present in 25%–75% of all suicide victims (Roy 1989). Sanders (1988) reviewed six studies of patients who committed suicide while admitted to a general hospital. Most of these patients had chronic or terminal illnesses that were painful, debilitating, or both. Some had multiple illnesses.

As in the general population, completed

Table 4–1. Attempted versus completed suicide in the general population

Risk category	Attempted	Completed
Male:female ratio	1:3	3:1
Most common methods	Wrist slashing Overdosing	Hanging Jumping Shooting
Most common psychiatric diagnoses	Personality disorder	Depression
Most common affect	Impulsive anger	Hopelessness
Most common precipitant	Acute relationship difficulty or loss	Chronic painful or disfiguring illness
Most common goal	Manipulation of others	Annihilation of self

suicides usually occur in medically ill patients who have comorbid, often unrecognized, psychiatric or neurological illness (Davidson 1993; Kellner et al. 1985) (Table 4–2).

It must be emphasized that regardless of how horrific the medical condition, significant suicide risk is not the rule. According to Brown et al. (1986), in a study of 44 terminally ill patients, only 10, all of whom had major depression, were at risk for suicide. The investigators concluded that "the majority of fatally ill people do not develop a severe depression" and "suicidal thoughts and desire for death appear in our patient group to be linked exclusively to the presence of mental disorder" (p. 210).

Table 4–2. Factors associated with suicide in medical-surgical patients

Completed suicide
  Chronic or terminal illness
  Painful or disfiguring illness
  Dyspnea
  Ostomy
  Comorbid psychiatric pathology
  Depression
  Dependent-dissatisfied personality
  Agitated delirium
  Hopelessness

Attempted suicide
  Distinguishing characteristics
    Impaired impulse control due to personality disorder, psychosis, functional disorder (schizophrenia or bipolar disorder), organic brain syndrome
  Method
    Lower lethality, greater reversibility
  Affect
    Anger, not depression
  Precipitant
    Loss of emotional support/interpersonal struggles with staff or family

Source. Adapted from Reich P, Kelly MJ: "Suicide Attempts by Hospitalized Medical and Surgical Patients." *New England Journal of Medicine* 294:298–301, 1976. Copyright 1976, Massachusetts Medical Society. Used with permission.

Hospitalized Medical-Surgical Patients

Suicidal hospitalized patients, especially those who are impulsive, harm themselves by the most expedient means available. In modern, multilevel hospitals, the easiest and quickest method has proven to be jumping from a window. In Glickman's (1980) study of 22 completed and 23 attempted suicides in King's County Hospital, Brooklyn, NY, between 1963 and 1978, 19 of 22 suicide victims jumped, as did 9 of 23 patients who attempted suicide. Five additional patients who attempted suicide tried to jump. These findings confirm those of earlier studies by Pollack (1957) and Farberow and Litman (1970), who found that 10 of 11 patients and 10 of 12 general hospital patients, respectively, jumped to their deaths.

The high lethality of jumping from a significant height makes death usually inevitable regardless of whether the patient actually intends to die. In a sample of medical inpatients at Peter Bent Brigham Hospital, Boston, MA, between 1967 and 1973, Reich and Kelly (1976) studied 17 patients who attempted suicide and survived. Of these 17 patients, 7 overdosed, 7 cut themselves, 1 hung herself, 1 inhaled a poisonous agent, and only 1 jumped. They judged 15 of the 17 patients to have mental disorders, but the cardinal suicide characteristics of depression and hopelessness were not present in this sample. "All . . . were impulsive acts, none of the patients gave warnings, left notes, expressed suicidal thoughts or appeared to be seriously depressed" (p. 973). Reich and Kelly linked these 17 attempts to impulsive reactions to loss of emotional support, usually from staff. The primary affect was anger.

Impulsivity can be countered. Pisetsky and Brown (1979) calculated a suicide rate of 1.55 per 10,000 patient admissions at the Bronx Veterans Administration Hospital in New York from 1947 to 1958 but found a rate of only 0.32 per 10,000 from 1971 to 1975. Between the two data collection periods, the authors successfully persuaded the hospital to implement programs to secure the windows and have the staff pay more careful attention to disruptions in the doctor-patient relationship. As a result of their recommendations, a fivefold drop in suicide rate occurred (Sanders 1988).

SUICIDE RISK FACTORS AMONG MEDICAL-SURGICAL PATIENTS

Medical Factors

Certain medical disorders that the psychiatric consultant will encounter in both inpatient and outpatient settings are associated with increased suicide risk. Three of these disorders are discussed in the following sections.

Cancer. In the most comprehensive study of the relation between cancer and suicide, Allebeck and colleagues (1985) gathered statistics on 963 suicides between 1962 and 1979 among 424,127 Swedish people with a diagnosis of cancer and found a 1.9 relative risk for men and a 1.6 relative risk for women. Gastrointestinal tumors (excluding colon and rectum) in men (relative risk 3.1) and lung tumors in either sex (relative risk 3.1 in men, 3.5 in women) were associated with the highest mortality from suicide. Allebeck and colleagues also made the important discovery that the longer the time from diagnosis, the lower the relative risk. In the first year after diagnosis, the relative risk is 16.0 for men and 15.4 for women. From 1 to 2 years, the ratio declines to 6.5 for men and 7.0 for women. By 3–6 years, the ratio is 2.1 for men and 3.2 for women. By 10 years after diagnosis, the rate, at 0.4, is actually less than one-half that in the general population.

The pain, disfigurement, and loss of function that cancer evokes in the popular imagination can precipitate suicide, especially early in patients' courses. The high relative risk of suicide just after diagnosis corresponds to a time of great fear. However, the data also suggest that as cancer patients live longer with their dis-

ease, they become less frightened and less susceptible to suicide as an escape from the terror.

Chronic renal failure. More formidable than the suicide risk among cancer patients is the relative suicide risk elevation in chronic renal failure patients. Abrams et al. (1971) reported very high rates of suicide and suicidal behavior among 3,478 renal dialysis patients studied at 127 dialysis centers. In their sample, 20 deaths were a result of suicide; 17 suicide attempts were unsuccessful; 22 patients withdrew from the program, knowing that doing so would hasten their deaths; and 117 deaths were attributed to noncompliance with treatment regimens. Although the authors claim a widely quoted suicide incidence rate of 400 times that of the general population, they do not make clear in their paper the time frame during which the dialysis patients committed suicide. Thus, their suicide figure is a prevalence rate. They also used an extremely broad definition of suicide that encompassed death caused by a wide range of causes, from willful acts of self-destruction to noncompliance. Nonetheless, suicidal behavior as defined by the authors occurred in approximately 5% of this large group of dialysis patients.

Acquired immunodeficiency syndrome. AIDS patients also have a high relative risk for suicide, even though the risk may be declining. Marzuk and associates (1988) found a suicide rate 36 times that of an age-matched sample of men without AIDS and 66 times that of the general population in New York City in 1985. In California, in 1986, the rate was 21 times higher than that in the general population (Kizer et al. 1988). In the largest study to date, Cote et al. (1991) charted a continuous decline of suicide rates, year by year, among AIDS patients in 45 states and the District of Columbia. In 1987, 1988, and 1989, 165 suicides among AIDS patients were reported to the National Center for Health Statistics. Of these, 164 were men. The relative suicide risk calculated for AIDS patients was 10.5 in 1987, 7.4 in 1988, and 6.0 in 1989. The authors attribute the decline to advances in medical care, diminishing social stigma, and improved psychiatric services; they also noted underreporting of deaths due to both AIDS and suicide.

Psychiatric Risk Factors

If a patient has a long-standing psychiatric diagnosis that predates a medical or surgical condition, the psychiatric consultant must be more suspicious about the possibility of suicide (Table 4–3). Patients with psychiatric disorders kill themselves at rates 3–12 times higher than other patients (Evenson et al. 1982). Male patients who have ever had a psychiatric admission die as a result of suicide at 5.7 times the rate for men in the general population. For men identified as psychiatric patients but never actually hospitalized, the rate is 3.4 times that of the general population. For women, the respective rates are 10 times and 4 times that of the general population.

History of a suicide attempt appears to be an important predictor of future suicide risk (Pokorny 1983). One of every 100 suicide attempt survivors will die by suicide within 1 year of their index attempt, a suicide risk approximately 100 times that of the general population (Hawton 1992).

Litman (1989) estimated that based on psychological autopsies, 95% of patients who completed suicide had psychiatric diagnoses, including 40% with mood disorders (bipolar or unipolar), 20%–25% with chronic alcoholism, 10%–15% with schizophrenia, and 20%–25% with severe personality disorder (Table 4–4).

An estimated 15% of patients with mood disorders eventually commit suicide, with the risk highest early in the illness course (Guze and Robins 1970). The Epidemiologic Catchment Area study revealed a lifetime suicide attempt rate of 7.0% among patients with uncomplicated panic disorder and 7.9% among patients with uncomplicated major depression.

With comorbid panic disorder and depression, the lifetime rate of suicide attempts rose to 19.5% (Johnson et al. 1990). Ten percent of patients with schizophrenia will eventually kill themselves, with the risk also greatest early in the illness course (Miles 1977).

One-quarter of all suicides occur in patients with active alcohol use disorders. Miles (1977) estimated that 15% of alcoholic patients will eventually commit suicide; they tend to succumb decades into their drinking, after family and social relationships have been ravaged and after work performances and health have been adversely affected. Murphy and Weitzel (1990) estimated that only 3.4% of alcoholic patients kill themselves, a rate that is nevertheless 60–120 times the lifetime risk in the general population. Klerman (1987) suggested that most of the higher suicide rates in men may be accounted for by the higher rates of alcoholism in men.

Familial Risk Factors

Persons with a family history of suicide appear to have an increased risk of suicide (Egeland and Sussex 1985). Roy (1983) studied 243 consecutive psychiatric inpatients with a family history of suicide and found that 48.6% of the patients had attempted suicide and 56.4% received a diagnosis of major depression at least once. In a control population of 5,602 psychiatric inpatients without a family history of suicide, only 21.0% had ever attempted suicide, and only 26.6% had a history of major depression.

Psychological and Psychosocial Risk Factors

Suicide is frequently a response to a loss, real or imagined. To help assess the meaning of suicidal ideation or behavior, the consultation-liaison psychiatrist must inquire about recent or anticipated losses and coping strategies that the patient has used with past losses (Davidson 1993). Fantasies of revenge, punishment, rec-

Table 4–3. Suicide relative risk: psychiatric factors

Target group	Incidence per 100,000	Control group	Relative risk (target group/ control group)	Source
Patients with history of psychiatric admission				
Men		General population	5.7	Roy 1985
Women		General population	10	
Patients never admitted				
Men		General population	3.4	
Women		General population	4	
Suicide attempters within a year of attempt		General population	100	Hawton 1992
Psychiatric inpatients	106	General ward patients	7	Kellner et al. 1985
Male Veterans Administration patients with suicidal behavior		General population	35	Pokorny 1983
Depression				
Men	400	General population	22	
Women	180	General population	30	
Dysthymia				
Men	190	General population	10	Roy 1989
Women	70	General population	12	
Schizophrenia				
Men	210	General population	11	
Women	90	General population	15	
Alcoholism				
Men	180	General population	10	
Women	130	General population	22	

Table 4–4. Psychiatric diagnoses and lifetime suicide risk

Diagnosis	Control group	Lifetime risk of suicide (%)	Source
Primary mood disorders	General population	15–30	Guze and Robins 1970
Schizophrenia	General population	10–20	Miles 1977
Psychopathology	General population	5–10	Miles 1977
Alcoholism	General population	3–7	Murphy and Weitzel 1990
Panic disorder	General population	7	Johnson et al. 1990
Panic disorder and depression	General population	7.9	Johnson et al. 1990

onciliation with a rejecting object, relief from the pain of loss, or reunion with a dead loved one may be evident (Furst and Ostow 1979).

A patient's degree of autonomy and extent of dependency on external sources of emotional support will shed light on the level of psychic resilience (Buie and Maltsberger 1989). A recent loss of a loved one or a parental loss during childhood increases suicide risk. Holidays and anniversaries of important days in the life and death of the deceased person, when the loved one's absence is experienced more intensely, also increase suicide risk. Glickman (1980) believes that a suicidal patient cannot be judged safe until he or she has either regained the lost object, accepted its loss, or replaced it with a new object.

■ SUICIDE RISK FACTOR SCALES

A great deal of research has been done in the attempt to develop clinical predictor scales for suicide risk. Unfortunately, scales developed to date have only been correlational, predicting groups at risk rather than identifying individuals within groups (Pokorny 1983). The main utility of such scales may be in increasing the likelihood that the clinician will ask about suicidal ideation and behaviors and other known risk factors (Davidson 1993).

Patterson et al. (1983) devised one of the most popular of these scales—the SAD PERSONS Scale for assessing the risk of sui-

cide—which is summarized in Table 4–5. This 10-point mnemonic includes **S**ex, **A**ge, **D**epression, **P**revious attempt, **E**thanol abuse, **R**ational thinking loss, **S**ocial supports lacking, **O**rganized plan, **N**o spouse, and **S**ickness as categories that should be surveyed. The higher scores on this scale correspond to greater suicide risk. The device, like all mnemonics, is useful to remind the examiner to address pertinent areas in a clinical interview, but the scale has not been demonstrated to have validity in specific assessments (Goldberg 1987). The

Table 4–5. The SAD PERSONS Scale for assessing the risk of suicide

Sex

Age

Depression

Previous attempt

Ethanol abuse

Rational thinking loss

Social supports lacking

Organized plan

No spouse

Sickness

One point is scored for each factor deemed present. The total score thus ranges from 0 (very little risk) to 10 (very high risk).

Source. Reprinted from Patterson WM, Dohn HH, Bird J, et al: "Evaluation of Suicidal Patients: The SAD PERSONS Scale." *Psychosomatics* 24:343–349, 1983. Copyright 1983, Academy of Psychosomatic Medicine. Used with permission.

SAD PERSONS Scale may have both sensitivity and specificity problems. There may be both false positives and false negatives. Nevertheless, this scale provides a summary of current knowledge about suicide epidemiology, a body of information that borrows from biological, psychological, and social sources of data in attempting to identify suicide risk.

■ PATIENT ASSESSMENT

The purpose of a suicide evaluation is to integrate an individual's feelings and thoughts in a moment of crisis with the aforementioned demographic and social variables. It is difficult to garner adequate information in enough spheres in a brief interview or two with a complex patient, then contextualize it using unwieldy epidemiological data fraught with inconsistencies and lacunae.

The ultimate problem with sifting through extensive clinical and demographic data is that it does not inform the consultant whether the person is at immediate risk for suicide. Once the medical inpatient, outpatient, or emergency department patient at high risk has been identified, the psychiatric consultant must decide what to do based on the clinical examination.

The consultation-liaison psychiatrist's first task is to create a clinical situation in which the patient feels free to reveal the unacceptable thoughts that may be driving his or her present suicidality.

All patients seen by consultation-liaison psychiatrists in medical, surgical, and emergency settings should be asked about suicidality. Inquiring about suicidality does not increase suicide risk, although not asking may increase both patient mortality and physician liability if the patient commits suicide. The psychiatric consultant must realize that there is something special and salvageable about people who survive their suicidal urges long enough to bring them to medical attention, and the consultant must address the ambivalence

that is central to the patient's suicidality. The psychiatrist must ally with the parts of these patients that want to survive.

A psychodynamic formulation weaves together the precipitating events, the conscious and unconscious motives driving the suicidality, and the characteristics of the patient's personality that propel him or her toward acting on suicidal thoughts (Gabbard 1990). Formulating the unfolding drama and identifying the crisis draw on a different set of concepts and clinical skills than epidemiological prediction (Pokorny 1983). Suicidality is a dynamic entity that waxes and wanes with the patient's circumstances. A patient's membership in a high-risk group is neither necessary nor sufficient to conclude that the patient is in suicidal crisis. The clinician must discern the individual variables that will ultimately determine the time of highest risk (Fawcett et al. 1987). Most suicidal episodes occur in patients with psychiatric diagnoses, but the diagnosis itself does not drive suicidality; rather, it is a crisis imposed on the substrate of the diagnosis (Klerman 1987).

Litman (1989) described a *presuicidal syndrome,* which characterizes lethal attempts and completed suicides. The presuicidal patient in crisis has constricted choices, constricted perception, a tunnel vision of the world as hopeless, physical tension, and emotional perturbation. The tension and distress may be relieved by a fantasy of death. The hopelessness is combined with help rejection and distrust. Often in the background, the patient has a long-term disposition toward impulsive action, an all-or-nothing approach to problems, and the characterological attitude "my way or no way."

Klerman (1987) framed the presuicidal crisis in terms of a medical model: there is an underlying condition that intermittently flares. The clinician must look for signs in the mental status examination that the patient has lost the capacity to think rationally. The hopelessness and helplessness of severe depression can reach irrational proportions. Hallucinations may command self-harm. Clouded sensorium;

impaired judgment; disinhibition; and misperceptions of delirium, intoxication, or substance withdrawal—all may cause a patient to act in self-destructive or dangerous ways.

Shneidman (1989) identified "10 commonalities of suicide" that may help the consultation-liaison psychiatrist to narrow a broad epidemiological suicide risk assessment so that it is relevant to an individual patient (Table 4–6). Hopelessness is a common finding reported by researchers who study psychological factors associated with suicide and suicide attempts (Fawcett et al. 1987; Shneidman 1989; Siomopoulous 1990).

The perspective of time appears to shift significantly among patients in suicidal crisis. Yufit (1991) found that suicidal persons typically have little interest in the future, much involvement in the past, and dissatisfaction with the present, unlike nonsuicidal control subjects, who were focused on the present and the future, with little interest in the past (Table 4–7). Litman (1989) reviewed 1,000 suicide notes from Los Angeles residents who had died and noted recurrent themes of regret over lost lovers or encroaching illness: "Often the communications describe fatigue, exhaustion and a need to escape. . . . The notes seldom (less than 10%) express anger or reproach. Humor is absent. The general mood of these notes that express feelings is one of hopelessness" (pp. 149–150).

Consultation-liaison psychiatrists who examine potentially suicidal patients must monitor themselves for reactions and countertransference feelings toward patients. A clinician may sense a patient's hopelessness and feel hopeless about the patient's prospects, identify with a patient's anger and become furious at the patient, or respond to haughty disdain with arrogant dismissal of the patient and his or her complaints. Particularly when evaluating patients with character disorders, the clinician must identify these feelings—what Maltsberger and Buie (1974) called *countertransference hate*—for what they are: something aroused in the consultant by the patient. The clinician must ensure that he or she does not act on these feelings and must regard them instead as further information about the state of the patient's

Table 4–6. Ten commonalities of suicide

1. The common purpose of suicide is to seek a solution.
2. The common goal of suicide is cessation of consciousness.
3. The common stimulus in suicide is intolerable psychological pain.
4. The common stressor in suicide is frustrated psychological needs.
5. The common emotion in suicide is hopelessness or helplessness.
6. The common cognitive state in suicide is ambivalence.
7. The common perceptual state in suicide is constriction.
8. The common action in suicide is aggression.
9. The common interpersonal act in suicide is communication of intention.
10. The common consistency in suicide is with lifelong coping patterns.

Source. Reprinted from Shneidman ES: "Overview: A Multidimensional Approach to Suicide," in *Suicide: Understanding and Responding.* Edited by Jacobs D, Brown HN. Madison, CT, International Universities Press, 1989, p. 16. Used with permission.

Table 4–7. Time perspective profiles

Time perspective profile of suicidal person
   High in the past (nostalgia, obsessions)
   Nominal, negative in the present
   Minimal or zero in the future

Time perspective profile of nonsuicidal person
   Very low in the past (except anniversaries)
   Moderately high in the present
   High in the future

Source. Reprinted from Yufit RI: "American Association of Suicidology Presidential Address: Suicide Assessment in the 1990s." *Suicide and Life-Threatening Behavior* 21:152–163, 1991. Copyright 1991, Guilford Publications. Used with permission.

mind and social relations. The clinician's unrecognized aversion to his or her patient can have dire consequences. If the clinician stops attempting to reach the buried rage and despair because of manifest antagonism, he or she can rationalize a relatively benign mental status examination in order to discharge a potentially lethal patient.

TREATMENT, MANAGEMENT, AND PREVENTION

Identify Risk Level

In one of the most practical approaches to suicide assessment, Goldberg (1987, p. 449) argued that, despite the lack of valid measures for predicting suicide risk, there are "issues that are considered so fundamental for suicide assessment that failure to obtain and record such information would practically constitute inadequate practice." He describes the minimum legal requirements for meeting the standard of care and enumerates what should become part of the medical record regardless of the consultant's theoretical stance. His recommendations for the fundamentals of suicide assessment are listed in Table 4–8.

Goldberg's approach is simple as well as sophisticated. The mental status examination, with its search for factors clouding insight, judgment, or consciousness, is the biological state of the art in the absence of any chemical or imaging test to characterize suicidality. Asking the patient to describe his or her ideas for disposition is a psychologically astute projective technique that provides a view of the patient's inner world and degree of hopelessness, which is correlated with self-destructiveness. Encouraging the patient's collaboration in negotiating a follow-up plan increases the chance of compliance after discharge (Hofmann and Dubovsky 1991). Including a third party helps the clinician both to evaluate the veracity of the patient's account and to gain other perspectives on the patient's situation. The responses

of both the patient and the third party to the intervention give some indication of the degree of the patient's social isolation and alienation, as well as of the social resources available to aid in recovery from the suicidal crisis. These diverse sources of information help the consultant to produce a global biopsychosocial formulation of risk level.

Until determined otherwise, a suicidal person is a patient in crisis from a life-threatening illness. In the absence of medical or surgical complications, such a patient is usually transferred from an emergency room to a secure psychiatric facility. In the general hospital, the patient's medical condition often prevents immediate transfer. Thus, a secure environment

Table 4–8. Fundamentals of suicide assessment

1. Determine whether delirium, psychosis, or depression is present.
2. Elicit the patient's statements about his or her suicidality.
3. Elicit the patient's ideas about what would help to mitigate his or her suicidality.
4. Confirm the patient's story with a third party.
5. Make a global formulation that includes acute and chronic management suggestions.
6. Ask a series of escalating questions addressing suicidality in medically hospitalized patients:

    - Are you discouraged about your medical condition?
    - Are there times when you think about your situation and feel like crying?
    - When you feel that way, what sort of thoughts go through your mind?
    - Did you ever feel that if your life were to go on like this, it would not be worth living?
    - Have you gotten to the point at which you've actually thought of a specific plan to end your life?
    - You say you've thought of shooting yourself. Do you have access to a gun?

Source. Adapted from Goldberg RJ: "The Assessment of Suicide Risk in the General Hospital." *General Hospital Psychiatry* 9:446–452, 1987. Copyright 1987, Elsevier Science. Used with permission.

must be created within the medical-surgical setting until the patient is stable enough for psychiatric transfer.

The patient's room must be secured—that is, anything that a patient could potentially use to injure himself or herself, such as sharp objects or material that could be fashioned into a noose, must be removed. Luggage and possessions should be searched with a suspicious eye and a morbid imagination. Staff must ferret out sharp objects, lighters, belts, caches of pills—anything that could inflict damage in either an impulsive or carefully planned way. Objects coming into the room (e.g., cutlery on the dinner tray, pop tops on soft drink cans) must be regarded as potential weapons.

The patient will need a sitter for constant observation, a process that must be truly constant. Social amenities may no longer apply. Patients permitted to use the bathroom unobserved have been known to leap from that window or maim themselves behind the closed door. A moment of privacy granted to the patient out of misplaced civility or a few minutes of inattention or absence by the sitter may be all the time a suicidal person needs to execute a suicide plan.

It should never be forgotten that given the right circumstances, any patient can overpower a sitter or staff member. All staff guarding suicidal patients should know how to summon security personnel as reinforcements when they perceive that they have lost control of the patient or the situation. In these days of cost-cutting measures, the consultant may feel pressure to limit the use of constant observation. The decision to employ constant observation must always be made on clinical grounds rather than on fiscal ones. The price of economizing on sitters could mean the life of the suicidal patient.

Remove or Treat Risk Factors

Underlying medical problems. The consulting psychiatrist must review the patient's chart to ensure that any underlying medical problem or condition is not contributing to a delirium or other secondary psychiatric disorder. The patient's alcohol and substance abuse history should be elicited to determine whether the agitation driving the patient's suicidality is the result of substance withdrawal.

Physical or chemical restraint. Agitation and overt suicidal behavior must be promptly treated with physical restraints, chemical restraints, or both. Neuroleptics should be used in patients with delirium, and neuroleptics and/or benzodiazepines should be given to agitated, anxious, or psychotic patients. Physical restraints may be required if a patient is believed to be unpredictable or impulsive.

Psychotherapy. A flexible approach to psychotherapy in medically ill patients who are potentially suicidal may include supportive therapy for dealing with the ravages of illness on the body or the sense of self. Family therapy should be employed, particularly when it will reinforce the patient's sense of connection to other people. To combat social isolation, efforts should be made to reestablish or strengthen connections to friends or community social service agencies.

Follow-up. The consultant's chart notes should identify the level of risk, clearly state the plan, and report the interval at which the consultant will return to continue the assessment and recommend modifications to the plan. The consultant must discuss his or her recommendations by telephone or in person with the referring physician and maintain close contact with the medical team throughout the hospitalization to ensure agreement and to minimize potentially life-threatening confusion about or deviation from the plan.

The consultant should also arrange follow-up care for the patient and detail it in the chart so that it becomes part of the inpatient's discharge plan. On discharge, in keeping with the idea that patients should not unwittingly be provided with the instruments of their own destruction, medication that could be lethal in overdose should be prescribed only in small quantities. The patient should only be given enough to last until the first outpatient appointment, and the consultant should keep in mind that the patient may hoard it anyway if absolutely intent on suicide. "Contracting for safety" may allow the patient and the consultation-liaison psychiatrist to anticipate dangerous situations and make plans for dealing with them by encouraging the patient to seek help rather than engage in self-destructive behavior.

In the emergency room or outpatient clinic setting, Davidson (1993) suggested that outpatient management may be an acceptable plan if the suicidal patient has 1) satisfactory impulse control, 2) absence of psychosis or intoxication, 3) absence of a specific plan and easily accessible means, 4) accessible social supports to which he or she is willing to turn, and 5) capacity for establishing rapport with the consultant. The converse of each of these points should prompt transfer to a psychiatric facility or medical-psychiatric unit: 1) poor impulse control; 2) psychosis, intoxication, or delirium; 3) a plan and the means to execute it; 4) isolation, exhaustion of family or friends, or changes in the network of support services that sustain the patient; and 5) a difficult interview on any grounds.

Psychiatric hospitalization. If the consultant has any doubts about a potentially suicidal patient in the emergency department or outpatient medical setting, he or she should admit first and ask questions later. The potential consequences of undertreating suicidality are deadly. A psychiatric or medical-psychiatric unit admission—even brief—may provide the opportunity to observe the patient further and the time and resources to construct the patient's formulation comprehensively enough to make a more appropriate disposition. The inpatient psychiatric or medical-psychiatric unit

is a place not only where the doctor can learn more about the patient but also where the patient can demonstrate what kind of care he or she might need.

REFERENCES

Abrams H, Moore GL, Westervelt FB: Suicidal behavior in chronic dialysis patients. Am J Psychiatry 127:1199–1204, 1971

Allebeck P, Bolund C, Ringback F: Increased suicide rate in cancer patients. J Clin Epidemiol 42:611–616, 1985

Brown J, Henteleff P, Barakat S, et al: Is it normal for terminally ill patients to desire death? Am J Psychiatry 143:208–211, 1986

Buie DH, Maltsberger JT: The psychological vulnerability to suicide, in Suicide: Understanding and Responding. Edited by Jacobs D, Brown HN. Madison, CT, International Universities Press, 1989, pp 59–71

Cote TR, Biggar RJ, Dannenberg AL: Risk of suicide among persons with AIDS: a national assessment. JAMA 268:2066–2068, 1991

Davidson L: Suicide and aggression in the medical setting, in Psychiatric Care of the Medical Patient. Edited by Stoudemire A, Fogel BS. New York, Oxford University Press, 1993, pp 71–86

Egeland JA, Sussex JN: Suicide and family loading for affective disorders. JAMA 254:915–918, 1985

Evenson RC, Wood JB, Nuttall EA, et al: Suicide rates among public mental health patients. Acta Psychiatr Scand 66:254–264, 1982

Farberow NL, Litman RE: Suicide prevention in hospitals, in The Psychology of Suicide. Edited by Shneidman ES, Farberow NL, Litman RE. New York, Science House, 1970, pp 423–458

Fawcett J, Shaughnessy R (eds): The suicidal patient, in Psychiatry: Diagnosis and Therapy. Norwalk, CT, Appleton & Lange, 1988, pp 49–56

Fawcett J, Scheftner W, Clark D, et al: Clinical predictors of suicide in patients with major affective disorders: a controlled prospective study. Am J Psychiatry 144:35–40, 1987

Furst S, Ostow M: The psychodynamics of suicide in Suicide: Theory and Clinical Aspects. Edited by Einsider B, Hankoff LD. Littleton, MA, PSG Publishing, 1979, pp 165–178

Gabbard GO: Affective disorders, in Psychodynamic Psychiatry in Clinical Practice. Washington, DC, American Psychiatric Press, 1990, pp 177–198

Glickman LS (ed): The suicidal patient, in Psychiatric Consultation in the General Hospital. New York, Marcel Dekker, 1980, pp 181–202

Goldberg RJ: The assessment of suicide risk in the general hospital. Gen Hosp Psychiatry 9:446–452, 1987

Guze SB, Robins E: Suicide and primary affective disorders. Br J Psychiatry 117:437–438, 1970

Havens L: Recognition of suicidal risk through the psychological examination. N Engl J Med 276:211–215, 1967

Hawton K: Suicide and attempted suicide, in Handbook of Affective Disorders, 2nd Edition. Edited by Paykel ES. New York, Guilford, 1992, pp 635–650

Hofmann D, Dubovsky S: Depression and suicide assessment. Emerg Med Clin North Am 9:107–121, 1991

Johnson J, Weissman MM, Klerman GL: Panic disorder, comorbidity, and suicide attempts. Arch Gen Psychiatry 47:805–808, 1990

Kaplan A, Klein R: Women and suicide, in Suicide: Understanding and Responding. Edited by Jacobs D, Brown HN. Madison, CT, International Universities Press, 1989, pp 257–282

Kellner CH, Best CL, Roberts JM, et al: Self-destructive behavior in hospitalized medical and surgical patients. Psychiatr Clin North Am 8:279–289, 1985

Kizer KW, Green M, Perkins CI, et al: AIDS and suicide in California (letter). JAMA 260:1881, 1988

Klerman GL: Clinical epidemiology of suicide. J Clin Psychiatry 48(suppl):33–38, 1987

Kontaxakis VP, Christodoulou GN, Mavreas VG, et al: Attempted suicide in psychiatric outpatients with concurrent physical illness. Psychother Psychosom 50:201–206, 1988

RE: Suicides: what do they have in mind? in ide: Understanding and Responding. by Jacobs D, Brown HN. Madison, CT, ional Universities Press, 1989, pp

Maltsberg
in the t. ie DH: Countertransference hate Psychiatry of suicidal patients. Arch Gen 633, 1974

Marzuk P, Tierney K, et al: Increased risk of suicide in AIDS. A 259:1333–1337, 1988

Miles CP: Conditions pre sing to suicide: a review. J Nerv Ment Dis 31–246, 1977
Epidemiol Rev
Monk M: Epidemiology of suic 9:51–69, 1987

Morgan AC: Special issues of assessm and treatment of suicide risk in the elderly, in Suicide: Understanding and Responding. Edited by Jacobs D, Brown HN. Madison, CT, International Universities Press, 1989, pp 239–255

Murphy GE, Weitzel RD: The lifetime risk of suicide in alcoholism. Arch Gen Psychiatry 47:383–392, 1990

Patterson WM, Dohn HH, Bird J, et al: Evaluation of suicidal patients: the SAD PERSONS Scale. Psychosomatics 24:343–349, 1983

Pisetsky JE, Brown W: The general hospital patient, in Suicide: Theory and Clinical Aspects. Edited by Hankoff LD, Einshidler B. Littleton, MA, PSG Publishing, 1979, pp 279–290

Pokorny AD: Prediction of suicide in psychiatric patients: report of a prospective study. Arch Gen Psychiatry 40:249–257, 1983

Pollack S: Suicide in a general hospital, in The Psychology of Suicide. Edited by Shneidman ES, Farberow NL. New York, McGraw-Hill, 1957, pp 152–176

Reich P, Kelly MJ: Suicide attempts by hospitalized medical and surgical patients. N Engl J Med 294:298–301, 1976

Roy A: Family history of suicide. Arch Gen Psychiatry 40:971–974, 1983

Roy A: Suicide: a multi-determined act. Psychiatr Clin North Am 8:243–250, 1985

Roy A: Emergency psychiatry: suicide, in Comprehensive Textbook of Psychiatry, 5th Edition. Edited by Kaplan HI, Sadock BJ. Baltimore, MD, Williams & Wilkins, 1989, pp 1414–1427

Sanders R: Suicidal behavior in critica   rat-
   cine: conceptual issues and mar dicine.
   egies, in Problems in Critical   PA, JB
   Edited by Wise MG. Phil
   Lippincott, 1988, pp 116 nensional ap-
Shneidman ES: Overview: a : Understanding
   proach to suicide, in Jacobs D, Brown
   and Responding. E national Universities
   HN. Madison, C
   Press, 1989, pp

Siomopoulos V: When patients consider suicide.
   Postgrad Med 88:205–213, 1990
Yufit RI: American Association of Suicidology presidential address: suicide assessment in the
   1990s. Suicide Life Threat Behav 21:152–163,
   1991

Chapter 5

Aggression and Agitation

Robert E. Hales, M.D.
Jonathan M. Silver, M.D.
Stuart C. Yudofsky, M.D.

Consultation-liaison psychiatrists are frequently called on to assess and treat patients who become aggressive. Overall, approximately 10% of patients admitted to a psychiatric unit in a general hospital exhibit violence toward others just before their admission (Tardiff and Swelliam 1982). Among patients who have neuropsychiatric disorders—such as those with posttraumatic brain injury, delirium, Alzheimer's disease, and other dementias—the prevalence is much higher.

DIAGNOSIS

Aggressive symptoms are assessed in an unusually broad and disparate fashion. Aggressive behavior is sometimes described as a symptom or as the central aspect of a distinct disorder. DSM-IV (American Psychiatric Association 1994) classification of primary aggressive disorders consists of two diagnoses: 1) intermittent explosive disorder (Table 5–1), and 2) personality change due to a general medical condition, aggressive type (Table 5–2). However, personality change due to a general medical condition, aggressive type, remains a catchall diagnosis that is overinclusive and indiscriminate with regard to the number and types of associated symptoms and does not describe the specific kinds of dyscontrol of rage and violence that occur secondary to brain lesions (Silver and Yudofsky 1987; Silver et al. 1992; Yudofsky et al. 1989).

DOCUMENTATION OF AGGRESSION

Accurate documentation of aggressive episodes is critical to assess the effectiveness of interventions and to conduct outcome research. To assess the effects of pharmacological agents in the treatment of aggressive behaviors, con-

Table 5–1. DSM-IV diagnostic criteria for intermittent explosive disorder

A. Several discrete episodes of failure to resist aggressive impulses that result in serious assaultive acts or destruction of property.

B. The degree of aggressiveness expressed during the episodes is grossly out of proportion to any precipitating psychosocial stressors.

C. The aggressive episodes are not better accounted for by another mental disorder (e.g., antisocial personality disorder, borderline personality disorder, a psychotic disorder, a manic episode, conduct disorder, or attention-deficit/hyperactivity disorder) and are not due to the direct physiological effects of a substance (e.g., a drug of abuse, a medication) or a general medical condition (e.g., head trauma, Alzheimer's disease).

Table 5–2. DSM-IV diagnostic criteria for personality change due to a general medical condition

A. A persistent personality disturbance that represents a change from the individual's previous characteristic personality pattern. (In children, the disturbance involves a marked deviation from normal development or a significant change in the child's usual behavior patterns lasting at least 1 year).

B. There is evidence from the history, physical examination, or laboratory findings that the disturbance is the direct physiological consequence of a general medical condition.

C. The disturbance is not better accounted for by another mental disorder (including other mental disorders due to a general medical condition).

D. The disturbance does not occur exclusively during the course of a delirium and does not meet criteria for a dementia.

E. The disturbance causes clinically significant distress or impairment in social, occupational, or other important areas of functioning.

Specify type:

Labile type: if the predominant feature is affective lability

Disinhibited type: if the predominant feature is poor impulse control as evidenced by sexual indiscretions, etc.

Aggressive type: if the predominant feature is aggressive behavior

Apathetic type: if the predominant feature is marked apathy and indifference

Paranoid type: if the predominant feature is suspiciousness or paranoid ideation

Other type: if the predominant feature is not one of the above, e.g., personality change associated with a seizure disorder

Combined type: if more than one feature predominates in the clinical picture

Unspecified type

sultation-liaison psychiatrists can use the Overt Aggression Scale (OAS) to document and to measure specific aspects of aggressive behavior based on observable criteria (Silver and Yudofsky 1991; Yudofsky et al. 1986). The OAS divides aggressive behaviors into four categories: 1) verbal aggression, 2) physical aggression against objects, 3) physical aggression against self, and 4) physical aggression against others. Within each category, descriptive statements define and numerical scores rate four levels of severity. All behaviors exhibited by the patient during an aggressive episode are checked off by an observer (such as the nursing staff or a family member). Therapeutic interventions used in response to these aggressive episodes are also listed, rated on the OAS, and checked off by the rater. These interventions are documented because they may reflect the observer's interpretation of the severity of the aggressive behaviors. Consulting psychiatrists may want to use the OAS to establish a baseline score for aggression before initiating psychopharmacological intervention and thereafter to document the efficacy, or lack thereof, of any therapeutic intervention.

DIFFERENTIAL DIAGNOSIS OF AGGRESSION

As with other symptoms or disorders in medicine and psychiatry, proper diagnosis is crucial because many psychiatric disorders are associated with aggressive behavior (Table 5–3). Organic brain disorders are strongly associated with dyscontrol of rage and violence. Table 5–4 summarizes common etiologies of medically and substance-induced aggression, and Table 5–5 reviews medications and drugs associated

with aggression (Yudofsky et al. 1990). Table 5–6 summarizes clinical features that alert the consultation-liaison psychiatrist to the potential presence of organically induced aggression. In soliciting the history of aggression, it is critical to interview family members, teachers, friends, and co-workers because patients with aggressive disorders—as opposed to their families—tend to minimize the presence and importance of the disorder (Silver and Yudofsky 1994). In addition, to develop a treatment plan, the clinician must learn from the patient and observers the context in which aggression occurs. Essential information includes the mental status of the patient before the aggressive event, the nature of precipitants, physical and social environment in which aggression occurs, ways in which the aggressive event is mitigated, and primary and secondary gains related to aggression. If the aggression occurs in the context of a psychiatric disorder, the clinician should obtain a thorough psychiatric his-

Table 5–3. DSM-IV diagnoses associated with violent behavior

Violent behavior as an essential feature
  Intermittent explosive disorder
  Conduct disorder
  Oppositional defiant disorder
  Antisocial personality disorder
  Borderline personality disorder
  Sexual sadism

Violent behavior as an associated feature
  Substance-related disorders
  Delirium, dementia, and other cognitive
    disorders
  Mental retardation
  Attention-deficit/hyperactivity disorder
  Brief psychotic disorder
  Schizoaffective disorder
  Delusional disorder
  Bipolar disorder
  Posttraumatic stress disorder

Violent behavior as an infrequent feature
  Atypical psychosis
  Major depressive disorder
  Dysthymic disorder
  Cyclothymic disorder
  Atypical depression
  Paranoid personality disorder
  Histrionic personality disorder
  Schizoid personality disorder
  Schizotypal personality disorder
  Dissociative fugue
  Adjustment disorder with disturbance of
    conduct

Source. Adapted from Reid WH, Balis GU: "Evaluation of the Violent Patient," in *American Psychiatric Association Annual Review,* Vol 6. Edited by Hales RE, Frances AJ. Washington, DC, American Psychiatric Press, 1987, pp. 491–509. Used with permission.

Table 5–4. Common etiologies of medically and substance-induced aggression

Alzheimer's disease

Brain tumors

Chronic neurological disorders (e.g., Huntington's disease, Wilson's disease, Parkinson's disease, multiple sclerosis, systemic lupus erythematosus)

Delirium (e.g., hypoxia, electrolyte imbalance, anesthesia and surgery, uremia)

Epilepsy (ictal, postictal, and interictal)

Infectious diseases (e.g., encephalitis, meningitis, AIDS)

Medications and drugs (see Table 5–5)

Metabolic disorders (e.g., hyperthyroidism or hypothyroidism, hypoglycemia, vitamin deficiencies, porphyria)

Stroke and other cerebrovascular disease

Traumatic brain injury

Source. Adapted from Yudofsky SC, Silver JM, Hales RE: "Pharmacologic Management of Aggression in the Elderly." *Journal of Clinical Psychiatry* 51 (10 suppl):22–28, 1990. Copyright 1990, Physicians Postgraduate Press. Used with permission.

Table 5–5. Drugs associated with aggression

Type of drug	Clinical effect or symptom
Alcohol	Intoxication and withdrawal
Analgesics	Delirium
Amphetamines	Intoxication or paranoia
Antianxiety agents	Disinhibition
Anticholinergic drugs	Delirium
Antidepressants	Delirium
Antipsychotics	Delirium and akathisia
Cocaine	Intoxification or paranoia
Hypnotics	Disinhibition
Steroids	Mania or delirium

Source. Adapted from Yudofsky SC, Silver JM, Hales RE: "Pharmacologic Management of Aggression in the Elderly." *Journal of Clinical Psychiatry* 51 (10 suppl):22–28, 1990. Copyright 1990, Physicians Postgraduate Press. Used with permission.

Table 5–6. Characteristic features of the organic aggression syndrome

Reactive	Triggered by modest stimuli
Nonreflective	Usually does not involve premeditation
Nonpurposeful	Aggression serves no obvious short- or long-term aims or goals
Explosive	Buildup is NOT gradual
Periodic	Brief outbursts of rage and aggression punctuated by long periods of relative calm
Ego-dystonic	After outbursts, patients are upset or embarrassed

Source. Adapted from Yudofsky SC, Silver JM, Hales RE: "Pharmacologic Management of Aggression in the Elderly." *Journal of Clinical Psychiatry* 51 (10 suppl):22–28, 1990. Copyright 1990, Physicians Postgraduate Press. Used with permission.

tory for the individual and the family. For *all* patients with aggression, the consultation-liaison psychiatrist must conduct a thorough review of physical symptoms, obtain a detailed review of neurological signs and symptoms,

and conduct a thorough physical examination. The neurological examination deserves emphasis; relevant laboratory tests should be ordered based on information from history and physical and neurological examinations. Neuropsychological batteries, such as the Halstead-Reitan or the Luria-Nebraska tests, are more useful than psychological tests like the Minnesota Multiphasic Personality Inventory (MMPI) or projective psychological tests for evaluating patients with aggressive symptoms or disorders.

TREATMENT

Treatment of aggressive symptoms and disorders is guided by the four D's (see Table 5–7). Almost without exception, treatment of aggressive disorders requires a multifaceted approach that often combines pharmacological treatments, behavioral treatments, psychodynamically informed psychotherapy, family treatment, and, as indicated, other specific approaches such as spiritual counseling, occupational therapy, and couples treatment. Although psychopharmacological management of aggression is the main focus of this chapter, other approaches have considerable efficacy in the treatment of aggression.

Pharmacological Treatment of Aggression

In conceptualizing an approach to the pharmacological treatment of aggression, the consultation-liaison psychiatrist must separate the management of acute aggression (that often constitutes a medical emergency) from the pharmacological treatment of chronic aggression. Currently, no medication is approved by the Food and Drug Administration (FDA) for the treatment of aggression. When medications are administered to treat aggression, frequently it is their sedating side effects and not their direct pharmacological actions that are being used.

Table 5–7. Four D's in the treatment of aggressive symptoms and disorders

Determine the etiologies of the psychological and/or central nervous system dysfunction that contributes to the aggression.

Delineate the biopsychosocial context in which the aggressive events occur.

Document and rate the aggression with the Overt Aggression Scale.

Develop a multifaceted treatment plan.

Source. Adapted from Silver JM, Yudofsky SC: "The Overt Aggression Scale: Overview and Guiding Principles." *Journal of Neuropsychiatry and Clinical Neurosciences* 3 (suppl 1):S22–S29, 1991. Used with permission.

Acute Aggression and Agitation

Physicians commonly utilize the sedative side effects of neuroleptics and benzodiazepines for the management of acute aggressive behavior and agitation. These agents are not specific in their capacities to inhibit aggressive behaviors but rather "cover over" the respective behaviors and symptoms. Therefore, the clinician must establish time limitations when prescribing medications for their sedative properties.

Neuroleptics. Consultation-liaison psychiatrists often prescribe neuroleptic medications to treat acute and chronic aggression. These agents are appropriate and effective in the treatment of aggression that is a result of psychosis. For example, a physically aggressive patient who presents in the emergency room with acute, manic psychosis with irritability would benefit from neuroleptic medication. Neuroleptic medication is also appropriate to treat a patient with paranoid schizophrenia who uses physical force to protect himself or herself from nurses because they are "agents sent from another planet to kidnap me." It is unfortunate that neuroleptic medications are also commonly used to treat chronic aggression associated with organic brain disorders. Unless aggressive behavior is clearly related to

psychotic ideation that responds to treatment with neuroleptic agents, consultation-liaison psychiatrists should limit the use of neuroleptics to a maximum of 4 weeks. After this period of time, the psychiatrist should determine whether the aggression is chronic and, accordingly, alter the treatment plan to utilize anti-aggression medications.

The essence of managing acute episodes of aggression with neuroleptics is to increase the dose of the neuroleptic, often every 1–2 hours, to establish the lowest dose that will produce the sedation necessary to control the aggressive or violent behaviors. Despite the disadvantages of haloperidol in the management of chronic aggression, it is often used because it can be administered in oral, intramuscular, and intravenous forms and has few cardiovascular side effects compared with other classes of neuroleptics. Table 5–8 summarizes guidelines for the use of haloperidol in the management of acute aggression.

Table 5–8. Use of haloperidol in the management of acute aggression

1. Initially administer 1 mg (po) or 0.5 mg (iv or im) q1h.

2. Increase dose by 1 mg q1h until control of aggression is achieved.

3. Maintain dosage of 2 mg (po) or 1 mg (iv or im) q8h.

4. When patient is not agitated or violent for 48 hours, decrease highest total daily dose at rate of 25% per day.

5. If violent behavior reemerges on tapering drug, reassess etiology and consider changing to a more specific medication to manage chronic aggression.

6. Do not maintain patient on haloperidol for more than 6 weeks—except for aggression secondary to psychosis.

Note. im = intramuscular; iv = intravenous; po = per os (oral); q1h = every hour, q8h = every 8 hours.
Source. Adapted from Yudofsky SC, Silver JM, Hales RE: "Pharmacologic Management of Aggression in the Elderly." *Journal of Clinical Psychiatry* 51 (10 suppl):22–28, 1990. Copyright 1990, Physicians Postgraduate Press. Used with permission.

Benzodiazepines. Benzodiazepines are also used to manage acute agitation and aggression. Intramuscular lorazepam has advantages over other benzodiazepines as an effective medication in the emergency treatment of the violent patient (Bick and Hannah 1986). Like haloperidol, lorazepam has flexible routes of administration (intravenous, intramuscular, or oral). In addition, lorazepam has a relatively brief duration of action and elimination half-life compared with other benzodiazepines, such as diazepam or chlordiazepoxide, which oversedate the patient through the buildup of active metabolites. Table 5–9 summarizes guidelines for the use of lorazepam in the management of acute aggression. Other medications such as paraldehyde, chloral hydrate, or diphenhydramine are also used to sedate patients who exhibit acute aggressive behaviors; however, in general, benzodiazepines and neuroleptics are preferable because they are safe and convenient, and psychiatrists and hospital staff are more familiar with their benefits and risks.

Chronic Aggression and Agitation

When a patient's agitation and aggression persist beyond several weeks, clinicians should consider treating aggression with medications that have more selective activity against aggression. When selecting a specific psychopharmacological agent, consultation-liaison psychiatrists must determine the underlying cause of the chronic aggression (e.g., aggression or irritability secondary to another psychiatric disorder such as mania or depression). Table 5–10 outlines an approach in the pharmacological treatment of chronic aggression.

Neuroleptics. The use of antipsychotic medications should be restricted to the treatment of aggression that is directly associated with psychosis. At regular intervals, the medication should be tapered to gauge the efficacy of the agent in treating the psychosis and the associated agitation and aggression.

Table 5–9. Use of lorazepam in the management of acute aggression

1. Initially administer 1–2 mg (po or im).
2. Repeat every hour until control of aggression is achieved.
3. If iv dose is given, push slowly! Do not exceed 2 mg (1 mL) per minute to avoid respiratory depression and laryngospasm; repeat in 30 minutes if required.
4. When patient is no longer violent or agitated, maintain at maximum of 2 mg (po or im) q4h.
5. When patient is not agitated or violent for 48 hours, decrease highest total daily dose at rate of 10% per day.
6. If violent behavior reemerges on tapering drug, reassess etiology and consider changing to a more specific medication to manage chronic aggression.
7. If lorazepam cannot be tapered without reemergence of aggression after 6 weeks, reevaluate and revise treatment plan to include a more specific medication to manage chronic aggression.

Note. im = intramuscular; iv = intravenous; po = per os (oral); q4h = every 4 hours.
Source. Adapted from Yudofsky SC, Silver JM, Hales RE: "Pharmacologic Management of Aggression in the Elderly." *Journal of Clinical Psychiatry* 51 (10 suppl):22–28, 1990. Copyright 1990, Physicians Postgraduate Press. Used with permission.

Antianxiety medications. In several case reports, buspirone, a 5-HT$_{1A}$ (serotonin) partial agonist, was effective in the management of aggression and agitation associated with traumatic brain injury (Gualtieri 1991), dementia (Colenda 1988; Tiller et al. 1988), and developmental disabilities and autism (Ratey et al. 1989; Realmuto et al. 1989). Because some patients become more aggressive in the initial phases of treatment with buspirone, the consultation-liaison psychiatrist may need to begin treatment at low dosages (i.e., 5 mg bid) and increase the dose by 5 mg every 3–5 days. Dosages ranging from 45 to 60 mg/day are sometimes required for effective treatment; a latency

Table 5–10. Psychopharmacological treatment of chronic aggression

Agent	Indications	Special clinical considerations
Antipsychotics	Psychotic symptoms	Oversedation and multiple side effects
Benzodiazepines	Anxiety symptoms	Paradoxical rage
Buspirone	Persistent, underlying anxiety and/or depression	Delayed onset of action
Carbamazepine	Seizure disorder	Bone marrow suppression and hepatotoxicity
Valproic acid	Seizure disorder	Hepatotoxicity
Lithium	Manic excitement or bipolar disorder	Neurotoxicity and confusion
Propranolol (and other β-blockers)	Chronic or recurrent aggression	Latency of 4–6 weeks
Serotonergic anti-depressants	Depression or mood lability with irritability	May need usual doses

Source. Adapted from Yudofsky SC, Silver JM, Hales RE: "Pharmacologic Management of Aggression in the Elderly." *Journal of Clinical Psychiatry* 51 (10 suppl):22–28, 1990. Copyright 1990, Physicians Postgraduate Press. Used with permission.

period of 3–6 weeks before therapeutic effects are observed is common.

Although no double-blind, controlled studies have examined the use of clonazepam in the management of chronic aggression, several case reports have indicated that it has benefits in the treatment of agitation in elderly patients (Freinhar and Alvarez 1986) and in a patient with schizophrenia and seizures (Keats and Mukherjee 1988).

Clonazepam is also used when aggression is associated with pronounced anxiety or when aggression is present with neurologically induced tics and disinhibited motor behavior. Dosages are initiated at 0.5 mg twice a day and rarely exceed a total daily dose of 6 mg.

Anticonvulsant medications. The consultation-liaison psychiatrist should consider using anticonvulsant medications, particularly carbamazepine, to treat patients whose chronic aggression is associated with seizure disorders or whose chronic aggression is related to diffuse neuronal destruction (such as that which occurs subsequent to traumatic brain injury, middle cerebral artery stroke, and Alzhei-

mer's disease). No double-blind, placebo-controlled studies have demonstrated the efficacy of carbamazepine in the treatment of aggression; however, several open studies indicate carbamazepine may be effective in reducing aggressive behavior associated with brain disorders (Mattes 1988), schizophrenia (Hakoloa and Laulumaa 1982; Luchins 1983), developmental disabilities (Folks et al. 1982), and dementia (Gleason and Schneider 1990; Leibovici and Tariot 1988). Carbamazepine should be prescribed in the same doses, aiming for the same blood levels, as those used to treat patients with bipolar disorder.

An anticonvulsant used to treat chronic aggression is valproic acid, particularly in patients with aggression secondary to central nervous system disorders (Gaikas et al. 1990; Mattes 1992).

Antimanic medications. Several authors suggest that lithium is effective in the treatment of aggressive patients without bipolar disorder, such as patients with mental retardation who exhibit self-directed aggression (Luchins and Dojka 1989) or aggression toward others (Dale

1980) and patients with traumatic brain injury (Haas and Cope 1985). In addition, children and adolescents (Vetro et al. 1985) and prison inmates (Sheard et al. 1976) with aggression reportedly respond to lithium. The consultation-liaison psychiatrist should consider using lithium in manic patients with aggression; in general, the same dosage of lithium and blood level monitoring that is recommended for patients with bipolar disorder without aggression should be used. One caveat, however, is that patients with brain injury have increased sensitivity to the neurotoxic effects of lithium (Hornstein and Seliger 1989) and therefore must be observed much more closely with neuropsychiatric evaluations and serum lithium levels.

Antidepressant medications. Many antidepressants are suggested for the treatment of aggression, especially those agents that act either preferentially or specifically on the serotonergic system of the brain. Amitriptyline (Szlabowicz and Stewart 1990) and trazodone (Pinner and Rich 1988) are reported to be useful in the treatment of aggression; however, most recent reports focus on the use of selective serotonin reuptake inhibitors. Fluoxetine, sertraline, and paroxetine have been used successfully in patients whose aggression is associated with brain lesions (Bass and Beltis 1991; Coccaro et al. 1990). Treatment should begin at relatively low doses (e.g., 10 mg of fluoxetine, 25 mg of sertraline, 10 mg of paroxetine). If antiaggressive effects are not achieved over several weeks, the dose should be increased gradually at 1- or 2-week intervals to relatively high ranges (80–100 mg/day of fluoxetine, 200–300 mg/day of sertraline, 60–80 mg/day of paroxetine).

β-Blockers. Since the first report of the use of β-adrenergic receptor antagonists to treat aggression appeared in 1977, more than 25 articles in both the neurological and the psychiatric literature reported on the use of β-blockers for this purpose (Yudofsky et al. 1987). Be-

Table 5–11. Clinical use of propranolol

1. Conduct a thorough medical evaluation.

2. Exclude patients with bronchial asthma, chronic obstructive pulmonary disease, insulin-dependent diabetes mellitus, congestive heart failure, persistent angina, significant peripheral vascular disease, hyperthyroidism.

3. Avoid sudden discontinuation of propranolol (particularly in patients with hypertension).

4. Begin with a single test dose of 20 mg/day in patients who may be at risk for hypotension or bradycardia. Increase dose by 20 mg/day every 3 days.

5. For patients without cardiovascular or cardiopulmonary disorder, begin propranolol on a 20-mg tid schedule.

6. Increase the dosage by 60 mg/day as often as every 3 days.

7. Increase medication unless the pulse rate is reduced to below 50 beats per minute or systolic blood pressure is less than 90 mm Hg.

8. Do not administer medication if severe dizziness, ataxia, or wheezing occurs. Reduce or discontinue propranolol if such symptoms persist.

9. Increase dose to 12 mg/kg or until aggressive behavior is under control.

10. Doses of greater than 800 mg are not usually required to control aggressive behavior.

11. Maintain the patient on the highest dose that he or she can tolerate for 4–8 weeks before concluding that the patient is not responding to propranolol. Some patients, however, respond rapidly.

12. Utilize concurrent medications with caution. Monitor plasma levels of all antipsychotic and anticonvulsant medications.

Source. Adapted from Silver JM, Hales RE, Yudofsky SC: "Neuropsychiatric Aspects of Traumatic Brain Injury," in *The American Psychiatric Press Textbook of Neuropsychiatry,* 2nd Edition. Edited by Yudofsky SC, Hales RE. Washington, DC, American Psychiatric Press, 1992, pp. 363–395. Used with permission.

cause a growing body of evidence suggests that β-adrenergic receptor antagonists are specific and effective agents for the treatment of aggression and violent behaviors in patients with central nervous syndromes, this approach is accepted as first-line treatment of organically induced aggression.

Guidelines for the use of propranolol in patients with chronic aggression are summarized in Table 5–11. Key clinical points related to the use of propranolol are that the peripheral effects of β-blockage (e.g., lowered blood pressure, bradycardia) are frequently saturated when the patient achieves a dosage of about 280 mg/day. Thereafter, increasing the dose of the β-blocker is not usually associated with cardiovascular side effects. Second, because of the long latency of 6–8 weeks before a therapeutic response is achieved, consultation-liaison psychiatrists should remind the family and other members of the treatment team that their support is an essential component of care. Third, despite reports that depression is commonly associated with the use of β-blockers, controlled trials and clinical experience indicate that depression is a rare side effect of β-blocker use (Yudofsky 1992). Finally, because the use of propranolol is associated with a significant increase in plasma levels of thioridazine, which has an absolute dosage ceiling of 800 mg/day, the combination of these two medications should be avoided whenever possible (Silver et al. 1986).

CONCLUSION

Aggression occurs commonly in the general hospital setting and has serious and far-reaching consequences for patients whom consultation-liaison psychiatrists evaluate. Although pharmacological intervention is often highly effective in the treatment of aggression, medications are used in the context of a carefully crafted treatment plan involving a full range of biopsychosocial approaches.

REFERENCES

American Psychiatric Association: Diagnostic and Statistical Manual of Mental Disorders, 4th Edition. Washington, DC, American Psychiatric Association, 1994

Bass JN, Beltis J: Therapeutic effect of fluoxetine on naltrezone-resistant self-injurious behavior in an adolescent with mental retardation. Journal of Child and Adolescent Psychopharmacology 1:331–340, 1991

Bick PA, Hannah AL: Intramuscular lorazepam to restrain violent patients (letter). Lancet 1:206, 1986

Coccaro EF, Astill JL, Herbert JL, et al: Fluoxetine treatment of impulsive aggression in DSM-III-R personality disorder patients. J Clin Psychopharmacol 10:373–375, 1990

Colenda CC: Buspirone in treatment of agitated demented patients (letter). Lancet 1:1169, 1988

Dale PG: Lithium therapy in aggressive mentally subnormal patients. Br J Psychiatry 137:469–474, 1980

Folks DG, King LD, Dowdy SB, et al: Carbamazepine treatment of selective affectively disordered inpatients. Am J Psychiatry 139:115–117, 1982

Freinhar JP, Alvarez WA: Clonazepam treatment of organic brain syndromes in three elderly patients. J Clin Psychiatry 47:525–526, 1986

Gleason RP, Schneider LS: Carbamazepine treatment of agitation in Alzheimer's outpatients refractory to neuroleptics. J Clin Psychiatry 51:115–118, 1990

Giakas WJ, Seibyl JP, Mazure CM: Valproate in the treatment of temper outbursts (letter). J Clin Psychiatry 51:525, 1990

Gualtieri CT: Buspirone for the behavior problems of patients with organic brain disorders (letter). J Clin Psychopharmacol 11:280–281, 1991

Haas JF, Cope N: Neuropharmacologic management of behavior sequelae in head injury: a case report. Arch Phys Med Rehabil 66:472–474, 1985

Hakoloa HP, Laulumaa VA: Carbamazepine in treatment of violent schizophrenics (letter). Lancet 1:1358, 1982

Hales RE: Introduction to psychiatric systems interface disorders (PSID), in DSM-IV Source Book, Vol 2. Washington, DC, American Psychiatric Press, pp 871–884

Hornstein A, Seliger G: Cognitive side effects of lithium in closed head injury (letter). J Neuropsychiatry Clin Neurosci 1:446–447, 1989

Keats MM, Mukherjee S: Antiaggressive effect of adjunctive clonazepam in schizophrenia associated with seizure disorder. J Clin Psychiatry 49:117–118, 1988

Leibovici A, Tariot PN: Carbamazepine treatment of agitation associated with dementia. J Geriatr Psychiatry Neurol 1:110–112, 1988

Lion JR, Reid WH: Assaults With Psychiatric Facilities. New York, Grune & Stratton, 1983

Luchins DJ: Carbamazepine for the violent psychiatric patient (letter). Lancet 2:755, 1983

Luchins DJ, Dojka D: Lithium and propranolol in aggression and self-injurious behavior in the mentally retarded. Psychopharmacol Bull 25:372–375, 1989

Mattes JA: Carbamazepine vs propranolol for rage outbursts. Psychopharmacol Bull 24:179–182, 1988

Mattes JA: Valproic acid for nonaffective aggression in the mentally retarded. J Nerv Ment Dis 180:601–602, 1992

Pinner E, Rich CL: Effects of trazodone on aggressive behavior in seven patients with organic mental disorders. Am J Psychiatry 145:1295–1296, 1988

Ratey JJ, Sovner R, Mikkelsen E, et al: Buspirone therapy for maladaptive behavior and anxiety in developmentally disabled persons. J Clin Psychiatry 50:382–384, 1989

Realmuto FM, August GJ, Garfinkle BD: Clinical effect of buspirone in autistic children. J Clin Psychopharmacol 9:122–124, 1989

Sheard MH, Marini JL, Bridges C, et al: The effects of lithium in impulsive aggressive behavior in man. Am J Psychiatry 133:1409–1413, 1976

Silver JM, Yudofsky SC: Aggressive behavior in patients with neuropsychiatric disorders: the scope of the problem. Psychiatric Annals 17:367–370, 1987

Silver JM, Yudofsky SC: The Overt Aggression Scale: overview and guiding principles. J Neuropsychiatry Clin Neurosci 3 (suppl 1):S22–S29, 1991

Silver JM, Yudofsky SC: Aggressive disorders, in Neuropsychiatry of Traumatic Brain Injury. Edited by Silver JM, Yudofsky SC, Hales RE. Washington, DC, American Psychiatric Press, 1994, pp 313–356

Silver JM, Yudofsky SC, Kogan M, et al: Elevation of thioridazine plasma levels by propranolol. Am J Psychiatry 143:1290–1292, 1986

Silver JM, Hales RE, Yudofsky SC: Neuropsychiatric aspects of traumatic brain injury, in The American Psychiatric Press Textbook of Neuropsychiatry, 2nd Edition. Edited by Yudofsky SC, Hales RE. Washington, DC, American Psychiatric Press, 1992, pp 363–395

Szlabowicz JW, Stewart JT: Amitriptyline treatment of agitation associated with anoxic encephalopathy. Arch Phys Med Rehabil 71:612–613, 1990

Tardiff K, Swelliam A: The occurrence of assaultive behavior among chronic psychiatric inpatients. Am J Psychiatry 139:212–215, 1982

Tiller JWG, Dakis JA, Shaw JM: Short-term buspirone treatment in disinhibition with dementia (letter). Lancet 2:510, 1988

Vetro A, Szentistvanyi L, Pallag M, et al: Therapeutic experience with lithium in childhood aggressivity. Pharmacopsychiatry 14:121–127, 1985

Yudofsky SC: β-Blockers and depression: the clinician's dilemma. JAMA 267:1826–1827, 1992

Yudofsky SC, Silver JM, Jackson M, et al: The Overt Aggression Scale: an operationalized rating scale for verbal and physical aggression. Am J Psychiatry 143:35–39, 1986

Yudofsky SC, Silver JM, Schneider SE: Pharmacologic treatment of aggression. Psychiatric Annals 17:397–407, 1987

Yudofsky SC, Silver J, Yudofsky B: Organic personality disorder, explosive type, in Treatments of Psychiatric Disorders, Vol 2: A Task Force Report of the American Psychiatric Association. Washington, DC, American Psychiatric Association, 1989, pp 839–852

Yudofsky SC, Silver JM, Hales RE: Pharmacologic management of aggression in the elderly. J Clin Psychiatry 51 (suppl 10):1–58, 1990

Chapter 6

Legal and Ethical Issues

Robert I. Simon, M.D.

Consultation-liaison psychiatrists encounter numerous thorny medicolegal issues in their practice. The delivery of competent mental health services requires a knowledgeable psychiatrist who is comfortable with the legal requirements surrounding consultation-liaison duties.

The consultation-liaison psychiatrist may have an increased risk for legal liability, particularly in the evaluation and treatment of violent patients. Appropriate risk assessment and intervention for suicidal patients or potentially violent patients will reduce significantly the likelihood of a successful malpractice claim (Simon 1992a).

ETHICAL ISSUES

Ethical issues arise daily for psychiatrists who are involved in consultations on patients who are medically ill. Medical decision making, informed consent, resuscitation, "brain death," organ transplantation, the withholding or with-

drawing of life support, and the allocation of medical resources all give rise to complex ethical and legal problems (Luce 1990). Moreover, what is considered ethical in clinical practice today may become a legal requirement tomorrow.

Since the late 1950s and early 1960s, the medical profession has moved away from an authoritarian, physician-oriented stance toward more collaboration between physician and patient in health care decisions. This is reflected in contemporary ethical principles (American Psychiatric Association 1993).

The ethical principles of beneficence, nonmaleficence (no misconduct), and respect for the dignity and autonomy of the patient provide the moral-ethical foundation for the doctor-patient relationship. For example, the consultation-liaison psychiatrist or attending physician has a legal and ethical duty to obtain consent from substitute decision makers when a patient cannot make an informed decision. The rights of all patients are the same—only how these rights are exercised is different (Parry and Beck 1990).

◼ CONFIDENTIALITY AND TESTIMONIAL PRIVILEGE

Breaching Confidentiality

Once the doctor-patient relationship is created, the clinician assumes an automatic duty to safeguard a patient's disclosures. This duty is not absolute, and in some circumstances, breaching confidentiality is both ethical and legal (see Table 6–1).

The psychiatrist should obtain the competent patient's permission before speaking to the patient's family. When this is not possible, a note should be recorded that explains the reasons for not obtaining the patient's permission. Maintaining confidentiality in the hospital is a complex issue because various staff members need to have information in order to develop evaluation and treatment plans. Information should be provided that will enable the staff to function effectively on behalf of the patient. It is often unnecessary to disclose intimate details of the patient's mental life.

Testimonial Privilege

Testimonial privilege is privilege to withhold information that applies only to the judicial setting. The patient, not the psychiatrist, holds testimonial privilege that controls the release of confidential information. Privilege statutes represent the most common recognition by the

state of the importance of protecting information provided by a patient to a psychotherapist. This recognition moves away from the essential purpose of the American system of justice (e.g., "truth finding") by insulating certain information from disclosure in court.

Exceptions to Testimonial Privilege

There are specific exceptions to testimonial privilege. Although exceptions vary, the most common include

- Child abuse reporting
- Civil commitment proceedings
- Court-ordered evaluations
- Criminal proceedings
- Cases in which a patient's mental state is part of the litigation

Liability

An unauthorized or unwarranted breach of confidentiality can cause a patient considerable emotional harm. As a result, a physician typically can be held liable for such a breach based on at least four theories:

1. Malpractice (breach of confidentiality)
2. Breach of statutory duty
3. Invasion of privacy
4. Breach of (implied) contract

Table 6–1. Common statutory exceptions to confidentiality between psychiatrist and patient

Child abuse

Competency proceedings

Court-ordered examination

Danger to self or others

Patient-litigant exception

Intent to commit a crime or harmful act

Civil commitment proceedings

Communication with other treatment providers

◼ THE RIGHT TO REFUSE TREATMENT AND INFORMED CONSENT

The right to refuse treatment is intimately connected with the doctrine of informed consent. By withholding consent, patients express their right to refuse treatment except under certain circumstances. In rare situations, courts have authorized treatment against the wishes of a competent patient. Generally, these cases involve situations in which the life of a fetus is at risk, a patient is encumbered or responsible for the care of dependent children and can be restored to full health through the intervention in question (most often, blood transfusion), and a patient who has attempted suicide is otherwise considered to be healthy. The right to refuse treatment also reflects the exercise of basic constitutional rights.

Informed consent has three essential ingredients:

1. *Competency:* clinicians provide the first level of screening to establish patient competency and to decide whether to accept a patient's treatment decision.
2. *Information:* the patient or a bona fide representative must be given adequate information (see Table 6–2).
3. *Voluntariness:* the patient must voluntarily consent to or refuse the proposed treatment or procedure.

Exceptions and Liability

The four basic exceptions to the requirement of obtaining informed consent are emergencies, incompetency, therapeutic privilege, and waiver.

Table 6–2. Informed consent: reasonable information to be disclosed

Although no consistently accepted set of information to be disclosed for any given medical or psychiatric situation exists, as a rule, five areas of information are generally provided:

1. **Diagnosis:** description of the condition or problem
2. **Treatment:** nature and purpose of proposed treatment
3. **Consequences:** risks and benefits of the proposed treatment
4. **Alternatives:** viable alternatives to the proposed treatment, including risks and benefits
5. **Prognosis:** projected outcome with and without treatment

Source. Adapted from Simon 1992b.

When emergency treatment is necessary to save a life or prevent imminent serious harm, and it is impossible to obtain either the patient's consent or that of someone authorized to provide consent for the patient, the law will typically "presume" that consent is granted. Two qualifications are necessary to apply this exception. First, the emergency must be serious and imminent, and second, the patient's condition and not other circumstances (e.g., adverse environmental conditions) must determine that an emergency exists.

The second exception to informed consent exists when a patient lacks sufficient mental capacity to give consent or is legally incompetent. Under these circumstances, consent is obtained from a substitute decision maker.

The third exception, therapeutic privilege, is the most difficult to apply. Informed consent may not be required if a psychiatrist determines that a complete disclosure of possible risks and alternatives might have a deleterious effect on the patient's health and welfare. Jurisdictions vary in their application of this exception. When specific case law or statutes outlining the factors relevant to such a decision are absent, a doctor must substantiate a patient's inability to psychologically withstand being informed of the proposed treatment. Therapeutic privilege is not a means of circumventing the legal requirement for obtaining informed consent from the patient before initiating treatment.

Finally, a physician need not disclose risks of treatment when the patient has competently, knowingly, and voluntarily waived his or her right for information (e.g., when the patient does not want information on drug side effects).

Aside from these four exceptions, a physician who treats a patient without obtaining informed consent is subject to legal liability. As a rule, treatment without any consent or against a patient's wishes may constitute a battery (intentional tort), whereas treatment commenced with inadequate consent is treated as an act of medical negligence.

Prescribing Medication for Unapproved Uses

Prescribing a Food and Drug Administration (FDA)-approved medication for an unapproved purpose does not violate federal law (Tardiff 1984). The FDA abides by the principle that good medical practice requires that a physician prescribe medication according to the best information available. However, the physician who deviates from the package insert may have to explain such a departure should a lawsuit arise.

A consultation-liaison psychiatrist may prescribe a drug for use that is not yet approved by the FDA. For example, no drug is currently approved by the FDA for the treatment of aggression (Yudofsky et al. 1995). However, a number of drugs including neuroleptics, benzodiazepines, β-blockers, anticonvulsants, and lithium are used effectively to treat aggressive episodes. Consultation-liaison psychiatrists often use intravenous haloperidol to treat delirium and stimulants to treat depression. Nevertheless, the psychiatric literature and clinical experience validate the usefulness of these drugs in the clinical management of violence and mood disorders, respectively.

The decision to prescribe drugs for nonapproved uses is based on sound knowledge of the drugs backed by firm scientific rationale and established medical studies. The psychiatrist should have texts or journal articles available to substantiate that a nonapproved use is based on the accepted practice of psychiatry.

The standard for obtaining informed consent is correspondingly heightened when a medication is prescribed for an unapproved use. The patient or guardian must be informed that the patient will be taking a drug that has not been approved by the FDA for a particular use and should be warned of all possible, reasonably foreseeable risks. Although a consent form may provide added protection, the nature of the disclosure should be recorded in the patient's chart. Whether the disclosure is given orally or provided in a consent form, the chart notes should also contain an assessment indicating whether the information was understood by the patient, whether consent was freely given, and the rationale for using a medication for unapproved purposes. This procedure should also be followed when prescribing drugs at higher-than-recommended doses.

Consultation-liaison practice, however, presents unique clinical problems. Consultation-liaison psychiatrists are faced daily with patients with delirium who require medications. No medications are FDA-approved specifically for delirium. Yet neuroleptic drugs are used regularly and effectively.

The FDA does not have the power to control psychiatrists or to dictate the practice of psychiatry, particularly with regard to prescribing drugs. The use of a drug after it is marketed is the responsibility of physicians, and they prescribe it at their sole discretion. The *Physicians' Desk Reference* (PDR; 1995), official guidelines, or any other reference cannot serve as a substitute for the psychiatrist's sound clinical judgment, training, and experience.

COMPETENCY IN HEALTH CARE DECISION MAKING

Consultation-liaison psychiatrists frequently are asked to assess patients' competency. Nearly every area of human endeavor is affected by the law and, as a fundamental condition, requires that the patient be mentally competent. Essentially, competency is defined as "having sufficient capacity, ability . . . (or) possessing the requisite physical, mental, natural, or legal qualifications. . . . " (Black 1990, p. 284). This definition is deliberately vague and ambiguous because the term *competency* is a broad concept encompassing many different legal issues and contexts. As a result, its definition, requirements, and application can vary widely depending on the circumstances (e.g., health care decisions, executing a will, or confessing to a crime).

The determination of incompetency requires a judicial decision. In this regard, it is clinically useful to distinguish the terms *incompetence* and *incapacity*. Incompetence refers to a court decision, whereas incapacity refers to a clinical determination (Mishkin 1989). Legally, only competent persons may give informed consent. An adult patient is considered legally competent unless adjudicated incompetent or temporarily incapacitated due to a medical condition. Incapacity does not prevent treatment. It merely means the clinician must obtain substitute consent.

Competency is not a scientifically determinable state; it is situation specific. The issue of competency arises in a number of legal contexts. Although there are no hard and fast rules, germane to determining competency is the patient's ability to

- Understand the particular treatment choice being proposed
- Make a treatment choice
- Be able to verbally or nonverbally communicate that choice

The above standard, however, acquires only a simple consent from the patient rather than an informed consent because alternative treatment choices are not provided.

A review of case law and scholarly literature reveals four standards for determining incompetency in decision making (Appelbaum et al. 1987). In the order of levels of mental capacity required, these standards include

1. Communication of choice
2. Understanding of information provided
3. Appreciation of options available
4. Rational decision making

Psychiatrists are generally most comfortable with a rational decision-making standard in determining incompetency. Most courts, however, prefer the first two standards. A truly informed consent that considers the patient's autonomy, personal needs, and values occurs when rational decision making is applied by the patient to the risks and benefits of appropriate treatment options provided by the clinician.

A valid consent is either expressed (orally or in writing) or implied from the patient's actions. The issue of competency, whether in a civil or criminal context, is commonly raised in two situations: when the person is a minor or is mentally disabled and lacks the requisite cognitive capacity for health care decision making. In many situations, minors are not considered legally competent, and therefore, the consent of a parent or designated guardian is required. However, there are exceptions to this general rule, such as minors who are considered emancipated (Smith 1986) or mature (*Gulf S I R Co. v. Sullivan* 1928), or in some cases of medical need, such as abortion (*Planned Parenthood v. Danforth* 1976) or mental health counseling (*Jehovah's Witnesses v. King County Hospital* 1968).

Mentally disabled patients, including mentally impaired psychiatric patients and psychiatrically impaired medically ill patients, present a slightly different problem in evaluating competency. Lack of capacity or competency *cannot* be presumed from either treatment for mental illness (*Wilson v. Lehman* 1964) or institutionalization of such persons (*Rennie v. Klein* 1978). Mental disability or illness does *not* in itself render a person incompetent in all areas of functioning. Instead, the patient must be examined to determine whether specific functional incapacities render a person incapable of making a particular kind of decision or performing a particular type of task. The legal designation of "incompetent" is applied to an individual who fails one of the mental tests of capacity and is therefore considered by law not mentally capable of performing a particular act or assuming a particular role. In other words, the fact that a patient is adjudicated incompetent to execute a will does not automatically mean that patient is incompetent to do other things, such as consent to treatment, testify as a witness, marry, drive a car, or make a legally binding contract.

Medically ill patients who are found to lack the requisite functional mental capacity to make a treatment decision, except in cases of an emergency (*Frasier v. Department of Health and Human Resources* 1986), must have an authorized representative or guardian appointed to make health care decisions on their behalf (*Aponte v. United States* 1984). Table 6–3 lists several consent options available (depending on the jurisdiction) for patients who lack mental capacity for health care decisions.

RIGHT TO DIE

Legal decisions addressing the issue of a terminally ill patient's "right to die" fall into one of two categories: 1) patients who are incompetent (i.e., removal of life-support systems) (*In re Conroy* 1985; *In re Quinlin* 1976) or 2) patients who are competent.

Incompetent Patients

On the very difficult and personal question of patient autonomy, the U.S. Supreme Court ruled in *Cruzan v. Director, Missouri Department of Health* (1990) that the state of Missouri may refuse to remove a food and water tube surgically implanted in the stomach of Nancy Cruzan without clear and convincing evidence of her wishes. The state has the right to maintain that individual's life, even to the exclusion of the family's wishes.

The importance of the *Cruzan* decision for physicians treating severely or terminally impaired patients is that they must seek clear and competent instructions from the patient regarding foreseeable treatment decisions. For example, physicians treating patients with progressive degenerative brain diseases should attempt to obtain the patient's wishes regarding the use of life-sustaining measures while that patient can still competently articulate those

Table 6–3. Common consent options for patients who lack the mental capacity for health care decisions

Proxy consent of next of kin

Adjudication of incompetence; appointment of a guardian

Institutional administrators or committees

Treatment review panels

Substituted consent of the court

Advance directives (living will, durable power of attorney, health care proxy)

Statutory surrogates (spouse or court-appointed guardian)[a]

[a]Medical Statutory Surrogate Laws (when treatment wishes of the patient are unstated).
Source. Reprinted from Simon RI: *Clinical Psychiatry and the Law,* 2nd Edition. Washington, DC, American Psychiatric Press, 1992a. Copyright 1992, American Psychiatric Press. Used with permission.

wishes. This information is best provided in the form of a living will, durable power of attorney agreement, or health care proxy. However, any written document that clearly and convincingly sets forth the patient's wishes would serve the same purpose.

Although physicians fear civil or criminal liability for stopping life-sustaining treatment, legal liability may occur for providing unwanted treatment to a competent patient or treatment that is against the best interests of an incompetent patient.

Competent Patients

A small but growing body of cases has emerged involving competent patients who usually have excruciating pain and terminal diseases and seek to stop further medical treatment. The single most significant influence in the development of this body of law is the doctrine of informed consent. Beginning with the fundamental tenet that "no right is held more sacred . . . than the right of every individual to the possession and control of his own person" (*Union Pacific Ry Co v. Botsford* 1891, pp. 250–251; *Schloendorff v. Society of New York Hospi-*

tal 1914, pp. 92–93), courts have fashioned the present-day informed consent doctrine and applied it to right-to-die cases.

Notwithstanding these principles, the right to decline life-sustaining medical intervention, even for a competent person, is not absolute. As noted in *In re Conroy* (1985), four countervailing interests may limit the exercise of that right: 1) preservation of life, 2) prevention of suicide, 3) safeguarding the integrity of the medical profession, and 4) the protection of innocent third parties.

As a result of the *Cruzan* decision, courts will focus on primarily the reliability of the evidence presented to establish the patient's competence—specifically, the clarity and certainty with which a decision to withhold medical treatment was made. Assuming that a terminally ill patient chose to forego any further medical intervention *and* the patient was competent at the time of the decision, courts are unlikely to overrule or subvert the patient's right to privacy and autonomy.

Do-Not-Resuscitate (DNR) Orders

Cardiopulmonary resuscitation (CPR) is a medical lifesaving technology. Immediate initiation of CPR at the time of a cardiac arrest leaves no time to think about the consequences of reviving a patient. Usually, patients requiring CPR have not thought about or expressed a preference for or against its use.

The ethical principle of patient autonomy justifies the position that the patient or substitute decision maker should make the decision regarding the use of CPR. The competent patient's decision about DNR should be followed. Malpractice liability for withholding unwanted and futile care is unlikely, whereas the psychiatrist is exposed to greater liability if care is provided against the patient's wishes (March and Staver 1991).

Schwartz (1987) noted that two key principles have emerged concerning DNR decisions:

1. DNR decisions are reached consensually by the attending physician and the patient or substitute decision maker.
2. DNR orders, including date and time, are written on the doctor's order sheet, and the reasons for the DNR order are documented in the chart.

Psychiatrists should become familiar with the specific hospital policy whenever a DNR order is written.

ADVANCE DIRECTIVES

Advance directives such as a living will, health care proxy, or a durable medical power of attorney are recommended in order to avoid ethical and legal complications associated with requests to withhold life-sustaining treatment measures (Simon 1992a; Solnick 1985). The Patient Self-Determination Act that became effective on December 1, 1991, requires all hospitals, nursing homes, hospices, managed care organizations, and home health care agencies to advise patients or family members of their right to accept or refuse medical care in the form of an advance directive (LaPuma et al. 1991). Advance directives provide a method for individuals, while they are competent, to choose alternative health care decision makers in the event of future incompetency.

Generally, durable power of attorney is construed to empower an agent to make health care decisions. Such a document is much broader and more flexible than a living will, which covers just the period of a diagnosed terminal illness and specifies only that no "extraordinary treatments" be used to prolong the act of dying (Mishkin 1985). The health care proxy is a legal instrument akin to the durable power of attorney but is specifically created for the delegation of health care decisions.

In a durable power of attorney or health care proxy, general or specific directions are set forth about how future decisions are to be made in the event that one becomes unable to make these decisions. The determination of a patient's competence, however, is not specified in most durable power of attorney and health care proxy statutes. Because this is a medical or psychiatric question, an examination by two physicians to determine the patient's ability to understand the nature and consequences of the proposed treatment or procedure, ability to make a choice, and ability to communicate that choice usually is sufficient. This information, like all significant medical observations, is clearly documented in the patient's chart.

Because durable power of attorney agreements or health care proxies are easily revoked, the treating psychiatrist or institution has no choice but to honor the patient's refusal, even if there is reasonable evidence that the patient is incompetent. If this situation occurs, legal consultation should be considered. If the patient is grossly confused and is an immediate danger to self and others, the physician or hospital is on firmer ground, both medically and legally, to temporarily override the patient's treatment refusal. Otherwise, it is generally better to seek a court order for treatment than to risk legal entanglement with the patient by attempting to enforce the advance directive's original terms. Typically, unless there are compelling medical reasons to do otherwise, courts will generally honor the patient's original treatment directions.

GUARDIANSHIP

Guardianship is a method of substitute decision making for individuals who are judicially determined to be unable to act for themselves (Parry 1985). In some states, there are separate provisions for the appointment of a "guardian of one's person" (e.g., health care decision making) and for a "guardian of one's estate" (e.g., authority to make contracts to sell one's property) (Sales et al. 1982). The latter guardian

is frequently referred to as a *conservator,* although this designation is not uniformly used throughout the United States. Two further distinctions—*general (plenary)* and *specific* guardianship—are made in some jurisdictions (Sales et al. 1982). As the name implies, the latter guardian is restricted to making decisions about a particular subject area. For instance, the specific guardian is authorized to make decisions about major or emergency medical procedures, and the disabled person retains the freedom to make decisions about all other medical matters. The general guardian, by contrast, has total control over the disabled individual's person, estate, or both (Sales et al. 1982).

Guardianship arrangements are increasingly utilized with patients who have dementia, particularly AIDS-related dementia and Alzheimer's disease (Overman and Stoudemire 1988). Under the Anglo-American system of law, however, an individual is presumed to be competent unless adjudicated incompetent. Thus, incompetence is a legal determination made by a court of law based on evidence from health care providers and others that the individual's functional mental capacity is significantly impaired.

Generally, the appointment of a guardian is limited to situations in which the individual's decision-making capacity is so impaired that he or she is unable to care for personal safety or provide necessities such as food, shelter, clothing, and medical care (*In re Boyer* 1981). The standard of proof required for a judicial determination of incompetency is clear and convincing evidence. Although the law does not assign percentages to proof, clear and convincing evidence is in the range of 75% certainty (Simon 1992a).

SUBSTITUTED JUDGMENT

Psychiatrists often find that the process required to obtain an adjudication of incompetence is unduly burdensome, is costly, and frequently interferes with the provision of quality treatment. Moreover, families are often reluctant to face the formal court proceedings necessary to declare their family member incompetent, particularly when sensitive family matters are disclosed. A common solution to both of these problems is to seek the legally authorized proxy consent of a guardian when the patient refusing treatment is believed to be incompetent. Proxy consent, however, is not available in every state (Simon 1992a).

Clear advantages are associated with having the family serve as decision makers (Perr 1984). First, use of responsible family members as surrogate decision makers maintains the integrity of the family unit and relies on the sources who are most likely to know the patient's wishes. Second, it is more efficient and less costly. There are some disadvantages, however. Proxy decision making requires synthesizing the diverse values, beliefs, practices, and prior statements of the patient for a specific circumstance (Emanuel and Emanuel 1992). As one judge characterized the problem, any proxy decision made in the absence of specific directions is at best only an optimistic approximation (*In re Jobes* 1987). Ambivalent feelings, conflicts within the family and with the patient, and conflicting economic interests may make certain family members suspect as guardians (Gutheil and Appelbaum 1980). Some family members are more impaired than the patient for whom proxy consent is being sought. In addition, relatives may not be available or may not want to get involved.

A number of states permit proxy decision making by statute, mainly through their informed consent statute (Solnick 1985). Some state statutes specify that another person (e.g., specific relatives) may authorize consent on behalf of the incompetent patient.

Unless proxy consent by a relative is provided by statute or by case law authority within the state, the consultation-liaison psychiatrist should not rely on the good faith consent by next of kin in treating a patient believed to be incompetent (Klein et al. 1983). The legally appropriate procedure is to seek judicial recognition of the family member as the substitute decision maker.

Some patients recover competency within a few days. As soon as the patient is competent, consent for further treatment should be obtained directly from the patient. For the patient who continues to lack mental capacity for health care decisions, an increasing number of states have statutes that permit involuntary treatment of incompetent mentally ill patients who refuse treatment, even if the patient does not meet current standards for involuntary civil commitment (Hassenfeld and Grumet 1984; Zito et al. 1984). As noted above, in most jurisdictions, a durable power of attorney permits the next of kin to consent (Solnick 1985). In some instances, however, this procedure may not meet judicial challenge. To avoid this problem, certain states created health care proxies specifically for health care decision making.

VOLUNTARY HOSPITALIZATION

The medical-surgical patient who is transferred to a psychiatric unit may want to leave. Because these patients were originally admitted for a medical or surgical problem, transfer to a psychiatric unit can be a bewildering experience. If the psychiatric unit is active with disturbed, noisy, or threatening patients, the medical-surgical patient may become terrified and demand immediate release. The consultation-liaison psychiatrist must understand the clinical and legal issues surrounding voluntary and involuntary hospitalization and discharge.

Although an expressed or implied contract may be lacking, it is well established legally that a doctor is not obligated to accept a patient who simply seeks medical or psychiatric treatment (*Salas v. Gamboa* 1988). In some situations, however, an implied contractual arrangement does exist, even between a physician and patient who have had no contact. The most common situation is a hospital's emergency room doctor, who is generally expected to provide services to all who seek treatment. This principle may extend to include physicians and psychiatrists who are on call as backup or support to the emergency room staff (*Dillon v. Silver* 1987). Once a patient is admitted to a hospital, whether through voluntary or involuntary admission, the hospital is responsible to provide reasonable care to that patient.

Depending on the circumstances surrounding the admission or potential admission, liability issues associated with patient admission may arise. The most common cause of legal action involves the psychiatrists' failure to comply with civil commitment requirements. This situation typically gives rise to a lawsuit based on the theories of false imprisonment (*Gonzalez v. New York* 1983), malicious prosecution, or assault (*St. Vincent's Medical Center v. Oakley* 1979).

Grounds for a lawsuit may exist when a voluntary patient seeks to leave a hospital and is then coerced to remain in the hospital by threat of civil commitment. In addition, a lawsuit may result when actual commitment proceedings are initiated without appropriate evidence for such an action (*Plumadore v. State* 1980). Another admission of liability may also occur if a patient represents a foreseeable risk of danger to self or others and the hospital does not hospitalize such a patient (*Clark v. State* 1985).

To protect a patient's civil rights, he or she should be informed of the types of voluntary admission. Pure or informal voluntary admission permits the patient to leave the hospital at any time. Only moral suasion is available to encourage the patient to stay. Conditional or formal voluntary admissions require that the patient stay for a period of time after giving written notice of intention to leave. The latter provision is used when the patient appears to be a danger to self or others.

In reality, the distinction between voluntary and involuntary admissions is not always clear. Patients are often induced or pressured into accepting voluntary admissions. If voluntary admission were maintained as truly voluntary, involuntary admissions would likely increase. The situation is analogous to plea bargaining in criminal cases. The criminal justice system would have to accommodate an increased number of cases if plea bargaining were eliminated.

In a U.S. Supreme Court case, *Zinermon v. Burch* (1990), a mentally ill patient who was unable to give informed consent was permitted to proceed with a civil rights action against state officials who committed him to a state hospital using voluntary commitment procedures. The court held that Florida must have procedures to screen all voluntary patients for competency and exclude incompetent persons from the voluntary admission process. For the few states that require competent consent to voluntary admission, screening procedures to exclude incompetent patients are needed.

Voluntary patients may want to leave the hospital against medical advice. If the patient is not a danger to self or others and is competent, the psychiatrist cannot do much more than try to deal with the discharge as a treatment issue. Regardless of whether the patient signs an AMA (against medical advice) form, a notation should be made in the record detailing the recommendations made to the patient about the need for further hospitalization as well as the possible risks of premature discharge. Voluntary patients who are incompetent but are not dangerous or gravely disabled cannot be kept in the hospital against their will, even if they have been adjudicated incompetent and a guardian gives consent for hospitalization. Under these circumstances, family or another responsible party should be involved at the time of a premature discharge.

INVOLUNTARY HOSPITALIZATION

The consultation-liaison psychiatrist may need to transfer medically ill patients involuntarily to a psychiatric unit. Three main substantive criteria serve as the foundation for all statutory commitment requirements. These criteria require that the individual is 1) mentally ill, 2) dangerous to self or others, and/or 3) unable to provide for basic needs. Generally, each state determines which criteria are required and defines each criterion. Because terms such as mentally ill are often loosely described, the proper definition relies on the clinician's judgment.

In addition to determining and defining criteria for committing individuals with mental illness to a psychiatric hospital, certain states have enacted legislation that permits the involuntary hospitalization of three other distinct groups: 1) people with developmental disabilities (mental retardation), 2) people addicted to substances such as alcohol and drugs, and 3) minors with mental disabilities. Special commitment provisions may exist governing requirements for the admission and discharge of mentally disabled minors as well as numerous due process rights of these individuals (*Parham v. J.R.* 1979).

Clinicians must remember that they cannot legally commit patients. This process is solely under the court's jurisdiction. The psychiatrist merely initiates a medical certification that brings the patient before the court, which usually occurs after a brief evaluation in the hospital. Psychiatrists who use reasonable professional judgment and act in good faith when requesting involuntary hospitalization are granted immunity from liability in many states.

Commitment statutes do not mandate involuntary hospitalization (Appelbaum et al. 1987). The statutes are permissive and enable mental health professionals and others to seek involuntary hospitalization for persons who meet certain criteria. On the other hand, the duty to seek involuntary hospitalization is a standard-of-care issue. That is, patients who are mentally ill and pose an imminent, serious threat to themselves or others may require involuntary hospitalization as a primary psychiatric intervention.

SECLUSION AND RESTRAINT

The psychiatric-legal issues surrounding seclusion and restraint are complex. There are both indications for and contraindications to the use of seclusion and restraint (see Tables 6–4 and 6–5). However, what the general psychiatrist believes are contraindications to the use of restraints are often viewed as indications by the consultation-liaison psychiatrist. A consultation-liaison psychiatrist frequently recommends restraint in confused, medically unstable patients. These patients usually have delirium and sometimes have dementia. If restraints are not used in such patients, they pull out their endotracheal tubes, arterial lines, and in some instances, intraaortic balloon pumps. Moreover, confused medically ill patients also climb over bed rails and fall onto the floor. Such falls frequently result in fractures and subdural hematomas.

Stringent legal regulation of seclusion and restraint has increased during the past decade, as have legal challenges on the use of seclusion and restraint in institutionalized mentally ill and mentally retarded patients. These lawsuits usually are part of a challenge to a wide range of alleged abuses within a hospital. Generally,

Table 6–4.   Indications for seclusion and restraint

To prevent clear, imminent harm to patient or others

To prevent significant disruption to treatment program or physical surroundings

To assist in treatment as part of ongoing behavior therapy

To decrease sensory overstimulation[a]

To respond to patient's voluntary reasonable request for intervention

[a]Seclusion only.
Source.   Reprinted from Simon RI: *Clinical Psychiatry and the Law,* 2nd Edition. Washington, DC, American Psychiatric Press, 1992a. Copyright 1992, American Psychiatric Press. Used with permission.

Table 6–5. Contraindications to seclusion and restraint

Extremely unstable medical and psychiatric conditions[a,b]

Patients with delirium or dementia who are unable to tolerate decreased stimulation[a,b]

Overtly suicidal patients[a,b]

Patients with severe drug reactions or overdoses,[b] or those who require close monitoring of drug dosages[a]

Punishment of the patient or convenience of staff

[a]Unless close supervision and direct observation are provided.
[b]May be indications for restraint in medically ill patients in the general hospital.
Source. Adapted from Simon RI: *Clinical Psychiatry and the Law,* 2nd Edition. Washington, DC, American Psychiatric Press, 1992a. Copyright 1992, American Psychiatric Press. Used with permission.

courts hold that restraints and seclusion are appropriate only when a patient presents a risk of harm to self or others, and a less restrictive alternative is not available. Additional considerations include the following:

- Restraint and seclusion must be implemented by a written order from an appropriate medical official. However, a physician on call at night can give a verbal order for restraint, as long as the patient is examined soon thereafter and an order is written.
- Orders must be confined to specific, time-limited periods.
- A patient's condition must be regularly reviewed and documented.
- Extension of the original order must be reviewed and reauthorized.

COLLABORATIVE, CONSULTATIVE, AND SUPERVISORY RELATIONSHIPS WITH NONMEDICAL THERAPISTS

The American Psychiatric Association formulated guidelines for psychiatrists who work with nonmedical mental health therapists (American Psychiatric Association 1980). The American Psychiatric Association Guidelines for Psychiatrists in Consultative Supervisory or Collaborative Relationships with Nonmedical Therapists is now more than a decade old (American Psychiatric Association 1980). Despite significant changes during this time, the guidelines have not been revised. Today, the relationship between psychiatrists and nonmedical therapists is infinitely more complex (Kleinman 1991). Furthermore, an important caveat that accompanies the guidelines states "that they do not represent official policy but rather a 'living document' to be adapted to local custom and practice." As mental health care is delivered increasingly by nonmedical therapists, psychiatrists will practice more within the framework of an organized health delivery system. Thus, the capacity to provide mental health care is enhanced. However, an obvious limit exists to nonmedical mental health professionals' ability to appropriately consult on medically ill patients (e.g., patients with delirium).

In a collaborative relationship, responsibility for the patient's care is shared according to the qualifications and limitations of each discipline (American Psychiatric Association 1980). The patient is informed of the separate responsibilities of each therapist. The responsibilities of each discipline do not diminish the other. Periodic evaluation of the patient's clinical condition and needs by the psychiatrist and the nonmedical therapist is necessary to determine whether the collaboration should continue. On termination of the collaborative relationship, the health care providers should inform the patient either separately or jointly.

When performing single consultations, the consultation-liaison psychiatrist ordinarily does not enter into a treatment relationship with the patient and does not assume responsibility for care. Because most consultation-liaison psychiatrists do follow-up care in hospitals, a doctor-patient treatment relationship may be construed by a court from the consultation-liaison psychiatrist's continuing relationship with the patient, regardless of whether actual orders are written. However, when orders are written about a patient, courts will likely find a doctor-patient relationship.

The consultation-liaison psychiatrist is not the primary physician. The consultation-liaison psychiatrist has a relationship with the consulting physician, not the patient. The consulting physician is free to accept or reject the findings and recommendations of the consultation-liaison psychiatrist. Consultation-liaison psychiatrists are not likely to be found ultimately liable for adverse outcomes when their suggestions are not acted on. They may, nonetheless, be sued along with the consulting physician. Follow-up and discussion with the consulting physician are important to avoid miscommunications, which facilitates a collaborative relationship that benefits the patient. The consultation-liaison psychiatrist relies on information provided by the physician. The risk of liability for the consultation-liaison psychiatrist will arise only if the consultative advice provided is negligently based on inadequate or limited information. When the consultation-liaison psychiatrist sees the patient directly, liability may be assessed for a negligent consultation.

The practice of psychiatry has changed a great deal since the guidelines were adopted, so that certain guidelines may no longer be applicable. Moreover, with the advent of biological treatments, guidelines do not help to define the scope of nonsupervisory responsibilities of psychiatrists who may provide medication backup for nonmedical professionals (Goldberg et al. 1991). The psychiatrist's liability in cases in which the nonmedical professional is found to have practiced outside of the scope of his or her practice will likely depend on the nature and extent of the psychiatrist's relationship with the nonmedical professional and the patient. Appelbaum (1991, p. 282) recommends that "all responsibilities should be clearly specified, preferably in a written agreement among the patient, the psychiatrist, and the nonmedical therapist."

MANAGED CARE

Health maintenance organizations (HMOs), independent practice associations (IPAs), and preferred provider organizations (PPOs) may create additional ethical and legal dilemmas for psychiatrists. Such managed care systems interject cost and contractual pressures into treatment and dispositional decisions. Psychiatrists must not allow themselves to be put in the position of choosing between a patient's need for quality care and the economic and administrative requirements of the health plan.

In *Wickline v. California* (1986), the treating physician, Dr. Polonsky, requested an extended stay of 8 days for his patient following surgery for Leriche's syndrome (occlusion of the terminal aorta). The Medi-Cal reviewer granted 4 days. Mrs. Wickline experienced complications following the premature release, resulting in amputation of her leg. She sued Medi-Cal. The jury ruled in her favor, but a California appellate court decided that the treating physician was liable, not Medi-Cal.

In his testimony, Dr. Polonsky stated that he believed "that Medi-Cal had the power to tell him, as a treating doctor, when a patient must be discharged from the hospital." The appellate court noted that third-party payers of health care services can be held liable when appeals on the behalf of the patients for medical care "are arbitrarily ignored or unreasonably disregarded or over-ridden." The court added that "the physician who complies without protest with the limitations imposed by a third party payor, when his medical judgment dictates otherwise, cannot avoid his ultimate responsibility for his patient's care. He cannot point to the health care payor as the liability scapegoat when the consequences of his own determinative medical decision go sour."

Accordingly, when a physician's decision and the position of a third-party payer conflict, it is the physician's duty to protest any compromise in patient care that might be presented by a third-party payer. All channels should be pursued to ensure that the physician's medical judgment (e.g., continued hospitalization) is carried out. Only after a physician has exhausted all options in an attempt to act in the patient's best medical interest can an argument likely be made that no liability attaches to the physician or affiliate hospital.

In a subsequent case, *Wilson v. Blue Cross of Southern California et al.* (1990), a California appeals court chose not to follow the specific language of the *Wickline* case. In the *Wilson* case, a patient with anorexia, drug dependency, and major depression was hospitalized at College Hospital in Los Angeles, California. The treating physician determined that the patient required 3–4 weeks of hospitalization. After approximately 1½ weeks, utilization review determined that further hospitalization was unnecessary. The patient's insurance company refused to pay for further inpatient treatment. The patient was discharged and committed suicide a few weeks later.

The Appellate Division of the California Court of Appeals heard that third-party payers are not immune from lawsuits in regard to utilization review activities. The court determined that the insurer may be subject to liability for harm caused to the patient by premature termination of hospitalization. Although the fact pattern of this case differs from that of the *Wickline* case, it is clear from the *Wilson* decision that a third-party payer may be held legally liable for a negligent decision to discharge the patient either separately or along with the patient's physician, depending on the facts of the case. Although *Wickline* and *Wilson* are California cases only, they offer insight and, perhaps, precedence concerning future reasoning by other courts who will be increasingly confronted by complex liability issues associated with utilization review decisions.

RISK MANAGEMENT

Psychiatric Malpractice

Psychiatric malpractice is medical malpractice. Malpractice is the delivery of substandard professional care that causes a compensable injury to a person (Simon and Sadoff 1992). Although this definition may seem relatively clear and simple, confusion may exist. For example, the essential issue is *not* the existence of substandard care per se but whether actual compensable liability exists. In order for a psychiatrist to be found liable to a patient for malpractice, the four fundamental elements listed in Table 6–6 must be established by a preponderance of the evidence (e.g., more likely than not). Unless all of these four elements are met, the physician is not liable, even if negligence occurred. A psychiatrist may be negligent but is still not liable. For example, if the patient had no real injuries because of the negligence or if he or she had an injury but it was not directly due to the psychiatrist's negligence, then a claim of malpractice would be defeated.

CONCLUSION

Myriad clinical-legal issues arise in the practice of consultation-liaison psychiatry. In particular, the consultation-liaison psychiatrist must understand legal issues surrounding the competency of patients to make health care decisions. Informed consent, substitute decision making, advance directives, and guardianship are areas in which frequent clinical-legal dilemmas arise.

Table 6–6. Four D's of malpractice

Duty—a duty of care was owed by the physician

Deviation—the duty of care was breached

Damages—the patient experienced actual damages

Direct causation—the deviation was the direct cause of the damages

Although the consultation-liaison psychiatrist does not need to be a lawyer, a thorough understanding of commonly encountered clinical-legal issues is essential for effective practice.

REFERENCES

American Psychiatric Association: Official actions: guidelines for psychiatrists in consultative, supervisory, or collaborative relationships with nonmedical therapists. Am J Psychiatry 137: 1489–1491, 1980

American Psychiatric Association: The Principles of Medical Ethics: With Annotations Especially Applicable to Psychiatry. Washington, DC, American Psychiatric Press, 1993

Appelbaum PS: General guidelines for psychiatrists who prescribe medication for patients treated by nonmedical therapists. Hosp Community Psychiatry 42:281–282, 1991

Appelbaum PS, Lidz CW, Meisel A: Informed Consent: Legal Theory and Clinical Practice. New York, Oxford University Press, 1987

Black HC: Black's Law Dictionary, 6th Edition. St. Paul, MN, West, 1990

Emanuel EJ, Emanuel LL: Proxy decision making for incompetent patients-an ethical and empirical analysis. JAMA 267:2067–2071, 1992

Goldberg RS, Riba M, Tasman A: Psychiatrists' attitudes toward prescribing medication for patients treated by nonmedical psychotherapists. Hosp Community Psychiatry 42:276–280, 1991

Gutheil TG, Appelbaum PS: Substituted judgment and the physician's ethical dilemma: with special reference to the problem of the psychiatric patient. J Clin Psychiatry 41:303–305, 1980

Hassenfeld IN, Grumet B: A study of the right to refuse treatment. Bull Am Acad Psychiatry Law 12:65–74, 1984

Joint Commission on Accreditation of Healthcare Organizations: Consolidated Standards Manual. Chicago, IL, Joint Commission on Accreditation of Healthcare Organizations, 1991, SC. 2.1-SC. 2.10, pp 146–147

Klein J, Onek J, Macbeth J: Seminar on Law in the Practice of Psychiatry. Washington, DC, Onek, Klein and Farr, 1983

Kleinman CC: Psychiatrists' relationships with nonmedical professionals, in American Psychiatric Press Review of Clinical Psychiatry and the Law, Vol 2. Edited by Simon RI. Washington, DC, American Psychiatric Press, 1991, pp 241–257

LaPuma J, Orentlicher D, Moss RJ: Advance directives on admission: clinical implications and analysis of the Patient Self-Determination Act of 1990. JAMA 266:402–405, 1991

Luce JM: Ethical principles in critical care. JAMA 263:696–700, 1990

March FH, Staver A: Physician authority for unilateral DNR orders. J Leg Med 12:115–165, 1991

Mishkin B: Decisions in Hospice. Arlington, VA, The National Hospice Organization, 1985

Mishkin B: Determining the capacity for making health care decisions, in Issues in Geriatric Psychiatry (Advances in Psychosomatic Medicine Series, Vol 19). Edited by Billig N, Rabins PV. Basel, Karger, 1989, pp 151–166

Overman W, Stoudemire A: Guidelines for legal and financial counseling of Alzheimer's disease patients and their families. Am J Psychiatry 145:1495–1500, 1988

Parry J: Incompetency, guardianship, and restoration, in The Mentally Disabled and the Law, 3rd Edition. Edited by Brakel SJ, Parry J, Weiner BA. Chicago, IL, American Bar Foundation, 1985, p 370

Parry JW, Beck JC: Revisiting the civil commitment/involuntary treatment stalemate using limited guardianship, substituted judgment and different due process considerations: a work in progress. Medical and Physical Disability Law Reporter 14:102–114, 1990

Perr IN: The clinical considerations of medication refusal. Legal Aspects of Psychiatric Practice 1:5–8, 1984

Physicians' Desk Reference, 46th Edition. Oradell, NJ, Medical Economics Company, 1995

Sales BD, Powell DM, Van Duizend R: Disabled Persons and the Law: Law, Society, and Policy Services, Vol 1. New York, Plenum, 1982, p 461

Schwartz HR: Do not resuscitate orders: the impact of guidelines on clinical practice, in Geriatric Psychiatry and the Law. Edited by Rosner R, Schwartz HR. New York, Plenum, 1987, pp 91–100

Simon RI: Clinical Psychiatry and the Law, 2nd Edition. Washington, DC, American Psychiatric Press, 1992a

Simon RI: Concise Guide to Psychiatry and Law for Clinicians. Washington, DC, American Psychiatric Press, 1992b

Simon RI, Sadoff RL: Malpractice law: an introduction, in Psychiatric Malpractice: Cases and Comments for Clinicians. Washington, DC, American Psychiatric Press, 1992, pp 23–55

Smith JT: Medical Malpractice: Psychiatric Care. Colorado Springs, CO, Shephards McGraw-Hill, 1986

Solnick PB: Proxy consent for incompetent non-terminally ill adult patients. J Leg Med 6:1–49, 1985

Tardiff K (ed): The Psychiatric Uses of Seclusion and Restraint. Washington, DC, American Psychiatric Press, 1984

Yudofsky SC, Silver JM, Hales RE: Treatment of Aggressive Disorders, in The American Psychiatric Press Textbook of Psychopharmacology. Edited by Schatzberg AF, Nemeroff CB. Washington, DC, American Psychiatric Press, 1995, pp 735–751

Zito JM, Lentz SL, Routt WW, et al: The treatment review panel: a solution to treatment refusal? Bull Am Acad Psychiatry Law 12:349–358, 1984

LEGAL CITE REFERENCES

Aponte v United States, 582 FSupp 555, 566–69 (D PR 1984)

Clark v State, No. 62962 Albany Court of Claims (NY 1985)

Cruzan v Director, Missouri Department of Health, 110 S Ct 284 (1990)

Dillon v Silver, 134 AD 2d 159, 520 NYS 2d 751 (1987)

Frasier v Department of Health and Human Resources, 500 So2d 858, 864, La Ct App (1986)

Gonzalez v New York, 121 Misc 2d 410, 467 NYS 2d 538 (1983), rev'd on other grounds, 110 AD 2d 810 488 NYS 2d 231

Gulf S I R Co. v Sullivan, 155 Miss 1, 119 So 501 (1928)

In re Boyer, 636 P2d 1085, 1089, Utah (1981)

In re Conroy, 98 NJ 321, 486 A2d 1209, 1222–23 (1985)

In re Jobes, 108 NJ 365, 529 A2d 434 (1987)

In re Quinlin, 70 NJ 10, 355 A2d 647, cert denied, 429 US 922 (1976)

Jehovah's Witnesses v King County Hospital, 278 FSupp 488 (WD Wash 1967), affd, 390 US 598 (1968)

Natanson v Kline, 186 Kan 393, 350 P2d 1093 (1960)

Parham v J.R., 442 US 584 (1979)

Planned Parenthood v Danforth, 428 US 52, 74 (1976)

Plumadore v State, 75 AD 2d 691, 427 NYS 2d 90 (1980)

Rennie v Klein, 462 FSupp 1131 (D NJ 1978), remanded, 476 FSupp 1294 (D NJ 1979) aff'd in part, modified in part and remanded, 653 F2d 836, 3rd Cir (1980), vacated and remanded, 458 U.S. 1119 (1982), 720 F2d 266, 3rd Cir (1983)

Salas v Gamboa, 760 SW2d 838, Tex App (1988)

Schloendorff v Society of New York Hospital, 211 NY 125, 105 NE 92 (1914), overruled, Bing v Thunig, 2 NY2d 656, 143 NE2d 3, 163 NYS2d 3 (1957)

St. Vincent's Medical Center v Oakley, 371 So2d 590, Fla App (1979)

Union Pacific Ry Co v Botsford, 141 US 250, 251 (1891)

Wickline v California, 183 Cal App 3d 1175, 228 Cal RpTr 661 (CAL Ct. App 1986)

Wilson v Blue Cross of Southern California et al., 222 CAL App 3d 660 (1990)

Wilson v Lehman, 379 SW2d 478, 479, Ky (1964)

Zinermon v Burch, 110 S Ct 975 (1990)

Section II

Psychiatric Disorders in General Hospital Patients

Chapter 7

Delirium (Confusional States)

Michael G. Wise, M.D.
Paula T. Trzepacz, M.D.

Delirium occurs in about 15%–18% of patients on medical and surgical wards, based on both referral and consecutive samples. Its prevalence is even higher in certain populations—30% in post–coronary artery bypass graft (CABG) (Smith and Dimsdale 1989) surgery and 50% in post–hip surgery patients (Gustafson et al. 1988). The prevalence increases with advanced age and in individuals with existing or progressive brain disease (e.g., dementia of the Alzheimer's type) (Kolbeinsson and Jonsson 1993; Lipowski 1990). The mortality associated with this psychiatric disorder is significant. In addition to an increased risk of mortality, patients with delirium have longer lengths of hospital stay (Francis et al. 1990; Marcantonio et al. 1994), will face future cognitive decline (Francis and Kapoor 1992), have increased utilization of hospital resources (Kane et al. 1993), have an increased frequency of major postsurgical complications (Marcantonio et al. 1994), and experience poor functional recovery (Cole and Primeau 1993; Marcantonio et al. 1994; Murray et al. 1993). Delirium is commonly diagnosed by consultation psychiatrists and underdiagnosed by nonpsychiatric physicians.

A wide variety of physiological and central nervous system (CNS) insults produce delirium, which helps to explain its high prevalence and extensive differential diagnosis. Accurate diagnosis must precede the etiological assessment and treatment. Without proper diagnosis and treatment, the prognosis for the patient with delirium is poor.

DEFINITION AND DIAGNOSTIC CRITERIA

DSM-IV (American Psychiatric Association 1994) diagnostic criteria for delirium are listed in Table 7–1. When delirium is present, a specific diagnosis is made based on etiology. If an etiology is determined, the diagnosis is delirium due to a general medical condition (e.g., delirium due to hepatic encephalopathy or delirium due to hypoglycemia), substance-induced delirium (including medication side effects), or delirium due to multiple etiologies. If the clinician is unable to determine a specific etiology, a diagnosis of delirium not otherwise specified is made.

Some neurologists divide the concept of delirium into two different types—an acute confusional state and an acute agitated delirium (R. D. Adams and Victor 1989; Mesulam 1985; Mori and Yamadori 1987). Delirium tremens is an example of hyperactive delirium. In patients who are acutely confused, incoherent, and disoriented but who do not have auto-nomic instability and hallucinations, some neurologists diagnose their condition as "acute confusional states" rather than delirium. This unfortunate disparity in the concept of delirium has historical roots, which are discussed by Lipowski (1980, 1990) and Berrios (1981).

EPIDEMIOLOGY AND RISK FACTORS

The prevalence of delirium across many studies ranges from 11% to 16%, and the incidence, which has a much larger variation, ranges from 4% to 31%.

Patients who are at increased risk for delirium include the elderly (who often also have dementia and medical morbidity), patients with CNS dysfunction (e.g., dementia), postsurgical patients (e.g., postcardiotomy, posttransplant, post–hip surgery), burn patients, and drug-dependent patients who are experiencing withdrawal. Advancing age increases the risk; the highest risk group is usually patients age 60 years and older (Lipowski 1980, 1990). Increasing age is also associated with an increasing prevalence of dementia, which is an independent risk factor for delirium. The aging brain has less "cerebral reserve" and flexibility in the face of external perturbations, including changes in vasculature, decreased cholinergic activity, and increased monoamine oxidase activity; all of these may increase an individual's vulnerability to delirium. Even with a relatively minor physiological stress such as a urinary tract infection, elderly demented patients are more likely than younger adults to develop delirium. Koponen and Riekkinen (1993, p. 103) found that 81% of patients with delirium in their study had "coexistent structural brain disease."

Brain damage related to HIV similarly increases the risk for delirium. Symptomatic HIV-1-seropositive individuals typically have significant cognitive deficits (Maj et al. 1994) that are consistent with a subcortical dementia. Perry (1990) reported that 90% of patients with

---

Table 7–1. DSM-IV diagnostic criteria for delirium

A. Disturbance of consciousness (i.e., reduced clarity of awareness of the environment) with reduced ability to focus, sustain, or shift attention.

B. A change in cognition (such as memory deficit, disorientation, language disturbance) or the development of a perceptual disturbance that is not better accounted for by a preexisting, established, or evolving dementia.

C. The disturbance develops over a short period of time (usually hours to days) and tends to fluctuate during the course of the day.

D. There is evidence from the history, physical examination, or laboratory findings of [*] judged to be etiologically related to the disturbance.
   [*]
   A general medical condition, diagnose delirium due to a general medical condition.

   Substance intoxication or withdrawal, diagnose substance-induced delirium.

   More than one etiology (e.g., more than one etiological general medical condition, a general medical condition plus substance intoxication or medication side effect), diagnose delirium due to multiple etiologies.

   A medical condition or substance use that is suspected but specific evidence is lacking, diagnose delirium not otherwise specified.

advanced acquired immunodeficiency syndrome (AIDS) have organic mental disorders. In another study, delirium was the most frequent neuropsychiatric complication of AIDS (Fernandez et al. 1989).

In drug-dependent patients, discontinuation or rapid tapering of drugs, particularly alcohol and sedative-hypnotics, is a common cause of delirium and is often unsuspected in hospitalized patients. (For a more detailed discussion of substance-induced delirium, please refer to Franklin and Frances, Chapter 13, in this volume.)

Low serum albumin predisposes to delirium, largely because of a reduction in drug-carrying capacity for protein-bound drugs, whose free serum levels then rise to cause toxicity despite total serum levels measured in the normal therapeutic range (Trzepacz and Francis 1990). Malnutrition, chronic disease, aging, nephrotic syndrome, and hepatic insufficiency are common causes of low serum albumin.

DSM-IV states that "children may be more susceptible to delirium than adults, especially when it is related to febrile illness and certain medications (e.g., anticholinergics)" (p. 126); however, delirium in children is vastly understudied. Prugh et al. (1980) described the only systematic, controlled study of delirium in children using electroencephalograms (EEGs), cognitive tests, and neurological and psychiatric examinations. They found the same constellation of symptoms as has been described for adult delirium. In Kornfeld and colleagues' (1965) sample of 119 unselected patients who had open heart surgery, none of the 20 children developed delirium, whereas 30% of the adults did.

Although sleep deprivation and sensory deprivation may contribute to the severity of delirium, based on the evidence, these conditions are not sufficient to cause delirium independently (Francis 1993). Sleep-wake abnormalities are a frequent component of delirium. Harrell and Othmer (1987) found that sleep disturbance developed after the onset of cognitive impairment (based on Mini-Mental State Exam; Folstein et al. 1975), which suggests that the disturbance was a symptom, rather than the cause, of delirium.

Despite investigations, no personality or premorbid psychological variables, such as depression or anxiety, are associated with delirium or predict its behavioral presentation (Dubin et al. 1979; Lipowski 1980).

■ CLINICAL FEATURES

Prodrome

Some patients manifest subclinical symptoms such as restlessness, anxiety, irritability, distractibility, or sleep disruption immediately before the onset of an overt delirium. Review of the patient's hospital medical chart, particularly the nursing notes, may reveal prodromal features.

Temporal Course

Two features of the temporal course of delirium are characteristic and assist in differential diagnosis: 1) abrupt/acute onset of symptoms and 2) fluctuation in symptom severity during an episode.

Diffuse Cognitive Impairment

Attentional deficits. Patients with delirium have difficulty sustaining attention and may be distractible or unable to focus. Poor performance on Trail Making Tests reflects poor concentration, visuomotor impairment, and difficulty switching mental sets (Trzepacz et al. 1988a).

Memory impairment. Both short- and long-term memory are impaired in patients with delirium. When impaired registration is present, memory difficulties may be secondary to attention deficits. After recovering from delirium, some patients are amnestic for the entire episode; others have islands of memory for certain experiences. These experiences are generally remembered negatively; therefore, patients must be reassured that delirium is transient and occurs commonly in medically ill patients.

Disorientation.   Disorientation to time and place is common in patients with delirium, with some fluctuation during relatively lucid intervals. Disorientation to person occurs often for doctors and nurses, less often for immediate family members, and rarely for one's own iden-

tity. It is not unusual for a patient with delirium to feel that he or she is in a familiar place (e.g., a room in his or her home) instead of in the hospital.

Visuoconstructional impairment.   Visuoconstructional impairment occurs often in patients with delirium. Patients may be unable to copy simple geometric designs or to draw more complex figures such as a clock face (see Figure 7–1). Instructions and scoring of clock face drawing are described elsewhere (Trzepacz and Baker 1993).

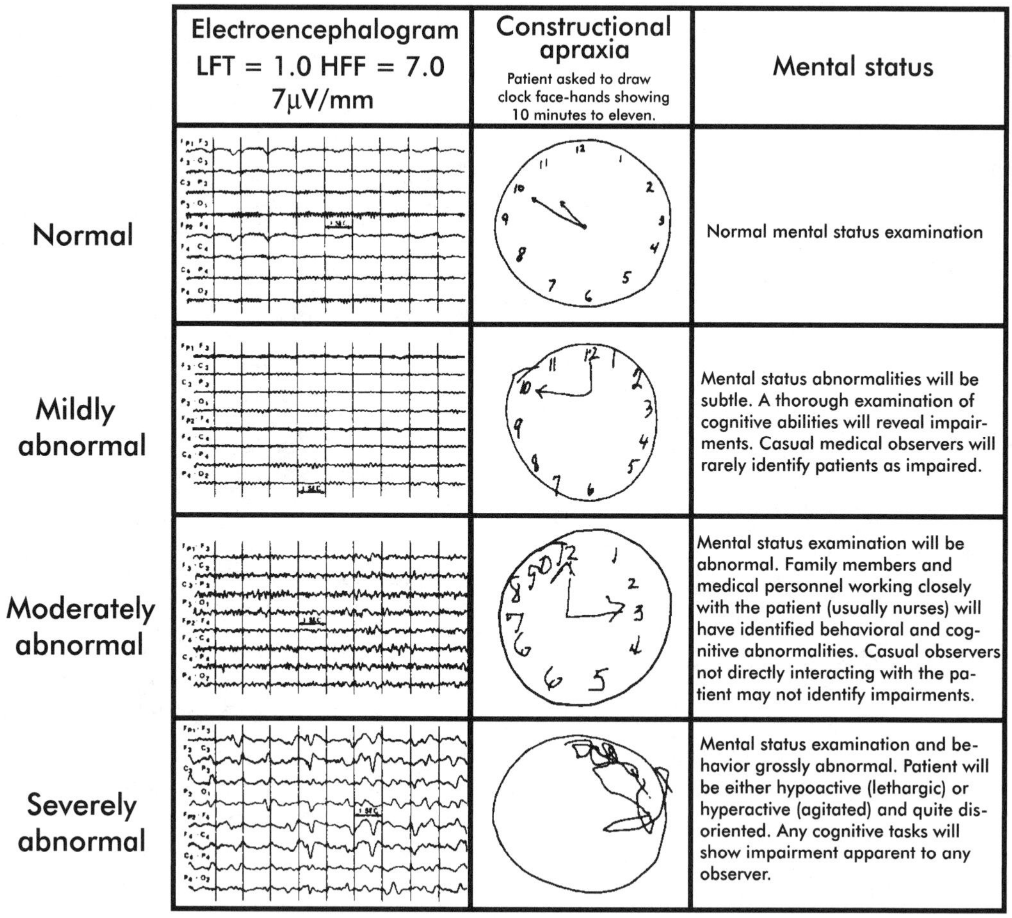

	Electroencephalogram LFT = 1.0 HFF = 7.0 7μV/mm	Constructional apraxia Patient asked to draw clock face–hands showing 10 minutes to eleven.	Mental status
Normal			Normal mental status examination
Mildly abnormal			Mental status abnormalities will be subtle. A thorough examination of cognitive abilities will reveal impairments. Casual medical observers will rarely identify patients as impaired.
Moderately abnormal			Mental status examination will be abnormal. Family members and medical personnel working closely with the patient (usually nurses) will have identified behavioral and cognitive abnormalities. Casual observers not directly interacting with the patient may not identify impairments.
Severely abnormal			Mental status examination and behavior grossly abnormal. Patient will be either hypoactive (lethargic) or hyperactive (agitated) and quite disoriented. Any cognitive tasks will show impairment apparent to any observer.

Figure 7–1.   Comparison of electroencephalogram, constructional apraxia, and mental status.
Source.   Reprinted from Wise MG, Brandt GT: "Delirium," in *The American Psychiatric Press Textbook of Neuropsychiatry,* 2nd Edition. Edited by Yudofsky SC, Hales RE. Washington, DC, American Psychiatric Press, 1992, p. 298. Copyright 1992, American Psychiatric Press, Inc. Used with permission.

Prefrontal executive functions. These functions are impaired in delirium (Trzepacz 1994) and include switching mental sets, abstraction, sequential thinking, verbal fluency, temporal memory, and judgment. Patients with delirium experience perseveration, concrete thinking, distractibility, and impaired performance on Trail Making Tests.

Thought and Language Disturbances

Patients with delirium often have disorganized thought patterns. The severity of the disorganization can range from tangentiality and circumstantiality to loose associations. When thought disturbance is at its most severe level of disorganization, speech may resemble a fluent aphasia. Dysnomia and dysgraphia are not specific to delirium, however, but impairment in the semantic content of writing may be more specific to delirium (Patten and Lamarre 1989).

Perceptual Disturbances

Patients with delirium often experience misperceptions, usually illusions or hallucinations, and infrequently experience metamorphopsias or delusional misidentifications. Illusions and hallucinations can be auditory or visual, but the latter are more common and therefore raise the suspicion of "organicity" whenever they occur. Tactile, gustatory, and olfactory hallucinations are less common.

Hallucinations can be simple visual or complex. Delirium tremens is classically associated with often vivid visual hallucinations and misperceptions.

Psychomotor Disturbances

Many patients with delirium have changes in psychomotor behavior—either hypoactive or hyperactive, or some combination. Hypoactive patients appear apathetic, somnolent, and quietly confused and usually receive a misdiagnosis of "depression" by nonpsychiatric physicians and nurses. Koponen and Riekkinen (1993) found that those patients with the "silent," or hypoactive, form of delirium had the most severe cognitive impairment compared with patients with hyperactive or mixed forms. However, Ross et al. (1991) found comparable cognitive impairment in hypoactive and hyperactive subtypes. In hyperactive delirium, the patient is agitated and hypervigilant and exhibits psychomotor hyperactivity.

Disturbance of Sleep-Wake Cycle

Sleep-wake disturbance is common in patients with delirium and ranges from insomnia to total disintegration of the sleep-wake cycle throughout a 24-hour period, with multiple periods of napping or drowsiness during day and night. Restoration of the normal diurnal sleep cycle is an important goal in treatment.

Delusions

Delusions are generally of a paranoid type and are not as well systematized as those that occur in patients with schizophrenia, nor are they mood congruent as typically seen in patients with depression or mania. Delusions occur in about one-fifth of patients with delirium. Persecutory ideas can lead to violent behavior and inadvertent harm to medical staff.

Affective Lability

Patients with delirium can exhibit rapid fluctuations in their emotional state (e.g., from fear to incongruent crying to irritability) over the course of minutes that are consistent with affective lability characteristic of "organicity." Emotional responses seen in patients with delirium include anxiety, panic, fear, anger, rage, sadness, apathy, and—rarely except in steroid-induced delirium—euphoria. In a recent study by Valan and Hilty (1995), 23% of patients referred to a consultation-liaison service for depression by staff-level physicians were subsequently given a diagnosis of delirium by the psychiatrist.

Neurological Abnormalities

Physical examination. Neurological abnormalities that occur in delirium are indicative of the underlying etiology because no focal motor or sensory signs are specific to delirium as a syndrome. Motor findings include tremor, myoclonus, asterixis, and reflex or muscle tone changes. The tremor associated with delirium, particularly toxic-metabolic, is generally absent at rest but apparent during movement (action or intention tremors).

EEG abnormalities. Engel and Romano (1959), in their classic paper, "Delirium, a Syndrome of Cerebral Insufficiency," proposed that the basic etiology of delirium was a derangement in metabolism manifested clinically by diffuse disturbances in cognitive functions and physiologically by generalized slowing of the EEG background rhythm. Pro and Wells (1977) reported that EEG changes virtually always accompany delirium. Hepatic encephalopathy is classically associated with severe slowing including triphasic delta waves. The EEG slowing illustrated in Figure 7–1 is an example of delirium caused by toxic-metabolic etiologies. Less typically, the EEG pattern in delirium is characterized by excess low-voltage beta waves, as seen most typically in delirium tremens (Kennard et al. 1945).

Spectral EEG analyses, which quantify by use of computers the relative proportions of beta, alpha, theta, and delta activity, support Engel and Romano's proposed correlation between EEG slowing and cognitive deterioration (Koponen et al. 1989b). Serial quantitative electroencephalographic (QEEG) studies are more sensitive to subtle shifts in EEG frequency and may help distinguish delirium from dementia (Jacobson et al. 1993).

Unfortunately, a given individual's normal dominant posterior rhythm could be slowed but still be in the alpha range and therefore be read as "normal."

DIAGNOSIS

The diagnosis of delirium requires recognition of the clinical features of the syndrome, as discussed in the previous section of this chapter, and a thorough evaluation of the patient's mental and physical status. In addition to conducting a routine bedside mental status examination, the examiner should test a broad range of cognitive functions in order to document the diffuse impairment necessary for a delirium diagnosis. Cognitive functions being tested include attention and concentration, short- and long-term memory, visuoconstructional ability (see Figure 7–1), abstraction, and language such as writing and confrontational naming.

The gold standard for diagnosis is a clinical evaluation using DSM criteria, and the most useful diagnostic laboratory measure is the EEG. In addition to cognitive tests (e.g., Mini-Mental State Exam; Folstein et al. 1975), which document some symptoms of delirium but cannot alone distinguish delirium from dementia, several instruments measure a broader range of symptoms of delirium and can be used for screening purposes or to quantitate symptom severity. The Delirium Rating Scale (DRS; Trzepacz et al. 1988b) and the Confusion Assessment Method (CAM; Inouye et al. 1990) are two more recently developed tests.

DIFFERENTIAL DIAGNOSIS

Because the differential diagnosis of delirium is extensive, a reluctance to carefully search for etiologies sometimes exists. Confusional states, particularly in critically ill and elderly patients, often have multiple causes (Trzepacz et al. 1985). When no apparent etiology exists at the time of consultation, one often becomes apparent within a few days. Not uncommonly, unrecognized medication use or substance abuse is the cause of an intoxication or withdrawal delirium.

Laboratory and radiological evaluation of patients with delirium has two levels: "basic" and "additional" tests (see Table 7–2). The basic battery is ordered in virtually every patient with delirium. Additional tests are ordered based on the specifics of a particular case. When information about the patient's mental and physical status is combined with the basic laboratory battery, the specific etiology (etiologies) is often apparent. If not, the clinician should review the case and consider ordering further diagnostic studies.

Terms such as *intensive care unit psychosis* are inappropriately used to explain delirium because they imply that no attempt at specific diagnosis is necessary because the environment is to blame. Koponen et al. (1989a) found clear organic etiologies in 87% of patients with delirium. They also found that the few patients who became confused because of psychological and environmental events actually had severe dementia.

Organizing the large number of potential causes for delirium into a usable differential diagnosis might be enhanced by using the following two-tiered differential diagnostic system.

Emergent Items (WHHHHIMP)

"Emergent diagnoses" (mnemonic WHHHHIMP), the first level of this diagnostic system, must be made by the physician early in the course of a delirium. Failure to do so can result in irreversible injury to the patient. We describe each letter of this mnemonic below:

W—Wernicke's encephalopathy or **W**ithdrawal: Patients with Wernicke's encephalopathy typically have the triad of confusion, ataxia, and ophthalmoplegia (usually lateral gaze paralysis). If Wernicke's encephalopathy is not immediately treated with parenteral thiamine, the patient develops a permanent amnestic disorder called Korsakoff's psychosis, which is termed *alcohol-induced persisting amnestic disorder* in DSM-IV. Sedative-

Table 7–2. Assessment of the patient with delirium

Physical status

History
Physical and neurological examination
Review of vital signs and anesthesia record if postoperative
Review of medical records
Careful review of medications and correlation with behavioral changes

Mental status

Interview
Cognitive tests (e.g., clock face, Trail Part A and B)

Basic laboratory—*consider in every patient with delirium*

Blood chemistries (electrolytes, glucose, calcium, albumin, blood urea nitrogen, creatinine, serum glutamic-oxaloacetic transaminase [SGOT], bilirubin, alkaline phosphatase, magnesium, PO_4—, Venereal Disease Research Laboratory [VDRL])
Complete blood count
Serum drug levels (e.g., digoxin, theophylline, phenobarbital, cyclosporine)
Arterial blood gases or oxygen saturation
Urinalysis and collection for culture and sensitivity (C&S)
Urine drug screen
Electrocardiogram
Chest X ray

Additional laboratory tests—*order as indicated by clinical condition*

Electroencephalogram
Lumbar puncture
Brain computed tomography (CT) or magnetic resonance imaging (MRI)
Blood chemistries (e.g., heavy metal screen, B_{12} and folate levels, lupus erythematosus [LE] Prep, antinuclear antibody [ANA] urinary porphyrins, human immunodeficiency virus)

hypnotic drugs are associated with delirium during withdrawal more than are other classes of drugs.

H—Hypoxemia, **H**ypertensive encephalopathy, **H**ypoglycemia, or **H**ypoperfusion: Arterial blood gases or oxygen saturation and current and past vital signs should be checked to establish whether hypoxemia or hypertensive encephalopathy is present. Patients with hypoglycemic-induced delirium usually have insulin-dependent diabetes mellitus, except for those who engage in factitious use of hypoglycemic agents. Hypoperfusion or hypoxemia of the brain can result from many causes, such as decreased cardiac output, cardiac arrhythmias, pulmonary failure, carbon monoxide poisoning, and severe anemia.

I—Intracranial bleeding or **I**nfection: Subarachnoid or intraparenchymal hemorrhage or subdural hematoma can present as delirium. If the patient had a brief period of unconsciousness, with or without headache, and now has delirium, or if the patient had or now has focal neurological signs, intracranial bleeding should be suspected. Infectious processes (e.g., elevated white blood cell count, fever) that cause delirium via systemic or CNS etiologies should be investigated.

M—**M**eningitis or Encephalitis: These are typically acute febrile illnesses (vital signs should be checked for fever) and usually have either nonspecific localizing neurological signs (e.g., meningismus with stiff neck) or more focal neurological signs.

P—**P**oisons or Medications: Probably the most common causes of delirium are exogenous substances—prescribed and over-the-counter medications or illicit substances and toxins. A less common cause is pesticide or solvent poisoning. In the emergency room, a toxicology screen should be ordered. Drug-drug interactions are common in delirium. The importance of taking a thorough medication history, including calling the family, caregivers, or pharmacist, cannot be overemphasized. Drugs with anticholinergic activity, including meperidine and fentanyl, are especially deliriogenic (Tollefson et al. 1991; Tune et al. 1993). Nurses' medication lists most clearly document doses and times of administration.

Critical Items (I WATCH DEATH)

Table 7–3 (I WATCH DEATH mnemonic) lists many of the insults that can cause delirium. Delirium, indicating acute brain failure, should marshal the same medical forces as failure of any other vital organ that is associated with substantial morbidity and mortality.

TREATMENT AND MANAGEMENT

The treatment of delirium has two separate and important aspects. The first is critical and bears directly on the survival of the patient: identify

Table 7–3. Differential diagnosis for delirium using mnemonic "I WATCH DEATH"

Infection	Encephalitis, meningitis, syphilis, HIV, sepsis
Withdrawal	Alcohol, barbiturates, sedative-hypnotics
Acute metabolic	Acidosis, alkalosis, electrolyte disturbance, hepatic failure, renal failure
Trauma	Closed-head injury, heatstroke, postoperative, severe burns
CNS pathology	Abscess, hemorrhage, hydrocephalus, subdural hematoma, infection, seizures, stroke, tumors, metastases, vasculitis
Hypoxia	Anemia, carbon monoxide poisoning, hypotension, pulmonary or cardiac failure
Deficiencies	Vitamin B_{12}, folate, niacin, thiamine
Endocrinopathies	Hyper/hypoadrenocorticism, hyper/hypoglycemia, myxedema, hyperparathyroidism
Acute vascular	Hypertensive encephalopathy, stroke, arrhythmia, shock
Toxins or drugs	Medications, illicit drugs, pesticides, solvents
Heavy metals	Lead, manganese, mercury

Note.   CNS = central nervous system; HIV = human immunodeficiency virus.

and reverse, when possible, the reason(s) for the delirium (discussed earlier in this chapter). The second aspect of treatment is to reduce psychiatric symptoms of delirium with medications and environmental manipulations regardless of whether psychosis or agitation is present.

Because of the high mortality and morbidity associated with delirium, proper medical management is important. The patient should be placed in a room near the nursing station so that he or she can be observed for medical deterioration and dangerous behaviors, such as attempting to crawl over bed rails or to pull out an intravenous line. If necessary, a sitter should be employed. Vital signs and fluid input and output should be monitored and good oxygenation ensured. All nonessential medications should be discontinued. If an etiology for the confusional state is not immediately identified, further laboratory, radiological, and physical examinations are recommended.

Haloperidol is the drug of first choice to treat a patient with delirium (Lipowski 1980, 1990) because it is a potent antipsychotic with virtually no anticholinergic or hypotensive properties, does not suppress respirations, has minimal cardiotoxicity, and can be given parenterally. Its safety profile is illustrated by the use of intravenous haloperidol in "mega" doses (e.g., 1,200 mg in a 24-hour period) in seriously ill patients without harmful side effects (Levenson 1995; Sanders and Cassem 1993; Sos and Cassem 1980; Tesar et al. 1985). Intravenous haloperidol can be given as a bolus injection or by continuous infusion drip. Continuous intravenous infusion of haloperidol is occasionally required to control severe refractory agitation and confusion (Fernandez et al. 1988; Riker et al. 1994). (Note: Haloperidol is not approved by the Food and Drug Administration [FDA] for intravenous use.) When extrapyramidal symptoms following oral versus intravenous haloperidol were measured in a blind fashion, intravenous administration of haloperidol was associated with fewer severe

extrapyramidal symptoms (Menza et al. 1987). However, patients with HIV dementia and Lewy body dementia are more sensitive to extrapyramidal side effects from haloperidol that is used to treat delirium. In small numbers of vulnerable patients who have a history of alcohol abuse or cardiomyopathy, intravenous haloperidol caused lengthening of the Q-T interval and torsades de pointes ventricular tachycardia (Hunt and Stern 1995; Metzger and Friedman 1993).

Droperidol is used by anesthesiologists as a preanesthetic agent and by other physicians to control nausea and vomiting. Like haloperidol, it is a butyrophenone and has comparable antidopaminergic potency but seems to have lower antipsychotic activity. Although droperidol is approved for intravenous use, it is more sedating, has a faster onset of action, has a shorter half-life, and has significantly greater α_1-adrenergic activity, thereby inducing hypotension, compared with haloperidol. Droperidol has been given as a continuous intravenous infusion for severe delirium without complications (Frye et al. 1995). Antipsychotic medications that are less potent, such as chlorpromazine and thioridazine, are more likely to cause hypotension and anticholinergic and quinidine-like side effects; therefore, they are not routinely recommended for delirium. Although risperidone is not available in parenteral formulation, it is clinically useful in treating delirium (personal clinical observation, 1995).

Regardless of the route of administration, the usual initial dosage of haloperidol in younger adult patients is 0.5–1 mg for mild, 2–5 mg for moderate, and 5–10 mg for severe confusion/agitation when given intravenously; the clinician should check the electrocardiogram (ECG) for Q-T prolongation. The initial dosage for frail or elderly patients is 0.5 mg for mild, 1 mg for moderate, and 2 mg for severe confusion/agitation. The dose is repeated at regular intervals, but not before 30 minutes, until the patient is calmer. Often only twice-a-day or three-times-a-day dosing is needed in patients whose level of agitation does not mandate more emergent care. After the confusion has cleared, haloperidol is continued and tapered over 1–5 days, depending on the severity of the episode. Abrupt discontinuation of medication immediately following improvement may, within 24 hours, be followed by recurrence of the delirium. A larger bedtime dose or the addition of lorazepam can be used in patients whose sleep-wake cycle has not normalized with haloperidol alone.

The use of benzodiazepines in patients with delirium is most appropriate in sedative-hypnotic or ethanol withdrawal delirium. In other cases, the sedation and mild cognitive impairment associated with benzodiazepines may further compromise the patient's sensorium or disinhibit his or her behaviors. Benzodiazepines have been used successfully as adjuncts to high-potency neuroleptics such as haloperidol in a subset of patients with severe delirium (F. Adams 1984; Garza-Trevino et al. 1989). Small doses of intravenous lorazepam, particularly in patients who have not responded to haloperidol alone, help to decrease agitation. A fluctuation in symptom severity is inherent to delirium; thus, one assessment will evoke management and medical recommendations that are time-limited in efficacy, and follow-up monitoring and dose adjustments are recommended.

Environmental interventions are sometimes helpful but are not a primary treatment for delirium. Both nurses and family members can frequently reorient patients to date and surroundings. It may help to place a clock, calendar, and familiar objects in the room. Adequate light in the room during the night may decrease frightening illusions or hasten reorientation during awakenings. A private room for the patient with delirium is not recommended unless adequate supervision is provided. Rooms with windows assist in orientation with diurnal cues (Wilson 1972). Returning devices such as eyeglasses or a hearing aid to patients who normally use them may improve the quality of sensory input and help patients better understand their surroundings.

Psychological support during and after a delirium episode is important. The presence of a calm family member can reassure the paranoid, agitated patient. In lieu of a family member, close supervision by reassuring nursing staff is essential. After the delirium has cleared, it is therapeutic to help the patient understand the bizarre experience (MacKenzie and Popkin 1980) and reassure him or her about its transience and frequent occurrence among hospitalized medically ill patients to prevent the belief that he or she is "going crazy." Family education also helps.

COURSE (PROGNOSIS)

The clinical outcome for a patient with delirium varies. The possibilities are full recovery; progression to stupor, coma, or death; seizures; chronic brain injury; and associated injuries (e.g., fracture or subdural hematomas from falls). Research has found that full recovery is unlikely at the time of hospital discharge for elderly patients (Levkoff et al. 1992) and that persistent cognitive deficits are common (Rockwood 1993), although these deficits may be due to previously unrecognized dementia that was heralded by the delirium. Seizures can accompany delirium but are more likely to occur with drug withdrawal, particularly alcohol, and burn encephalopathy (Antoon et al. 1972).

Morbidity

Delirium in patients who undergo orthopedic surgery is a harbinger of poor recovery and long-term outcome. Some behaviors in patients with delirium, such as striking caregivers, can interfere with ongoing medical care. These patients may pull out intravenous lines, urinary catheters, nasogastric tubes, arterial lines, nasopharyngeal tubes, and intraaortic balloon pumps. Inouye et al. (1989) reported that the risk of complications, such as decubiti and aspiration pneumonia, was more than six times greater in patients with delirium.

Mortality

Most psychiatrists, and physicians in general, are unaware of the mortality associated with delirium. Of 77 patients who received a DSM-III (American Psychiatric Association 1980) diagnosis of delirium from a consultation psychiatrist, 19 (25%) died within 6 months (Trzepacz et al. 1985). Furthermore, the elderly patient who develops delirium in the hospital has a 22% (Rabins and Folstein 1982) to 76% (Flint and Richards 1956) chance of dying during that hospitalization. Patients who survive hospitalization have a very high death rate during the months immediately after discharge.

SUMMARY

Delirium is a ubiquitous, underrecognized clinical syndrome that accompanies potentially life-threatening medical conditions. Delirium is especially common in patients who are elderly, have impaired cognition or structural brain disorders, are seriously burned, have HIV-related illness, or are dependent on sedative-hypnotics or alcohol. Psychiatrists must be able to correctly diagnose delirium based on specific signs and symptoms, organize a prioritized differential diagnosis, assist the primary physician in identifying the probable cause(s) for the delirium, and recommend and monitor treatment for symptoms. Correct management and treatment of delirium is lifesaving and can reduce hospital costs associated with the increased length of stay for patients with delirium (Thomas et al. 1988).

REFERENCES

Adams F: Neuropsychiatric evaluation and treatment of delirium in the critically ill cancer patient. The Cancer Bulletin 36:156–160, 1984

Adams RD, Victor M: Principles of Neurology. New York, McGraw-Hill, 1989

American Psychiatric Association: Diagnostic and Statistical Manual of Mental Disorders, 3rd Edition. Washington, DC, American Psychiatric Association, 1980

American Psychiatric Association: Diagnostic and Statistical Manual of Mental Disorders, 4th Edition. Washington, DC, American Psychiatric Association, 1994

Antoon AY, Volpe JJ, Crawford JD: Burn encephalopathy in children. Pediatrics 50:609–616, 1972

Berrios GE: Delirium and confusion in the 19th century: a conceptual history. Br J Psychiatry 139:439–449, 1981

Cole MG, Primeau FJ: Prognosis of delirium in elderly hospital patients. Can Med Assoc J 149:41–46, 1993

Dubin WR, Field NL, Gastfriend DR: Postcardiotomy delirium: a critical review. J Thorac Cardiovasc Surg 77:586–594, 1979

Engel GL, Romano J: Delirium, a syndrome of cerebral insufficiency. Journal of Chronic Disease 9:260–277, 1959

Fernandez F, Holmes V, Adams F, et al: Treatment of severe, refractory agitation with a haloperidol drip. J Clin Psychiatry 49:239–241, 1988

Fernandez F, Levy J, Mansell P: Management of delirium in terminally ill AIDS patients. Int J Psychiatry Med 19:165–172, 1989

Flint FJ, Richards SM: Organic basis of confusional states in the elderly. BMJ 2:1537–1539, 1956

Folstein MF, Folstein SE, McHugh PR: Mini-Mental State: a practical method for grading the cognitive state of patients for the clinician. J Psychiatr Res 12:189–198, 1975

Francis J: Sensory and environmental factors in delirium. Paper presented at a Conference "Delirium: Current Advancements in Diagnosis, Treatment and Research" sponsored by the VA Medical Center, Minneapolis, MN, September 1993

Francis J, Kapoor WN: Prognosis after hospital discharge of older medical patients with delirium. J Am Geriatr Soc 40:601–606, 1992

Francis J, Martin D, Kapoor W: A prospective study of delirium in hospitalized elderly. JAMA 263:1097–1101, 1990

Frye MA, Coudreaut MF, Hakeman SM, et al: Continuous droperidol drip infusion for management of agitated delirium in an ICU. Psychosomatics 36:301–305, 1995

Garza-Trevino E, Hollister L, Overall J, et al: Efficacy of combinations of intramuscular antipsychotics and sedative-hypnotics for control of psychotic agitation. Am J Psychiatry 146:1598–1601, 1989

Gustafson Y, Berggren D, Brannstrom B, et al: Acute confusional states in elderly patients treated for femoral neck fracture. J Am Geriatr Soc 36:525–530, 1988

Harrell R, Othmer E: Postcardiotomy confusion and sleep loss. J Clin Psychiatry 48:445–446, 1987

Hunt N, Stern TA: The association between intravenous haloperidol and torsades de pointes. Psychosomatics 36:541–549, 1995

Inouye S, Horwitz R, Tinetti M, et al: Acute confusional states in the hospitalized elderly: incidence, factors, and complications (abstract). Clin Res 37:524A, 1989

Inouye S, van Dyck C, Alessi C, et al: Clarifying confusion: the Confusion Assessment Method. Ann Intern Med 113:941–948, 1990

Jacobson SA, Leuchter AF, Walter DO: Conventional and quantitative EEG in the diagnosis of delirium among the elderly. J Neurol Neurosurg Psychiatry 56:153–158, 1993

Kane FJ, Remmell R, Moody S: Recognizing and treating delirium in patients admitted to general hospitals. South Med J 86:985–988, 1993

Kennard MA, Bueding E, Wortis WB: Some biochemical and electroencephalographic changes in delirium tremens. Quarterly Journal of Studies on Alcohol 6:4–14, 1945

Kolbeinsson H, Jonsson A: Delirium and dementia in acute medical admissions of elderly patients in Iceland. Acta Psychiatr Scand 87:123–127, 1993

Koponen HJ, Riekkinen PJ: A prospective study of delirium in elderly patients admitted to a psychiatric hospital. Psychol Med 3:103–109, 1993

Koponen H, Stenback U, Mattila E, et al: Delirium among elderly persons admitted to a psychiatric hospital: clinical course during the acute stage and one-year follow-up. Acta Psychiatr Scand 79:579–585, 1989a

Koponen H, Partanen J, Paakkonen A, et al: EEG spectral analysis in delirium. J Neurol Neurosurg Psychiatry 52:980–985, 1989b

Kornfeld DS, Zimberg S, Malm JR: Psychiatric complications of open-heart surgery. N Engl J Med 273:287–292, 1965

Levenson JL: High-dose intravenous haloperidol for agitated delirium following lung transplantation. Psychosomatics 36:66–68, 1995

Levkoff SE, Evans DA, Liptzin B, et al: Delirium: the occurrence and persistence of symptoms among elderly hospitalized patients. Arch Intern Med 152:334–340, 1992

Lipowski ZJ: Delirium: Acute Brain Failure in Man. Springfield, IL, Charles C Thomas, 1980

Lipowski ZJ: Delirium: Acute Confusional States. New York, Oxford University Press, 1990

MacKenzie TB, Popkin MK: Stress response syndrome occurring after delirium. Am J Psychiatry 137:1433–1435, 1980

Maj M, Satz P, Janssen R, et al: WHO neuropsychiatric AIDS study, cross-sectional phase II. Arch Gen Psychiatry 51:51–61, 1994

Marcantonio ER, Goldman L, Mangione CM, et al: A clinical prediction rule for delirium after elective noncardiac surgery. JAMA 271:134–139, 1994

Menza M, Murray G, Holmes V, et al: Decreased extrapyramidal symptoms with intravenous haloperidol. J Clin Psychiatry 48:278–280, 1987

Mesulam M-M (ed): Patterns in behavioral neuroanatomy: association areas, the limbic system, and hemispheric specialization, in Principles of Behavioral Neurology. Philadelphia, PA, FA Davis, 1985, pp 1–70

Metzger E, Friedman R: Prolongation of the corrected QT and torsades de pointes cardiac arrhythmia associated with intravenous haloperidol in the medically ill. J Clin Psychopharmacol 13:128–132, 1993

Mori E, Yamadori A: Acute confusional state and acute agitated delirium. Arch Neurol 44:1139–1143, 1987

Murray AM, Levkoff SE, Wetle TT, et al: Acute delirium and functional decline in the hospitalized elderly patient. J Gerontol 48:M181–M186, 1993

Patten S, Lamarre C: Dysgraphia (letter). Can J Psychiatry 34:746, 1989

Perry S: Organic mental disorders caused by HIV: update on early diagnosis and treatment. Am J Psychiatry 147:696–710, 1990

Pro JD, Wells CE: The use of the electroencephalogram in the diagnosis of delirium. Diseases of the Nervous System 38:804–808, 1977

Prugh DG, Wagonfeld S, Metcalf D, et al: A clinical study of delirium in children and adolescents. Psychosom Med 42(suppl):177–197, 1980

Rabins PV, Folstein MF: Delirium and dementia: diagnostic criteria and fatality rates. Br J Psychiatry 140:149–153, 1982

Riker RR, Fraser GL, Cox PM: Continuous infusion of haloperidol controls agitation in critically ill patients. Crit Care Med 22:433–440, 1994

Rockwood K: The occurrence and duration of symptoms in elderly patients with delirium. J Gerontol 48:M162–M166, 1993

Ross CA, Peyser CE, Shapiro I, et al: Delirium: phenomenologic and etiologic subtypes. Int Psychogeriatr 3:135–147, 1991

Sanders KM, Cassem EH: Psychiatric complications in the critically ill cardiac patient. Tex Heart Inst J 20:180–187, 1993

Smith L, Dimsdale J: Postcardiotomy delirium: conclusions after 25 years? Am J Psychiatry 146:452–458, 1989

Sos J, Cassem NH: Managing postoperative agitation. Drug Therapy 10:103–106, 1980

Tesar GE, Murray GB, Cassem NH: Use of high-dose intravenous haloperidol in the treatment of agitated cardiac patients. J Clin Psychopharmacol 5:344–347, 1985

Thomas RI, Cameron DJ, Fahs MC: A prospective study of delirium and prolonged length of hospital stay. Arch Gen Psychiatry 45:937–940, 1988

Tollefson GD, Montague-Clouse J, Lancaster SP: The relationship of serum anticholinergic activity to mental status performance in an elderly nursing home population. J Neuropsychiatry Clin Neurosci 3:314–319, 1991

Trzepacz PT: A review of delirium assessment instruments. Gen Hosp Psychiatry 16:397–405, 1994

Trzepacz PT, Baker RW: The Psychiatric Mental Status Examination. New York, Oxford University Press, 1993

Trzepacz PT, Francis J: Low serum albumin and risk of delirium (letter). Am J Psychiatry 147:675, 1990

Trzepacz P, Teague G, Lipowski Z: Delirium and other organic mental disorders in a general hospital. Gen Hosp Psychiatry 7:101–106, 1985

Trzepacz PT, Brenner R, Coffman G, et al: Delirium in liver transplantation candidates: discriminant analysis of multiple test variables. Biol Psychiatry 24:3–14, 1988a

Trzepacz P, Baker R, Greenhouse J: A symptom rating scale for delirium. Psychiatry Res 23:89–97, 1988b

Tune L, Carr S, Cooper T, et al: Association of anticholinergic activity of prescribed medications with postoperative delirium. J Neuropsychiatry Clin Neurosci 5:208–210, 1993

Valan MN, Hilty D: Incidence of delirium in patients referred for evaluation of depression (abstract). Proceedings of the 42nd annual meeting of the Academy of Psychosomatic Medicine, November 9–12, 1995, Palm Springs, CA, p 20

Wilson LM: Intensive care delirium. Arch Intern Med 130:225–226, 1972

Wise MG, Brandt GT: Delirium, in The American Psychiatric Press Textbook of Neuropsychiatry, 2nd Edition. Edited by Yudofsky SC, Hales RE. Washington, DC, American Psychiatric Press, 1992, p 298

Chapter 8

Dementia

Kevin F. Gray, M.D.
Jeffrey L. Cummings, M.D.

Changes in mental status and behavior are among the most frequently encountered phenomena in a general medical hospital setting, especially in elderly or postoperative patients (Lipowski 1990). The emergence of delirium in a hospitalized patient may be the first indication of an undiagnosed dementing illness. The detection of dementia by the psychiatric consultant becomes critical when considering treatment, prognosis, placement, rehabilitation, or even the patient's ability to comply with a medication regimen.

DEFINITIONS

Dementia

Dementia is a syndrome of acquired persistent impairment in intellectual function. Multiple spheres of mental activity such as memory, language, visuospatial skills, emotion or personality, and cognition must be compromised for a diagnosis of dementia to be considered (Cummings et al. 1980). The notion of acquired impairment removes congenital retardation from the realm of dementia; persistent impairment distinguishes dementia from delirium; and impairment in multiple spheres separates dementia from unitary disorders such as amnesia and aphasia. Although some dementias are chronic, irreversible, and progressive conditions, the term *dementia* does not automatically imply irreversibility. The principal causes of dementia are listed in Table 8–1.

Dementia reflects the effect of pathological processes on the brain and is not the result of normal aging. The "normal elderly" are a heterogeneous group in whom intrinsic age-related processes may be complicated by the effects of illness and medications. Studies on optimally healthy elderly demonstrate only slowed information processing and some signs of inefficiency in generating problem-solving strategies (Boone et al. 1990). Naming, attention, and predominantly verbal neuropsychological tasks are all unaffected by age.

Table 8–1. Etiological classification of the principal dementia syndromes

Degenerative disorders
  Cortical
    Alzheimer's disease
    Lewy body disease
    Pick's disease
    Frontal-lobe degeneration of non-Alzheimer's type
  Subcortical
    Parkinson's disease
    Huntington's disease
    Progressive supranuclear palsy
    Spinocerebellar degenerations
    Idiopathic basal ganglia calcification
    Striatonigral degeneration
    Wilson's disease
    Thalamic dementia

Vascular dementias
  Multiple large vessel occlusions
  Strategic infarct dementia
  Lacunar state (multiple subcortical infarctions)
  Binswanger's disease (white matter ischemic injury)
  Mixed cortical and subcortical infarctions

Myelinoclastic disorders
  Demyelinating
    Multiple sclerosis
    Marchiafava-Bignami disease
  Dysmyelinating
    Metachromatic leukodystrophy
    Adrenoleukodystrophy
    Cerebrotendinous xanthomatosis

Traumatic conditions
  Posttraumatic encephalopathy
  Subdural hematoma
  Dementia pugilistica

Neoplastic dementias
  Meningioma (particularly subfrontal)
  Glioma
  Metastatic deposits
  Meningeal carcinomatosis

Hydrocephalic dementias
  Communicating
    Normal-pressure hydrocephalus
  Noncommunicating
    Aqueductal stenosis
    Intraventricular neoplasm
    Intraventricular cyst
    Basilar meningitis

Inflammatory conditions
  Systemic lupus erythematosus
  Antiphospholipid antibody syndrome
  Temporal arteritis
  Sarcoidosis
  Granulomatous arteritis

Infection-related dementias
  Syphilis
  Chronic meningitis
  Postencephalitic dementia syndrome
  Whipple's disease
  Acquired immunodeficiency syndrome (AIDS)
  Creutzfeldt-Jakob disease
  Subacute sclerosing panencephalitis
  Progressive multifocal leukoencephalopathy

Toxic conditions
  Alcohol-related syndrome
  Polydrug abuse
  Iatrogenic dementias
    Anticholinergic agents
    Antihypertensive drugs
    Psychotropic agents
    Anticonvulsant agents
    Miscellaneous agents
  Metals
  Industrial solvents

Metabolic disorders
  Cardiopulmonary failure
  Uremia
  Hepatic encephalopathy
  Endocrine disorders
    Thyroid
    Adrenal
    Parathyroid
  Anemia and hematological conditions
  Deficiency states (vitamin B_{12}, folate)
  Porphyria

Psychiatric disorders
  Depression
  Mania
  Schizophrenia
  Conversion disorder
  Malingering

Source. Adapted from Cummings JL: "Dementia Syndromes: Neurobehavioral and Neuropsychiatric Features." *Journal of Clinical Psychiatry* 48 (no 5, suppl):3–8, 1987. Copyright 1987, Physicians Postgraduate Press. Used with permission.

Cortical Dementia

Cortical dementias are disorders producing dysfunction of the cerebral cortex, as characterized by the A's: amnesia, aphasia, apraxia, and agnosia. Dementia of the Alzheimer's type (DAT) is the classic example of a cortical dementia. The "cortical" designation is a clinical concept that emphasizes the predominance of cortical dysfunction in these disorders despite coexisting pathology in subcortical regions (Cummings and Benson 1984).

Subcortical Dementia

Subcortical dementias reflect pathological processes primarily involving the deep gray and deep white matter structures. The clinical findings in subcortical dementia reflect the disruption of fundamental cerebral functions such as arousal, attention, motivation, and rate of information processing. The dementias due to human immunodeficiency virus (HIV) infection,

Huntington's disease (HD), and Parkinson's disease (PD) are all considered examples of subcortical dementias (Mandell and Albert 1990). Table 8–2 illustrates the features that distinguish cortical and subcortical dementias.

Mixed Dementia

Mixed dementia includes disease processes that produce a mixed clinical syndrome with both cortical and subcortical features. The most common entity in this category is vascular dementia, the syndrome of multiple strokes producing cognitive dysfunction. Vascular disease not only affects several brain regions but can coexist with other pathological processes.

Dementia Associated With Psychiatric Disorders: "Pseudodementia"

The term *pseudodementia* is commonly used to refer to cognitive deficits caused by clinical depression and other psychiatric disorders that

Table 8–2. Distinguishing features of cortical and subcortical dementias

Characteristic	Subcortical	Cortical
Language	No aphasia	Aphasia early
Memory	Recall impaired; recognition is better preserved than recall	Amnesia: recall and recognition impaired
Visuospatial skills	Impaired	Impaired
Calculation	Preserved until late	Involved early
Frontal systems	Disproportionately affected	Impaired to the same degree as other abilities
Cognitive processing speed	Slowed early	Response time normal until late in disease course
Personality	Apathetic, inert	Unconcerned or disinhibited
Mood	Depressed	Euthymic
Speech	Dysarthric	Normal articulation[a]
Posture	Bowed or extended	Normal, upright[a]
Coordination	Impaired	Normal[a]
Gait	Abnormal	Normal[a]
Motor speed	Slowed	Normal[a]
Movement disorders	Common (chorea, tremor, tics, rigidity)	Absent[a]

[a]Motor system involvement occurs late in the course of the cortical dementias.
Source. Adapted from Cummings JL: *Subcortical Dementia*. New York, Oxford University Press, 1990, pp. 1–16. Copyright 1990, Oxford University Press. Used with permission.

produce a reversible syndrome of cognitive impairment indistinguishable from primary dementia (Caine 1981; Wells 1979). However, because there is nothing "pseudo" about the cognitive impairment seen in patients with depression, the term *dementia syndrome of depression* (DSD) is preferable (M. F. Folstein and McHugh 1978).

EPIDEMIOLOGY

Estimates suggest that up to 4 million Americans have severe dementia, and an additional 1–5 million patients have mild to moderate dementia. Furthermore, based on the growing number of elderly persons in the population, the number of Americans with severe dementia is projected to increase 60% by the year 2000 and 100% by 2020 if current trends continue (U.S. Congress Office of Technology Assessment 1987).

Prevalence

The most commonly occurring dementia is DAT, which accounts for approximately 50% of patients evaluated for progressive cognitive decline. Perhaps another 15%–20% display a combination of Alzheimer's disease and vascular pathology at autopsy (Tomlinson et al. 1970).

Vascular dementia is the second most common cause of dementia. It occurs in 17%–29% of patients with dementia, with an additional 10%–23% of patients exhibiting vascular dementia mixed with DAT.

Together, DAT and vascular dementia account for 70%–90% of patients with dementia, whereas all the other syndromes listed in Table 8–1 account for the remaining 10%–30%. This latter group invites the special attention of the consultant because it contains the potentially reversible causes of dementia such as metabolic, structural, or psychiatric conditions (Rabins 1983). The consultant must also be mindful that the prevalence, severity, and

likely etiology of dementia are all variable, depending on whether a patient resides at home, in an institution, in a hospital, or in a nursing home.

Predisposition/Risk Factors

An age-associated risk for the development of DAT clearly exists, but whether this risk ultimately plateaus, continues to increase, or finally declines in the oldest population is unknown. A family history for dementia is also convincingly associated with DAT; individuals with dementia are three to four times more likely to have an affected relative than are control subjects (Mendez et al. 1992). Low level of education as well as head trauma with loss of consciousness appear to be associated with an increased risk for the development of DAT (Cummings 1995b; Van Duijn et al. 1992). It has recently been shown that inheritance of the apolipoprotein-e-4 allele, a gene involved in cholesterol metabolism, is also a risk factor for DAT (Corder et al. 1993; Roses 1995). The risk for cerebrovascular disease increases with age. Vascular dementia is most commonly encountered in patients who are older than 60 years; men are affected more often than women. Typically, vascular dementia is associated with stroke risk factors: age, hypertension, heart disease, cigarette smoking, diabetes mellitus, excessive alcohol consumption (more than three drinks per day), and hyperlipidemia. Female gender, age over 50, and continuous rather than periodic drinking may all predispose to the syndrome of alcoholic dementia (Cutting 1982).

Familial Associations

Various researchers have explored the association between DAT and a family history of dementia and have identified possible genetic loci for familial DAT on chromosomes 21, 19, 14, and 1 (Levy-Lahad et al. 1995; Schellenberg et al. 1992; Whatley and Anderton 1990). As with heart disease, however, these loci do not account for the majority of DAT cases in the general population (Whatley and Anderton 1990).

More directly familial is HD, which is inherited as an autosomal dominant trait with complete penetrance, so that half the offspring of HD patients are affected (S. E. Folstein et al. 1990). Wilson's disease (WD) is inherited as an autosomal recessive trait (Dening and Berrios 1989).

CLINICAL FEATURES

Cortical Dementia

Dementia of the Alzheimer's type. According to DSM-IV (American Psychiatric Association 1994), the clinical diagnosis of DAT requires the gradual, progressive development of multiple cognitive deficits, including both memory impairment and nonmemory cognitive disturbances.

The memory impairment found in DAT is manifested by disorientation for time and place and failure to remember three unrelated words for 3 minutes, even with cues (Petersen et al. 1994). The typical language disturbance is a fluent aphasia with anomia; speech has an empty quality and lacks specific content words. Naming and comprehension are progressively impaired, whereas the ability to repeat is relatively preserved; paraphasic errors are common (Cummings and Benson 1986). The gradual development of an isolated, progressive aphasia may be the precursor of a more generalized dementia syndrome in some patients (Green et al. 1990). Patients retain the ability to recognize objects and to use them appropriately at a time when they can no longer name them accurately (Rapcsak et al. 1989). Disturbances in executive cognitive functions include abnormalities of planning, organizing, sequencing, and abstracting. Clinically, these executive functions help to orchestrate and to

maintain goal-directed behavior. Apathy, distractibility, purposeless stereotypy, overreliance on environmental cues, agitation, and a tendency to perseverate may all arise from disturbed executive cognitive systems (Royall et al. 1992). DAT is relentlessly progressive, advancing through mild, moderate, and severe stages.

Pick's disease. Pick's disease is a progressive, degenerative disorder of the frontal lobes and is perhaps the best known of several frontal-lobe degenerations (FLDs), which preferentially affect the frontal or frontal and temporal lobes. Pick's disease, FLD with nonspecific histological changes, and FLD with motor neuron disease are the major types of FLD. The several FLD syndromes are indistinguishable clinically and present with marked personality changes that may precede the development of overt cognitive decline by at least 2 years. Disinhibition and irritability are common, as are wandering, impulsivity, and poor judgment. Social withdrawal, loss of drive, and even major depression may be the first symptoms in some patients. Features of the Klüver-Bucy syndrome, such as hyperorality, hypersexuality, compulsive exploration of the environment, and visual agnosia, are not uncommon. Disproportionate impairment of frontal/executive skills is present on neuropsychological testing. Aphasia is present in some patients. The clinical presentation plus the relatively late onset of memory and visuospatial disturbances in FLD help to distinguish FLD from DAT (Baldwin and Forstl 1993).

Subcortical Dementia

Huntington's disease. The clinical triad of dementia, chorea, and a "positive" family history should suggest the diagnosis of HD to the consultant. HD is a typical subcortical dementia, with diminished cognitive speed, a memory retrieval deficit (characterized by poor spontaneous recall but preserved recognition memory), poor executive functions, and motor symptoms. The absence of aphasia and other cortical features distinguishes HD from DAT (S. E. Folstein et al. 1990). Personality changes such as irritability or apathy are common and may antedate the onset of chorea (Cummings 1995a). Depression is common in HD, and the risk of suicide is increased; mania and a syndrome with persecutory delusions resembling schizophrenia are seen as well (McHugh and Folstein 1975).

Wilson's disease.   WD is a recessively inherited defect in the copper-carrying serum protein ceruloplasmin. Although WD is an uncommon cause of dementia, the consultant must be aware of this diagnosis because the progression of this disease can be halted by treatment with chelating agents. Onset of WD is usually during adolescence or early adulthood. Dementia in WD is variable but tends to be mild; additional neurological findings include dysarthria, dystonia, rigidity, cerebellar abnormalities, tremor, and gait and postural disturbances (Starosta-Rubinstein et al. 1987). Psychiatric symptoms of WD include personality and behavioral changes such as irritability, aggression, disinhibition, and recklessness. Depressive features are common, whereas psychosis is infrequently seen.

Parkinson's disease.   Assessment of dementia in PD is complex because the effects of aging, depression (in perhaps half of all PD patients), and chronic disability must be considered in addition to the profound motor deficits. Although PD dementia is generally classified as a subcortical dementia, the presentation and course of cognitive decline in PD are highly variable, and cortical-type deficits may occur.

Progressive supranuclear palsy.   Progressive supranuclear palsy (PSP) is a progressive extrapyramidal syndrome usually beginning in the sixth decade of life. PSP is characterized by supranuclear gaze paresis, pseudobulbar palsy, axial rigidity, and a dementia with subcortical features (Albert et al. 1974; J. C. Steele et al. 1964). In addition to the loss of volitional down gaze, the most common presenting symptoms are postural instability and falling, gait abnormalities, depression, dysarthria, and memory disturbances (Maher and Lees 1986).

Limbic encephalopathy.   Limbic encephalopathy is a relatively rare, nonmetastatic complication of carcinoma. This dramatic paraneoplastic syndrome usually is associated with small cell lung cancer and is characterized by cognitive, affective, and behavioral changes. Central nervous system (CNS) pathological changes include extensive neuronal loss, perivascular infiltration, astrocytosis, and glial nodules. The earliest and most prominent feature is the sudden onset of memory loss that is often severe. Limbic encephalopathy should be considered in any patient who presents with a pure amnestic syndrome. Other common symptoms include spells of confusion or disorientation, seizures, depression, bizarre behaviors, hallucinations, paranoia, and anxiety. These symptoms may precede the diagnosis of cancer by as many as 6 years; therefore, it is important for the consultant to recognize limbic encephalopathy because it may be the first sign of a malignancy that is still at an early, possibly curable stage (Camara and Chelune 1987).

Mixed Dementia

Vascular dementia.   Although ischemia, hemorrhage, and anoxia can all cause vascular dementia, this disorder is most often associated with ischemic vascular disease. There is considerable heterogeneity in both the pathological and the clinical expression of vascular dementia. The accumulation of cerebral infarctions can produce the progressive cognitive impairment termed *multi-infarct dementia*. Chronic ischemia without frank infarction can impair cognition, focal infarcts in critical areas subserving multiple cognitive functions can produce the syndrome of strategic infarct dementia, and ischemic injury can coexist with other dementias such as DAT (Chui et al. 1992; Roman et al. 1993; Tatemichi et al. 1995).

Vascular dementia is characterized by abrupt onset, stepwise progression, fluctuating course, depression, pseudobulbar palsy, a history of hypertension, a history of strokes, evidence of associated atherosclerosis, focal neurological symptoms, and focal neurological signs on examination. These features together constitute an ischemia score (Table 8–3) that is valuable in differentiating vascular dementia from DAT (Hachinski et al. 1975; Molsa et al. 1985; Rosen et al. 1980). The ischemia score does not differentiate vascular dementia from vascular dementia plus DAT (Erkinjuntti et al. 1988).

The clinical presentation of vascular dementia depends on the mechanism of cerebral injury. Deep hemispheric infarction, ischemia causing a lacunar state, or Binswanger's disease will produce a subcortical dementia associated with pseudobulbar palsy, spasticity, and weakness (Fisher 1989). Superficial cortical infarctions will produce a cortical dementia associated with hemimotor and hemisensory dysfunction. Psychotic features are common in vascular dementia, although neither the nature and prevalence of delusions nor the occurrence of hallucinations distinguishes vascular dementia from DAT (Cummings et al. 1987). Depression is common following stroke and occurs most often with left cortical and subcortical lesions. The severity of depression is correlated with proximity of the lesion to the left frontal pole. A history of stroke or preexisting cortical atrophy may be an important risk factor for the subsequent development of poststroke depression (Robinson and Starkstein 1990).

Trauma.   Serious head trauma can cause dementia. Amnesia and personality alterations are the most common neurobehavioral deficits following traumatic brain injury (TBI). Posttraumatic amnesia includes a variable period of unconsciousness caused by the injury, a period of retrograde amnesia for information acquired from a few minutes to a few years before the injury, and a period of anterograde amnesia lasting from hours to months after recovery from unconsciousness (Levin et al. 1982). Recovery is not always complete, and a degree of permanent anterograde memory disturbance may persist (Levin 1989). Aphasia can occur in up to 30% of TBI patients (Jennett and Teasdale 1981). TBI increases the risk for developing secondary psychiatric syndromes, including depression, mania, and psychosis (McAllister 1992). Subjective symptoms such as headache, dizziness, easy fatigability, and disordered sleep persist in some patients for several months, even after mild head trauma; this *postconcussional syndrome* is a complex blend of physiological and psychological factors that results in significant chronic disability for a small proportion of patients (Lishman 1988).

Three other important dementia syn-

Table 8–3.   Hachinski Ischemia Score

Abrupt onset	2
Stepwise progression	1
Fluctuating course	2
Nocturnal confusion	1
Relative preservation of personality	1
Depression	1
Somatic complaints	1
Emotional incontinence	1
History of hypertension	1
History of strokes	2
Evidence of associated atherosclerosis	1
Focal neurological symptoms	2
Focal neurological signs	2

Alzheimer's disease scores   4 or less
Vascular dementia scores   7 or more

Source.   Adapted from Hachinski VC, Iliff LD, Zilhka E, et al: "Cerebral Blood Flow in Dementia." *Archives of Neurology* 32:632–637, 1975. Used with permission.

dromes are associated with head trauma. The chronic, repeated head trauma experienced by boxers can lead to dementia pugilistica, a syndrome characterized by ataxia and dysarthria that progresses to dementia with parkinsonian-type extrapyramidal features (Jordan 1987). A potentially reversible cause of dementia following head trauma is subdural hematoma, a condition that may present as dementia, delirium, or psychosis (Black 1984). Finally, an uncommon but potentially treatable dementia associated with head trauma is normal-pressure hydrocephalus (NPH), a condition that may also occur following subarachnoid hemorrhage or intracranial infection or may have no known precipitant. NPH produces a triad of clinical symptoms: 1) a gait disturbance, often described as "magnetic," that appears early; 2) a subcortical dementia; and 3) urinary incontinence that may not appear until late in the course (Benson 1985). This triad is not specific to NPH; vascular dementia more commonly causes this triad.

Dementias associated with infectious diseases. Infection with HIV-1 produces a dementing illness initially termed the *AIDS (acquired immunodeficiency syndrome) dementia complex* (Navia et al. 1986) and more recently designated HIV-1-associated cognitive/motor complex (American Academy of Neurology AIDS Task Force 1991). Two clinical categories are recognized: 1) a more severe form known as *HIV-1-associated dementia complex* and 2) a less severe form termed *HIV-1-associated minor cognitive/motor disorder,* in which only the most demanding activities of daily living are impaired despite the presence of demonstrable cognitive, motor, or behavioral abnormalities.

Primary HIV-1-associated dementia complex is now the most common dementia associated with infectious diseases, but several other clinically important conditions deserve mention. Creutzfeldt-Jakob disease is an uncommon dementia characterized by extremely

rapid progressive deterioration and death, usually within 1 year. Patients show intellectual devastation, myoclonic jerks, muscle rigidity, and ataxia (Brown et al. 1986).

Progressive multifocal leukoencephalopathy (PML) is a subacute viral disorder that occurs in adults with chronic systemic illness. The lesions of PML are distributed randomly in the nervous system, which results in highly variable clinical manifestations. PML usually progresses to death in 2–4 months, with dementia, blindness, and impaired motility present in the advanced stages.

Chronic meningitis caused by fungal, parasitic, or chronic bacterial infections can present as dementia. Slow, progressive compromise of intellectual function, with fluctuations in arousal, apathy, lethargy, disorientation, and poor memory, is typical; cranial nerve abnormalities are common, and focal signs may be present. The consultant must consider this diagnosis when evaluating immunocompromised or debilitated patients (Luby 1992).

Acute herpes simplex encephalitis preferentially damages the medial, temporal, and orbitofrontal regions of the cortex, and neurological sequelae are often seen among survivors of the acute illness. Although amnesia is the most common residual deficit, aphasia or other cognitive deficits can occur. Recovery of intellect is variable, and dementia can be a long-term consequence of the disease (Skoldenberg 1991).

Syphilitic infection of the CNS ultimately can manifest as dementia in a variety of ways. All forms of neurosyphilis begin as a meningitis that is usually asymptomatic but if left untreated may evolve into meningovascular syphilis or general paresis. Meningovascular syphilis usually occurs 6–7 years after the original infection and should always be considered in a young person who has one or more cerebrovascular accidents. General paresis usually becomes evident 15–20 years after infection, beginning with the insidious onset of a memory defect, inattention, and indifference;

facial quivering, hand tremor, and myoclonus may be present.

Toxic-metabolic dementias. This category is especially important for the consultant because toxic-metabolic dementias are particularly common in the hospital setting, and many are potentially treatable or reversible to some extent. Whereas acute, overwhelming toxic-metabolic states present as delirium, more chronic, insidious toxic-metabolic conditions produce a slowly progressive dementia that has subcortical features (Cummings and Benson 1992).

Although cognitive disturbances in toxic-metabolic dementias vary with the specific etiology of the dementia, these patients generally show impaired attention and concentration, forgetfulness, and disturbed executive functioning. Probably the largest single group of patients with toxic-metabolic dementia are those with alcoholism, a diagnosis that is often unrecognized in elderly patients (Beresford et al. 1988). Traditionally, Wernicke-Korsakoff syndrome (WKS) is considered to be an isolated amnesia rather than a true dementia. It is produced by dietary thiamine deficiency. The acute phase of WKS—Wernicke's encephalopathy—is characterized by ophthalmoplegia, ataxia, and confusion. Only 25% of patients who eventually develop the chronic amnesia of WKS have a prior clinical diagnosis of Wernicke's encephalopathy (Blansjaar et al. 1992). Korsakoff's syndrome is the chronic amnestic phase of WKS and is characterized by a severe disability in learning new material and by a retrograde amnesia with relative sparing of remote memories. Confabulation is common in the early phases of Korsakoff's syndrome, and variable degrees of apathy, loss of insight, and diminished initiative frequently accompany the amnesia. With abstinence, a significant proportion of WKS patients show improvement in cognitive deficits, usually within the first year, refuting the widespread view that WKS is permanent and irreversible.

Neoplastic dementias. In addition to the paraneoplastic syndromes noted previously, brain tumors can present clinically as dementia. As many as 1%–2% of patients given a psychiatric diagnosis may have undiagnosed CNS tumors (Keschner et al. 1938; Selecki 1965). Tumors may cause a variety of behavioral changes, but no mental syndromes are strictly characteristic of tumors located in specific areas of the brain. Psychiatric symptom formation is influenced greatly by the extent of tumor involvement, the rapidity of tumor growth, and the propensity of a given tumor to cause increased intracranial pressure; tumor location plays a less important role. Nevertheless, psychiatric disturbances are more commonly associated with frontal- and temporal-lobe tumors than with tumors of the parietal or occipital lobes. When elaborating a differential diagnosis in the patient with dementia, the consultant must keep in mind that frontal-lobe tumors may produce executive cognitive dysfunction as well as apathetic and akinetic syndromes, whereas temporal-lobe tumors may affect memory and language functions (Price et al. 1992).

Dementia Associated With Psychiatric Disorders: "Pseudodementia"

Depression. Depression is often encountered among patients evaluated for impaired cognition. In one large series, 27% of patients referred to a dementia clinic met criteria for a depressive disorder (Reding et al. 1985). Several potential relations exist between depression and dementia: 1) depression can occur in response to the onset of cognitive impairment; 2) depression and dementia can be produced by the same underlying condition, as in stroke or PD; 3) clinical symptoms of dementing illnesses overlap with those of depression and can lead to the misdiagnosis of either; and 4) dementia is a syndrome that can be caused by depression (i.e., DSD). Currently, DSD can only be established with certitude retrospectively because the patient recovers intellectual function after successful antidepressant therapy (Cummings 1989).

Several salient clinical features are associated with DSD: 1) the elapsed time between onset and seeking medical help is shorter than is typical for degenerative dementias; 2) in many patients, a history of primary mood disorder exists; 3) a high frequency of current depressed mood and delusions is present; and 4) severe early morning awakening is common (Emery and Oxman 1992). The consultant should keep in mind that nearly half of all patients with an initial diagnosis of DSD will develop irreversible dementia within 3 years; recommendations for thorough evaluation and close follow-up of the patient with DSD are essential (Alexopoulos et al. 1993).

Conversion disorder. Conversion ("hysterical") dementia is a rare syndrome. Marked disparity between the ability to answer questions on mental status testing and abilities demonstrated in casual or unstructured situations should suggest this diagnosis to the consultant. Caution must be exercised because despite the presence of apparent primary gain, secondary gain, or bizarre symptoms, between 50% and 70% of patients who are given a diagnosis of conversion disorder eventually manifest a physical etiology (McEvoy and Wells 1979; Merskey and Buhrich 1975; B. L. Miller et al. 1986).

Acute psychosis. During the acute psychotic phase, both mania and schizophrenia may be mistaken for primary dementia syndromes, especially in elderly patients.

Malingering. Entirely conscious simulation of dementia is quite rare, and careful observation usually reveals much that is inconsistent with genuine cognitive impairment. Isolated symptoms, such as loss of speech or memory, are produced more commonly than a full dementia syndrome. An underlying disorder should always be sought, but the absence of obvious disease and accompanying motive and evidence of awareness on the part of the patient serve to alert the consultant to the diagnosis of malingering (Lishman 1987).

PATHOPHYSIOLOGY

Dementia of the Alzheimer's Type

On gross inspection, the brain in DAT is characterized by cortical atrophy, with widened sulci and ventricular enlargement. Microscopic examination reveals neuronal loss, neurofibrillary tangles, neuritic plaques, granulovacuolar degeneration, and amyloid angiopathy. Tangles are located within neurons and are composed of primarily paired helical filaments that contain abnormally phosphorylated microtubule-associated tau proteins. Plaques are located extracellularly and consist of a core of amyloid peptide and aluminosilicates surrounded by dystrophic nerve processes, terminals, and organelles (Matsuyama and Jarvik 1989). Granulovacuolar degeneration consists of intracytoplasmic vacuoles, particularly in neurons of the hippocampus. Amyloid angiopathy is present in nearly all cases of DAT; this cerebrovascular amyloid is identical to that found in neuritic plaques and is also present in extracerebral vessels in skin, subcutaneous tissue, and intestine (Mirra et al. 1993; Vinters et al. 1988). Virtually all of these neuropathological changes are found in the brains of individuals without dementia; the location and density of these lesions determine the postmortem histological diagnosis of DAT (Khachaturian 1985; Vinters 1991).

Pick's Disease

Perhaps 20% of the FLDs are Pick's disease, diagnosed by the presence of distinctive intraneuronal Pick bodies and ballooned Pick cells on microscopic examination; the remaining 80% are designated as FLD of the non-Alzheimer's type and lack the distinctive histological features of Pick's disease (Brun 1987).

Huntington's Disease

Pathologically, in HD, atrophy of the caudate nucleus and loss of the γ-aminobutyric acid (GABA)–ergic interneurons—cells with an inhibitory function in movement mechanisms—from the striatum occur.

Wilson's Disease

The primary biochemical defect in WD is unknown; however, an abnormality on chromosome 13 results in diminished synthesis of ceruloplasmin. When the ability of the liver to handle copper and excrete it into the bile is impaired, unbound copper accumulates in the CNS, liver, cornea, and kidneys, where levels reach toxic proportions (Starosta-Rubinstein et al. 1987).

Parkinson's Disease

PD is an idiopathic disorder characterized by progressive loss of dopaminergic neurons in the substantia nigra and other pigmented brain stem nuclei. PD represents an example of a long-latency neurological disease because tremor, rigidity, and bradykinesia emerge only when a 70%–80% reduction in dopamine occurs. The pathological hallmark of PD is the presence of Lewy bodies in the cytoplasm of the remaining nigral neurons, where they are considered to represent a marker for neuronal cell degeneration (Gibb 1989).

Progressive Supranuclear Palsy

In PSP, neurofibrillary tangles, granulovacuolar degeneration, cell loss, and gliosis are found in the subthalamic nucleus, red nucleus, substantia nigra, and dentate nucleus, but the cortex is unaffected (J. C. Steele et al. 1964). Both the nigrostriatal dopaminergic and the cholinergic systems are impaired (Ruberg et al. 1985).

HIV-Associated Dementia

The severity of clinical deterioration generally correlates with the severity of brain pathology. Some degree of cerebral atrophy is present in almost all HIV-infected patients with dementia. Histological examination demonstrates diffuse pallor of the centrum semiovale with a mononuclear inflammatory response in the white matter and the deep gray nuclei (Navia 1990).

Vascular Dementia

Several mechanisms for dementia caused by stroke are recognized, including the location of cerebral injury, the volume of cerebral tissue involved, the number of cerebral insults, and the co-occurrence of vascular dementia and DAT (Tatemichi 1990). Subcortical lacunar infarctions are found in approximately 70% of patients with vascular dementia. This so-called lacunar state is produced by multiple small infarctions involving the basal ganglia, thalamus, and internal capsule and is the most frequent cause of vascular dementia. Vascular dementia may also result from the cumulative effects of watershed or border zone infarctions that are caused by critical reductions in cerebral perfusion in association with severe extracranial atherosclerosis; this pathology is seen in up to 40% of patients with vascular dementia (Meyer et al. 1988). A diagnosis of Binswanger's disease is made on the basis of extensive ischemic white matter damage in the subcortical periventricular regions of the centrum semiovale. These periventricular areas are susceptible to damage produced by occlusion or hypoperfusion of the blood vessels supplying the deep white matter (Tatemichi 1990). Vascular dementia may also result from the cumulative effects of multiple cerebral emboli; these embolic infarcts are found in approximately 20% of patients with vascular dementia and represent the third most frequent cause of vascular dementia. Embolic infarcts are usually larger than lacunae and have a bilateral hemispheric distribution. An identifiable cardiac source for emboli is found in one-fourth of these patients. Combinations of two or more different types of strokes are common and occur in nearly one-third of patients with vascular dementia (Meyer et al. 1988). An additional cause of vascular dementia to consider is the hypercoagulable state associated with the antiphospholipid antibody syndrome, especially in young stroke patients and in older stroke patients with few vascular risk factors (Gorman and Cummings 1993).

Trauma

Rapid acceleration or deceleration of the brain produces stretching and twisting of neuronal axons. The resulting spectrum of diffuse axonal injury ranges from brief disruption of physiological function without obvious anatomical disruption to frank axonal tearing (Graham et al. 1987).

Creutzfeldt-Jakob Disease

Creutzfeldt-Jakob disease is caused by a transmissible infectious agent—the "prion." Prions are proteinaceous particles containing little or no nucleic acid. Most cases of Creutzfeldt-Jakob disease arise sporadically, without any infectious source identified. Direct transmission of Creutzfeldt-Jakob disease has only occurred iatrogenically, as from contaminated neurosurgical instruments (Hsiao and Prusiner 1990). Microscopic neuropathology includes neuronal loss, astrocytic proliferation, and spongiform change in the cells of the cortex, striatum, and thalamus (Masters and Richardson 1978).

Toxic-Metabolic Dementias

Anoxia causes a breakdown of energy-dependent membrane functions, with loss of ionic homeostasis and neuronal death (Espinoza and Parer 1991). Hippocampal neurons appear to be most vulnerable to anoxic injury (Zola-Morgan et al. 1986).

Alcoholic dementia. At autopsy, the brains of chronic alcohol abusers show cortical atrophy and nerve fiber disintegration with dissolution of myelin sheaths (Lishman 1981). The characteristic pathology of WKS involves punctate lesions of the gray nuclei in the periventricular regions surrounding the third and fourth ventricles and the Sylvian aqueduct (Victor et al. 1989).

Chronic drug intoxications. Benzodiazepines are among the most widely prescribed medications in the world. Despite having valuable sedative, hypnotic, and anxiolytic properties, benzodiazepines negatively affect memory in two distinct ways: 1) anterograde amnesia after benzodiazepine administration and 2) impairment of memory consolidation and subsequent memory retrieval (American Psychiatric Association Task Force 1990). High-potency, short half-life benzodiazepines are more likely to impair memory, even after a single dose (Scharf et al. 1987). Memory impairment depends on the dose and the route of benzodiazepine administration, with higher doses and intravenous administration causing the greatest impairment. Duration of benzodiazepine treatment is also a significant factor; this is especially true in elderly patients, who may experience an insidious, gradual decrease in memory function, even at a constant benzodiazepine dose (American Psychiatric Association Task Force 1990).

Endocrine-related dementias. Repeated or severe episodes of hypoglycemia can produce permanent amnesia; therefore, poorly controlled insulin-dependent diabetic patients are at risk for this complication of their illness (Sachon et al. 1992). Hypoglycemia has its greatest effect on hippocampal neurons and thus affects cognitive processes much more than motor or sensory processes (Blackman et al. 1990; Chalmers et al. 1991).

Pernicious anemia.   In the elderly, atrophy of the gastric mucosa with loss of intrinsic factor secretion predisposes to vitamin B_{12} deficiency and subsequent development of pernicious anemia. Pathological lesions found in the CNS consist of focal areas of myelin degeneration scattered throughout the cortical white matter, the optic tracts, and the cerebellar peduncles. Low serum B_{12} levels are common in the elderly but are unlikely to be associated with dementia in the absence of macrocytosis and anemia or a significant neurological disorder (Crystal et al. 1994).

Neoplastic Dementias

Approximately 80% of all brain tumors are primary brain tumors, and the remaining 20% are metastatic.

◼ DIFFERENTIAL DIAGNOSIS

Clinical Examination

Mental status examination (MSE).   Using the MSE for effective cognitive screening is the cornerstone of neuropsychiatric assessment and diagnosis. The MSE serves as a probe of brain function and may be conceptualized as a structure built on a solid foundation of intact attentional systems.

The entire MSE depends on the integrity of attentional systems, and a patient with poor attention can be expected to demonstrate deficits in other domains. Attention is a complex and multifaceted ability that includes two primary components—*arousal* and *concentration* (directed attention). Arousal should be tested by inspection, and the forward digit span should be used (i.e., the patient's ability to hear and repeat correctly at least five random numbers presented in a steady monotone at the rate of one per second) (G. A. Miller 1956). Directed

attention should be tested by having the patient spell "WORLD" backward (or, alternatively, reciting the days of the week or the months of the year in reverse order) after the patient first performs the task forward correctly (M. F. Folstein et al. 1975).

For screening purposes, the three chief language domains are fluency, comprehension, and repetition. The consultant can use these three basic elements to distinguish among the major aphasia syndromes (Figure 8–1).

Recent or short-term memory is tested by stating three to five words and then asking the patient to recall them in 5–10 minutes. This task may be structured along a spectrum of difficulty (depending on the patient's expected level of performance) by giving more words with a longer time interval before recall is tested. Failure to encode and store the words may be distinguished from failure to recall learned material by providing recall cues; the clinician should give categorical prompts (e.g., "One of the words was a color."), then three choices to determine whether the patient has retrieval problems or a true amnesia. The patient with DAT is not reliably aided by cues on memory testing (Petersen et al. 1994).

Constructional tasks are useful clinical tools because they provide information about right-hemispheric and visuospatial function. Drawing a three-dimensional cube is a good screening item, as is clock drawing (Strub and Black 1993).

The frontal/executive cognitive domain includes planning, anticipation, sequencing, abstraction, and goal-directed activity. *Patients may be substantially impaired clinically by subtle dysfunction in this domain.* The consultant should remain alert for the patient who appears to be intact but who requires constant prompting, cuing, and supervision because frontal-system dysfunction may be the culprit.

Neurological examination.   The extent of the neurological examination will vary, but im-

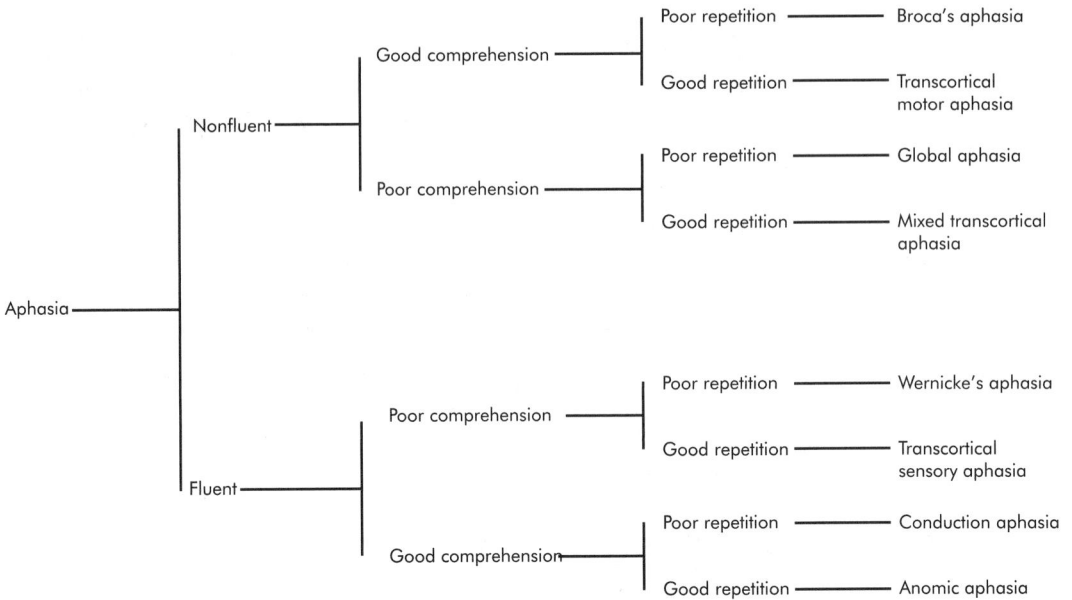

Figure 8–1. Systematic approach to differential diagnosis and localization of common aphasia syndromes.
Source. Reprinted from Cummings JL: *Clinical Neuropsychiatry.* Boston, MA, Allyn & Bacon, 1985, pp. 17–35. Copyright 1985, Allyn & Bacon. Used with permission.

portant elements to include in a dementia workup are cranial nerve testing; observation of gait, posture, and motor speed; testing muscle strength and tone; inspecting for tremor or other abnormal movements such as dyskinesias or myoclonus; testing muscle stretch reflexes and extensor plantar responses; and noting pathological signs such as the grasp, snout, jaw jerk, or glabellar reflexes. Sensory examination also should be included when warranted by clinical information (Paulson 1977; Quality Standards Subcommittee of the American Academy of Neurology 1994; Thomas 1994).

Longitudinal History

Clinical history is invaluable to the consultant who must evaluate the patient with dementia; the history should be obtained or corroborated through reliable caregivers. The consultant must inquire about quality of onset (gradual versus sudden) and pattern of progression (re-

lentless versus "stepwise"). The consultant must understand the typical features of an illness such as DAT in order to address potentially reversible supervening processes and to avoid the therapeutic nihilism that sometimes accompanies the dementias.

Reversible Etiologies

Of the dementia syndromes listed in Table 8–1, many are reversible to some degree (Barry and Moskowitz 1988). When rare or complicated dementia syndromes are encountered, a systematic approach to diagnosis is essential; additional neuroimaging studies, specific enzymatic or immunological assays, or biopsy of brain or extraneural tissues may be required for diagnosis (Reichman and Cummings 1990).

Laboratory Data

The laboratory evaluation in dementia is used to detect possibly reversible causes of cognitive compromise or to identify common conditions that may be amplifying intellectual deficits. Laboratory assessment is particularly valuable in consultation-liaison psychiatry because a disproportionate number of patients with dementia will have adverse cognitive consequences of systemic medical illnesses or drug effects. A battery of tests commonly used to assess patients with dementia is shown in Table 8–4 (Cummings and Benson 1992). The consultant should recommend lumbar puncture as part of the dementia workup in cases of suspected metastatic cancer, CNS infection or

Table 8–4. Laboratory tests in the assessment of dementia

Screening battery
  Complete blood count
  Erythrocyte sedimentation rate
  Blood glucose
  Blood urea nitrogen (BUN)
  Electrolytes
  Serum calcium and phosphorus
  Thyroid-stimulating hormone
  Vitamin B_{12} and folate levels
  Fluorescent treponemal antibody absorption
    (FTA-ABS)

If unexplained fever or urinary symptoms present
  Urinalysis
  Urine culture and sensitivity

If unexplained fever or pulmonary symptoms present
  Chest X ray

If cardiovascular symptoms present or evidence of vascular dementia
  Electrocardiogram (ECG)

If risk factors for HIV encephalopathy present
  Serum HIV test

If drug intoxication suspected
  Serum drug level

Tests selected on the basis of specific symptoms or history
  Blood gases
  Heavy metals
  Disease-specific tests (e.g., serum copper and
    ceruloplasmin for Wilson's disease)

Note. HIV = human immunodeficiency virus.

vasculitis, hydrocephalus, immunosuppression, and positive syphilis serology. Lumbar puncture should also be considered for patients with early onset, unusually rapid progression, or atypical features (Corey-Bloom et al. 1995).

Additional Diagnostic Studies

Imaging. Because no laboratory test is yet available for DAT, diagnosis is aided by the use of neuroimaging techniques. Some patients with dementia will have normal computed tomography (CT) scans, whereas some control subjects without dementia will have atrophic changes similar to those associated with dementia (DeCarli et al. 1990). In general, correlations between ventricular enlargement and cognitive function are stronger than those between cortical atrophy and cognition (Burns 1990; Giacometti et al. 1994).

Neuroimaging plays an especially important role in diagnosing vascular dementia. CT detects actual infarctions in fewer than half of patients with clinical evidence of vascular dementia (Radue et al. 1978). Nonetheless, areas of decreased lucency in the white matter— "leuko-araiosis"—are seen on CT scans in the majority of patients with vascular dementia. Enlargement of the lateral and third ventricles correlates significantly with severity of cognitive impairment in vascular dementia (Aharon-Peretz et al. 1988). Magnetic resonance imaging (MRI) is the most sensitive structural imaging technique for diagnosing vascular dementia (Kertesz et al. 1987).

Imaging is also variably helpful in evaluating other forms of dementia. Frontal atrophy on CT or MRI is usually apparent late in the course of FLD (B. L. Miller et al. 1991). CT or MRI can demonstrate gross atrophy of the caudate nucleus in HD (Gray and Cummings 1994). MRI studies have not demonstrated any specific pattern of abnormalities in patients with dementia and PD (Huber et al. 1989). MRI is becoming the primary diagnostic instrument in NPH and demonstrates enlarged ventricles, increased signal adjacent to the ventricles, and evidence of cerebrospinal fluid (CSF) flow disturbances within the ventricular system (Kunz et al. 1989).

In HIV-1 dementia, structural imaging studies using CT or MRI show atrophy and evidence for demyelination of subcortical white matter. CT imaging in abstinent chronic alcohol abusers demonstrates lateral ventricular enlargement with widening of the cortical sulci; this atrophy does not correlate with intellectual impairment and may improve in some patients with abstinence (Carlen 1978).

Structural imaging studies in patients with DSD show diminished brain density and increased ventricular brain ratio values more similar to those of patients with dementia than to age-matched control subjects (Pearlson et al. 1989). The prognostic significance of these findings is unclear. Application of newer techniques such as polysomnographic sleep studies may eventually prove useful in this regard because diminished rapid eye movement (REM) sleep latency is a common feature of depression (Buysse et al. 1992).

The electroencephalogram (EEG) in patients with Creutzfeldt-Jakob disease frequently shows a characteristic intermittent periodic burst pattern (Brown et al. 1986). Neuroimaging is nondiagnostic, although functional imaging techniques may be useful for directing brain biopsy (Holthoff et al. 1990; Jibiki et al. 1994).

Although the yield of potentially treatable conditions found with routine CT or MRI is low, the consultant should always recommend imaging in patients with impaired cognition for less than 3 months; rapid onset of impairment over 48 hours or less; head trauma during the week before the decline in mental state; a clinical history of stroke, seizures, or malignant tumor; urinary or fecal incontinence; and neurological abnormalities such as headache, visual field deficit, papilledema, abnormal gait, postural instability, or any focal findings on neurological examination (Alexander et al. 1995; Dietch 1983).

Neuropsychological testing. Neuropsychological testing can be a useful adjunct to mental status testing of patients with known or suspected intellectual impairment (Zec 1993). It does not replace a thorough MSE and should be used to amplify the results of clinical testing or to clarify questions that have arisen. Neuropsychological testing is particularly valuable as a means of 1) distinguishing between mild dementia and normal aging in elderly individuals, 2) differentiating mild dementia from the effects of low educational level or limited natural cognitive capacities, 3) providing detailed quantitative information that may help to differentiate among types of dementias, and 4) establishing a baseline description of cognitive function that may be followed over time to determine whether the patient is undergoing progressive decline. Neuropsychological test performance can be affected by anxiety, depression, delirium, low educational level, or sociocultural influences, and interpretation must take these factors into account (Levin 1994).

CLINICAL COURSE AND PROGNOSIS

DAT usually begins after age 50, with an insidious and gradually progressive decline in mental abilities. The patient and family members often are unaware of the evolving cognitive impairment, and the onset of the illness is identified only in retrospect. Memory difficulties are manifest by forgetting tasks, repeating questions, or losing the thread of a telephone conversation or a television program. The patient may complain about memory problems very early in the course of the disease, but insight is rapidly lost. In fact, the patient's lack of insight in the face of gross cognitive impairments is characteristic of DAT. Typically, the patient's daily responsibilities increasingly are assumed by colleagues and family members, who do not yet recognize the presence of a progressive disease and may think only that the patient is "slipping" with age. Other common early findings include bungled finances or getting lost while driving. Alcohol may produce an exaggerated emotional response, whereas a family vacation or trip to visit relatives often will reveal problems with orientation and memory. Intercurrent illness that requires hospitalization or anesthesia may provoke episodes of "sundowning" or delirium (Bliwise 1994).

Delusional beliefs often develop (Burns et al. 1990). Patients commonly are convinced that others are trying to steal from them or harm them, that their spouse is unfaithful, that family members are not who they claim to be (Capgras' syndrome), that their house is not really their home, or that family members are plotting to abandon them. The patient often will pace around the house without apparent purpose ("touring"), engage in repetitive, stereotyped activities such as opening and closing drawers, or wander from the house and get lost in formerly familiar surroundings.

The patient's responses become increasingly erratic and exaggerated, and well-intentioned attempts by family members or caregivers to insist or "force" the patient to perform tasks such as bathing or getting into a car may precipitate "catastrophic reactions."

Eventually, patients become unable to recognize close family members, and they may even misidentify their own reflection in a mirror. Primitive reflexes, such as the grasp, snout, and suck emerge, and new-onset seizures may appear (Romanelli et al. 1990). In the final stage of the illness, the patient becomes incontinent of urine and feces, loses all intelligible vocabulary, and is unable to walk or to sit up (Reisberg 1988). Death from pneumonia or another infectious process frequently occurs after a period of total confinement to bed.

Studies of patients with DAT consistently show an annual rate of decline on mental status testing approximately equivalent to three points per year on the Mini-Mental State Exam (MMSE). Although individual patients vary in their rate of decline, dramatic deviations from this rate warrant investigation. Currently, DAT is the fourth leading cause of death among the elderly.

Patients with PD survived an average 9–10 years after diagnosis in the pre-L-dopa era and now survive for 13–14 years (Martilla 1992). Treatment with penicillamine before irreversible hepatic or neurological injury has occurred will allow a normal life span in many individuals with WD (Patten 1993). This outcome contrasts with 8- to 12-year survival typical of patients with WD before the advent of efficacious treatment. HD symptoms typically begin at about age 40; the disease course tends to last about 15 years (S. E. Folstein et al. 1990).

Vascular dementia has a poor prognosis. Patients generally succumb to cardiovascular events (myocardial infarction, congestive heart failure) rather than their brain disease, but it is not unusual for them to sustain additional strokes before death. Mean survival in patients with vascular dementia is 5–7 years (Nielsen et al. 1991).

Infectious dementias have disease-specific prognoses. Patients with CNS syphilis or chronic meningitis that is detected early and properly treated may have a complete reversal of intellectual changes. The course of HIV encephalopathy is highly variable; some patients survive for several years after the onset of cognitive deficits, whereas others survive only 2–9 months after the onset of the dementia. Ninety percent of patients with Creutzfeldt-Jakob disease die within 1 year of the onset of symptoms, and 50% die within 6 months (Brown et al. 1986).

TREATMENT AND MANAGEMENT

Medical Therapy

Treatment and management of dementia aim to control the underlying disease and to manage the associated cognitive and behavioral manifestations. No current interventions halt the underlying disease process of degenerative disorders, but many other types of dementing processes can be effectively treated. Halting the progression of cognitive deterioration and optimizing the function of remaining cognitive capacity are the goals of treatment in vascular dementia. Medical and surgical treatments are focused on management of associated risk factors and disease-specific interventions for associated medical conditions (Skoog 1994). Individual patients may benefit from speech therapy or physical therapy. Use of daily aspirin therapy (325 mg/day) to inhibit platelet aggregation is recommended (Meyer et al. 1989). Ticlopidine may ameliorate progressive ischemic injury in patients who cannot tolerate or do not respond to aspirin (Flores-Runk and Raasch 1993).

Surgical shunting of CSF produces improvement in 40%–50% of patients with NPH; dementia is the least likely of the NPH triad to improve with shunting, whereas gait disturbance has the best outcome. Although no absolute guidelines define accurately those patients who are most responsive to surgery, as a rule, patients with good surgical prognosis present with the full clinical triad, with a short duration of symptoms, and have a known cause of their NPH (Clarfield 1989; Friedland 1989; Vanneste 1994).

Given the insidious course of WKS and the high prevalence of undiagnosed WKS, all alcohol-dependent patients should be treated with thiamine (Blansjaar and van Dijk 1992).

Pharmacotherapy

Therapy for DAT is divided into two main categories: control of behavioral manifestations of the illness and attempts to restore cognitive function. Behavioral disturbances, such as agitation, wandering, suspiciousness, hallucinations, and hostility, that arise during the course of dementia are generally treated with low-dose neuroleptic medications (Schneider et al. 1990). Initial treatment with low doses of a high-potency agent (haloperidol 0.5–2 mg/day) is usually recommended. If troublesome extrapyramidal side effects emerge, dose reduction or changing to a midpotency agent such as loxapine is preferable to the use of anticholinergic drugs (Carlyle et al. 1993). If more sedation is required, a trial with the low-potency agent thioridazine may prove efficacious. In doses up to 50 mg/day, this medication is generally free from anticholinergic effects (C. Steele et al. 1986). Avoid the use of neuroleptic medications on an "as-needed" basis that far too often treats episodes of agitation "after the fact." Instead, consultants should help caregivers to recognize times when problems regularly arise so that they can medicate the patient in anticipation of agitation. This helps to minimize the total amount of medication required. The cautious, adjunctive use of low doses of short-acting benzodiazepines such as lorazepam or oxazepam may also prove beneficial. Clonazepam (0.5 mg) can be used to maintain sleep in patients with frequent awakening or nocturnal wandering; trazodone (50–150 mg) is useful for agitation and for patients with difficulty falling asleep (Pinner and Rich 1988). Other medications recently reported to help modify agitated behavior include buspirone, carbamazepine, valproate, fluoxetine, estrogen, and leuprolide (Kunik et al. 1994; Kyomen et al. 1991; Mazure et al. 1992; Rich and Ovsiew 1994; Schneider and Sobin 1991; Sobin et al. 1989; Tiller et al. 1988). Control of unwanted behavioral symptoms is a key to helping patients with dementia remain with their families (Zubenko et al. 1992).

Attempts to find an effective treatment for DAT have largely focused on augmentation of cerebral cholinergic neurotransmission (Davis and Mohs 1982). Various cholinomimetic strategies have been tried, including acetylcholine precursors, cholinergic agonists, and cholinesterase inhibitors; however, the therapeutic potential of these agents is limited by potentially toxic side effects and poor penetration across the blood-brain barrier. Tacrine, a centrally active, reversible cholinesterase inhibitor, has produced modest cognitive improvement in controlled trials (Davis et al. 1992; Farlow et al. 1992). Reversible hepatotoxicity requires blood tests every 1–2 weeks (alanine aminotransferase [ALT]/serum glutamic-pyruvic transaminase [SGPT]) during the dose-escalation phase of treatment.

Nonsedating antidepressants and psychostimulants are useful for treating the dysphoric mood symptoms, irritability, and labile affect commonly seen in patients with vascular dementia, PD, HIV/AIDS, or other CNS disease (Cummings 1994; Holmes et al. 1989; Panzer and Mellow 1992). Use of antidepressant or electroconvulsive therapy for DSD should be initiated on the basis of intrapsychic depressive symptoms and characteristic sleep disturbance rather than for the mere complaint or presence of cognitive impairment (Emery and Oxman 1992). Evidence of confusion on low doses of tricyclic antidepressants may identify patients with DSD at high risk for development of primary dementia (Reding et al. 1985). However, the availability of newer antidepressant agents (with more favorable side-effect profiles) should prompt a medication trial in cognitively impaired patients whenever the relative contribution of depression to the overall clinical picture is uncertain (Jones and Reifler 1994).

Ward Management

The consultant must pay attention to the patient's environment; too much or too little stimulation may result in withdrawal or agitation. Patients with dementia do best in familiar and constant surroundings with regular daily routines. Caregivers must learn the patient's (and their own) limitations. Caregivers should be encouraged to simplify tasks and to avoid rushing the patient or forcing the patient to do things beyond his or her ability (Mace and Rabins 1991; Small 1989).

Family Therapy/Support

The consultant's most crucial allies in working with patients who have dementia are family members because they provide most of the care for these progressively dependent individuals. Family members of patients with dementia frequently become depressed, experience an enormous burden in the course of providing care, and need referral to psychological, social, and legal services (Overman and Stoudemire 1988). They may be sufficiently depressed or anxious to require pharmacotherapy and psychiatric care, but more frequently, support groups or family therapy to help families respond with mutual support is indicated. Social service referrals help to inform the family about community resources such as home health services, day care, respite care, and nursing home care. Advice from an attorney is helpful for establishing wills, establishing trusts, and dealing with other estate management issues. Families should also be encouraged to provide advance directives regarding the care of hospitalized patients with dementia and should be counseled about the importance of autopsy (Raia 1994).

REFERENCES

Aharon-Peretz J, Cummings JL, Hill MA: Vascular dementia and dementia of the Alzheimer type. Arch Neurol 45:719–721, 1988

Albert ML, Feldman RG, Willis AL: The "subcortical dementia" of progressive supranuclear palsy. J Neurol Neurosurg Psychiatry 37:121–130, 1974

Alexander EM, Wagner EH, Buchner DM, et al: Do surgical brain lesions present as isolated dementia? A population-based study. J Am Geriatr Soc 43:138–143, 1995

Alexopoulos GS, Meyers BS, Young RC, et al: The course of geriatric depression with "reversible dementia": a controlled study. Am J Psychiatry 150:1693–1699, 1993

American Academy of Neurology AIDS Task Force: Nomenclature and research case definitions for neurologic manifestations of human immunodeficiency virus-type 1 (HIV-1) infection. Neurology 41:778–785, 1991

American Psychiatric Association: Diagnostic and Statistical Manual of Mental Disorders, 4th Edition. Washington, DC, American Psychiatric Association, 1994, pp 133–155

American Psychiatric Association Task Force: Benzodiazepine Dependence, Toxicity, and Abuse. Washington, DC, American Psychiatric Press, 1990, pp 42–44

Baldwin B, Forstl H: "Pick's disease"—101 years on—still there, but in need of reform. Br J Psychiatry 163:100–104, 1993

Barry PP, Moskowitz MA: The diagnosis of reversible dementia in the elderly: a critical review. Arch Intern Med 148:1914–1918, 1988

Benson DF: Hydrocephalic dementia, in Handbook of Clinical Neurology, Vol 46: Neurobehavioral Disorders. Edited by Vinken PJ, Bruyn GW, Klawans HL. New York, Elsevier, 1985, pp 323–333

Beresford TP, Blow FC, Brower KJ, et al: Alcoholism and aging in the general hospital. Psychosomatics 29:61–72, 1988

Black DW: Mental changes resulting from subdural haematoma. Br J Psychiatry 145:200–203, 1984

Blackman JD, Towle VL, Lewis GF, et al: Hypoglycemic thresholds for cognitive dysfunction in humans. Diabetes 39:828–835, 1990

Blansjaar BA, van Dijk JG: Korsakoff minus Wernicke syndrome. Alcohol Alcohol 27:435–437, 1992

Blansjaar BA, Takens H, Zwinderman AH: The course of alcohol amnestic disorder: a three-year follow-up study of clinical signs and social disabilities. Acta Psychiatr Scand 86:240–246, 1992

Bliwise DL: What is sundowning? J Am Geriatr Soc 42:1009–1011, 1994

Boone KB, Miller BL, Lesser IM, et al: Performance on frontal lobe tests in healthy, older individuals. Developmental Neuropsychology 6:215–223, 1990

Brown P, Cathala F, Castaigne P, et al: Creutzfeldt-Jakob disease: clinical analysis of a consecutive series of 230 neuropathologically verified cases. Ann Neurol 20:597–602, 1986

Brun A: Frontal lobe degeneration of non-Alzheimer type, I: neuropathology. Archives of Gerontology and Geriatrics 6:193–208, 1987

Burns A: Cranial computerized tomography in dementia of the Alzheimer's type. Br J Psychiatry 157 (suppl 9):10–15, 1990

Burns A, Jacoby R, Levy R: Psychiatric phenomena in Alzheimer's disease, I: disorders of thought content; II: disorders of perception. Br J Psychiatry 157:72–81, 1990

Buysse DJ, Reynolds CF III, Hoch CC, et al: Rapid eye movement sleep deprivation in elderly patients with concurrent symptoms of depression and dementia. J Neuropsychiatry Clin Neurosci 4:249–256, 1992

Caine ED: Pseudodementia: current concepts and future directions. Arch Gen Psychiatry 38:1359–1364, 1981

Camara EG, Chelune GJ: Paraneoplastic limbic encephalopathy. Brain Behav Immun 1:349–355, 1987

Carlen PL, Wortzman G, Holgate RC, et al: Reversible cerebral atrophy in recently abstinent chronic alcoholics measured by computed tomography scans. Science 200:1076–1078, 1978

Carlyle W, Ancill RJ, Sheldon L: Aggression in the demented patient: a double-blind study of loxapine versus haloperidol. Int Clin Psychopharmacol 8:103–108, 1993

Chalmers J, Risk MT, Kean DM, et al: Severe amnesia after hypoglycemia: clinical, psychometric, and magnetic resonance imaging correlations. Diabetes Care 14:922–925, 1991

Chui HC, Victoroff JI, Margolin D, et al: Criteria for the diagnosis of ischemic vascular dementia proposed by the state of California Alzheimer's Disease Diagnostic and Treatment Centers. Neurology 42:473–480, 1992

Clarfield AM: Normal-pressure hydrocephalus: saga or swamp? JAMA 262:2592–2593, 1989

Corder EH, Saunders AM, Strittmatter WJ, et al: Gene dose of apolipoprotein E type 4 allele and the risk of Alzheimer's disease in late onset families. Science 261:921–923, 1993

Corey-Bloom J, Thal LJ, Galasko D, et al: Diagnosis and evaluation of dementia. Neurology 45: 211–218, 1995

Crystal HA, Ortof E, Frishman WH, et al: Serum vitamin B12 levels and incidence of dementia in a healthy elderly population: a report from the Bronx Longitudinal Aging Study. J Am Geriatr Soc 42:933–936, 1994

Cummings JL: Dementia and depression: an evolving enigma. J Neuropsychiatry Clin Neurosci 1:236–242, 1989

Cummings JL: Depression in neurologic diseases. Psychiatric Annals 24:525–531, 1994

Cummings JL: Behavioral and psychiatric symptoms associated with Huntington's disease. Adv Neurol 65:179–186, 1995a

Cummings JL: Dementia: the failing brain. Lancet 345:1481–1484, 1995b

Cummings JL, Benson DF: Subcortical dementia: review of an emerging concept. Arch Neurol 41:874–879, 1984

Cummings JL, Benson DF: Dementia of the Alzheimer's type: an inventory of diagnostic clinical features. J Am Geriatr Soc 34:12–19, 1986

Cummings JL, Benson DF: Dementia: A Clinical Approach. Boston, MA, Butterworth-Heinemann, 1992

Cummings JL, Benson DF, LoVerme S Jr: Reversible dementia. JAMA 243:2434–2439, 1980

Cummings JL, Miller B, Hill MA, et al: Neuropsychiatric aspects of multi-infarct dementia and dementia of the Alzheimer's type. Arch Neurol 44:389–393, 1987

Cutting J: Alcoholic dementia, in Psychiatric Aspects of Neurologic Disease, Vol 2. Edited by Benson DF, Blumer D. New York, Grune & Stratton, 1982, pp 149–165

Davis KL, Mohs RC: Enhancement of memory processes in Alzheimer's disease with multiple-dose intravenous physostigmine. Am J Psychiatry 139:1421–1424, 1982

Davis KL, Thal LJ, Gamzu ER, et al: A double-blind, placebo-controlled multicenter study of tacrine for Alzheimer's disease. N Engl J Med 327:1253–1259, 1992

DeCarli C, Kaye JA, Horowitz B, et al: Critical analysis of the use of computer-assisted transverse axial tomography to study human brain in aging and dementia of the Alzheimer's type. Neurology 40:872–883, 1990

Dening DC, Berrios GE: Wilson's disease: psychiatric symptoms in 195 cases. Arch Gen Psychiatry 46:1126–1134, 1989

Dietch JT: Computerized tomographic scanning in cases of dementia. West J Med 138:835–837, 1983

Emery VO, Oxman TE: Update on the dementia spectrum of depression. Am J Psychiatry 149:305–317, 1992

Erkinjuntti T, Haltia M, Palo J, et al: Accuracy of the clinical diagnosis of vascular dementia: a prospective clinical and post-mortem neuropathological study. J Neurol Neurosurg Psychiatry 51:1037–1044, 1988

Espinoza MT, Parer JT: Mechanisms of asphyxial brain damage and possible pharmacologic interventions in the fetus. Am J Obstet Gynecol 164:1582–1591, 1991

Farlow M, Gracon SI, Hershey LA, et al: A controlled trial of tacrine in Alzheimer's disease. JAMA 268:2523–2529, 1992

Fisher CM: Binswanger's encephalopathy: a review. J Neurol 236:65–79, 1989

Flores-Runk P, Raasch RH: Ticlopidine and antiplatelet therapy. Ann Pharmacother 27:1090–1098, 1993

Folstein MF, McHugh PR: Dementia syndrome of depression, in Alzheimer's Disease: Senile Dementia and Related Disorders. Edited by Katzman R, Terry RD, Bick KL. New York, Raven, 1978, pp 87–93

Folstein MF, Folstein SE, McHugh PR: Mini-Mental State: a practical method for grading the cognitive state of patients for the clinician. J Psychiatr Res 12:189–198, 1975

Folstein SE, Brandt J, Folstein MF: Huntington's disease, in Subcortical Dementia. Edited by Cummings JL. New York, Oxford University Press, 1990, pp 87–107

Friedland RP: "Normal"-pressure hydrocephalus and the saga of the treatable dementias. JAMA 262:2577–2581, 1989

Giacometti AR, Davis PC, Alazraki NP, et al: Anatomic and physiologic imaging of Alzheimer's disease. Clin Geriatr Med 10:277–298, 1994

Gibb WRG: Dementia and Parkinson's disease. Br J Psychiatry 154:596–614, 1989

Gibb WRG, Luthert PJ, Janota I, et al: Cortical Lewy body dementia: clinical features and classification. J Neurol Neurosurg Psychiatry 52:185–192, 1989

Gorman DG, Cummings JL: Neurobehavioral presentations of the antiphospholipid antibody syndrome. J Neuropsychiatry Clin Neurosci 5:37–42, 1993

Graham DI, Adams JH, Gennarelli TA: Pathology of brain damage in head injury, in Head Injury, 2nd Edition. Edited by Cooper PR. Baltimore, MD, Williams & Wilkins, 1987, pp 72–88

Gray KF, Cummings JL: Neuroimaging in dementia, in Localization and Neuroimaging in Neuropsychology. Edited by Kertesz A. San Diego, CA, Academic Press, 1994, pp 621–651

Green J, Morris JC, Sandson J, et al: Progressive aphasia: a precursor of global dementia? Neurology 40:423–429, 1990

Hachinski VC, Iliff LD, Zilhka E, et al: Cerebral blood flow in dementia. Arch Neurol 32:632–637, 1975

Holmes VF, Fernandez F, Levy JK: Psychostimulant response in AIDS-related complex patients. J Clin Psychiatry 50:5–8, 1989

Holthoff VA, Sandmann J, Pawlik G, et al: Positron emission tomography in Creutzfeldt-Jakob disease. Arch Neurol 47:1035–1038, 1990

Hsiao K, Prusiner SB: Inherited human prion diseases. Neurology 40:1820–1827, 1990

Huber SJ, Shuttleworth EC, Christy JA, et al: Magnetic resonance imaging in dementia of Parkinson's disease. J Neurol Neurosurg Psychiatry 52:1221–1227, 1989

Jennett B, Teasdale G: Management of Head Injuries. Philadelphia, PA, FA Davis, 1981, pp 271–288

Jibiki I, Fukushima T, Kobayashi K, et al: Utility of 123I-IMP SPECT brain scans for the early detection of site-specific abnormalities in Creutzfeldt-Jakob disease (Heidenhain type): a case study. Neuropyschobiology 29:117–119, 1994

Jones BN, Reifler BV: Depression coexisting with dementia: evaluation and treatment. Med Clin North Am 78:823–840, 1994

Jordan BD: Neurologic aspects of boxing. Arch Neurol 44:453–459, 1987

Kertesz A, Black SE, Nicholson L, et al: The sensitivity and specificity of MRI in stroke. Neurology 37:1580–1585, 1987

Keschner M, Bender MB, Strauss I: Mental symptoms associated with brain tumor: a study of 530 verified cases. JAMA 110:714–718, 1938

Khachaturian ZS: Diagnosis of Alzheimer's disease. Arch Neurol 42:1097–1105, 1985

Kunik ME, Yudofsky SC, Silver MJ, et al: Pharmacologic approach to management of agitation associated with dementia. J Clin Psychiatry 55(suppl):13–17, 1994

Kunz U, Heintz P, Ehrenheim C, et al: MRI as the primary diagnostic instrument in normal pressure hydrocephalus? Psychiatry Res 29:287–288, 1989

Kyomen HH, Nobel KW, Wei JY: The use of estrogen to decrease aggressive physical behavior in elderly men with dementia. J Am Geriatr Soc 39:1110–1112, 1991

Levin HS: Memory deficit after closed-head injury. J Clin Exp Neuropsychol 12:129–153, 1989

Levin HS: A guide to clinical neuropsychological testing. Arch Neurol 51:854–859, 1994

Levin HS, Benton AL, Gassman RG: Neurobehavioral Consequences of Closed Head Injury. New York, Oxford University Press, 1982, pp 73–122

Levy-Lahad E, Wijsman EM, Nemens E, et al: A familial Alzheimer's disease locus on chromosome 1. Science 269:970–973, 1995

Lipowski ZJ: Delirium: Acute Confusional States. New York, Oxford University Press, 1990, pp 47–53

Lishman WA: Cerebral disorder in alcoholism: syndromes of impairment. Brain 104:1–20, 1981

Lishman WA: Organic Psychiatry. Oxford, Blackwell Scientific, 1987, pp 404–413

Lishman WA: Physiogenesis and psychogenesis in the "post-concussional syndrome." Br J Psychiatry 153:460–469, 1988

Luby JP: Infections of the central nervous system. Am J Med Sci 304:379–391, 1992

Mace NL, Rabins PV: The 36-Hour Day. Baltimore, MD, Johns Hopkins University Press, 1991, pp 116–143

Maher ER, Lees AJ: The clinical features and natural history of the Steele-Richardson-Olszewski syndrome (progressive supranuclear palsy). Neurology 36:1005–1008, 1986

Mandell AM, Albert ML: History of subcortical dementia, in Subcortical Dementia. Edited by Cummings JL. New York, Oxford University Press, 1990, pp 17–30

Martilla RJ: Epidemiology, in Handbook of Parkinson's Disease, 2nd Edition. Edited by Koller WC. New York, Marcel Dekker, 1992, pp 35–57

Masters CL, Richardson EP Jr: Subacute spongiform encephalopathy (Creutzfeldt-Jakob disease)—the nature and progression of spongiform change. Brain 101:333–344, 1978

Matsuyama SS, Jarvik LJ: Hypothesis: microtubules, a key to Alzheimer disease. Proc Natl Acad Sci U S A 86:8152–8156, 1989

Mazure CM, Druss BG, Cellar JS: Valproate treatment of older psychotic patients with organic mental syndromes and behavioral dyscontrol. J Am Geriatr Soc 40:914–916, 1992

McAllister TW: Neuropsychiatric sequelae of head injuries. Psychiatr Clin North Am 15:395–413, 1992

McEvoy JP, Wells CE: Case studies in neuropsychiatry, II: conversion pseudodementia. J Clin Psychiatry 40:447–449, 1979

McHugh PR, Folstein MF: Psychiatric syndromes of Huntington's chorea: a clinical and phenomenologic study, in Psychiatric Aspects of Neurologic Disease. Edited by Benson DF, Blumer D. New York, Grune & Stratton, 1975, pp 267–286

Mendez MF, Underwood KL, Zander BA, et al: Risk factors in Alzheimer's disease. Neurology 42:770–775, 1992

Merskey H, Buhrich NA: Hysteria and organic brain disease. Br J Med Psychol 48:359–366, 1975

Meyer JS, McClintic KL, Rogers RL, et al: Aetiological considerations and risk factors for multi-infarct dementia. J Neurol Neurosurg Psychiatry 51:1489–1497, 1988

Meyer JS, Rogers RL, McClintic K, et al: Randomized clinical trial of daily aspirin therapy in multi-infarct dementia: a pilot study. J Am Geriatr Soc 37:549–555, 1989

Miller BL, Benson DF, Goldberg MA, et al: The misdiagnosis of hysteria. Am Fam Physician 34:157–160, 1986

Miller BL, Cummings JL, Villanueva-Meyer J, et al: Frontal lobe degeneration: clinical, neuropsychological, and SPECT characteristics. Neurology 41:1374–1382, 1991

Miller GA: The magic number seven, plus or minus two: some limits on our capacity for processing information. Psychol Rev 63:81–97, 1956

Mirra SS, Hart MN, Terry RD: Making the diagnosis of Alzheimer's disease: a primer for practicing pathologists. Arch Pathol Lab Med 117:132–144, 1993

Molsa PK, Paljarvi L, Rinne JO, et al: Validity of clinical diagnosis in dementia: a prospective clinicopathological study. J Neurol Neurosurg Psychiatry 48:1085–1090, 1985

Navia BA: The AIDS dementia complex, in Subcortical Dementia. Edited by Cummings JL. New York, Oxford University Press, 1990, pp 181–198

Navia BA, Jordan BD, Price RW: The AIDS dementia complex, I: clinical features. Ann Neurol 19:517–524, 1986

Nielsen H, Lolk A, Pederson I, et al: The accuracy of early diagnosis and predictors of death in Alzheimer's disease and vascular dementia—a follow-up study. Acta Psychiatr Scand 84:277–282, 1991

Overman W Jr, Stoudemire A: Guidelines for legal and financial counseling of Alzheimer's disease patients and their families. Am J Psychiatry 145:1495–1500, 1988

Panzer MJ, Mellow AM: Antidepressant treatment of pathologic laughing or crying in elderly stroke patients. J Geriatr Psychiatry Neurol 5:195–199, 1992

Patten BM: Wilson's disease, in Parkinson's Disease and Movement Disorders, 2nd Edition. Edited by Jankovic J, Tolosa E. Baltimore, MD, Williams & Wilkins, 1993, pp 217–233

Paulson GW: The neurological examination in dementia, in Dementia, 2nd Edition. Edited by Wells CE. Philadelphia, PA, FA Davis, 1977, pp 169–188

Pearlson GD, Rabins PV, Kim WS, et al: Structural brain CT changes and cognitive deficits in elderly depressives with and without reversible dementia ("pseudodementia"). Psychol Med 19:573–584, 1989

Petersen RC, Smith GE, Ivnik RJ, et al: Memory function in very early Alzheimer's disease. Neurology 44:867–872, 1994

Pinner E, Rich CL: Effects of trazodone on aggressive behavior in seven patients with organic mental disorders. Am J Psychiatry 145:1295–1296, 1988

Price TRP, Goetz KL, Lovell MR: Neuropsychiatric aspects of brain tumors, in The American Psychiatric Press Textbook of Neuropsychiatry, 2nd Edition. Edited by Yudofsky SC, Hales RE. Washington, DC, American Psychiatric Press, 1992, pp 473–497

Quality Standards Subcommittee of the American Academy of Neurology: Practice parameters for diagnosis and evaluation of dementia (summary statement). Neurology 44:2203–2206, 1994

Rabins PV: Reversible dementia and the misdiagnosis of dementia: a review. Hosp Community Psychiatry 34:830–835, 1983

Radue EW, duBoulay GH, Harrison MJG, et al: Comparison of angiographic and CT findings between patients with multi-infarct dementia and those with dementia due to primary neuronal degeneration. Neuroradiology 16:113–115, 1978

Raia PA: Helping patients and families to take control. Psychiatric Annals 24:192–196, 1994

Rapcsak SZ, Croswell SC, Rubens AB: Apraxia in Alzheimer's disease. Neurology 39:664–668, 1989

Reding M, Haycox J, Blass J: Depression in patients referred to a dementia clinic: a three-year prospective study. Arch Neurol 42:894–896, 1985

Reichman WE, Cummings JL: Diagnosis of rare dementia syndromes: an algorithmic approach. J Geriatr Psychiatry Neurol 3:73–84, 1990

Reisberg B: Functional assessment staging (FAST). Psychopharmacol Bull 24:653–659, 1988

Rich S, Ovsiew F: Leuprolide acetate for exhibitionism in Huntington's disease. Mov Disord 9:353–357, 1994

Robinson RG, Starkstein SE: Current research in affective disorders following stroke. J Neuropsychiatry Clin Neurosci 2:1–14, 1990

Roman GC, Tatemichi TK, Erkinjuntti T, et al: Vascular dementia: diagnostic criteria for research studies. Report of the NINDS-AIREN international workshop. Neurology 43:250–260, 1993

Romanelli MF, Morris JC, Ashkin K, et al: Advanced Alzheimer's disease is a risk factor for late-onset seizures. Arch Neurol 47:847–850, 1990

Rosen WG, Terry RD, Fuld PA, et al: Pathological verification of ischemic score in differentiation of dementias. Ann Neurol 7:486–488, 1980

Roses AD: Apolipoprotein E genotyping in the differential diagnosis, not prediction, of Alzheimer's disease. Ann Neurol 38:6–14, 1995

Royall DR, Mahurin RK, Gray KF: Bedside assessment of executive cognitive impairment: the Executive Interview. J Am Geriatr Soc 40:1221–1226, 1992

Ruberg RM, Javoy-Agid F, Hirsh E, et al: Dopaminergic and cholinergic lesions in progressive supranuclear palsy. Ann Neurol 18:523–529, 1985

Sachon C, Grimaldi A, Digy JP, et al: Cognitive function, insulin-dependent diabetes and hypoglycaemia. J Intern Med 231:471–475, 1992

Scharf MB, Saskin P, Fletcher K: Benzodiazepine-induced amnesia: clinical laboratory findings. J Clin Psychiatry 5 (monograph):14–17, 1987

Schellenberg GD, Bird TD, Wijsman EM, et al: Genetic linkage evidence for a familial Alzheimer's disease locus on chromosome 14. Science 258:668–671, 1992

Schneider LS, Sobin PB: Non-neuroleptic medications in the management of agitation in Alzheimer's disease and other dementia: a selective review. International Journal of Geriatric Psychiatry 6:691–708, 1991

Schneider LS, Pollock VE, Lyness SA: A meta-analysis of controlled trials of neuroleptic treatment in dementia. J Am Geriatr Soc 38:553–563, 1990

Selecki BR: Intracranial space-occupying lesions among patients admitted to mental hospitals. Med J Aust 1:383–390, 1965

Skoldenberg B: Herpes simplex encephalitis. Scand J Infect Dis Suppl 80:40–46, 1991

Skoog I: Risk factors for vascular dementia: a review. Dementia 5:137–144, 1994

Small GW: Dementia and amnestic syndromes, in Treatments of Psychiatric Disorders: A Task Force Report of the American Psychiatric Association. Washington, DC, American Psychiatric Association, 1989, pp 815–831

Sobin P, Schneider L, McDermott H: Fluoxetine in the treatment of agitated dementia (letter). Am J Psychiatry 146:1636, 1989

Starosta-Rubinstein S, Young AB, Kluin K, et al: Clinical assessment of 31 patients with Wilson's disease. Arch Neurol 44:365–370, 1987

Steele C, Lucas MJ, Tune L: Haloperidol versus thioridazine in the treatment of behavioral symptoms in senile dementia of the Alzheimer's type: preliminary findings. J Clin Psychiatry 47:310–312, 1986

Steele JC, Richardson JC, Olszewski J: Progressive supranuclear palsy: a heterogeneous degeneration involving the brain stem, basal ganglia, and cerebellum with vertical gaze and pseudobulbar palsy, nuchal dystonia and dementia. Arch Neurol 10:333–359, 1964

Strub RL, Black FW: The Mental Status Examination in Neurology, 3rd Edition. Philadelphia, PA, FA Davis, 1993

Tatemichi TK: How acute brain failure becomes chronic: a view of the mechanisms of dementia related to stroke. Neurology 40:1652–1659, 1990

Tatemichi TK, Desmond DW, Prohovnik I: Strategic infarcts in vascular dementia: a clinical and brain imaging experience. Arzneimittelforschung 45:371–385, 1995

Thomas RJ: Blinking and the release reflexes: are they clinically useful? J Am Geriatr Soc 42:609–613, 1994

Tiller JWG, Dakis JA, Shaw JM: Short-term buspirone treatment in disinhibition with dementia (letter). Lancet 2:510, 1988

Tomlinson BE, Blessed G, Roth M: Observations on the brains of demented old people. J Neurol Sci 11:205–242, 1970

U.S. Congress Office of Technology Assessment: Losing a Million Minds: Confronting the Tragedy of Alzheimer's Disease and Other Dementias (OTA-BA-323). Washington, DC, U.S. Government Printing Office, 1987, pp 3–55

Van Duijn CM, Tanja TA, Haaxma R, et al: Head trauma and the risk of Alzheimer's disease. Am J Epidemiol 135:775–782, 1992

Vanneste JA: Three decades of normal pressure hydrocephalus: are we wiser now? J Neurol Neurosurg Psychiatry 57:1021–1025, 1994

Victor M, Adams RD, Collins GH: The Wernicke-Korsakoff Syndrome and Related Neurologic Disorders Due to Alcoholism and Malnutrition, 2nd Edition. Philadelphia, PA, FA Davis, 1989

Vinters HV: Pathologic issues in the diagnosis of Alzheimer disease. Bulletin of Clinical Neurosciences 56:39–47, 1991

Vinters HV, Miller BL, Pardridge WM: Brain amyloid and Alzheimer disease. Ann Intern Med 109:41–54, 1988

Wells CE: Pseudodementia. Am J Psychiatry 136:895–900, 1979

Whatley SA, Anderton BH: The genetics of Alzheimer's disease. International Journal of Geriatric Psychiatry 5:145–159, 1990

Zec RF: Neuropsychological functioning in Alzheimer's disease, in Neuropsychology of Alzheimer's Disease and Other Dementias. Edited by Parks RW, Zec RF, Wilson RF. New York, Oxford University Press, 1993, pp 3–80

Zola-Morgan S, Squire LR, Amaral DG: Human amnesia and the medial temporal region: enduring memory impairment following a bilateral lesion limited to the CA1 field of the hippocampus. J Neurosci 6:2950–2967, 1986

Zubenko GS, Rosen JR, Sweet RA, et al: Impact of psychiatric hospitalization on behavioral complications of Alzheimer's disease. Am J Psychiatry 149:1484–1491, 1992

Chapter 9

Depression

Alvin M. Rouchell, M.D.
Richard Pounds, M.D.
John G. Tierney, M.D.

Depression in medically ill patients is an important clinical entity (Cassem 1991; Rodin et al. 1991). Although major depressive disorder occurs in 3.7%–6.7% of the general population (Robins et al. 1984), the prevalence of major depression is 10%–14% among general medical inpatients and 9%–16% among general medical outpatients (Katon 1987; Katon and Schulberg 1992; Perez-Stable et al. 1990; Schulberg et al. 1985).

UNDERDIAGNOSIS AND UNDERTREATMENT

Even though depression occurs commonly in medically ill patients, it is underdiagnosed and undertreated (Katon 1987; Perez-Stable et al. 1990; Sliman et al. 1992). Fewer than one-half of all depressed patients are identified and adequately treated by primary care physicians (Prestidge and Lake 1987). The most common cause for the underdiagnosis and undertreat-

ment of depression in medical patients is the mistaken notion that if a depression is understandable, explainable, and reactive to environmental circumstances, then it is neither pathological nor requires treatment (Rifkin 1992).

MORBIDITY AND MORTALITY

The presence of major or minor depression in a medically ill patient has a significant effect on the patient's morbidity and mortality. In one study, the presence of major depressive disorder was the best predictor of myocardial infarction, angioplasty, and death during the 12 months following cardiac catheterization (Carney et al. 1988). In another study, major depression in patients hospitalized following a myocardial infarction was an independent risk factor for mortality at 6-month follow-up (Frasure-Smith et al. 1993). Morris et al. (1993) reported that patients with either major or minor depression following a stroke were 3.4 times more likely to die during a 10-year period than patients without depression. Patients with poststroke depression and few social contacts were particularly vulnerable—more than 90% died. Silverstone (1990) examined the effect of depressive mood on patients with acute, life-threatening medical illnesses (myocardial infarction, subarachnoid hemorrhage, pulmonary embolus, and upper gastrointestinal hemorrhage). He reported that 47% of these depressed patients either died or had further life-threatening complications, whereas only 10% of the nondepressed patients died or had further complications. Depressed mood is also associated with an increased risk of death in home dialysis patients. In addition to depressed mood, these high-risk patients typically exhibit preoccupation with somatic complaints, degradation of self, despondency, and pessimism (Burton et al. 1986).

ECONOMICS

Adverse economic consequences occur when depression complicates the inpatient or outpatient course of a medical illness. Von Korff et al. (1992) estimated that high utilizers of medical resources, who were 15% of their health maintenance organization (HMO) patient population, accounted for 64% of the total health care costs. Moreover, in this same HMO patient population, 23.5% of the high utilizers had current major depression, and 16.8% had dysthymic disorder (Katon et al. 1990). Among patients in one family practice clinic, depressed high utilizers scheduled nearly twice as many visits, placed more telephone calls, and had more laboratory testing than the remainder of the patients in the clinic population (Katon 1991). Successful treatment of depressed high utilizers significantly reduced disability days and scores on disability scales at 1-year follow-up (Von Korff et al. 1992).

DEPRESSION AS THE INITIAL MANIFESTATION OF PHYSICAL ILLNESS

Depression may precede the other signs and symptoms of many medical conditions. Depressive and other psychological symptoms were the initial manifestations of cancer of the pancreas in 22 of one series of 46 patients; furthermore, the psychological symptoms preceded the physical symptoms by as many as 43 months (Fras et al. 1967). Major depression is sometimes present in patients with Cushing's disease, Addison's disease, hyperthyroidism, and hypothyroidism even before the classic endocrine signs and symptoms are evident (Fava et al. 1987). In Huntington's disease (HD), primary or secondary depression may appear decades before the neurological symptoms (Folstein et al. 1983).

DIAGNOSIS

History of Present Illness

A thorough history of the present illness is essential to properly evaluate depression in a medically ill patient. The history confirms the presence of depressive symptoms and excludes other psychiatric disorders. Suicidal potential must be assessed. In addition, the clinician should identify psychosocial factors that contribute to the depression. Furthermore, the history and review of systems may provide the first clues to an underlying medical condition (Rodin and Voshart 1986). A complete list of drugs—prescribed, over-the-counter, and illicit—may help to identify substances that exacerbate or cause depression (Cassem 1991).

Neurovegetative symptoms of depression are often difficult to differentiate from the physical symptoms of medical conditions and the side effects from the treatment of those medical disorders. At times, however, careful exploration of the vegetative symptoms may suggest a medical etiology, especially if the consultation-liaison psychiatrist is knowledge-able about these effects. Vegetative symptoms in the medically ill patient with depression are usually multiple and more severe than symptoms arising solely from the medical condition (Cameron 1990).

Mental Status Examination

When Winokur (1990) compared depressive syndromes that followed medical conditions with those that were preceded by other psychiatric disorders, he found that subtle cognitive changes were more common in the medically ill group. Minor changes in speech production, fluency, or word finding are often the only mental status findings indicative of general medical or substance-related organic mood disorder (Dietch and Zetin 1983).

Past History

Past history is an important consideration in the differential diagnosis of the patient's current condition. Most patients with primary depression have a positive history for mood disorders (Wise and Rundell 1994). In contrast, only 20% of patients with a DSM-III-R (American Psychiatric Association 1987) organic mood disorder have a history of depression (Yates et al. 1991).

Family History

The family history in patients with secondary depression is often negative for mood disorders (Popkin et al. 1987). A positive family history of depression increases the likelihood that the patient's current difficulties are due to a primary depression (Cameron 1990).

Physical Examination

The physical examination, with emphasis on the neurological portion, is crucial in detecting medical conditions that are sometimes missed by the referring physician (Koranyi 1979). Table 9–1 outlines pertinent physical findings in depressed patients that might indicate a concurrent medical illness.

Routine Laboratory Studies

A complete blood count (CBC), blood chemistries, thyroid function tests, and urinalysis with toxicology screen identify many toxic and medically induced depressions. In addition, some clinicians routinely obtain chest X ray, electrocardiogram (ECG), and cortisol levels. With newer, more accurate assaying techniques, thyroid-stimulating hormone (TSH) levels are usually sufficient for thyroid disorder screening (Goldman 1992). Arterial blood gases or oxygen saturation measurements are sometimes necessary to rule out respiratory causes of fatigue and weakness (Dietch and Zetin 1983). An electroencephalogram (EEG) is needed when the history suggests a diagnosis of epilepsy or a hypoactive delirium misdiagnosed as depression. Toxicology and blood levels are helpful in the diagnosis of drug abuse and medication-induced depression. Computed tomography (CT) and magnetic resonance imaging (MRI) scans are sometimes necessary to evaluate depressed patients with central nervous system (CNS) disorders.

SPECIFIC MEDICAL CONDITIONS AND DEPRESSION

Major depression is seen more commonly in patients with certain medical conditions (Table 9–2). Several possible relations exist between depression and medical illnesses. The depression can predate the medical condition and thus represent a contributing cause or an early manifestation of that illness. At other times, the depression may occur after the medical condition. In these cases, the depression can be a pathophysiological result of the medical illness and/or a psychological reaction to the physical disorder. In some patients, depression and a medical illness can coexist but are etiologically

Table 9–1.   Physical findings and possible diagnoses in medically ill patients with depressive symptoms

System	Physical findings	Possible diagnoses	System	Physical findings	Possible diagnoses
General appearance	Weight loss	Depression		Scar	Thyroid surgery
		Cancer			
		Hyperthyroidism	Eyes	Pinpoint pupils	Opiate intoxication
		AIDS		Dilated pupils	Anticholinergic drugs
		Cocaine abuse			
	Weight gain	Atypical depression			Cocaine abuse
		Hypothyroidism		Nystagmus	Multiple sclerosis
		Cushing's syndrome			Drug toxicity
		Psychotropic drugs		Exophthalmos	Hyperthyroidism
		Antihistaminic drugs	Throat	Tongue scar	Epilepsy
	Jaundice	Hepatitis	Heart	Tachycardia	Hyperthyroidism
		Alcoholism			Withdrawal syndromes
		Drug abuse			Cocaine abuse
	Pallor	Anemia		Bradycardia	Hypothyroidism
	Motor activity				
	Tremor	Parkinson's disease	Abdomen	Red striae	Cushing's syndrome
		Huntington's chorea		Hepatomegaly	Alcoholism
		Hyperthyroidism			
		Withdrawal syndromes	Extremities	Pretibial edema	Hypothyroidism
	Hemiparesis	Stroke			
	Agitation/ retardation	Depression	Neurological	Facial asymmetry, hemiparesis	Stroke
		Withdrawal syndromes		Masklike facies, tremor, shuffling gait	Parkinsonism Neuroleptics
	Truncal obesity	Cushing's syndrome			
Skin	Hyperpigmentation	Addison's disease		Scanning speech, ataxia, nystagmus	Multiple sclerosis
	Needle tracks	Drug abuse		Choreiform movements	Huntington's disease
	Pigmented lesions	Kaposi's sarcoma		Delayed deep tendon reflexes	Hypothyroidism
Head	Masklike facies	Parkinson's disease		Asymmetrical reflexes	Stroke
	Moon facies	Cushing's syndrome			
Neck	Goiter	Hyperthyroidism			
		Hypothyroidism			

Note.   AIDS = acquired immunodeficiency syndrome.
Source.   Adapted from Summers et al. 1981.

Table 9–2. Likelihood of developing major depression following diagnosis of specific medical conditions

Condition	Prevalence (%)	Reference
Hemodialysis	6.5	Hinrichsen et al. 1989
Coronary artery disease	18	Carney et al. 1987
	19	Forrester et al. 1992
	18	Schleifer et al. 1989
	16	Frasure-Smith et al. 1993
Cancer	25–38	Kathol et al. 1990
	20	Massie and Holland 1990
Chronic pain	32	Katon et al. 1985
	21	Sullivan et al. 1992
Neurological disorders		
Stroke	27	Robinson et al. 1990
Parkinson's disease	28.6	Mayeux et al. 1986
	51	Sano et al. 1989
Multiple sclerosis	6–57	Minden and Schiffer 1990
	37	Schiffer et al. 1983
Epilepsy	55	Mendez et al. 1986
Huntington's disease	41	Folstein et al. 1983
Dementia	11	Greenwald et al. 1989
Endocrine conditions		
Hyperthyroidism	31	Kathol et al. 1986
Diabetes mellitus	24	Popkin et al. 1988
Cushing's syndrome	66.6	Haskett 1985
HIV disease	30.3	Atkinson et al. 1988
Chronic fatigue	17.2	Cathebras et al. 1992
	46.4	Kreusi et al. 1989

Note. HIV = human immunodeficiency virus.

unrelated (Dietch and Zetin 1983; Rodin et al. 1991).

End-Stage Renal Disease/Dialysis

Hinrichsen et al. (1989) utilized the Research Diagnostic Criteria (RDC; Spitzer et al. 1978) to evaluate 124 patients with end-stage renal disease and found a prevalence rate for current major depression of 6.5% and for minor depression of 17.7% (see also Cohen, "Renal Disease" section, Chapter 17, in this volume). The presence of suicidal ideation, depressed mood, and discouragement helped to discriminate depressed from nondepressed dialysis patients. The importance of identifying depressed dialysis patients is indicated by a suicide rate that may be 100–400 times that of the general population (Burton et al. 1986).

Coronary Artery Disease

Depression in patients with coronary artery disease (CAD) is associated with poor psychosocial rehabilitation and increased mortality (see also Halperin, "Heart Disease" section, Chapter 17, and Pasnau et al., Chapter 18, in this volume). Carney et al. (1987) found that

18% of patients with coronary angiograms that proved CAD met DSM-III (American Psychiatric Association 1980) criteria for major depression. Forrester et al. (1992) found similar results in 129 patients following myocardial infarction; 19% of these patients met DSM-III criteria for major depression. The depressed group was characterized by a positive history for depression, female gender, large infarcts, severe functional physical impairment, and poor social relationships. Three months after myocardial infarction, most patients with major depression were still depressed and had not returned to work (Schleifer et al. 1989). In a prospective study, Frasure-Smith and colleagues (1993) evaluated 222 patients within 1 week following myocardial infarction. Thirty-five (16%) met DSM-III-R criteria for major depression. Six months later, 17% of the depressed, and only 3% of the nondepressed, patients had died. This difference in mortality rates was independent of cardiac factors.

Cancer

The frequency of depressive disorders reported in cancer patients varies widely, depending on tumor type, patient population, and diagnostic criteria (see also Fawzy and Greenberg, Chapter 20, in this volume). The diagnosis of depression in cancer patients is further complicated by the presence of physical symptoms of the cancer or its treatment that are difficult to distinguish from the vegetative symptoms of depression.

Massie and Holland (1990) diagnosed DSM-III-R major depression in 20% and adjustment disorder with depressed mood in 27% of 546 inpatient and outpatient psychiatric consultations on cancer patients. They indicated that risk factors for depressive disorders in cancer patients include history of mood disorder; alcoholism; advanced stages of cancer; poorly controlled pain; and concurrent medical illnesses or medications, such as chemotherapy agents, known to cause depression.

Chronic Pain

Pain is a frequent complaint in patients in medical settings and is often comorbid with major depression and alcoholism (see also Bouckoms, Chapter 31, in this volume). Katon et al. (1985) diagnosed DSM-III major depressive disorder in 32.4% of 37 patients with chronic pain; 43.2% of all the chronic pain patients had a history of major depression, and 40.5% of the total were concurrently abusing alcohol. In a review of the literature, Sullivan et al. (1992) concluded that cognitive-behavior therapy and tricyclic antidepressants were effective treatments for both depression and pain in patients with chronic low back pain.

CNS and Neurological Disorders

Stroke. Among CNS disorders, depression subsequent to stroke is the most extensively studied (see also Fricchione et al., Chapter 21, in this volume). Much of these data were gathered in the last 10 years by Robinson and colleagues (Robinson and Price 1982; Robinson et al. 1983, 1984a, 1984b, 1985, 1987, 1990).

Estimates of depression prevalence among poststroke patients range from 30% to 50% (mean, 38%) (Robinson and Price 1982; Robinson et al. 1983, 1984a, 1987). At the time of initial in-hospital evaluation, 26% of the 103 patients examined met the examiner's criteria for major depression, whereas 20% had minor depression. At the 6-month follow-up, 34% had symptoms of major depression, and 26% had symptoms of minor depression; thus, 60% of the sample received a diagnosis of a depressive syndrome.

Over the years, the Robinson group reported differences in clinical features of poststroke depression based on neuroanatomical location of the stroke and the time of onset of the depressive syndrome. They reported a higher frequency and severity of depression among patients with left- versus right-hemisphere lesions. They also reported the highest frequency of major depression with left anterior lesions (Robinson and Price 1982; Robinson et al. 1983, 1984a). Some of the clinical features of poststroke depression reported by the Robinson group to date are listed in Table 9–3.

Four studies to date report the benefit of psychiatric treatment of patients with poststroke depression. Two of these studies were double-blind, prospective trials. First, Lipsey et al. (1984) showed that nortriptyline was more effective than placebo; second, Reding et al. (1986) showed that trazodone was more effective than placebo. The other two studies were retrospective chart reviews that demonstrated the efficacy of electroconvulsive therapy (ECT) (Murray et al. 1986) and methylphenidate compared with placebo (Lingham et al. 1988). Studies that demonstrate how psychiatric interventions alter the rehabilitation, course, and prognosis of patients after stroke remain to be done.

Studies of the course and prognosis of poststroke depression reveal that 1) the high-risk period for depression extends for 2 years after the stroke; 2) major depression, left

Table 9–3. Clinical features of poststroke depression

Of patients with left frontal stroke, 70% had diagnosable depressive disorders when lesions were anterior (i.e., <40% of anterior-posterior distance from the frontal pole).

The closer the lesion is to the left frontal pole, the more severe the depression.

The larger the lesion is in the left frontal pole, the more severe the depression.

Severity of depression in bilateral stroke patients is more dependent on proximity of the stroke to the left frontal pole than on proximity to the right frontal or posterior pole.

Proximity to the left frontal pole is more important to severity of depression than is motor dominance (handedness) or language dominance.

During a 6-month follow-up period, the correlation between functional impairment, cognitive impairment, and social functioning is increased in the depressed patient.

untreated, has a natural course of about 1 year; and 3) minor depression, left untreated, has a chronic course of about 2 years (Lipsey et al. 1984; Robinson et al. 1984b, 1987). In a 10-year follow-up of stroke patients, Morris et al. (1993) reported that the presence of depression during acute phase poststroke recovery was associated with a more than threefold greater mortality during this 10-year period. This study highlighted the importance of psychiatric treatment to reduce morbidity and mortality after a stroke and the need for research into the relative efficacy of various interventions, including psychotherapy.

Dementia. In a literature review, Greenwald et al. (1989) cited prevalence estimates of depression as a complication of dementia ranging from 0% to 85%. The prevalence of depression varies between dementia of the Alzheimer's type (DAT) and multi-infarct dementia (MID). In a study of 30 patients with DAT and 15 patients with MID, Cummings et al. (1987) reported that 0% of patients with DAT had major depression and 17% had depression symptoms, whereas 26% of patients with MID had major depression and 60% had depression symptoms.

The biochemical underpinnings of depression in patients with DAT are similar to those of primary depression. Zubenko et al. (1990) compared depressed patients who had dementia with nondepressed patients who had dementia and reported a 10- to 20-fold reduction in the level of norepinephrine in the cortex, as well as relative preservation of choline acetyl transferase activity in subcortical regions, of the depressed patients. According to Cummings et al. (1987), the marked decrease in cholinergic function found in DAT may have clinical and biological implications; the cholinergic deficit in patients with DAT may offer some protection from severe depression and may help to explain the relative increase in occurrence of depression syndromes in patients with MID.

The same problems that complicate the diagnosis of depression and dementia hamper treatment studies. However, in one study, Greenwald et al. (1989) concluded that although initial treatment failures and intolerance of side effects were common, syndromal depressions that complicate dementia are treatable. They compared 10 patients with depression and dementia, 10 nondepressed patients with dementia, and 30 age-matched, depressed control subjects without dementia. All depressed patients were treated with conventional somatic antidepressant therapy (i.e., antidepressant medications or ECT). Seventy percent of the patients with depression and dementia responded to antidepressant treatment, and 73% of the depressed control group without dementia responded.

Parkinson's disease (PD).   Estimates of the prevalence of depression in patients with PD range from 25% to 70% (Cummings 1992); Cummings found that the average prevalence across nine studies was approximately 40%. Two 1990 studies also found that about half of the patients with depression met criteria for major depression and the other half met criteria for minor depression (Mayeux 1990; Starkstein et al. 1990).

Patients with PD at increased risk for depressive illness have a history of depression (Mayeux et al. 1981; Starkstein et al. 1990) and greater functional disability (Cummings 1992). Depression seems to be more common among patients with dopamine responsive signs (i.e., gait changes, akinesia, and rigidity) (Cummings 1992).

Four studies demonstrated the efficacy of psychopharmacological interventions in depressed patients with PD (Cummings 1992). Imipramine (Strang 1965) and desipramine (Laitinen 1969) decreased both depression and motor symptoms below baseline. Bupropion (Goetz et al. 1984) reportedly reduced depression in fewer than one-half and motor symptoms in fewer than one-third of depressed patients with PD. In a study of nortriptyline (Andersen et al. 1980), features of depression decreased but PD symptoms were unchanged. According to the Cummings review (1992), ECT relieved both mood and motor symptoms of PD in patients with depressive syndromes. However, reduction in the motor symptoms is usually short-lived (Burke et al. 1988; Cummings 1992; Douyon et al. 1989).

Huntington's disease.   HD is a genetically transmitted autosomal dominant disorder (with 100% penetrance) first described by George Huntington in 1872 (Whitehouse et al. 1992). The patients develop chorea and dementia; depression and behavioral changes can occur well before the movement disorder begins (Cummings and Benson 1992b; Folstein 1989).

HD is a rare disorder; consequently, estimates of the disorder's prevalence vary, and estimates of the occurrence of depression are even less precise. In a monograph, Folstein (1989) estimated the point prevalence of HD among Caucasians to be from 5 to 7 per 100,000. In a series of 88 patients with HD, Folstein et al. (1983) reported a prevalence of 41% for "major affective disorder" (p. 537). A retrospective study of suicide deaths among patients with HD revealed a suicide rate 2–23 times greater than that for age-matched groups without HD (Schoenfeld et al. 1984).

The duration of HD varies from 17 to 30 years (Martin and Gusella 1986), and to date there is no known treatment (Folstein 1989; Martin and Gusella 1986; Whitehouse et al. 1992). However, some success has been reported for the treatment of depressive syndromes associated with HD. Folstein (1989) and Folstein et al. (1983) reported efficacy of tricyclic antidepressants and ECT but called for formal trials of somatic therapies. Ford (1986) reported efficacy of monoamine oxidase inhibitors (MAOIs) in the treatment of three patients with HD and affective syndromes. Based on the high rate of suicide among these patients, vigilance for depression is clearly indicated.

Epilepsy. Epilepsy is common and affects approximately 1% of the population (Cummings 1985). Among patients with epilepsy, depression is the most common and important psychiatric disorder (Blumer 1991; Mendez et al. 1986).

Although the actual prevalence is unknown, a retrospective survey by Currie et al. (1971) of 666 patients with temporal-lobe epilepsy (TLE) reported depression in 11%. In a study of suicide among patients with epilepsy, Matthews and Barabas (1981) reported a suicide rate of 5% compared with 1.4% in the general population.

Multiple sclerosis. The prevalence of multiple sclerosis (MS) in the general population varies from 1 to 80 per 100,000 depending on the latitude (Adams and Victor 1989). The likelihood of developing clinical major depression following a diagnosis of MS is 27%–54% (Joffe et al. 1987; Minden and Schiffer 1990; Minden et al. 1987; Schiffer et al. 1983; Whitlock and Siskind 1980). In 1987, Minden et al. (1987) conducted a study of 50 outpatients with MS and found that 54% of patients had at least one major depressive episode since onset of their illness.

The etiology of depression in patients with MS is unknown. However, several studies add to the growing body of evidence that the brain injury associated with MS directly contributes to the prevalence of depression. In the same study cited in the previous paragraph, Minden et al. (1987) observed that the severity of depressive symptoms in MS was not associated with disability, type of disability, duration of illness, type of MS, clinical status, fatigability, sex, age, or socioeconomic status. Higher rates of depression were reported among patients with CNS lesions when patients with "cerebral" MS were compared with patients with "non-cerebral" MS and non-CNS disorders (Schiffer

et al. 1983; Whitlock and Siskind 1980). In summary, research suggests that

- Patients with MS have more depressive disturbances than does the general population (Minden et al. 1987).
- Patients with MS have more depressive syndromes than do patients with similarly disabling non-CNS lesions (Rabins et al. 1986).
- Patients with MS who have predominantly cerebral disease have increased rates of depression compared with patients with MS who have predominantly spinal disease (Schiffer et al. 1983).

HIV disease. The challenge for the consultation-liaison psychiatrist is to differentiate depressive syndromes from human immunodeficiency virus (HIV) encephalopathy (Cummings and Benson 1992a), CNS lymphoma, HIV-associated dementia, and constitutional features of HIV-related infections (Price et al. 1988) (see also Worth and Halman, Chapter 26, in this volume).

Although systematic data are not yet available, existing studies suggest that major depression, adjustment disorder, and suicide attempts are common in HIV-infected patients. For example, in a retrospective review, Perry and Tross (1984) reported that 17.3% of patients with acquired immunodeficiency syndrome (AIDS) met DSM-III criteria for major depression (Holmes et al. 1989). Suicide rates are considerably higher among HIV-seropositive individuals than in the general population. Marzuk and associates (1988) reported that men ages 20–59 years with a diagnosis of AIDS are approximately 36 times more likely to commit suicide than age-matched men in the general population.

Endocrine Disorders

Hyperthyroidism. Major depressive episodes are seen in as many as 31% of patients with hyperthyroidism (Kathol et al. 1986). Depressed patients with hyperthyroidism tend to be older, appear more ill, and lose more weight than nondepressed patients with hyperthyroidism. Depressed thyrotoxic patients should be treated with care because antidepressant medications may exacerbate the symptomatology of hyperthyroidism (Folks 1984). Fortunately, major depression in these patients almost always responds favorably to antithyroid therapy alone (Kathol et al. 1986).

Hypothyroidism. Hypothyroidism is usually the result of ablation of the thyroid gland, autoimmune thyroiditis, or lithium therapy. Hypothyroidism may occur in as many as 10% of patients taking lithium and is much more likely to occur in women (Goldman 1992). The association between clinical hypothyroidism and depression is well known. In addition to depression, subclinical hypothyroidism also causes cognitive dysfunction and rapid-cycling mood in patients with bipolar disorder (Haggerty et al. 1990). A corollary to the hypothesis that decreased levels of thyroid functioning cause depression is the concept that supplemental thyroid hormone favors recovery from depression. This is the rationale for the augmentation of tricyclic antidepressants with thyroid hormone in the treatment of drug-resistant depression (Joffe 1990).

In many patients with hypothyroidism, the depression responds to thyroid hormone replacement alone, but the response may take a prolonged time. When that is the case, antidepressants are indicated and efficacious (Goldman 1992; Joffe 1990).

Hyperparathyroidism. Depression occurs in about 30% of patients with primary hyperparathyroidism and is the most common neuropsychiatric clinical feature (Palmer 1983; Stewart and Broadus 1987). The severity of the cognitive and depressive symptoms parallels elevations in the serum calcium. Depression in patients with hyperparathyroidism usually abates quickly after correction of the calcium level. Occasionally, an antidepressant is necessary (Fava et al. 1987).

Diabetes mellitus. The point prevalence of DSM-III major depression in patients with insulin-dependent, type I diabetes mellitus is about 24% (Popkin et al. 1988). The level of depression correlates with the severity of the complications of the diabetes (Leedom et al. 1991) and the length of the illness (Palinkas et al. 1991).

Cushing's syndrome. *Cushing's syndrome* refers to hypercortisolism from any cause. *Cushing's disease* is the term used specifically for hypercortisolism due to adrenocorticotropic hormone (ACTH)-secreting tumors of the pituitary gland. Other causes of Cushing's syndrome are paraneoplastic, nonpituitary tumors that produce ACTH; adrenal adenomas; and corticosteroid medication. Exogenous steroids are more commonly linked to manic syndromes, especially with doses of prednisone greater than 40 mg/day, but Cushing's disease is highly associated with depression (Goldman 1992). Haskett (1985), in a series of 30 patients with Cushing's syndrome, reported that two-thirds met RDC for endogenous depression. These patients with Cushing's syndrome and depression were more irritable and emotionally labile compared with patients who had primary mood disorders.

Hyperprolactinemia. Although seizure disorder is the most common cause of transient hyperprolactinemia (Lishman 1987), sustained elevated levels of prolactin are usually due to hormone-secreting tumors, neuroleptic medication, pregnancy, oral contraceptives, renal failure, hypothyroidism, or cirrhosis (Goldman 1992). The depression among women with hyperprolactinemia is often severe enough to meet DSM-III criteria for major depression (Mastrogiacomo et al. 1983), whereas men usually have milder forms of depression with complaints of sadness, demoralization, and apathy.

Bromocriptine often reverses both the amenorrhea and the depression in hyperprolactinemic women (Fava et al. 1987).

Chronic fatigue syndrome. Fatigue is common in patients in primary care settings. Cathebras et al. (1992) studied 686 patients who presented to a family practice clinic and noted that 13.6% complained of fatigue. Almost half of these fatigued patients had a previous diagnosis of anxiety or depression during their lives. At the time of the complaint of fatigue, 17.2% fulfilled DSM-III criteria for major depression.

Kreusi et al. (1989) reviewed the case histories of 28 patients who met the Centers for Disease Control (CDC) criteria for chronic fatigue syndrome. The lifetime prevalence of major depression was 46.4% among these 28 patients with chronic fatigue. The physical symptoms of chronic fatigue preceded the psychiatric disorder in only 2 of 21 patients. Thus, the authors concluded that the psychiatric problems were more likely a cause of, not only a psychological reaction to, chronic fatigue syndrome.

MEDICATIONS AND SUBSTANCES ASSOCIATED WITH DEPRESSION

Consultation-liaison psychiatrists must be cautious in implicating medications as a cause for clinical depression. Although more than 100 medications are associated with depression, only a few have been clearly shown to cause depressive syndromes (Zelnik 1987) (Table 9–4). Many studies, especially the older ones, have serious methodological flaws.

Antihypertensive Medications

Reserpine. Depressive syndromes occur in 20% of patients taking reserpine; an additional 7% have a psychotic depression (Goodwin et al. 1972). Patients with psychotic depression

Table 9–4. Medications and psychoactive substances associated with depression

Antihypertensive medications
  Reserpine
  Methyldopa
  β-Blockers (in predisposed individuals)
Oral contraceptives
Steroids
Benzodiazepines
Histamine$_2$ receptor antagonists
  Cimetidine
  Ranitidine
Cancer chemotherapeutic agents
  Vincristine
  Vinblastine
  Procarbazine
  L-Asparaginase
  Amphotericin B
  Interferon
Psychoactive substances
  Alcohol
  Opiates
  Amphetamine or cocaine withdrawal

have a severely depressed mood, psychomotor changes, and diurnal worsening of the mood in the morning (Hall et al. 1980). In contrast to primary depression, anxiety, lack of guilt, and lack of self-deprecation are typical of reserpine-induced depression (Beers and Passman 1990). The depression is dose related and is more prevalent at doses greater than 0.5 mg/day (Ganzini et al. 1993). The latency period between exposure to reserpine and onset of the depression is generally 4–6 months (Zelnik 1987). This period may be the length of time required for depletion of serotonin, norepinephrine, and dopamine from CNS presynaptic storage vesicles (Hall et al. 1980).

Methyldopa. Ten percent of patients taking methyldopa become mildly to moderately depressed, and 7% develop a severe depression (Hall et al. 1980). In an extensive review of the literature, Paykel and colleagues (1982) identified 83 depressed patients out of 2,320 taking methyldopa, for a prevalence of only 3.6%. The onset of the depressive symptoms was fairly rapid; they occurred within a few days of starting the drug. Once the methyldopa was stopped, the depressive symptoms resolved within a week in most patients.

Propranolol and other β-blockers. Whether propranolol and the other β-blockers cause depression is controversial. Hall et al. (1980) indicated that some degree of depression occurred in 30%–50% of patients taking significant doses of propranolol. Petrie and associates (1982) established that propranolol can cause nonspecific fatigue and lassitude and cautioned against the use of these nonspecific symptoms to diagnose depression. These investigators also concluded that there was a dose-response relation between the severity of the depression and the dose of the β-blocker. Zelnik (1987) concluded that patients taking β-blockers who became depressed often had past histories or family histories of depression. The depressive symptoms typically cleared within a week after the medication was stopped.

Other antihypertensives. Fewer than 2% of patients taking clonidine or guanethidine become depressed (Paykel et al. 1982). Calcium channel blockers and angiotensin-converting enzyme (ACE) inhibitors are rarely associated with depression. On the contrary, ACE inhibitors may elevate mood, and caution is recommended when using them in patients with bipolar disorder (Rauch et al. 1991). Diuretics can cause weakness and apathy because of electrolyte changes. These symptoms are sometimes confused with depression (Beers and Passman 1990).

Oral Contraceptives

Shortly after the introduction of oral contraceptives into clinical practice, depressive symptoms were a frequently reported side effect; they occurred in 7%–34% of users (Herzberg and Coppen 1970). Depressive symptoms were associated with the amount of estrogen compared with progesterone (Hall et al. 1980). Modern low-dose estrogen preparations usually do not cause mood changes that satisfy DSM-III-R criteria for major depression (Patten and Lamarre 1992).

Steroids

Steroid reactions are diverse; of patients with steroid-related psychiatric syndromes, 40% have depression, 28% have hypomania, 8% have mixed manic and depressive features, 14% have psychosis, and 10% have delirium (Lewis and Smith 1983). The overall prevalence of steroid side effects is 6% (Kershner and Wang-Cheng 1989). The most discriminating factor is dose. Fewer than 2% of patients who receive less than 40 mg/day of prednisone develop psychiatric symptoms, compared with 4%–6% who receive 41–80 mg/day and 18.4% who receive more than 80 mg/day (Boston Collaborative Drug Surveillance Program 1972). Steroid reactions begin within the first week of treatment but may require 4–6 weeks to resolve after cessation of the medication (Hall et al. 1979). Low-dose neuroleptic medication is the treatment of choice for the acute episode; lithium prophylaxis can be useful in patients requiring high doses of steroids (Kershner and Wang-Cheng 1989).

Benzodiazepines

Smith and Salzman (1991) reviewed the relation between benzodiazepines and depression and concluded that 1) benzodiazepines occasionally are associated with depression and even suicide, 2) no one benzodiazepine is more likely to cause depression than any other, 3) higher doses of the medication are associated with greater risk for depression, and 4) decreasing the dose or stopping the benzodiazepine eliminates the depression in most cases. In contrast, Tiller and Schweitzer (1992) proposed that the benzodiazepines do not induce depression but rather unmask the depressive symptomatology in agitated patients with depression.

Cimetidine and Ranitidine

Even though delirium is the most common psychiatric side effect of the H_2-receptor antagonists, case reports of depression are also described (Pascualy and Veith 1989).

Cancer Chemotherapy Medications

Depression is reportedly seen with a variety of chemotherapy medications: vincristine, vinblastine, procarbazine, L-asparaginase, amphotericin B, and interferon (see also Chapter 20).

Psychoactive Substances

Depression is common among people who abuse drugs (Dackis and Gold 1992; Dorus and Senay 1980; see also Franklin and Frances, Chapter 13, in this volume). In particular, alcohol (K. M. Davidson and Ritson 1993), opiates (Rounsaville et al. 1982), amphetamine withdrawal (Kramer et al. 1967), or cocaine withdrawal (Gawin and Kleber 1986) can cause a substance-induced mood disorder with depressive features (American Psychiatric Association 1994; see Table 9–5).

Alcohol. The ingestion of alcohol at low doses enhances mood; however, at higher doses, alcohol causes dysphoric mood states (K. M. Davidson and Ritson 1993). According to various rating scales, more than half of alcoholic patients have symptoms of depression (Schuckit 1983). Some alcoholic patients develop an alcohol-induced depression that is indistinguishable from DSM-III major depression (Dackis et al. 1986; Schuckit 1983).

Most alcohol-induced depressions resolve between 2 days and 2 weeks following abstinence (Schuckit 1983). The focus of treatment is on sobriety (Dackis and Gold 1992). Antidepressants are usually not necessary unless the patient has a history of major depression that occurred during a period of abstinence (Dackis and Gold 1992; K. M. Davidson and Ritson 1993).

Opiates. Opiate addicts have high rates of depression. In a study of 157 patients who were addicted to opiates, 17% met RDC for major depression, and 60% had depressive symptoms (Rounsaville et al. 1982). Because opiate-induced depressions generally persist after abstinence, antidepressants are indicated and are usually effective (Dackis and Gold 1992; Rounsaville et al. 1982).

Cocaine withdrawal. People who are addicted to cocaine typically binge until their supply of cocaine is exhausted. The resulting "crash" begins within hours of abstinence, lasts for about 3 days, and is characterized by depressive symptoms, irritability, and anxiety (Satel et al. 1991). Gawin and Kleber (1986) evaluated 30 chronic cocaine abusers during withdrawal and determined that 13% fulfilled DSM-III criteria for major depression and 20% for dysthymic disorder. Even though symptoms are usually mild (Satel et al. 1991) and the emphasis in treatment is on abstinence (Dackis and Gold 1992), bromocriptine (Giannini et al. 1989), amantadine (Tennant and Sagherian 1987), and desipramine (Gawin and Kleber 1984) can attenuate the depressive symptoms and drug craving that occur in patients undergoing cocaine withdrawal.

COURSE AND PROGNOSIS

When depression accompanies a medical illness, each complicates the other. Katon and Schulberg (1992) showed that the severity of the initial depressive symptoms and the presence of a comorbid medical condition were the best predictors of persistence of depression.

Table 9–5. Comparison of DSM-IV mood disorder due to general medical condition or substance abuse with prior diagnostic categories[a]

DSM-III (1980) Organic affective syndrome	DSM-III-R (1987) Organic mood syndrome	DSM-IV (1994) Mood disorder due to a general medical condition	DSM-IV (1994) Substance-induced mood disorder
A. Predominant disturbance is in mood, with at least symptoms from criterion B for manic or major depressive episode	A. Prominent and persistent depressed, elevated, or expansive mood	A. Prominent and persistent disturbance in mood characterized by either (or both): 1. Depressed mood or markedly diminished interest or pleasure in all, or almost all, activities 2. Elevated, expansive, or irritable mood	A. Prominent and persistent disturbance in mood characterized by either (or both): 1. Depressed mood or markedly diminished interest or pleasure in all, or almost all, activities 2. Elevated, expansive, or irritable mood
B. Evidence from history, physical examination, or laboratory tests of a specific organic factor that is judged to be etiologically related to the disturbance	B. Evidence from the history, physical examination, or laboratory tests of a specific organic factor (or factors) judged to be etiologically related to the disturbance	B. Evidence from the history, physical examination, or laboratory findings that the disturbance is the direct physiological consequence of a general medical condition	B. Evidence from the history, physical examination, or laboratory findings of substance intoxication or withdrawal, and the symptoms in criterion A developed during, or within a month of, substance intoxication or withdrawal
C. No clouding of consciousness, as in delirium; no loss of intellectual abilities, as in dementia; no hallucinations or delusions, as in organic delusional syndrome or organic hallucinosis	C. Not occurring exclusively during the course of delirium	C. Disturbance is not better accounted for by another mental disorder	C. Disturbance is not better accounted for by a mood disorder that is not substance induced
		D. Disturbance does not occur exclusively during the course of a delirium	D. Disturbance does not occur exclusively during the course of a delirium
		E. Symptoms cause significant distress or impairment in social, occupational, or other important areas of functioning	E. Symptoms cause significant distress or impairment in social, occupational, or other important areas of functioning

[a]DSM-I and DSM-II did not list a comparable diagnosis.

The presence of depression is associated with higher morbidity and mortality in patients with CAD (Carney et al. 1988), myocardial infarction (Frasure-Smith et al. 1993), stroke (Morris et al. 1993; Robinson et al. 1990), acute life-threatening illnesses (Silverstone 1990), renal failure (Burton et al. 1986), and cancer (Shekelle et al. 1981).

◼ TREATMENT

Underlying Medical Conditions

Treatment of depression in medically ill patients is complex. Once the diagnosis of depression is established, the initial step in treatment is the identification of causative toxic or medical factors. All medical conditions should be treated. If the medical condition is chronic, then the depression should be treated in a manner similar to that for primary depression. Clinicians should reduce or discontinue medications thought to contribute to the depression. If the medical condition requires continued treatment, then the offending medication should be replaced with another medication that has comparable pharmacological activity but does not cause depression (Cameron 1990; Fava et al. 1987).

Psychopharmacology

As new agents join the established antidepressant drugs, the clinician has more flexibility in the pharmacological treatment of depression (see also Jachna et al., Chapter 30, in this volume). Selecting the correct medication is particularly important in treating depression in medically ill patients. Proper selection depends on side-effect profile, concurrent conditions and medications, target symptoms, and previous treatment responses.

Tricyclic and related agents. This group includes the tricyclic agents imipramine, amitriptyline, desipramine, nortriptyline, doxepin, clomipramine, and protriptyline. Trazodone and amoxapine are also included in this group. These agents are equally efficacious when given at therapeutically equivalent doses. The differences among these medications lie in the relative activity of each agent at the muscarinic, histaminic, noradrenergic, and serotonergic receptors.

Each of these compounds, except trazodone, has significant anticholinergic activity (Table 9–6); amitriptyline and clomipramine are particularly potent. Therapeutic doses of these agents are equivalent to several milligrams of atropine. Symptoms of anticholinergic action such as dry mouth, blurred vision, and constipation are often tolerated and may subside with time. More severe symptoms such as urinary retention, ileus, and anticholinergic delirium are particularly troublesome. Elderly patients and individuals taking other medications that have anticholinergic side effects are especially vulnerable to these complications.

Orthostatic hypotension is another serious potential complication of the tricyclic agents. The ability of an antidepressant to block the α_1 receptor is partially responsible for orthostasis. The resulting increased risk of falls in medically ill patients, especially the elderly, is a significant problem. Although the secondary amine nortriptyline is not entirely free of orthostatic properties, it is less likely to result in orthostasis than are other tricyclic antidepressants (Chutka 1990). The consultant must monitor supine and standing blood pressures at the initiation of treatment because significant changes typically begin at low doses.

Sedation is another common side effect that results in complications and noncompliance. Amitriptyline, clomipramine, doxepin, and trazodone are highly sedating. This effect is often advantageous in the early stages of treatment because it decreases insomnia, but early morning "hangover" at higher doses can significantly interfere with a patient's function-

Table 9–6. Affinities[a] for muscarinic acetyl cholinergic receptors

Drug	Affinity[b]	Affinity[c]
Antidepressants		
Amitriptyline (Elavil, Endep)	5.5	10.4
Protriptyline (Vivactil)	4.0	
Clomipramine (Anafranil)	2.7	
Trimipramine (Surmontil)	1.7	
Doxepin (Adapin, Sinequan)	1.3	4.3
Nortriptyline (Aventyl, Pamelor)	0.7	2.7
Imipramine (Tofranil)		2.1
Desipramine (Norpramin, Pertofrane)	0.5	1.5
Paroxetine (Paxil)	0.93	
Maprotiline (Ludiomil)	0.2	
Amoxapine (Asendin)	0.1	
Fluoxetine (Prozac)	0.05	0.17
Sertraline (Zoloft)	0.05	0.16
Nefazodone (Serzone)		0.009
Bupropion (Wellbutrin)	0.002	<0.003
Trazodone (Desyrel)	0.0003	<0.0003
Antipsychotics		
Thioridazine (Mellaril)	5.6	
Chlorpromazine (Thorazine)	1.4	
Mesoridazine (Serentil)	1.4	
Loxapine (Loxitane)	0.22	
Prochlorperazine (Compazine)	0.18	
Trifluoperazine (Stelazine)	0.15	
Perphenazine (Trilafon)	0.067	
Fluphenazine (Permitil, Prolixin)	0.053	
Thiothixene (Navane)	0.034	
Haloperidol (Haldol)	0.0042	
Molindone (Moban)	0.00026	
Atropine[d]	48	

[a]A higher number means greater antagonism.
[b]These values come from El-Fakahany and Richelson 1983 and J. L. Black et al. 1985.
[c]These values come from Cusack and Richelson 1993.
[d]Listed for comparison.
Source. Reprinted from El-Fakahany E, Richelson E: "Antagonism by Antidepressants of Muscarinic Acetylcholinergic Receptors in Human Brain." *British Journal of Pharmacology* 78:97–102, 1983; and Black JL, Richelson E, Richardson JW: "Antipsychotic Agents: A Clinical Update." *Mayo Clinic Proceedings* 60:777–789, 1985. Used with permission.

ing. Sedation and appetite stimulation relate to the antidepressant's activity at the CNS histamine$_1$ receptor.

The other major problem is that tricyclic agents possess a quinidine-like antiarrhythmic activity. This activity slows conduction and can prolong the QRS duration and the Q-T and P-R intervals. These effects are often evident at therapeutic levels and are of great concern in overdose. The use of tricyclic agents in patients with first-degree heart block or bundle-branch block could result in a higher-degree heart block. Tricyclic agents should be avoided in patients with second- and third-degree heart block or bifascicular or trifascicular block (Chutka 1990). Patients with hereditary prolongation of the Q-T intervals are also at risk (Moss and Robinson 1992); because 90% of these cases are familial, a good family history that explores sudden death and syncope is necessary. The ultimate evaluation of cardiac conduction is an ECG. The use of tricyclic antidepressants should be avoided when the corrected Q-T is greater than 440 msec. The antiarrhythmic activity of the tricyclic antidepressants and their lack of effect on left ventricular function in congestive heart failure (Roose et al. 1986) led to the conclusion that tricyclic antidepressants were safe in post–myocardial infarction patients, aside from the increased risk of orthostasis. Recent research raises concern because of reports of increased mortality when antiarrhythmics are prescribed to post–myocardial infarction patients and possibly even patients with cardiac ischemia (Glassman et al. 1993).

Selective serotonin reuptake inhibitors. The selective serotonin reuptake inhibitors (SSRIs) are a class of agents with a unique side-effect profile. Overall, these agents are well tolerated by medically ill patients with depression. The most common complaints are gastrointestinal upset, nervousness, sexual dysfunction, and insomnia. There is little clinical difference between the frequency of these side effects among the different SSRIs (Table 9–7). SSRIs do differ in the presence of active metabolites and elimination half-life. For example, fluoxetine, which has an elimination half-life of 1–3 days, is converted to norfluoxetine, which is an SSRI with a half-life of 7–9 days. Therefore, steady-state plasma levels are not reached for 5–6 weeks; a similar amount of time is required to eliminate norfluoxetine from the patient's system after discontinuation. Sertraline and paroxetine do not have this liability (Nemeroff 1993).

A troublesome aspect of many SSRIs is their inhibition of the cytochrome P450 II D6 system. Fluoxetine, paroxetine, and sertraline each inhibit this system to some degree. This enzyme system metabolizes antiarrhythmics, antidepressants, neuroleptics, codeine, oxycodone, and hydroxycodone (Ottson et al. 1993). In addition, as many as 7% of the Caucasian population are deficient in this enzyme and are considered slow metabolizers (Ottson et al. 1993). When SSRIs are used in medically ill patients, drugs metabolized by the P450 system can accumulate to toxic levels and must be monitored. Codeine and other similar opiates that require biotransformation for full activity are less effective (Ottson et al. 1993).

Newer antidepressants. Bupropion is a monocyclic phenylbutamine of the aminoketone type that is structurally similar to amphetamine (Weintraub and Evans 1989). Although the exact mechanism of action is unknown, bupropion inhibits the reuptake of dopamine at higher doses (Richelson 1988). After initial concerns about the incidence of seizures in bulimic patients (Horne et al. 1988), a subsequent study showed the actual risk to be 0.4% in depressed patients when the dose was less than 450 mg/day (Johnston et al. 1991). This incidence rate is comparable to that seen in patients receiving 200–300 mg/day of a tricyclic antidepressant (J. Davidson 1989). Nevertheless, patients who have a history of seizures or head trauma, have an epileptiform EEG, have anorexia or bulimia, or are on medications or have a neurological condition known to lower the seizure threshold should not receive bupropion (Stoudemire 1995). The advantages of bupropion are the result of its otherwise benign side-effect profile. Unlike the SSRIs, bupropion has a low incidence of sexual dysfunction (Walker et al. 1993). Additionally, bupropion is efficacious in patients with attention-deficit/hyperactivity disorder (Barrickman et al. 1995). The side effects of bupropion

Table 9–7. Side effects reported with selective serotonin reuptake inhibitors

	Fluoxetine/ Placebo (%)	Sertraline/ Placebo (%)	Paroxetine/ Placebo (%)
Nausea	21.1/10.1	26.1/11.8	25.7/9.3
Diarrhea	12.3/7.0	17.7/9.3	11.6/7.6
Dry mouth	9.5/6.0	16.3/9.3	18.1/12.1
Constipation	4.5/3.3	8.4/6.3	13.8/8.6
Nervousness	14.9/8.5	3.4/1.9	5.2/2.6
Agitation	9.4/5.5	2.6/1.3	2.1/1.9
Sexual dysfunction	1.9/0	Male 15.5/2.2	22.9/0
		Female 1.7/0.2	1.8/0
Insomnia	13.8/7.1	16.4/8.8	13.3/6.2
Drowsiness or somnolence	11.6/6.3	13.4/5.9	23.3/9.0
Headache	20.3/15.5	20.3/19.0	17.6/17.3

Source. Physicians' Desk Reference 1994.

are excessive stimulation, insomnia, tremor, and perceptual abnormalities in susceptible individuals (Weintraub and Evans 1989).

Venlafaxine is a phenylamine antidepressant that inhibits the presynaptic reuptake of serotonin, norepinephrine, and, to a lesser extent, dopamine without significant effects on the postsynaptic cholinergic, histaminic, or β-adrenergic receptors (Cunningham 1994). Like the other newer antidepressants, the more common side effects generally are not serious: nervousness, nausea, sweating, anorexia, dry mouth, and dizziness (Montgomery 1993). However, one potentially significant side effect is a dose-related elevation of the diastolic blood pressure; 19% of patients receiving 200 mg/day or more of venlafaxine had sustained hypertension (Feighner 1994). Venlafaxine has two unique pharmacological properties: only 30% of the medication is bound to plasma proteins, which allows safer administration with other medications that are highly protein bound such as warfarin and digoxin (Ereshefsky et al. 1995), and dosage adjustments are not necessary for elderly patients (Feighner 1994). The combination of venlafaxine with an MAOI, which can result in a serotonin syndrome, should be avoided (Ereshefsky et al. 1995).

Nefazodone is a phenylpiperazine antidepressant structurally similar to trazodone. Nefazodone is a selective serotonin (5-HT$_{2A}$) postsynaptic receptor antagonist that also blocks the presynaptic reuptake of serotonin and norepinephrine (Ayd 1995). In vitro studies indicate that nefazodone is devoid of affinity for the muscarinic, cholinergic, H$_1$ histaminic, and α$_1$-adrenergic receptors. Consequently, compared with tricyclic antidepressants, nefazodone less often causes dry mouth, constipation, urinary retention, exacerbation of glaucoma, excessive sedation, weight gain, or priapism (D. P. Taylor et al. 1995). Furthermore, nefazodone does not suppress REM sleep and improves overall sleep quality (Armitage et al. 1994). The more common adverse effects seen with nefazodone are mild se-

dation, dry mouth, nausea, headache, constipation, and dizziness (Ereshefsky et al. 1995). Because of nefazodone's inhibition of the cytochrome P450 III A4 isoenzyme, plasma levels of coadministered alprazolam, triazolam, ketoconazole, terfenadine, and astemizole increase. In particular, the combination of nefazodone with either terfenadine or astemizole should be avoided because of the risk of cardiotoxicity (Ayd 1995).

Monoamine oxidase inhibitors. MAOIs are the oldest of the antidepressants. Despite their longevity, they are poorly understood. Phenelzine, tranylcypromine, and isocarboxazid irreversibly inhibit both MAO-A and MAO-B. Deprenyl, used in PD, at low doses irreversibly inhibits MAO-B; it is not currently recommended for the treatment of depression. MAOIs have no significant anticholinergic activity, have no effect on cardiac conduction, and tend to be activating depressants. Orthostasis and hypotension are the only cardiovascular side effects associated with MAOIs. These side effects are particularly problematic in elderly patients because they are sensitive to these effects, and the consequences of falls are so devastating (Chutka 1990).

An important concern in using MAOIs is the hypertensive crisis that results from exposure to tyramine in the diet. Tyramine-containing foods such as aged fermented products, organ meats, overripe fruit, and broad beans are especially problematic (Shelman et al. 1989). Another source of difficulty is concomitant use of sympathomimetics, other psychotropic agents, and meperidine. The use of sympathomimetics with MAOIs can result in a hypertensive crisis; when tricyclic antidepressants, SSRIs, or meperidine are combined with MAOIs, a serotonergic syndrome can result, with symptoms similar to those of neuroleptic malignant syndrome (Nierenberg and Semprebon 1993). Despite these hazards, MAOIs are very effective in atypical depression and anxiety disorders, especially panic disorder.

Psychostimulants. The use of psychostimulants in medical settings to treat secondary mood disorder symptoms is well documented (Lazarus et al. 1992; Massand et al. 1991). Psychostimulants are fast-acting, well tolerated, and safe among the elderly and the medically ill.

Treatment-resistant depression (TRD). The clinician has several options when a patient does not respond adequately to an antidepressant. First, maximizing the current medication is necessary before changing agents. The clinician should increase the dose until either a response occurs or the patient is unable to tolerate side effects. The clinician can then change to a different medication, begin ECT, or augment the original antidepressant with lithium or thyroid hormone. A complete lack of response to an agent suggests a shift to a different class of antidepressant, whereas a partial response makes augmentation more attractive. Multiple drug failures, life-threatening severity of illness, or psychotic depression suggest ECT as an option.

The two agents most commonly used for antidepressant augmentation are lithium (Nemeroff 1991; Stein and Bernadt 1993) and thyroid hormone (Nemeroff 1991). Typically, lithium is used at full therapeutic doses; lithium augmentation is reported to be successful in 44%–66% of patients with TRD (Stein and Bernadt 1993). Thyroid augmentation is probably less effective but is worth consideration in cases of high-normal TSH or other indication of poor thyroid function. Carbamazepine has been little researched, but it may prove to be a useful augmenting agent (DeLaFuente and Mendlewicz 1992).

Electroconvulsive Therapy

ECT remains among the most effective treatments available for depression. Despite more than 60 years of experience, the mechanism of action for ECT is unknown (Lerer 1987). ECT is unfortunately considered a second-line treatment for depression; however, it is considered a first-line therapy in several clinical situations commonly encountered in consultation-liaison settings (Table 9–8). Psychotic depressions frequently are poorly responsive to medications. In addition, the patient with psychosis is at risk for self-injury or injuring others. The response rate to ECT is as high as 83% (Avery and Lubrano 1985), which is superior to the response rate to antidepressant medications seen in nonpsychotic depression. Another situation in which ECT deserves early consideration is depressed patients with unrelenting intense suicidality. Similarly, the rapid response to ECT in a malnourished, anorexic medically ill patient is lifesaving and avoids a more invasive stopgap intervention such as an enteral feeding tube.

ECT is an effective, often lifesaving, treatment for some of the medical causes of catatonia, such as lethal catatonia (Rummans 1993). The "functional" catatonias—primarily caused by depression, mania, or schizophrenia—are exquisitely sensitive to ECT. Once an organic etiology for the catatonia is ruled out (usually by EEG), ECT is the treatment of choice (M. Taylor 1990).

Table 9–8. Indications for electroconvulsive therapy as a first-line treatment

Psychotic/delusional depression

Intense suicidal tendencies associated with depression

Severe malnutrition/dehydration associated with depression

Catatonia of most functional and some organic etiologies

Severe manic excitement

Treatment failure with antidepressants

History of depression responsive to electroconvulsive therapy

Medical conditions in which exposure to antidepressant medication is problematic (e.g., severe coronary artery disease, pregnancy)

Treatment resistance, as defined earlier, is a frequent indication for ECT. Many studies about the efficacy of ECT report patients who have previously failed pharmacotherapy. The response rate is good, but the 1-year relapse rate, even with maintenance antidepressants following ECT, is as high as 50% (Sackeim et al. 1990). Most relapses occur within the first 2–4 months after ECT. Options to decrease the risk of relapse include maintenance ECT and lithium or carbamazepine augmentation and antidepressants.

There are no absolute contraindications to ECT (American Psychiatric Association Task Force on ECT 1990). Some conditions increase the morbidity associated with ECT and require thoughtful review of the risks versus benefits in a particular patient. These conditions are divided into three not mutually exclusive groups: 1) any condition that causes increased intracranial pressure, 2) any condition that increases risk of serious hemorrhage, and 3) any pathophysiological change that causes hemodynamic compromise, such as an acute myocardial infarction or malignant arrhythmia. The addition of β-blockers and antiarrhythmics before ECT reduces some of these risks.

Mortality associated with ECT is less than 0.05% and is essentially the risk of brief general anesthesia. Arrhythmias, myocardial infarction, and congestive heart failure are the most frequent causes of death (Selvin 1987).

Psychotherapy

Psychotherapy for depression in the medically ill patient requires a flexible, eclectic approach (see also Chapter 33 in this volume). Because of increasingly shorter lengths of stay in the hospital and the emergent nature of the medical situation, therapy, by necessity, is focused and brief. This approach demands a rapid assessment of the presenting problem, exploration of the precipitating events, and a comprehensive psychosocial history (Liberzon et al. 1992). The typical goals of the brief therapy are to improve self-esteem, correct misunderstandings about the illness, help the patient accept limitations imposed by the illness and hospital (Massie and Holland 1990), reduce isolation, assist the patient in coping with loss and disability, and facilitate the expression of fears and concerns (Haig 1992).

Therapy with a cognitive-behavioral emphasis is showing promise in the treatment of the depressed medical patient in the outpatient consultation-liaison setting. Larcombe and Wilson (1984), in a controlled study, demonstrated the effectiveness of cognitive-behavior therapy in 22 patients with depression and MS compared with similar patients on a waiting list. Cognitive therapy is particularly useful in patients with false assumptions about their illness.

Rodin (1984) reviewed the technical problems unique to conducting psychotherapy in an inpatient consultation-liaison setting. Therapy with medically ill patients is emotionally demanding on the therapist. The therapist is often too supportive too quickly. In addition, therapy is frequently interrupted by medical setbacks, tests, or medical procedures. The therapist must have an understanding of the medical situation and incorporate the limitations of the illness into a reasonable psychosocial treatment plan. Furthermore, therapy is conducted with little or no privacy. Finally, hospitalized patients and medically ill outpatients are often regressed, which makes even supportive psychotherapy more difficult.

In cancer patients, group therapy promotes support, improves interpersonal relationships, decreases loneliness, and helps the patient develop a sense of meaning in life (Haig 1992). Spiegel (1990) used psychoeducational group therapy to treat depressed women with metastatic breast cancer. He unexpectedly found that the patients in group therapy lived twice as long as the patients who received only routine oncological care. Also, a group of 68 distressed patients with malignant melanoma who participated in a 6-week structured psychiatric group had fewer metastases and a lower mortality rate 6 years later than a control group who received standard surgery alone (Fawzy et al. 1993). Levine et al. (1991) used a psychoeducational approach to treat depressed HIV-positive patients. This approach helped the patients function better in employment and social situations, alleviated abandonment issues, and improved social support.

The family of the medically ill patient with depression is also often in turmoil and may need care. Family therapy can provide emotional support, relieve guilt, expedite communications between the patient and the family, prepare the family for change, decrease alienation from the patient, and prevent displacement of anger toward the hospital staff (Haig 1992).

◼ REFERENCES

Adams RD, Victor M: Principles of Neurology, 4th Edition. New York, McGraw-Hill, 1989, pp 756–762

American Psychiatric Association: Diagnostic and Statistical Manual of Mental Disorders, 3rd Edition. Washington, DC, American Psychiatric Association, 1980

American Psychiatric Association: Diagnostic and Statistical Manual of Mental Disorders, 3rd Edition, Revised. Washington, DC, American Psychiatric Association, 1987

American Psychiatric Association: Diagnostic and Statistical Manual of Mental Disorders, 4th Edition. Washington, DC, American Psychiatric Association, 1994

American Psychiatric Association Task Force on ECT: The practice of ECT: recommendations for treatment, training and privileging. Convulsive Therapy 7:85–120, 1990

Andersen J, Aabro E, Gulmann N, et al: Antidepressive treatment in Parkinson's disease treated with L-dopa. Acta Neurol Scand 62: 210–219, 1980

Armitage R, Rush AJ, Trivedi M, et al: The effects of nefazodone on sleep architecture in depression. Neuropsychopharmacology 10:123–127, 1994

Atkinson H, Grant L, Kennedy CJ, et al: Prevalence of psychiatric disorders among men infected with human immunodeficiency virus. Arch Gen Psychiatry 45:859–864, 1988

Avery D, Lubrano A: Depression treated with imipramine and ECT: the DeCarolis study reconsidered. Am J Psychiatry 142:430–436, 1985

Ayd FJ: Nefazodone: the latest FDA approved antidepressant. International Drug Therapy Newsletter 30:17–20, 1995

Barrickman LL, Perry PJ, Allen AJ, et al: Bupropion versus methylphenidate in the treatment of attention deficit hyperactivity disorder. J Am Acad Child Adolesc Psychiatry 34:649–657, 1995

Beers MH, Passman LJ: Antihypertensive medications and depression. Drugs 40:792–799, 1990

Black JL, Richelson E, Richardson JW: Antipsychotic agents: a clinical update. Mayo Clin Proc 60:777–789, 1985

Blumer D: Epilepsy and disorders of mood. Adv Neurol 55:185–195, 1991

Boston Collaborative Drug Surveillance Program: Acute adverse reactions to prednisone in relation to dosage. Clin Pharmacol Ther 13:694–698, 1972

Burke WJ, Peterson J, Rubin EH: Electroconvulsive therapy in the treatment of combined depression and Parkinson's disease. Psychosomatics 29:341–346, 1988

Burton HJ, Kline SA, Lindsay RM, et al: The relationship of depression to survival in chronic renal failure. Psychosom Med 48:261–269, 1986

Cameron OG: Guidelines for diagnosis and treatment of depression in patients with medical illness. J Clin Psychiatry 51 (suppl 7):49–54, 1990

Carney RM, Rich MW, Tevelde A, et al: Major depressive disorder in coronary artery disease. Am J Cardiol 60:1273–1275, 1987

Carney RM, Rich MW, Freedland KE, et al: Major depressive disorder predicts cardiac events in patients with coronary artery disease. Psychosom Med 50:627–633, 1988

Cassem NH: Depression, in Massachusetts General Hospital Handbook of General Hospital Psychiatry, 3rd Edition. Edited by Cassem NH. St Louis, MO, Mosby Year Book, 1991, pp 237–268

Cathebras PJ, Robbins JM, Kirmayer LJ, et al: Fatigue in primary care: prevalence, psychiatric comorbidity, illness behavior and outcome. J Gen Intern Med 7:276–286, 1992

Chutka DS: Cardiovascular effects of the antidepressants: recognition and control. Geriatrics 45:55–67, 1990

Cummings JL: Ictal and interictal behavioral alterations, in Clinical Neuropsychiatry. Edited by Cummings JL. Boston, MA, Allyn & Bacon, 1985, pp 95–116

Cummings JL: Depression in Parkinson's disease: a review. Am J Psychiatry 149:443–454, 1992

Cummings JL, Benson DF: HIV encephalopathy, Jakob-Creutzfeldt disease, and other infectious dementias, in Dementia: A Clinical Approach, 2nd Edition. Boston, MA, Butterworth-Heinemann, 1992a, pp 177–188

Cummings JL, Benson DF: Subcortical dementias in the extrapyramidal disorders, in Dementia: A Clinical Approach, 2nd Edition. Boston, MA, Butterworth-Heinemann, 1992b, pp 95–152

Cummings JL, Miller B, Hill MA, et al: Neuropsychiatric aspects of multi-infarct dementia and dementia of the Alzheimer type. Arch Neurol 44:389–393, 1987

Cunningham LA: Depression in the medically ill: choosing an antidepressant. J Clin Psychiatry 55 (suppl A):90–100, 1994

Currie S, Heathfield G, Henson A, et al: Clinical course and prognosis of temporal lobe epilepsy, a survey of 666 patients. Brain 94:173–190, 1971

Cusack BM, Richelson E: Antagonism by antidepressants and some of their metabolites at 7 neurotransmitter receptors of normal human brain. FASEB J 7:A394, 1993

Dackis CA, Gold MS: Psychiatric hospitals for treatment of dual diagnosis, in Substance Abuse—A Comprehensive Textbook, 2nd Edition. Edited by Lowinson JH, Ruiz P, Millman RB, et al. Baltimore, MD, Williams & Wilkins, 1992, pp 479–485

Dackis CA, Pottash AL, Gold MS, et al: Evaluating depression in alcoholics. Psychiatr Res 17:105–109, 1986

Davidson J: Seizures and bupropion: a review. J Clin Psychiatry 50:256–261, 1989

Davidson KM, Ritson EB: The relationship between alcohol dependence and depression. Alcohol Alcohol 28:147–155, 1993

DeLaFuente JM, Mendlewicz J: Carbamazepine addition in tricyclic antidepressant-resistant unipolar depression. Biol Psychiatry 32:369–374, 1992

Dietch JT, Zetin M: Diagnosis of organic depressive disorders. Psychosomatics 24:971–979, 1983

Dorus W, Senay EC: Depression, demographic dimensions, and drug abuse. Am J Psychiatry 137:699–704, 1980

Douyon R, Serby M, Klutchko B, et al: ECT and Parkinson's disease revisited: a "naturalistic" study. Am J Psychiatry 146:1451–1455, 1989

El-Fakahany E, Richelson E: Antagonism by antidepressants of muscarinic acetylcholinergic receptors in human brain. Br J Pharmacol 78:97–102, 1983

Ereshefsky L, Benefield WH, Laird LK: Update on drug therapy for depression. Primary Psychiatry 2:28–36, 1995

Fava GA, Sonino N, Morphy MA: Major depression associated with endocrine disease. Psychiatric Developments 4:321–348, 1987

Fawzy FI, Fawzy NW, Hyun CS, et al: Malignant melanoma: effects of an early structured psychiatric intervention, coping, and affective state on recurrence and survival six years later. Arch Gen Psychiatry 50:681–689, 1993

Feighner JP: The role of venlafaxine in rational antidepressant therapy. J Clin Psychiatry 55 (suppl A):62–68, 1994

Folks DG: Organic affective disorder and underlying thyrotoxicosis. Psychosomatics 25:243–249, 1984

Folstein SE: Huntington's Disease: A Disorder of Families (A Monograph). Baltimore, MD, Johns Hopkins University Press, 1989

Folstein SE, Abbott MH, Chase GA, et al: The association of affective disorder with Huntington's disease in a case series and in families. Psychol Med 13:537–542, 1983

Ford MF: Treatment of depression in Huntington's disease with monoamine oxidase inhibitors. Br J Psychiatry 149:654–656, 1986

Forrester AW, Lipsey JR, Teitelbaum ML, et al: Depression following myocardial infarction. Int J Psychiatry Med 22:33–46, 1992

Fras L, Litin EM, Pearson JS: Comparison of psychiatric symptoms in carcinoma of the pancreas with those in some other intra-abdominal neoplasms. Am J Psychiatry 123:1553–1561, 1967

Frasure-Smith N, Lesperance F, Talajic M: Depression following myocardial infarction impact on 6-month survival. JAMA 270:1819–1825, 1993

Ganzini L, Walsh JR, Millar SM: Drug-induced depression in the aged. Drugs Aging 3:147–158, 1993

Gawin FH, Kleber HD: Cocaine abuse treatment: open pilot trial with desipramine and lithium carbonate. Arch Gen Psychiatry 41:903–909, 1984

Gawin FH, Kleber HD: Abstinence symptomatology and psychiatric diagnosis in cocaine abusers. Arch Gen Psychiatry 43:107–113, 1986

Giannini AJ, Folts DJ, Feather JN, et al: Bromocriptine and amantadine in cocaine detoxification. Psychiatry Res 29:11–16, 1989

Glassman AH, Roose SP, Bigger JT: The safety of tricyclic antidepressants in cardiac patients. JAMA 269:2673–2675, 1993

Goetz GG, Tanner CM, Klawans HL: Bupropion in Parkinson's disease. Neurology 34:1092–1094, 1984

Goldman MB: Neuropsychiatric features of endocrine disorders, in The American Psychiatric Press Textbook of Neuropsychiatry, 2nd Edition. Edited by Yudofsky SC, Hales RE. Washington, DC, American Psychiatric Press, 1992, pp 519–540

Goodwin FK, Ebert MH, Bunney WE: Mental effects of reserpine in man: a review, in Psychiatric Complications of Medical Drugs. Edited by Shader RI. New York, Raven, 1972, pp 73–101

Greenwald BS, Kramer-Gunsberg E, Marin DB, et al: Dementia with coexistent major depression. Am J Psychiatry 146:1472–1478, 1989

Haggerty JJ, Garbutt JC, Evans DL, et al: Subclinical hypothyroidism: a review of neuropsychiatric aspects. Int J Psychiatry Med 20:193–208, 1990

Haig RA: Management of depression in patients with advanced cancer. Med J Aust 156:499–503, 1992

Hall RC, Popkin MK, Stickney SK, et al: Presentation of steroid psychoses. J Nerv Ment Dis 167:229–236, 1979

Hall RC, Stickney SK, Gardner ER: Behavioral toxicity of non-psychiatric drugs, in Psychiatric Presentations of Medical Illness: Somatopsychic Disorders. Edited by Hall RC. New York, Spectrum Publications, 1980, pp 337–349

Haskett RF: Diagnostic categorization of psychiatric disturbance in Cushing's syndrome. Am J Psychiatry 142:911–916, 1985

Herzberg B, Coppen A: A change in psychological symptoms in women taking oral contraceptives. Br J Psychiatry 116:161–164, 1970

Hinrichsen GA, Lieberman JA, Pollack S, et al: Depression in hemodialysis patients. Psychosomatics 30:284–289, 1989

Holmes VF, Fernandez F, Levy JK: Psychostimulant response in AIDS-related complex patients. J Clin Psychiatry 50:5–8, 1989

Horne RL, Ferguson JM, Pope HG, et al: Treatment of bulimia with bupropion: a multi-center controlled trial. J Clin Psychiatry 49:262–266, 1988

Joffe RT: A perspective on the thyroid and depression. Can J Psychiatry 35:754–758, 1990

Joffe RT, Lippert GP, Gray TA, et al: Mood disorder and multiple sclerosis. Arch Neurol 44:376–378, 1987

Johnston JA, Lineberry CG, Ascher JA, et al: A 102-center prospective study of seizure in association with bupropion. J Clin Psychiatry 52:450–456, 1991

Kathol RG, Turner R, Delahunt J: Depression and anxiety associated with hyperthyroidism: response to antithyroid therapy. Psychosomatics 27:501–505, 1986

Kathol RG, Mulgi A, Williams J, et al: Diagnosis of major depression in cancer patients according to four sets of criteria. Am J Psychiatry 147:1021–1024, 1990

Katon W: The epidemiology of depression in medical care. Int J Psychiatry Med 17:93–112, 1987

Katon W: The development of a randomized trial of consultation-liaison psychiatry trial in distressed high utilizers of primary care. Psychiatr Med 9:577–591, 1991

Katon W, Schulberg H: Epidemiology of depression in primary care. Gen Hosp Psychiatry 14:237–247, 1992

Katon W, Egan K, Miller D: Chronic pain: lifetime psychiatric diagnoses and family history. Am J Psychiatry 142:1156–1160, 1985

Katon W, Von Korff M, Lin E, et al: Distressed high utilizers of medical care: DSM-III-R diagnoses and treatment needs. Gen Hosp Psychiatry 12:355–362, 1990

Kershner P, Wang-Cheng R: Psychiatric side effects of steroid therapy. Psychosomatics 30:135–139, 1989

Koranyi EK: Morbidity and rate of undiagnosed physical illnesses in a psychiatric clinic population. Arch Gen Psychiatry 36:414–419, 1979

Kramer JC, Fischman VS, Littlefield DC: Amphetamine abuse pattern and effects of high doses taken intravenously. JAMA 201:305–309, 1967

Kreusi MJ, Dale J, Straus SE: Psychiatric diagnoses in patients who have chronic fatigue syndrome. J Clin Psychiatry 50:53–56, 1989

Laitinen L: Desipramine in treatment of Parkinson's disease. Acta Neurol Scand 45:109–113, 1969

Larcombe NA, Wilson PH: An evaluation of cognitive-behavior therapy for depression in patients with multiple sclerosis. Br J Psychiatry 145:366–371, 1984

Lazarus LW, Winemiller DR, Lingam VR, et al: Efficacy and side effects of methylphenidate for poststroke depression. J Clin Psychiatry 53:447–449, 1992

Leedom L, Meehan WP, Procci W, et al: Symptoms of depression in patients with type II diabetes mellitus. Psychosomatics 32:280–286, 1991

Lerer B: Neurochemical and other neurobiological consequences of ECT: implications for the pathogenesis and treatment of affective disorders, in Psychopharmacology: The Third Generation of Progress. Edited by Meltzer HY. New York, Raven, 1987, pp 577–588

Levine SH, Bystritsky A, Baron D, et al: Group psychotherapy for HIV-seropositive patients with major depression. Am J Psychother 45:413–424, 1991

Lewis DA, Smith RE: Steroid-induced psychiatric syndromes: a report of 14 cases and a review of the literature. J Affect Disord 5:319–322, 1983

Liberzon I, Goldman RS, Hendrickson WJ: Very brief psychotherapy in the psychiatric consultation setting. Int J Psychiatry Med 22:65–75, 1992

Lingham VR, Lazarus LW, Groves L, et al: Methylphenidate in treating post-stroke depression. J Clin Psychiatry 49:151–153, 1988

Lipsey JR, Robinson RG, Pearlson GD, et al: Nortriptyline treatment of post-stroke depression: a double blind study. Lancet 84:297–300, 1984

Lishman WA: Epilepsy, in Organic Psychiatry, 2nd Edition. Oxford, Blackwell Scientific, 1987, pp 207–276

Martin JB, Gusella JF: Huntington's disease. N Engl J Med 315:1267–1276, 1986

Marzuk PM, Tierney H, Tardiff K, et al: Increased risk of suicide in persons with AIDS. JAMA 259:1333–1337, 1988

Massand P, Pickett P, Murray GB: Psychostimulants for secondary depression in medical illness. Psychosomatics 32:203–208, 1991

Massie MJ, Holland JC: Depression and the cancer patient. J Clin Psychiatry 51 (suppl 7):12–17, 1990

Mastrogiacomo I, Fava M, Fava GA, et al: Correlations between psychological symptoms in hyperprolactinemic amenorrhea. Neuroendocrinology Letters 5:117–122, 1983

Matthews WS, Barabas G: Suicide and epilepsy: a review of the literature. Psychosomatics 2:515–524, 1981

Mayeux R: Depression in the patient with Parkinson's disease. J Clin Psychiatry 52:20–23, 1990

Mayeux R, Stern Y, Rosen J, et al: Depression, intellectual impairment, and Parkinson disease. Neurology 31:645–650, 1981

Mayeux R, Stern Y, Williams JB, et al: Clinical and biochemical features of depression in Parkinson's disease. Am J Psychiatry 143:756–759, 1986

Mendez MF, Cummings JL, Benson F: Depression in epilepsy: significance and phenomenology. Arch Neurol 43:766–770, 1986

Minden SL, Schiffer RB: Affective disorders in multiple sclerosis. Arch Neurol 47:98–104, 1990

Minden SL, Orav J, Reich P: Depression in multiple sclerosis. Gen Hosp Psychiatry 9:426–434, 1987

Montgomery SA: Venlafaxine: a new dimension in antidepressant pharmacotherapy. J Clin Psychiatry 54:119–126, 1993

Morris PL, Robinson RG, Andrzejewski P, et al: Association of depression with 10 year post-stroke mortality. Am J Psychiatry 150:124–129, 1993

Moss AJ, Robinson J: Clinical features of the idiopathic long QT syndrome. Circulation 85(suppl):140–144, 1992

Murray GB, Shea VS, Conn DK: Electroconvulsive therapy for post-stroke depression. J Clin Psychiatry 47:258–260, 1986

Nemeroff CB: Augmentation regimens for depression. J Clin Psychiatry 52 (suppl 5):21–27, 1991

Nemeroff CB: Paroxetine: an overview of the efficacy and safety of a new selective serotonin reuptake inhibitor in the treatment of depression. J Clin Psychopharmacol 13 (suppl 2): 18–22, 1993

Nierenberg DW, Semprebon M: The central nervous system serotonin syndrome. Clin Pharmacol Ther 53:84–88, 1993

Ottson SV, Wu D, Joffe RT, et al: Inhibition by fluoxetine of cytochrome $P_{450}2D6$ activity. Clin Pharmacol Ther 53:401–409, 1993

Palinkas LA, Barrett-Connor E, Wingard DL: Type 2 diabetes and depressive symptoms in older adults: a population based study. Diabet Med 8:532–539, 1991

Palmer FJ: The clinical manifestations of primary hyperparathyroidism. Compr Ther 9:56–64, 1983

Pascualy M, Veith RC: Depression as an adverse drug reaction, in Aging and Clinical Practice: Depression and Coexisting Disease. Edited by Robinson RG, Rabins PV. New York, Igaku-Shoin, 1989, pp 132–151

Patten SB, Lamarre CJ: Can drug-induced depressions be identified by their clinical features? Can J Psychiatry 37:213–215, 1992

Paykel ES, Flemenger R, Watson JP: Psychiatric side effects of antihypertensive drugs other than reserpine. J Clin Psychopharmacol 2:14–39, 1982

Perez-Stable EJ, Miranda J, Munoz RF, et al: Depression in medical outpatients: underrecognition and misdiagnosis. Arch Intern Med 150:1083–1088, 1990

Perry SW, Tross S: Psychiatric problems of AIDS inpatients in the New York Hospital: preliminary report. Public Health Rep 99:200–205, 1984

Petrie WM, Maffucci RJ, Woosley RL: Propranolol and depression. Am J Psychiatry 139:92–93, 1982

Physicians' Desk Reference, 48th Edition. Oradell, NJ, Medical Economics, 1994, pp 879, 2002, 2269

Popkin MK, Callies AL, Colon EA: A framework for the study of medical depression. Psychosomatics 28:27–33, 1987

Popkin MK, Callies AL, Untz RD, et al: Prevalence of major depression, simple phobia, and other psychiatric disorders in patients with long-standing type I diabetes mellitus. Arch Gen Psychiatry 45:64–68, 1988

Prestidge BR, Lake CR: Prevalence and recognition of depression among primary care outpatients. J Fam Pract 25:67–72, 1987

Price RW, Brew B, Sidtis J, et al: The brain in AIDS: central nervous system HIV-1 infection and AIDS dementia complex. Science 239:586–592, 1988

Rabins PV, Brooks BR, O'Donnell P, et al: Structural brain correlates of emotional disorder in multiple sclerosis. Brain 109:585–597, 1986

Rauch SL, Stern TA, Zusman RM: Neuropsychiatric considerations in the treatment of hypertension. Int J Psychiatry Med 21:291–308, 1991

Reding MJ, Orto LA, Winter SW, et al: Antidepressant therapy after stroke—a double blind trial. Arch Neurol 43:763–765, 1986

Richelson E: Synaptic pharmacology of antidepressants: an update. McLean Hospital Journal 13:67–89, 1988

Rifkin A: Depression in physically ill patients. Postgrad Med 92:147–154, 1992

Robins LN, Helzer JE, Weissman MM, et al: Lifetime prevalence of specific psychiatric disorders in three sites. Arch Gen Psychiatry 41:949–958, 1984

Robinson RG, Price TR: Post-stroke depressive disorders: a follow-up study of 103 patients. Stroke 13:635–641, 1982

Robinson RG, Starr LB, Kubos KL, et al: A two year longitudinal study of post-stroke mood disorder: findings during the initial evaluation. Stroke 14:736–741, 1983

Robinson RG, Kubos KL, Starr LB, et al: Mood disorders in stroke patients—importance of lesion location. Brain 107:81–93, 1984a

Robinson RG, Starr LB, Price TR: A two year longitudinal study of mood disorders following stroke: prevalence and duration at six months follow-up. Br J Psychiatry 144:256–262, 1984b

Robinson RG, Lipsey JR, Price TR: Diagnosis and clinical management of post-stroke depression. Psychosomatics 26:769–778, 1985

Robinson RG, Bolduc P, Price TR: A two-year longitudinal study of post-stroke depression: diagnosis and outcome at one and two year follow-up. Stroke 18:837–843, 1987

Robinson RG, Morris PL, Federoff JP: Depression in cerebrovascular disease. J Clin Psychiatry 51 (suppl 7):26–31, 1990

Rodin G: Expressive psychotherapy in the medically ill: resistances and possibilities. Int J Psychiatry Med 14:99–108, 1984

Rodin G, Voshart K: Depression in the medically ill: an overview. Am J Psychiatry 143:696–705, 1986

Rodin G, Craven J, Littlefield C: Introduction, in Depression in the Medically Ill: An Integrated Approach. New York, Brunner/Mazel, 1991, p xi

Roose SP, Glassman AH, Giardina EV, et al: Nortriptyline in depressed patients with left ventricular impairment. JAMA 256:3253–3257, 1986

Rounsaville BJ, Weissman MM, Crits-Christoph K, et al: Diagnosis and symptoms of depression in opiate addicts. Arch Gen Psychiatry 39:151–156, 1982

Rummans TA: Medical indications for electroconvulsive therapy. Psychiatric Annals 23:27–32, 1993

Sackeim HA, Prudic J, Devanand DP, et al: The impact of medication resistance and continuation medication on relapse following response to electroconvulsive therapy in major depression. J Clin Psychopharmacol 10:96–104, 1990

Sano M, Stern Y, Williams J, et al: Coexisting dementia and depression in Parkinson's disease. Arch Neurol 46:1284–1286, 1989

Satel SL, Price LH, Palumbo JM, et al: Clinical phenomenology and neurobiology of cocaine abstinence: a prospective inpatient study. Am J Psychiatry 148:1712–1716, 1991

Schiffer RB, Caine ED, Bamford KA, et al: Depressive episodes in patients with multiple sclerosis. Am J Psychiatry 140:1498–1500, 1983

Schleifer SJ, Macari-Hinson MM, Coyle DA, et al: The nature and course of depression following myocardial infarction. Arch Intern Med 149:1785–1789, 1989

Schoenfeld M, Myers RH, Cupples LA, et al: Increased rate of suicide among patients with Huntington's disease. J Neurol Neurosurg Psychiatry 47:1283–1287, 1984

Schuckit M: Alcoholism and other psychiatric disorders. Hosp Community Psychiatry 34:1022–1027, 1983

Schulberg HC, Saul M, McClelland M, et al: Assessing depression in primary medical and psychiatric practices. Arch Gen Psychiatry 42:1164–1170, 1985

Selvin BL: Electroconvulsive therapy—1987. Anesthesiology 67:367–385, 1987

Shekelle RB, Raynor WJ, Ostfeld AM, et al: Psychological depression and 17 year risk of death from cancer. Psychosom Med 43:117–125, 1981

Shelman KI, Walker SE, MacKenzie S, et al: Dietary restriction, tyramine, and the use of monoamine oxidase inhibitors. J Clin Psychopharmacol 9:397–402, 1989

Silverstone PH: Depression increases mortality and morbidity in acute life threatening medical illness. J Psychosom Res 34:651–657, 1990

Sliman RJ, Donahue TA, Jarjoura D, et al: Recognition of depression by internal medicine residents. J Community Health 17:143–152, 1992

Smith BD, Salzman C: Do benzodiazepines cause depression? Hosp Community Psychiatry 42:1101–1102, 1991

Spiegel D: Can psychotherapy prolong cancer survival? Psychosomatics 31:361–366, 1990

Spitzer RL, Endicott J, Robins E: Research Diagnostic Criteria: rationale and reliability. Arch Gen Psychiatry 35:773–782, 1978

Starkstein SE, Preziosi TJ, Bolduc PL, et al: Depression in Parkinson's disease. J Nerv Ment Dis 178:27–31, 1990

Stein G, Bernadt M: Lithium augmentation therapy in tricyclic-resistant depression. Br J Psychiatry 162:634–640, 1993

Stewart AF, Broadus AE: Mineral metabolism, in Endocrinology and Metabolism. Edited by Felig P, Baxter JD, Broadus AE, et al. New York, McGraw-Hill, 1987, pp 1317–1453

Stoudemire A: Expanding psychopharmacologic treatment options for the depressed medical patient. Psychosomatics 36:519–526, 1995

Strang RR: Imipramine in treatment of parkinsonism: a double-blind placebo study. BMJ 2:33–34, 1965

Sullivan MJ, Reesor K, Mikail S, et al: The treatment of depression in chronic low back pain: review and recommendations. Pain 50:5–13, 1992

Summers WK, Munoz RA, Read MR: The psychiatric physical examination—part 1: methodology. J Clin Psychiatry 42:95–98, 1981

Taylor M: Catatonia: a review of a behavioral neurologic syndrome. Neuropsychiatry, Neuropsychology, and Behavioral Neurology 3:48–72, 1990

Taylor DP, Carter RB, Eison AS, et al: Pharmacology and neurochemistry of nefazodone, a novel antidepressant drug. J Clin Psychiatry 56 (no 6, suppl):3–11, 1995

Tennant FS, Sagherian AA: Double-blind comparison of amantadine and bromocriptine mesylate for ambulatory withdrawal from cocaine dependence. Arch Intern Med 147:109–112, 1987

Tiller JW, Schweitzer I: Benzodiazepines: depression or antidepressants. Drugs 44:165–169, 1992

Von Korff M, Ormel J, Katon W, et al: Disability and depression among high utilizers of health care: a longitudinal analysis. Arch Gen Psychiatry 49:91–100, 1992

Walker PW, Cole JQ, Gardiner EA, et al: Improvement in fluoxetine-associated sexual dysfunction in patients switched to bupropion. J Clin Psychiatry 54:459–465, 1993

Weintraub M, Evans P: Bupropion: a chemically and pharmacologically unique antidepressant. Hospital Formulary 24:254–259, 1989

Whitehouse PJ, Friedland RP, Strauss ME: Neuropsychiatric aspects of degenerative dementias associated with motor dysfunction, in The American Psychiatric Press Textbook of Neuropsychiatry, 2nd Edition. Edited by Yudofsky SC, Hales RE. Washington, DC, American Psychiatric Press, 1992, pp 585–604

Whitlock FA, Siskind MM: Depression as a major symptom of multiple sclerosis. J Neurol Neurosurg Psychiatry 43:861–865, 1980

Winokur G: The concept of a secondary depression and its relationship to comorbidity. Psychiatr Clin North Am 123:567–583, 1990

Wise MG, Rundell JR: Concise Guide to Consultation Psychiatry, 2nd Edition. Washington, DC, American Psychiatric Press, 1994, p 3

Yates WR, Wesner RB, Thompson R: Organic mood disorder: a valid psychiatry consultation diagnosis? J Affect Disord 22:37–42, 1991

Zelnik T: Depressive effects of drugs, in Presentations of Depression: Depressive Symptoms in Medical and Other Psychiatric Disorders. Edited by Cameron OG. New York, Wiley, 1987, pp 355–399

Zubenko GS, Mossy J, Kopp U: Neurochemical correlates of major depression in primary dementia. Arch Neurol 47:209–214, 1990

Chapter 10

Mania

J. Stephen McDaniel, M.D.
Karen M. Johnson, M.D.
James R. Rundell, M.D.

DEFINITIONS

In a *manic episode,* as defined by DSM-IV (American Psychiatric Association 1994), the essential feature is a distinct period lasting at least 1 week during which the predominant mood is either elevated, expansive, or irritable.

Manic episodes are sometimes phases of primary bipolar disorder (manic-depressive illness) or secondary to a particular medical or toxic etiology (i.e., secondary mania). *Bipolar disorder* is a mood syndrome characterized by one or more manic episodes usually accompanied by one or more major depressive episodes. Primary bipolar disorder has a prevalence of 0.4%–1.2% in the general adult population (American Psychiatric Association 1994). The prevalence of this disorder in the medically ill population is unknown.

Secondary mania is a diagnosis of particular importance to consultation-liaison psychiatrists. This condition resembles primary mania; however, it occurs secondary to specific identifiable medical or toxic factors. According to DSM-IV, secondary mania is called "mood disorder due to a general medical condition, with manic features," when caused by a medical illness, or "substance-induced mood disorder, with manic features," when caused by substance intoxication or withdrawal (American Psychiatric Association 1994). Like primary mania, the essential feature of this syndrome is a prominent and persistent elevated or expansive mood. According to DSM-IV, a secondary mania diagnosis is not made if the mood disturbance occurs in the context of delirium or dementia; however, mild cognitive impairment is often observed. Other characteristic features of secondary mania include irritability, mood lability, hallucinations, and delusions.

EPIDEMIOLOGY

Weissman et al. (1988) examined the Epidemiologic Catchment Area (Eaton et al.

1981) data to calculate lifetime prevalence rates for primary bipolar disorder. A lifetime prevalence rate of 1.2% was calculated. Using more recent diagnostic instruments, Goodwin and Jamison (1990) found the annual risk of having a manic episode to be 0.24%–0.77% in the general United States population. Unfortunately, available data reflect findings in the general population; therefore, translating these numbers to include medically ill populations is difficult. In their retrospective chart review of 755 patients who were seen by a psychiatric consultation-liaison service in a general hospital over a 1-year period, Rundell and Wise (1989) found that 13 out of 15 (87%) patients identified as having mania met criteria for secondary mania.

A number of associated features and risk factors have been identified for primary bipolar disorder. Understanding these risk factors can be helpful in attempting to differentiate primary and secondary mania. Patients with primary bipolar disorder have a mean age at onset of 30 years (Goodwin and Jamison 1990), and with increasing age, the interval between manic episodes tends to decrease and duration of episodes tends to increase (Krauthammer and Klerman 1978). Initial bipolar manic episodes rarely occur after age 50 (Wise and Rundell 1993). Several investigators reported that a positive family history of mood disorder is associated with an earlier age at onset of initial manic episode among bipolar patients (Stone 1989). In addition, earlier age at onset is associated with a higher total lifetime number of manic episodes (Angst 1978; Mendlewicz et al. 1972). Although early reports of manic patients suggested differences in prevalence among ethnic and socioeconomic categories, current evidence argues against demographic risk factors for developing bipolar disorder (Goodwin and Jamison 1990). Although precise genetic mechanisms elude investigators to date, bipolar disorder occurs at much higher rates in first-degree biological relatives of bipolar patients than in the general population (American Psychiatric Association 1994).

CLINICAL FEATURES

Manic syndromes in medical-surgical patients may be exacerbations of underlying bipolar disorder or secondary mania. The essential clinical feature of a manic episode is a distinctly expansive, elevated, or irritable mood. This disturbance is sufficiently severe to cause impairment in occupational or social functioning or to require hospitalization to prevent harm to oneself or others. Frequently, the manic person does not recognize that he or she is ill and resists treatment. When delusions or hallucinations are present, the content is usually consistent with the mania (mood-congruent).

Manic episodes often develop in stages, beginning with mild hypomania referred to by Jacobson (1965) as *hypomanic alert,* through moderate manic symptoms, including grandiose or paranoid delusions, to severe mania accompanied by profound psychosis (Goodwin and Jamison 1990). The time frame to progression of a full manic syndrome varies; it could take a few days or even a few hours. Manic episodes develop more abruptly than depressive episodes.

A sizable amount of literature has examined the possible role of psychosocial or physical stress in precipitating episodes of bipolar illness; however, it is now generally accepted that environmental conditions contribute more to the timing of an episode than to underlying vulnerability, which is largely genetic (Roy et al. 1985). Wehr and colleagues (1987) proposed that sleep reduction is the common denominator in many of the environmental stresses that precipitate mania.

Much less literature has described the course and prognosis of secondary mania. As in primary bipolar mania, manic symptoms caused by medical illness or a medication can occur rapidly within hours or days; secondary mania is not generally believed to be a chronic illness. Once the etiology is determined and treated, secondary mania usually resolves. However, some secondary manic syndromes, such as those attributed to the human immuno-deficiency virus (HIV) or structural brain insults, can become chronic because the underlying organic pathology cannot be eradicated. In considering a differential diagnosis of manic syndromes, a previous diagnosis of bipolar disorder is believed to increase the risk for secondary mania. Toxic and metabolic exacerbations of underlying mood disorders occur frequently and can occur simultaneously with a diagnosis of primary mood disorder. Even patients whose primary bipolar disorder is successfully managed with lithium carbonate therapy can develop secondary mania related to any of a number of medical or toxic etiologies (e.g., steroids).

Clinicians must be alert to the increased mortality in bipolar patients. Suicide attempts occur more frequently in bipolar patients, especially men. In bipolar patients, overall increased mortality is greater than that which is due to suicide (Winokur and Clayton 1986). The reason for this increased mortality is unclear. Patients with mania should be treated aggressively in the general hospital, including management of underlying medical or toxic etiologies.

PATHOPHYSIOLOGY

Interest in the neuropathology and anatomy of mania grew out of the observation that lesions of the central nervous system (CNS) are frequently accompanied by signs of abnormal cognitive, behavioral, or motor functioning. For example, structural lesions of the CNS are associated with secondary depression and mania. Lesions associated with a manic syndrome usually occur in the orbitofrontal and basotemporal cortices, the head of the caudate, and the thalamus.

It is now generally accepted that lesions in the frontal, limbic, and temporal lobes are more frequently associated with mood disor-

ders than lesions in other brain regions. Left-sided lesions are often associated with increased relative risk for depression, and right-sided lesions are associated with risk for mania (Cummings 1986; Starkstein and Robinson 1989). Goodwin and Jamison (1990) pointed out, however, that the left-right differences may be reversed in regions closer to the posterior poles. Thus, in right-handed patients, depression risk is relatively increased by left frontotemporal or right parietooccipital lesions, whereas manic symptoms are more likely to follow right frontotemporal or left parietooccipital lesions.

Because not every patient with right-hemisphere limbic lesions develops secondary mania, premorbid risk factors are believed to play a key role. Two such risk factors were identified through comparison studies. One factor is genetic predisposition to mood disorders (Robinson et al. 1988). The second risk factor is brain atrophy (Starkstein et al. 1987). Patients with secondary mania had significantly more subcortical atrophy than did other study patients. Moreover, among patients who developed secondary mania, those who had a family history of psychiatric disorders had significantly less atrophy than those without such a family history, which suggests that genetic predisposition to mood disorders and brain atrophy may be independent risk factors (Starkstein and Robinson 1992).

Neurochemical abnormalities associated with primary bipolar disorder involve ascending monoaminergic pathways that are also probably involved in secondary mania (Larson and Richelson 1988). Starkstein et al. (1988) have postulated that in the presence of certain risk factors for secondary mania (e.g., subcortical atrophy or family history of mood disorders), increases in biogenic amine turnover produced by right-hemisphere lesions may play an important role in the production of secondary mania.

Neurochemical theories of the etiology of mania focus on an association between increases in the functional output of baso-temporal cortex pathways resulting in excess catecholamines (norepinephrine or dopa-mine) or indoleamines (serotonin), whereas depression is associated with functional defi-cits of these neurotransmitters. Pharmacologi-cal studies support these associations, but asso-ciations do not necessarily infer a direct cause-and-effect relation. Other pathways and neurotransmitters are almost certainly involved in the etiologies of mood syndromes.

Many investigators believe that sleep dep-rivation is the final common pathway in the pathophysiology of mania. Patients with pri-mary bipolar disorder often shift from depres-sion to mania after they miss a night of sleep. Total sleep deprivation and sleep deprivation in the second half of the night can induce tem-porary remissions in depressed patients as well (Gillin 1983; Joffe and Brown 1984). Goodwin and Jamison (1990) reported that sleep depri-vation is probably an important precipitant in the manic states that occasionally accompany bereavement, postpartum states, and jet lag. It is worth remembering that sleep deprivation is a common characteristic of medical and surgi-cal hospitalization, particularly in intensive care units. Insomnia and/or decreased need for sleep is almost invariably present during mania.

In summary, data on the phenomenology of secondary mania suggest that several gen-eral principles hold true. Numerous studies of patients with brain damage have found that pa-tients who develop secondary mania have a significantly greater frequency of lesions in the right hemisphere than do patients with brain injury who become depressed or develop no mood disturbance at all. The right-hemisphere lesions associated with mania are in specific right-hemisphere structures that are connected to the limbic system. The right basotemporal cortex appears to be particularly important be-cause direct lesions of this cortical region are frequently associated with secondary mania (Starkstein and Robinson 1992).

■ DIFFERENTIAL DIAGNOSIS

The clinical presentation of secondary mania includes any of the symptoms found in primary bipolar mania. The clinical history, physical ex-amination, and laboratory evaluations are im-portant elements in differentiating primary and secondary mania in medical-surgical patients. Because at least one-third of bipolar manic pa-tients have either disorientation or some mem-ory blanks during a manic episode, the differ-ential diagnosis of primary and secondary mania is often difficult (Winokur and Clayton 1986). The distinction between the two is im-portant because eradication of the etiology is the treatment of choice for secondary mania. However, manic symptoms are treatable, so in-tervention need not be delayed while complet-ing the medical workups. Careful attention must be paid to past or family history of mood disorders. The onset of mania in a patient older than 35 years without a personal or family his-tory of mood disorders strongly suggests sec-ondary mania, as does the onset of mania dur-ing a hospitalization for a medical disorder. Patients with primary bipolar disorder usually have their first manic episode between late ad-olescence and early adulthood, with a mean age at onset of 30 years (Goodwin and Jamison 1990; Krauthammer and Klerman 1978).

Psychiatric disorders other than bipolar disorder can have symptoms that mimic a manic episode. Stimulant abuse, delirium, schizophrenia, schizoaffective disorder, anxi-ety disorders, some personality disorders (bor-derline personality disorder and histrionic per-sonality disorder), and adolescent conduct disorders should be considered before estab-lishing a diagnosis of secondary mania.

Several medical conditions are temporally associated with mania and hypomania syn-dromes. Among the multiple potential etiolo-gies reportedly associated with secondary ma-nia, several have proven to be consistent and frequent causes. These frequent conditions, listed in Table 10–1, have been temporally associated with onset of mania in series of patients or in clinical studies (i.e., more than single case reports).

Few studies of relative risks of all these potential causes have been done. As mentioned earlier in this chapter, patients with family or personal histories of mood disorders are at higher risk for mania. Many medications, particularly those that modulate central monoaminergic metabolism, are reported to produce mania. Corticosteroid use has long been associated with secondary mania. A recent addition to this list of etiologies is the group of drugs known as anabolic steroids, which are used by some athletes. Even patients who do not have specific risk factors are at risk for mania or hypomania when using such steroids.

Searching for potential causes of secondary manic states requires a thorough investigative assessment (Table 10–2), which should begin with a careful medical and psychiatric

Table 10–1. Most frequent causes of secondary mania[a]

Medications
  Levodopa
  Decongestants containing phenylephrine
  Sympathomimetics/bronchodilators
  Corticosteroids
  Adrenocorticotropic hormone
  Antidepressants
Metabolic abnormalities
  Hyperthyroidism
Neurological disorders
  Temporal-lobe seizures
  Multiple sclerosis
  Right-hemispheric strokes or injuries
Central nervous system tumors
  Gliomas
  Meningiomas
  Thalamic metastases

[a]These causes are temporally associated with mania in either a series of patients or in clinical studies.
Source. Adapted from Stoudemire GA: "Selected Organic Mental Disorders," in *The American Psychiatric Press Textbook of Neuropsychiatry.* Edited by Hales RE, Yudofsky SC. Washington, DC, American Psychiatric Press, 1987, pp. 125–140. Used with permission.

history; chart review, with special attention to medications prescribed or surreptitiously taken; and physical examination. The neurological examination should investigate possible focal deficits, especially findings associated with nondominant hemispheric lesions, such as left-sided hemiparesis with hyperactive deep tendon reflexes and Babinski sign, attention disturbance (left-sided neglect), anosognosia, and constructional dyspraxia. Other brain regions associated with manic symptoms include lesions of the anterior cerebral artery

Table 10–2. Evaluation of secondary mania

Medical-psychiatric history
  Current medical symptoms
  Recent infections
  Use of prescribed medications
  Use of drugs of abuse
  History of psychiatric disorders, especially mood disorders
  Family history of psychiatric disorders, especially mood disorders
Vital signs
Physical examination, with attention to focal neurological deficits
Mental status examination, with emphasis on mood, psychotic symptoms, and cognition
Laboratory evaluation
  Blood glucose
  Electrolytes
  Renal/hepatic function tests
  Complete blood count
  Serum calcium
  Serum cortisol
  Serum thyroxine
  Vitamin B_{12}
  Folate
  Toxicology screen
  Blood alcohol
  Pregnancy test
  Levels of antimanic drug(s) if already prescribed
Electrocardiogram
Computed tomography and magnetic resonance imaging scans
Cerebrospinal fluid examination
Electroencephalogram

and associated frontal-lobe dysfunction, as well as basal ganglia lesions that may also yield signs of movement disorders, such as athetosis, chorea, parkinsonism, or hemiballismus. When the etiology of mania is a stroke, lateralized focal lesions are found in the right hemisphere involving regions of the basal ganglia, thalamus, or midbrain nuclei or limbic portions of the frontal or temporal lobes (Starkstein and Robinson 1992). Mental status examination should carefully evaluate mood, level of psychosis, and cognitive impairment (see Wise and Strub, Chapter 2, in this volume).

Diagnostic laboratory evaluations should include basic screening (see Table 10–2) and toxicology screening to detect cocaine, amphetamines, phencyclidine (PCP), other hallucinogens, alcohol, sedative-hypnotics, and prescription medications such as antidepressants and corticosteroids that may produce manic symptoms (see Table 10–1). Brain imaging (computed tomography [CT] or magnetic resonance imaging [MRI]) should be done if neurological conditions with structural CNS changes are suspected. Similarly, an electroencephalogram (EEG) may indicate whether the diagnosis is a seizure or delirium. Because many of the systemic conditions related to secondary mania include cardiac manifestations, an electrocardiogram (ECG) is indicated; it is a necessary part of the pretreatment lithium evaluation as well. If a patient is taking lithium, carbamazepine, or valproic acid, the medication level should be checked.

■ TREATMENT AND MANAGEMENT

In all cases of secondary mania, the basic medical treatment focuses on elimination of the underlying medical etiology whenever possible and the attenuation of symptoms whenever elimination is not possible. A careful and thorough medical and neurological evaluation helps the conscientious clinician in his or her management strategy.

Even though removing remediable etiologies is the first line of treatment for secondary mania, pharmacological intervention is usually necessary to control manic symptoms while the clinician searches for an etiology. Antimanic drugs usually lead to rapid resolution of emotional symptoms (Starkstein and Robinson 1992). However, the treating clinician must be aware of the serious effect of mania on patients, particularly those patients who are medically ill. Complications such as sleep deprivation, dehydration, weight loss, and fatigue may make patients more vulnerable to medication side effects and more vulnerable to underlying medical illness.

A number of medication options (lithium, anticonvulsants, benzodiazepines, and neuroleptics) are available for treatment of secondary mania (see also Jachna et al., Chapter 30, in this volume). Table 10–3 describes dosing strategies and serum levels for some of these antimanic agents. For primary and sometimes for secondary mania, pharmacological intervention is recommended for up to 6 months beyond symptom resolution to prevent relapse.

The most important consideration in selecting a treatment for manic symptoms is the nature and severity of symptoms (Goodwin and Jamison 1990). Mild manic symptoms usually respond well to lithium alone. Hudson and colleagues (1989) reported that restoring a normal sleep pattern often averts escalation to more severe manic symptoms. Short-term adjunctive treatment with a bedtime dose of a benzodiazepine, such as clonazepam, also helps to normalize sleep. For more severe symptoms, especially gross hyperactivity and psychotic features, a neuroleptic is indicated. Interest in the role of anticonvulsants in the treatment of mania is growing, particularly for patients who are lithium intolerant or lithium nonresponders. Many clinicians consider anticonvulsants as first-line treatment modalities, especially for secondary mania. A discussion of pharmacological guidelines for the treatment of secondary mania follows.

Table 10–3. Antimania medications

Drug	Daily dosage (mg)	Half-life[a] (hours)	Serum level
Carbamazepine	400–1,200	25–65[a]	8–12 μg/mL
Lithium	300–1,800	18–36	0.6–1.2 mEq/L
Valproic acid	1,000–1,500	6–16	50–120 mg/mL
Clonazepam	1.5–6.0	18–58	[b]

[a]With repeated doses, half-life declines because carbamazepine usually induces its own metabolism.
[b]Serum levels less meaningful than for carbamazepine, lithium, or valproic acid.
Source. Adapted from Wise MG, Rundell JR: *Consultation Psychiatry,* 2nd Edition. Washington, DC, American Psychiatric Press, 1993. Used with permission.

Lithium Carbonate

All patients treated with lithium should have a pretreatment evaluation. Although contraindications are rare, an assessment of organ systems most often adversely affected (kidney, cardiovascular system, and CNS) is necessary. This assessment is particularly important in medically ill populations. Lithium is titrated within a rather narrow therapeutic range (i.e., toxic effects occur at doses only moderately higher than therapeutic levels). Serum levels are carefully monitored and are usually drawn 12 hours after the last dose. The half-life of lithium is 18–36 hours; therefore, steady-state serum levels are usually achieved 5–8 days after a dosage change. Because the therapeutic benefits of lithium may take 10–14 days to appear, concomitant neuroleptic use is usually necessary for acute management of mania.

Doses should begin at 300 mg/day and be increased gradually over several weeks to serum lithium levels of 0.8–1.2 mEq/L. If seizures are part of the clinical picture, anticonvulsants are preferable. Treatment should continue for several months beyond resolution of symptoms. The generally accepted therapeutic range of serum lithium concentrations is 0.6–1.2 mEq/L. Patients in an acute manic phase are best treated with lithium doses that achieve serum concentrations at the upper end of this therapeutic range. However, in severely ill medical patients, in elderly patients, or in those with renal disease, lower doses should be used when possible. Some elderly patients may be maintained adequately with satisfactory blood levels of the drug by administering 300–450 mg/day of lithium (Bernstein 1991). Elderly patients and patients with brain disease are particularly susceptible to developing confusion and tremor at therapeutic levels (A. Stoudemire et al. 1993). Therefore, dosage aiming for the lower end of the therapeutic range is recommended for elderly individuals and others susceptible to the neurological side effects of lithium. Furthermore, treating medically ill patients with lithium requires knowledge of potential drug-drug interactions.

The primary metabolic consideration in the use of lithium in medically ill patients is renal function (A. Stoudemire et al. 1993). Lithium is excreted by the kidney, and rates of excretion are affected by age and creatinine clearance. Therefore, pretreatment renal function screening is absolutely necessary. Thiazide diuretics, which act primarily at the distal tubule, enhance proximal reabsorption of lithium because they deplete sodium. Loop diuretics such as furosemide appear to have less effect on lithium clearance. Potassium-sparing diuretics such as spironolactone and triamterene also may reduce lithium clearance, although they are less studied than other diuretics.

A. Stoudemire and colleagues (1993) warned that patients taking thiazide diuretics usually need approximately half the amount of lithium to attain therapeutic levels, but there is considerable interindividual variation. When a patient is taking a diuretic agent, the lithium dose should be started low and increased slowly, and lithium levels should be monitored at least twice weekly. Thereafter, frequent monitoring should be resumed after any change in diuretic dosage or in diet.

Lithium is dialyzable and should therefore be given to patients on renal dialysis *after* their dialysis treatments; the usual dose is 300–600 mg/day (A. Stoudemire et al. 1993). The dose is typically not given until after the next dialysis. Serum levels of lithium are tested several hours after dialysis because plasma levels may actually rise in the postdialysis period when equilibration between tissue stores occurs (Bennett et al. 1980). The dialyzability of lithium makes dialysis the treatment of choice in cases of life-threatening lithium toxicity.

In almost all patients treated with lithium, the kidneys lose some ability to concentrate urine. Occasionally, this leads to symptomatic polyuria (nephrogenic diabetes insipidus). The mechanism is a direct effect of lithium on the loop of Henle and the distal tubule. This effect is dose related and, in rare cases, is irreversible. Recent research indicates that once-a-day dosing may partially mitigate this problem (A. Stoudemire et al. 1993). If the polyuria threatens lithium treatment and there are compelling clinical reasons to continue lithium instead of alternative agents, several options are available. First, thiazide diuretics are sometimes used—with the previously noted precautions—to enhance lithium reabsorption at the proximal tubule, thereby protecting the more distal nephron from high lithium concentrations. The total lithium dose is reduced by as much as 50% if this strategy is used. A second option is the use of potassium-sparing diuretics such as amiloride, which are reportedly helpful in managing polyuria; the usual dose is 10–20 mg/day (Kosten and Forrest 1986). In refractory cases, 50 mg/day of hydrochlorothiazide should be added. With or without adjunctive thiazide therapy, amiloride increases lithium levels, which may lead to lithium toxicity if levels are not monitored. If amiloride is used alone, hyperkalemia is a risk; electrolytes should be checked frequently after starting the drug. If amiloride is used with hydrochlorothiazide, the lithium dosage should be reduced.

Adverse effects. Although side effects of lithium are usually mild and transient, the clinician must monitor medically ill patients closely for adverse effects. The most common side effects are tremor, nausea, vomiting, diarrhea, polyuria, and polydipsia. Hypothyroidism, rashes, nephrogenic diabetes insipidus, interstitial nephritis, and weight gain are less common. Nonspecific ST segment and T-wave changes are commonly seen on the ECG; actual conduction defects and arrhythmias are rare. However, Cassem (1991) recommends the cautious use of lithium in elderly patients or patients with cardiac disease because lithium may have an inhibitory effect on impulse generation and transmission within the atrium. The most commonly reported adverse cardiac effects are sinus node dysfunction or first-degree atrioventricular block.

Many of lithium's side effects decrease with dosage reduction, but that is not always possible, especially in patients prone to relapse. β-Blockers (atenolol 50 mg/day) sometimes help to control lithium-induced tremor, and, as discussed above, diuretics may help control polyuria.

Lithium toxicity markedly affects the CNS and is a life-threatening emergency in consultation-liaison settings. Symptoms of lithium-induced CNS toxicity include ataxia, slurred speech, and nystagmus and can proceed to convulsions, coma, and death if lithium levels are greater than 2.5 mEq/L. The threshold for more serious side effects is lower in predisposed or medically ill patients.

Anticonvulsants

Carbamazepine and valproic acid are effective agents in the treatment of both primary and secondary mania, including lithium-unresponsive mania (Goodwin and Jamison 1990; Pope et al. 1991; Prien and Gelenberg 1989). Sometimes these agents are used in combination with lithium. Carbamazepine is a compound structurally similar to tricyclic antidepressants. Although the precise mechanism of action of carbamazepine in affective illness is not clear, it blocks the reuptake of norepinephrine, inhibits stimulation-induced release of norepinephrine at synaptic sites, and appears to decrease γ-aminobutyric acid (GABA) turnover in animals (Post 1982). Valproic acid, a widely used anticonvulsant, enhances GABA activity in the brain by inhibiting degradation, stimulating GABA synthesis and release, and enhancing its postsynaptic action. Both the anticonvulsant and the antimanic activity of valproic acid is believed to be dependent on its GABAergic effects (Bernstein 1991). Because these anticonvulsants are hepatically metabolized, a pretreatment liver function assessment is necessary. General dosage recommendations and therapeutic levels are outlined in Table 10–3. The therapeutic anticonvulsant levels listed in Table 10–3 are used for treating seizures; considerable variability in the appropriate levels for treating mania may exist. The clinician must monitor symptom response and side-effect profiles closely.

Carbamazepine

Adverse effects. When prescribing carbamazepine to medically ill patients, its potential hematological toxicity, quinidine-like effects on cardiac conduction, antidiuretic actions, and enzyme induction that alters the metabolism of other drugs must be considered. Particularly common problems in the consultation-liaison setting are carbamazepine's interaction with the calcium channel blockers diltiazem and verapamil—two agents that may elevate carbamazepine levels into the toxic range (A. Stoudemire et al. 1993).

Carbamazepine administration may result in two different hematological reactions. One is a predictable and usually transient drop in both red and white blood cell (WBC) counts when treatment is initiated; the other is aplastic anemia—a rare side effect that can occur at any time after initiation of therapy. Leukopenia (defined as WBC count < 50) occurs in 7%–12% of treated patients (Seetharam and Pellock 1991; Sobotka et al. 1990). Leukopenia is seemingly unrelated to aplastic anemia. The latter occurs in approximately 1 in 575,000 treated patients per year (Seetharam and Pellock 1991). Patients who have preexisting anemia or neutropenia do not appear to be at greater risk for the life-threatening complications of aplastic anemia or agranulocytosis (A. Stoudemire et al. 1993). A hematological consultation should be obtained before initiating carbamazepine therapy in any patient with a baseline hemoglobin level below 12 g/dL or a WBC count below 4,000/mm^3. Preexisting neutropenia is a relative but not an absolute contraindication to carbamazepine.

Hepatic side effects related to carbamazepine are usually limited to a benign, asymptomatic elevation of alanine aminotransferase or aspartate aminotransferase, usually less than twice the upper limit of normal values. This benign reaction occurs in no more than 5% of patients (Jeavons 1983). However, a rare, idiosyncratic, and life-threatening hepatotoxicity is reported to occur in fewer than 1 in 10,000 patients (Jeavons 1983). This complication is acute hepatic necrosis and occurs unpredictably, usually within the first month of therapy. Regular blood monitoring is suggested for patients with risk factors for liver disease or with abnormal baseline liver function. Prescribing carbamazepine to patients with preexisting liver disease has risks; therefore, significant liver disease is also a relative contraindication to carbamazepine.

The quinidine-like effects of carbamazepine are related to its tricyclic structure; therefore, precautions similar to those for tricyclics are indicated (Levenson 1993).

Carbamazepine has an antidiuretic action that is associated with both clinically significant hyponatremia and mild, asymptomatic hyponatremia. The effect is probably mediated via a direct action on the renal tubules. Risk factors that predispose a patient to hyponatremia include advanced age, diuretic use, and congestive heart failure. These patients should have weekly electrolyte determinations during the first month of therapy.

Because carbamazepine is a potent inducer of cytochrome P450 3A3/4, it influences the metabolism of many drugs that rely on that enzyme. Therefore, the blood levels of some drugs may drop if carbamazepine is added to a patient's medication regimen. Carbamazepine even induces its own metabolism, necessitating gradual increases in dosage over the first few weeks of treatment to maintain a steady blood level. This phenomenon is problematic for women taking oral contraceptives (which may have reduced effectiveness if taken concomitantly with carbamazepine). Furthermore, drug metabolites that are not usually clinically significant might be present in larger quantities as a result of carbamazepine induction of metabolic enzymes. Hydroxymetabolites of desipramine have been reported to cause ECG changes in a patient concurrently treated with carbamazepine and desipramine, despite a desipramine level in the therapeutic range (Baldessarini et al. 1988).

Valproic Acid

Adverse effects. When prescribing valproic acid to medically ill patients, the clinician must be alert to gastrointestinal side effects, hepatotoxicity, coagulation effects, and possible drug-drug interactions. The most troublesome side effect of valproic acid for most patients is nausea, often accompanied by vomiting. Medically ill patients, particularly those predisposed to nausea, are at increased risk. Depakote (divalproex sodium) is generally less

likely to cause gastrointestinal upset than Depakene (valproic acid), and more frequent dosing, preferably after meals, sometimes is better tolerated than larger doses taken fewer times a day. A substantial number of patients find valproic acid to be intolerable because of gastrointestinal toxicity (A. Stoudemire et al. 1993).

Although hepatic toxicity is a concern when prescribing valproic acid, it is relatively rare. Hepatic necrosis is a major risk factor for children under age 2 years, but in adults, it is an uncommon complication that occurs in only 1 in 10,000 patients (Eadie et al. 1988). Other investigators report the incidence of hepatic necrosis to be as low as 1 in 50,000, with 95% of patients developing symptoms within the first 6 months of therapy (Scheffner et al. 1988). Therefore, periodic liver function tests should be done during the first 6 months of therapy. Aside from this rare hepatic complication, a more common and benign hepatic effect of valproic acid is an increase in serum ammonia levels resulting from valproic acid's inhibition of urea synthesis. Although this elevation in serum ammonia usually does not cause any difficulties in patients, it can be problematic for patients with preexisting liver disease, especially those prone to hepatic encephalopathy. Therefore, significant liver disease is a relative contraindication to valproic acid therapy.

Valproic acid can adversely affect coagulation by increasing prothrombin time, decreasing fibrinogen levels, and reducing platelet counts. One or more of these findings occur in as many as one-third of patients treated with valproic acid (Rochel and Ehrenthal 1983). Therefore, clinicians must closely monitor patients with preexisting anticoagulation therapy or bleeding diatheses.

In contrast to carbamazepine, which is an enzyme inducer, valproic acid inhibits liver enzymes that metabolize drugs. Therefore, valproic acid can prolong the half-life of drugs that are hepatically metabolized. For example, prolonged and elevated benzodiazepine levels can cause increased sedation and ataxia. Valproic acid can increase the levels of other anticonvulsants. For example, valproic acid increases phenobarbital levels by inhibiting its metabolism (Redenbaugh et al. 1980) and raises the free fraction of phenytoin by displacing the drug from protein binding sites (Bruno et al. 1980). Valproic acid also increases the level of the 10,11-epoxide metabolite of carbamazepine, which is not usually measured with routine testing (Pisani et al. 1986). Thus, carbamazepine toxicity is sometimes produced at "therapeutic" levels when given concomitantly with valproic acid. The clinician must closely monitor the patient and drug levels when using combinations of anticonvulsants.

Benzodiazepines

Clonazepam, a benzodiazepine long used as an anticonvulsant, is increasingly popular among some clinicians for the rapid, although perhaps nonspecific, control of manic symptoms; it is relatively safe and easy to use (no blood monitoring). Clonazepam is often used in the dosage range of 2–5 mg/day to restore sleep in patients with acute mania. This medication is used safely and effectively in combination with the other antimanic agents.

Adverse effects. Like other benzodiazepines, clonazepam can potentiate CNS depression or disinhibition when used with other psychotropic agents. Tolerance can develop when clonazepam is used for maintenance therapy. In medically ill patients, clinicians must monitor for clonazepam's long half-life and hepatic metabolism, drug-drug interactions, and effects on respiratory drive.

Clonazepam has a long half-life (18–58 hours) in healthy adults (A. Stoudemire et al. 1993). Because it is metabolized in the liver, the half-life in elderly patients or in patients with impaired hepatic function, congestive heart failure, or metabolic inhibition from other

drugs is even longer. Therefore, the effects of drug accumulation such as ataxia, sedation, confusion, or stupor must be monitored closely in such patients. Clonazepam's discontinuation raises the potential for withdrawal symptoms. Clonazepam should be tapered as slowly as 0.25 mg every 2 weeks in patients who have had months or years of clonazepam therapy (A. Stoudemire et al. 1993). Like other benzodiazepines, clonazepam can decrease hypoxic respiratory drive; therefore, it is relatively contraindicated in patients with chronic obstructive pulmonary disease who are at risk for carbon dioxide retention. If used in such patients, clinicians must monitor blood oxygen levels to ensure that pulmonary function is not compromised.

Neuroleptics

For many years, neuroleptic agents were the mainstay for acute manic symptom management, especially if those symptoms included psychosis or hyperactivity. Psychosis and hyperactivity are potentially dangerous in hospitalized patients, particularly in critical care settings. Neuroleptics are frequently used while lithium or other antimanic drugs are started. Whether to choose a neuroleptic of high potency (e.g., haloperidol, thiothixine) or low potency (e.g., chlorpromazine, thioridazine) depends on the clinical setting. High-potency neuroleptics infrequently cause hypotension and sedation; thus, rapid dose escalation is possible. Low-potency neuroleptics, on the other hand, are more sedating—actually an advantage in achieving early control in acute mania if patients are healthy enough to tolerate side effects. However, low-potency neuroleptics have a higher frequency of anticholinergic and α-blockade side effects, which are particularly troublesome in elderly and medically compromised patients. To minimize the possibility of side effects, the neuroleptic dose should be reduced and gradually discontinued as manic symptoms begin to subside.

Other Treatments

Medications

Several other medications are occasionally used to treat mania. Calcium channel blockers (e.g., verapamil, diltiazem) may be effective treatment for some patients with mania, but further studies are needed (Dubvosky et al. 1985).

Electroconvulsive Therapy

Electroconvulsive therapy (ECT) is a valuable treatment alternative in managing acute mania. ECT is especially useful for severely manic patients who exhibit unremitting, frenzied physical activity. This behavior is especially dangerous in medically ill patients and is considered a medical emergency (Akiskal 1988). Other indications for ECT are acutely manic patients who are unresponsive to antimanic agents or who are at high risk for suicide. If ECT is used, lithium should not be administered; lithium can prolong neuromuscular blockade induced by succinylcholine (Blackwell and Schmidt 1984; Rudorfer and Linnoila 1986). Consultation-liaison psychiatrists who use ECT to treat primary and secondary mania in medical-surgical populations must maintain a firm understanding of medical contraindications to ECT, such as space-occupying intracerebral lesions, a recent myocardial infarction, and a leaky or otherwise unstable aneurysm (Weiner and Coffey 1987).

Psychotherapy

In many cases of primary and secondary mania in the general hospital setting, supportive psychotherapy is a powerful adjunct to pharmacotherapy. The behavioral and psychological manifestations of mania produce profound changes in perception, attitudes, personality, mood, and cognition. Psychological interventions are of unique value to patients undergoing such devastating changes in the way they perceive themselves and are perceived by others (Goodwin and Jamison 1990). Supportive psychotherapy also helps to develop a therapeutic alliance, which is an important tool in managing behavioral manifestations of mania. In addition, because manic patients frequently resist medications that will decrease euphoria, a strong alliance may help to enhance compliance. Clinicians may find it helpful to offer relief for symptoms that the patient finds bothersome and not to focus on symptoms the patient finds pleasurable or ego-syntonic. Supportive psychotherapy allows an open forum in which consultation-liaison psychiatrists can educate patients about mania, its underlying etiologies, and potential treatment measures. The psychotherapeutic relationship also is a safe environment to examine concerns about how the manic symptoms have affected the patient's family and to address fears of recurrence. Family therapy in the clinic and hospital settings can comfort the patient and family, particularly if they are attempting to cope with the stress of underlying medical illness.

Behavioral Management

When the patient is medically stable, psychiatric hospitalization is often required to manage acute manic symptoms, particularly if those symptoms include psychosis or suicidality. Transferring the patient to an inpatient psychiatric or medical-psychiatric unit provides a more controlled environment for treatment.

Because patients with secondary mania are often hospitalized for medical reasons at the time of symptom onset, consultation-liaison psychiatrists are typically called on to help manage the patients' symptoms. In such instances, close patient monitoring is essential. Psychiatric units are sometimes asked to provide staff or sitters experienced in working with psychiatric patients. The consultation-liaison psychiatrist must make clear treatment recommendations and openly communicate these to the referring clinicians. The ideal setting for treating patients with secondary mania is a medical-psychiatry unit, where patients can receive specialized care delivered by a staff accustomed to handling both the medical and the psychiatric sequelae of psychiatric illness.

SUMMARY

Mania, particularly in the general hospital patient, is a serious condition necessitating accurate diagnosis and treatment. Consultation-liaison psychiatrists are in a unique position to provide care for such patients. Diagnostic evaluations must carefully assess the multiple possible etiologies. Treatment options include a number of somatic therapies used alone or in combination. Supportive psychotherapy is a valuable tool, as is the treating clinician's liaison relationship with the staff of medical-surgical wards. For many manic patients in the general hospital setting, treatment is best rendered on inpatient psychiatric or medical-psychiatric units.

REFERENCES

Akiskal HS: The clinical management of affective disorders, in Psychiatry, Vol I. Edited by Michels R, Cavenar JO, Cooper AM, et al. Philadelphia, PA, JB Lippincott, 1988, pp 1–27

American Psychiatric Association: Diagnostic and Statistical Manual of Mental Disorders, 4th Edition. Washington, DC, American Psychiatric Association, 1994

Angst J: The course of affective disorders, II: typology of bipolar manic-depressive illness. Archives of Psychiatrie and Nervenartz 226: 65–73, 1978

Baldessarini RJ, Teicher MH, Cassidy JW, et al: Anticonvulsant cotreatment may increase toxic metabolites of antidepressants and other psychotropic drugs. J Clin Psychopharmacol 8:381–382, 1988

Bennett WM, Muther RS, Parker RA: Drug therapy in renal failure: dosing guidelines for adults, part II: sedatives, hypnotics, and tranquilizers; cardiovascular, antihypertensive, and diuretic agents; miscellaneous agents. Ann Intern Med 93:286–325, 1980

Bernstein JG: Psychotropic drug prescribing, in Massachusetts General Hospital Handbook of General Hospital Psychiatry, 3rd Edition. Edited by Cassem NH. St Louis, MO, Mosby Year Book, 1991, pp 527–570

Blackwell B, Schmidt GL: Drug interactions in psychopharmacology. Psychiatr Clin North Am 7:625–637, 1984

Bruno J, Gallo JM, Lee CS, et al: Interactions of valproic acid with phenytoin. Neurology 30: 1233–1236, 1980

Cassem NH: Depression, in Massachusetts General Hospital Handbook of General Hospital Psychiatry, 3rd Edition. Edited by Cassem NH. St Louis, MO, Mosby Year Book, 1991, pp 237–268

Cummings JL: Organic psychoses: delusional disorders and secondary mania. Psychiatr Clin North Am 9:293–311, 1986

Dubvosky SL, Franks RD, Schrier D: Phenelzine induced hypomania: effect of verapamil. Biol Psychiatry 20:1009–1014, 1985

Eadie MJ, Hooper WD, Dickinson RG: Valproate-associated hepatotoxicity and its biochemical mechanisms. Medical Toxicology and Adverse Drug Experiences 3:85–106, 1988

Eaton WW, Reigier DA, Locke BZ, et al: The Epidemiologic Catchment Area Program of the National Institute of Mental Health. Public Health Rep 96:319–325, 1981

Gillin JC: The sleep therapies of depression. Prog Neuropsychopharmacol Biol Psychiatry 7: 351–364, 1983

Goodwin FK, Jamison KR: Manic-Depressive Illness. New York, Oxford University Press, 1990

Hudson JI, Lipinski JF, Frankenburg FR, et al: Effects of lithium on sleep in mania. Biol Psychiatry 25:665–668, 1989

Jacobson JE: The hypomanic alert: a program designed for the greater therapeutic control. Am J Psychiatry 122:295–299, 1965

Jeavons PM: Hepatotoxicity in antiepileptic drugs, in Chronic Toxicity of Antiepileptic Drugs. Edited by Oxley J, Janz D, Meinardi H. New York, Raven, 1983, pp 201–246

Joffe RT, Brown P: Clinical and biological correlates of sleep deprivation in depression. Can J Psychiatry 29:530–536, 1984

Kosten TR, Forrest JN: Treatment of severe lithium-induced polyuria with amiloride. Am J Psychiatry 143:1563–1568, 1986

Krauthammer C, Klerman GL: Secondary mania: manic syndromes associated with antecedent physical illness or drugs. Arch Gen Psychiatry 35:1333–1339, 1978

Larson EW, Richelson E: Organic causes of mania. Mayo Clin Proc 63:906–912, 1988

Levenson JL: Cardiovascular disease, in Psychiatric Care of the Medical Patient. Edited by Stoudemire A, Fogel BS. New York, Oxford University Press, 1993, pp 539–564

Mendlewicz J, Fieve RR, Rainer J, et al: Manic-depressive illness: a comparative study of patients with and without a family history. Br J Psychiatry 120:523–530, 1972

Pisani F, Fazio A, Oteri G, et al: Sodium valproate and valpromide: differential interactions with carbamazepine in epileptic patients. Epilepsia 27:548–552, 1986

Pope HG, McElroy SL, Keck PE, et al: Valproate in the treatment of acute mania: a placebo-controlled study. Arch Gen Psychiatry 48:62–68, 1991

Post RM: Use of the anticonvulsant carbamazepine in primary and secondary affective illness: clinical and theoretical implications. Psychol Med 12:701–704, 1982

Prien RF, Gelenberg AJ: Alternatives to lithium for preventive treatment of bipolar disorder. Am J Psychiatry 146:840–848, 1989

Redenbaugh JE, Sato S, Penry JK, et al: Sodium valproate: pharmacokinetics and effectiveness in treating intractable seizures. Neurology 30:1–6, 1980

Robinson RG, Boston JD, Starkstein SE, et al: Comparison of mania with depression following brain injury: causal factors. Am J Psychiatry 145:172–178, 1988

Rochel M, Ehrenthal W: Haematological side effects of valproic acid, in Chronic Toxicity of Antiepileptic Drugs. Edited by Oxley J, Janz D, Meinardi H. New York, Raven, 1983, pp 101–104

Roy A, Breier A, Doran AR, et al: Life events in depression. J Affect Disord 9:143–148, 1985

Rudorfer MV, Linnoila M: Electroconvulsive therapy, in Lithium Therapy Monographs, Vol I: Lithium Combination Treatment. Edited by Johnson FN. Basel, Switzerland, Karger, 1986, pp 164–178

Rundell JR, Wise MG: Causes of organic mood disorder. J Neuropsychiatry Clin Neurosci 1:398–400, 1989

Scheffner D, Konig S, Rauterberg-Rutland I, et al: Fatal liver failure in 16 children with valproate therapy. Epilepsia 29:520–542, 1988

Seetharam MN, Pellock JM: Risk-benefit assessment of carbamazepine in children. Drug Saf 6:148–158, 1991

Sobotka JL, Alexander B, Cook BL: A review of carbamazepine's hematologic reactions and monitoring recommendations. DICP 24:1214–1217, 1990

Starkstein SE, Robinson RG: Affective disorders and cerebrovascular disease. Br J Psychiatry 154:170–182, 1989

Starkstein SE, Robinson RG: Neuropsychiatric aspects of cerebral vascular disorders, in The American Psychiatric Press Textbook of Neuropsychiatry. Edited by Yudofsky SC, Hales RE. Washington, DC, American Psychiatric Press, 1992, pp 449–472

Starkstein SE, Pearlson GD, Boston JD, et al: Mania after brain injury: a controlled study of causative factors. Arch Neurol 44:1069–1073, 1987

Starkstein SE, Moran TH, Bowersox JA, et al: Behavioral abnormalities induced by frontal cortical and nucleus accumbens lesions. Brain Res 473:74–80, 1988

Stone K: Mania in the elderly. Br J Psychiatry 155:220–224, 1989

Stoudemire A, Fogel BS, Gulley LR, et al: Psychopharmacology in the medical patient, in Psychiatric Care of the Medical Patient. Edited by Stoudemire A, Fogel B. New York, Oxford University Press, 1993, pp 155–206

Stoudemire GA: Selected organic mental disorders, in The American Psychiatric Press Textbook of Neuropsychiatry. Edited by Hales RE, Yudofsky SC. Washington, DC, American Psychiatric Press, 1987, pp 125–140

Wehr TA, Sack DA, Rosenthal NE: Sleep reduction as a final common pathway in the genesis of mania. Am J Psychiatry 144:201–204, 1987

Weiner RD, Coffey CE: Electroconvulsive therapy in the medically ill, in Principles of Medical Psychiatry. Edited by Stoudemire A, Fogel BS. Orlando, FL, Grune & Stratton, 1987, pp 113–134

Weissman MM, Leaf PJ, Tischler GL, et al: Affective disorders in five United States communities. Psychol Med 18:141–153, 1988

Winokur G, Clayton P: The Medical Basis of Psychiatry. Philadelphia, PA, WB Saunders, 1986

Wise MG, Rundell JR: Consultation Psychiatry, 2nd Edition. Washington, DC, American Psychiatric Press, 1993

Chapter 11

Somatization and Somatoform Disorders

Susan E. Abbey, M.D., F.R.C.P.C.

Somatization is poorly understood and has been defined as "one of medicine's blind spots" (Quill 1985, p. 3075). Somatization can be conceptualized as a way of responding or living. It is a ubiquitous human phenomenon that, at times, becomes problematic and warrants clinical attention. Somatization is extremely common in medical settings and among the patients referred to consultation-liaison psychiatrists (Katon et al. 1984). Not all patients who express somatic symptoms have a somatoform disorder. Many patients who somatize have another Axis I disorder or transiently somatize in the context of significant social stress.

■ SOMATIZATION AS A PROCESS

Definitions and Clinically Useful Theoretical Concepts

Somatization. *Somatization* has been used as a descriptive term for patients who have a tendency to experience and communicate psychological and interpersonal distress in the form of somatic distress and medically unexplained symptoms for which they seek medical help (Katon et al. 1984; Kleinman 1986). Everyone somatizes at times, but the frequency with which it is done, the intensity of the stressor required to elicit somatization, and the symptoms experienced vary. Most people have experienced somatic symptoms in response to the loss of an important relationship (e.g., the death of a loved one, a broken love affair), and everyone knows what is meant when someone refers to the sensation of a "broken heart." Experiencing headaches or stomachaches is common in many people who do not feel prepared for a task for which there is no acceptable excuse except illness.

Three components of somatization have been described (Lipowski 1988) for which interventions can be tailored: 1) experiential, 2) cognitive, and 3) behavioral (see Table 11–1).

Somatization has a variety of patterns. A study of 685 family practice patients described

Table 11–1. Clinical implications of the components of somatization

Component	Potential intervention
Experiential	Techniques to decrease somatic sensations (e.g., biofeedback, pharmacotherapy for concomitant psychiatric disorder)
Cognitive	Reattribution of sensation from sinister to benign
	Distraction techniques
Behavioral	Operant techniques to reduce medication consumption
	Contract to "save" symptoms for regular visit with primary care physician rather than visiting emergency room

three forms of somatization associated with different sociodemographic and illness behavior characteristics. Most patients met criteria for only one form of somatization (Kirmayer and Robbins 1991b). The three forms of somatization were

1. *Medically unexplained symptoms*—somatic symptoms not explained after appropriate assessment

2. *Hypochondriacal somatization*—bodily preoccupation and a tendency to worry about the possibility of or vulnerability to serious physical illness

3. *Somatic presentation of psychiatric disorder*—primary psychiatric disorders other than somatoform disorders in which somatic symptoms are the most prominent part of the clinical picture (e.g., major depression, panic disorder)

Medically unexplained symptoms. Medically unexplained symptoms are extremely common in patients in both community and clinic settings. In a study of 14 common symptoms in 1,000 patients in an ambulatory medical clinic, 74% were medically unexplained (Kroenke and Mangelsdorff 1989).

Somatosensory amplification. Symptoms are the result of bodily sensations and their subsequent cortical interpretation. *Somatosensory amplification* refers to the tendency to experience somatic sensations as intense, noxious, or disturbing (Barsky et al. 1988a). It is composed of three elements: 1) hypervigilance to bodily sensations, 2) predisposition to select out and concentrate on weak or infrequent bodily sensations, and 3) reaction to sensations with cognitions and affect that intensify them and make them more alarming (Barsky et al. 1988a). Somatosensory amplification has both trait and state components.

Illness behavior. The distinction between *illness* and *disease* (Eisenberg 1977) is a useful one for consultation-liaison psychiatrists. Illness has been described as the response of the individual and his or her family to symptoms. This contrasts with disease, which is defined by physicians and is associated with pathophysiological processes and documentable lesions. Mismatches between illness and disease are common and are at the root of many management problems. Patients with a disease such as hypertension may not perceive themselves as ill and thus may be noncompliant with treatment. Patients with somatoform disorder may view themselves as very ill despite not having a disease.

Illness behavior refers to "the manner in which individuals monitor their bodies, define and interpret their symptoms, take remedial action, and utilize sources of help as well as the more formal health care system. It also is concerned with how people monitor and respond to symptoms and symptom change over the course of an illness and how this affects behaviour, remedial actions taken, and response to treatment" (Mechanic 1986, p. 1). Illness behavior may be regarded as a syndrome, as a symptom, as a dimension, or as an explanation of behavior (Mayou 1989). Illness behavior is affected by a wide variety of social, psychiatric, and cultural factors (Kleinman 1986, 1988;

Mayou 1989; Mechanic 1986). Illness behavior can be used as a means of negotiating tensions in relationships (Mechanic 1986). As Mechanic (1986) noted, "illness is often used to achieve a variety of social and personal objectives having little to do with biological systems of the pathogenesis of disease" (p. 3).

Abnormal illness behavior is when a physician identifies "an inappropriate or maladaptive mode of perceiving, evaluating or acting in relation to one's own health status, which persists despite the fact that a doctor (or other appropriate social agent) has offered an accurate and reasonably lucid explanation of the nature of the illness and the appropriate course of management to be followed, based on a thorough examination of all parameters of functioning, and taking into account the individual's age, educational and sociocultural background" (Pilowsky 1987, p. 89). Abnormal illness behavior may be somatically or psychologically focused and may be either illness-affirming or illness-denying.

Psychological factors affecting a medical condition. This DSM-IV diagnostic category is used when psychological or behavioral factors adversely affect a general medical condition (American Psychiatric Association 1994). These psychological or behavioral factors include Axis I and II disorders, psychological symptoms that do not meet diagnostic criteria, personality traits or coping styles, and maladaptive health behaviors. The adverse effect may occur by 1) influencing the development or exacerbation of the medical condition, 2) interfering with the treatment, 3) increasing health risk, and 4) causing stress-related psychophysiological changes.

The problem of defining new diagnoses at the borderline of psychiatry and medicine. Consultation-liaison psychiatrists are asked to assess and manage disorders that exist at the interface of medicine and psychiatry and that are poorly understood, such as fibro-

myalgia (Kellner 1991), chronic fatigue syndrome (Abbey and Garfinkel 1990), functional gastrointestinal disorders (Walker et al. 1992), irritable bowel syndrome (IBS) (Guthrie 1992; Walker et al. 1990), noncardiac chest pain (Chambers and Bass 1992), chronic headache (Hopkins 1992), dizziness (Sullivan et al. 1993), medically unexplained syncope (Linzer et al. 1992), and chronic unexplained pelvic pain (Walker et al. 1988). All of these disorders appear to be characterized by increased current and lifetime prevalence of psychiatric disorders, increased nonspecific emotional distress, and increased psychosocial stressors. Multifactorial models for the etiology of these different conditions have been proposed. All of the models include factors such as psychiatric disorder, psychosocial stressors or trauma, and concepts related to somatosensory amplification and misattribution of symptoms.

Somatization as a Clinical Problem

Somatization is a ubiquitous phenomenon that in and of itself does not necessarily constitute a clinical problem. It becomes clinically significant when it is associated with significant occupational and social dysfunction or excessive health care use. Persistent somatization should be distinguished from transient somatization, which may occur as part of an acute response to a variety of significant life stressors, including bereavement (Lipowski 1988). Persistent somatization becomes a way of life and is a burden to patients, families, the health care system, employers, and society at large.

There is increasing concern about the economic burden of somatization (Shaw and Creed 1991). It has been estimated that somatization accounts for about 10% of total direct health care costs (Ford 1983). Patients with somatization disorder have higher average health costs than other patients: total charges 9 times greater, hospital charges 6 times greater, and physician services 14 times greater.

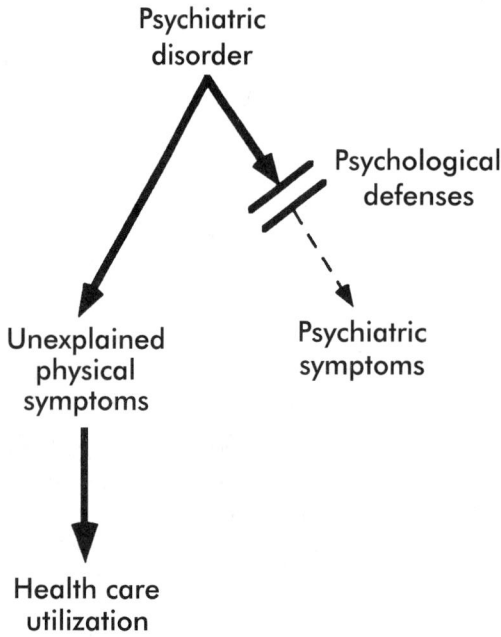

Somatization as a masked presentation of psychiatric illness.

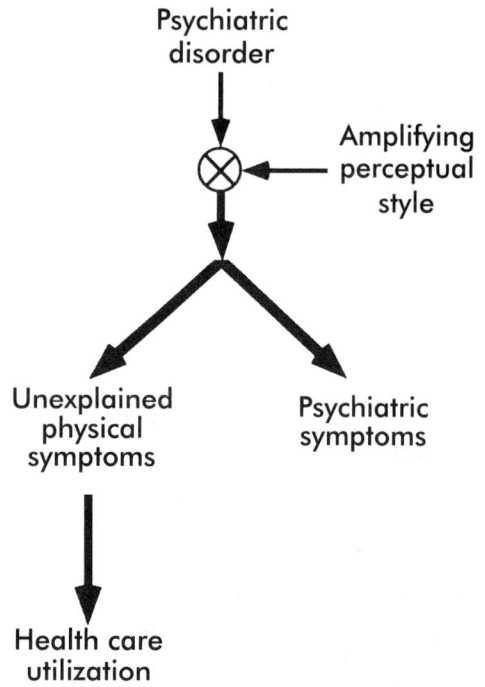

Somatization as an amplifying perceptual style.

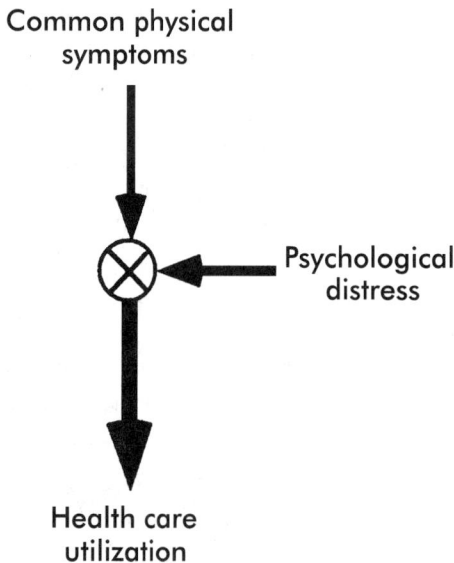

Somatization as a tendency to seek care for common symptoms.

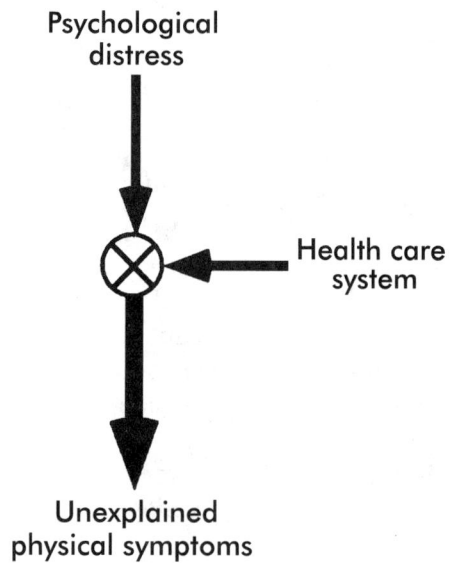

Somatization as a response to the incentives of the health care system.

Figure 11–1.   Four models of the relation between psychiatric symptomatology and psychiatric disorder. *Source.*   Reprinted from Simon GE: "Somatization and Psychiatric Disorders," in *Current Concepts of Somatization: Research and Clinical Perspectives.* Edited by Kirmayer LJ, Robbins JM. Washington, DC, American Psychiatric Press, 1991, pp. 37–62. Used with permission.

Relation Between Psychiatric Disorders and Somatization

Strong interrelations exist among somatization, psychiatric disorders, and health care utilization, with four models advanced to explain these relations (Simon 1991) (see Figure 11–1).

Somatization as a "masked presentation" of psychiatric illness. Physical symptom reporting and health care seeking may result from the physical symptoms that are an integral part of most psychiatric disorders. The somatizing patient focuses on these symptoms to the exclusion of the psychological symptoms and may in fact attribute the psychological symptoms to the distress of having the physical symptoms (e.g., "Yes, doctor, I am sad, but you would be too if you couldn't sleep or eat and had no energy!").

Somatization as an amplifying personal perceptual style. In this model, somatization is thought to result from an amplifying personal perceptual style, which is conceived of as a stable personality trait or a consequence of abnormal neuropsychological information processing (Barsky et al. 1988a).

Somatization as a tendency to seek care for common symptoms. This model posits that emotional distress prompts people to seek care for common symptoms for which they would not seek care in the absence of emotional distress. This model is supported by research in patients with IBS. Medical help seeking in patients with IBS is associated with higher levels of emotional distress despite levels of physical symptomatology similar to patients in the community with IBS who do not seek medical care (Drossman et al. 1988).

Somatization as a response to the incentives of the health care system. This model proposes that somatic symptom reporting is caused by the health care system, which tends to reinforce illness behavior and symptom reporting and may produce "iatrogenic somatization" (Simon 1991).

Etiological Factors in Somatization and Somatoform Disorders

Pathophysiological mechanisms (Table 11–2). Understanding and acknowledging physiological mechanisms underlying somatization help both the patient and the physician avoid dualistic "mind versus body" (i.e., "imaginary" versus "real") thinking and develop a therapeutic alliance.

Genetic factors. A number of studies have suggested that somatoform disorders have a genetic component (Torgersen 1986).

Developmental and social learning. Many cognitive appraisals patients make about somatic symptoms have their roots in early family experiences. For example, many patients with somatic symptoms report that their mothers were worried about health-related issues and

Table 11–2. Pathophysiological mechanisms of somatization

Physiological mechanisms
  Autonomic arousal
  Muscle tension
  Hyperventilation
  Vascular changes
  Cerebral information processing
  Physiological effects of inactivity
  Sleep disturbance
Psychological mechanisms
  Perceptual factors
  Beliefs
  Mood
  Personality factors
Interpersonal mechanisms
  Reinforcing actions of relatives and friends
  Health care system
  Disability system

Source. Adapted from Mayou 1993; Sharpe and Bass 1992.

had catastrophic interpretations for illness (e.g., every cough was likely to herald pneumonia). By the same token, physical symptoms are a major form of interpersonal communication in some families (Ford 1983; Kellner 1986).

Personality characteristics. Introspectiveness (i.e., the tendency to think about oneself) is associated with increased symptom reporting, greater physical and psychological distress, and more medical help seeking (Mechanic 1986). Negative affectivity is a construct based on negative mood, poor self-concept, and pessimism, which is associated with increased symptom reporting and greater worry about perceived symptoms (Pennebaker and Watson 1991).

Psychodynamics. Bodily symptoms may represent metaphors through which a patient expresses emotional distress or psychic conflict (McDougall 1989). Self psychologists argue that bodily preoccupation may develop in response to a sense of fragmentation of the self and can be understood as an attempt to restore a sense of integration. Rodin (1984) applied this paradigm and stated that somatization may arise from "a defective and fragile sense of self and from the relative inability to distinguish physical from psychological experiences" (p. 257). The theoretical construct of alexithymia refers to an impairment in the ability to verbalize affect and elaborate fantasies (Taylor 1984) and has been implicated in some forms of somatization.

Sexual abuse. A potential association exists between sexual abuse and childhood and adult somatoform disorders (Morrison 1989), chronic pelvic pain syndromes (Walker et al. 1988), "functional" gastrointestinal disorders (Drossman et al. 1990), and increased health care utilization (Drossman et al. 1990). Individuals who had been raped or molested before age 17 years were more likely to view common and benign symptoms as indicative of disease

than were individuals who had not experienced childhood sexual or physical trauma (Barsky et al. 1993). Consultation-liaison patients should be asked specifically about sexual abuse, particularly in gynecology and gastroenterology settings. The mechanism by which childhood sexual abuse and physical trauma are translated into somatization and adult somatoform disorders remains poorly understood.

Sociocultural factors. The ongoing stigmatization of psychiatric distress in American culture is a powerful factor promoting somatization. Organic or physical illnesses are seen as more real and less blameworthy than psychiatric disorders, which are often associated with connotations of malingering and weak moral fiber, or in some other way are seen as under the individual's voluntary control (Kirmayer and Robbins 1991a). Somatization may be the only form of communication permissible for the socially powerless (e.g., a headache that requires one to rest and remove oneself from the situation is more acceptable than openly expressing the view that the behavior of one's mate or employer is intolerable).

Iatrogenesis. The health care insurance and disability systems foster somatization by providing reinforcement and a substrate on which this psychopathology may thrive (Simon 1991). Insurance reimbursement patterns that provide coverage for physical but not psychiatric disorders foster somatization (Folks and Houck 1993).

Diagnostic Process

Examination for somatization or somatoform disorder is often difficult and requires technical skills in addition to those that are a standard part of a psychiatric assessment (Creed and Guthrie 1993; Sharpe et al. 1992).

Collaborate with referral sources. Collaboration with the referral source is essential for a clear understanding of the reason for referral and of what the patient has been told about it.

Review the medical records. The type, number, and frequency of the patient's symptoms as well as comments about the patient's prior attitude toward symptoms and behavior should be documented (Creed and Guthrie 1993). The importance of a thorough chart review cannot be overlooked because the consultation-liaison psychiatrist may be the first person to review thoroughly the typically thick chart and thus may be in a better position than any other member of the medical team to reach a diagnosis of either a general medical condition or a psychiatric disorder.

Collaborate with family and friends. This collaboration is almost always crucial to obtain an accurate assessment of the patient's history, current and past functional capacity, and current and past psychosocial stressors.

Build an alliance with the patient. The patient's ambivalence about seeing a psychiatrist must be addressed directly and early in the examination. It is essential to know what the patient has been told about the consultation process. The specific approach to the examination will vary according to the patient. For very resistant patients, the initial interview is often dominated by gaining sufficient cooperation to allow a more detailed assessment to take place at a later time. The initial phase of the examination focuses on the history of physical symptoms. Allowing the patient to report a detailed history of his or her physical symptoms and concerns gives him or her a sense that the consultation-liaison psychiatrist considers the symptoms to be serious. The question "How has this illness or symptom affected your life?" may go a long way toward answering the question "How has your life affected this illness?"

Perform a mental status examination. In addition to routine psychiatric observations, the assessment of the mental status of the patient with somatic symptoms should include the components shown in Table 11–3.

Complete a physical examination. A complete physical evaluation of the patient is a prerequisite for accurate diagnosis and treatment for several reasons. The consultation-liaison psychiatrist may be in the best position to diagnose a general medical condition because "something about the patient (personality, behavior, affect, odd cognition) has effectively distracted the primary physician and other consultants" (Cassem and Barsky 1991, p. 132).

The physical examination may help to establish a positive diagnosis of somatization disorder. For example, awareness of physical signs associated with stress (e.g., tender anterior chest wall, tender abdomen, spurious breathing, short breath-holding time) leads to a more confident diagnosis rather than a diagnosis of exclusion, which always has an implication of doubt associated with it (Sharpe and Bass 1992).

Clinical Management

The key to the clinical management of the patient with somatization disorder is to adopt

Table 11–3. Specific components of the mental status examination in the patient with somatic symptoms

Signs of abnormal illness behavior

Quality of the patient's descriptions of his or her symptoms

Thoughts, behaviors, and emotions associated with symptom occurrence

Range and depth of emotional response

Level of denial

Patient's explanations for his or her physical symptoms and the meaning of negative tests

Presence of abnormal hostility to physicians

Source. Adapted from Creed and Guthrie 1993; Sharpe et al. 1992.

"caring" rather than "curing" as a goal. "Management" is a much more realistic goal than "treatment" in this population (Bass and Benjamin 1993; Creed and Guthrie 1993; Sharpe et al. 1992). Three potential management approaches to the patient with somatization disorder have been described:

1. A *reattribution approach* that emphasizes helping the patient to link his or her physical symptoms with psychological or stressful factors in his or her life. This is accomplished via a three-step process that links psychosocial stressors (e.g., marital strife) through physiological mechanisms (e.g., increased muscle tension) to physical symptoms (e.g., headache) (Goldberg et al. 1989).
2. A *psychotherapeutic approach* in which the consultation-liaison psychiatrist concentrates on developing a close and trusting relationship with the patient.
3. A *directive approach* in which the patient is treated as though he or she has a physical problem and interventions are framed in a medical model (Benjamin 1989).

The three management approaches vary in their suitability for different patients. The reattribution approach is particularly useful in primary care settings, in medical or surgical inpatients with a fair degree of insight, and in psychiatric settings with patients who have less lengthy histories of somatization. The reattribution technique can be easily taught to primary care practitioners (Goldberg et al. 1989). The psychotherapeutic approach is most suitable for patients with persistent somatization who are willing to explore the effect of psychosocial factors on their symptoms. The directive approach is most useful for hostile patients who deny the importance of psychological or social factors in their symptomatology.

Principles of management.   The fundamental principles of management of patients

with somatization and somatoform disorders are shown in Table 11–4 and are discussed in detail in the following sections.

Emphasize explanation of symptoms.   In order to engage in treatment, patients require a sense that their primary physician and consultation-liaison psychiatrist are taking them seriously, appreciate the magnitude of their distress, and have a rationale for the proposed management plan. Reassurance, which is often thought of as helpful, may in fact be harmful in some patients. The appropriateness of reassurance must be evaluated for each patient (Warwick 1992). Confrontation is not a useful technique (Eisendrath 1989; Lazare 1981).

It is important to emphasize to patients that the psychiatrist is not dismissing their symptoms as "all in their head" but rather sees the symptoms as "real" and "in their body" and wants to explore all opportunities for symptom control. Physiological mechanisms underlying symptoms may be explained (see Table 11–2) (Sharpe and Bass 1992). Understanding the meaning of the symptom(s) to the patient and tailoring one's explanation in light of this meaning may improve the doctor-patient relationship.

Ensure regular follow-up.   The key to effective management is regular follow-up. It results in decreased health care utilization overall

Table 11–4.   Principles of management of somatization and somatoform disorders

Emphasize explanation

Arrange for regular follow-up

Treat mood or anxiety disorders

Minimize polypharmacy

Provide specific therapy when indicated

Change social dynamics

Recognize and control negative reactions and countertransference and is less stressful for patients and physicians. The best choice for most patients is management by their primary care practitioner in consultation with a consultation-liaison psychiatrist. The consultation-liaison psychiatrist may provide primary follow-up if significant comorbid Axis I or Axis II pathology is present or if the primary care physician cannot manage the symptoms.

Treat mood or anxiety disorders. Mood or anxiety disorders have significant morbidity in their own right and interfere with participation in rehabilitation and psychotherapy; also, their physiological concomitants may fuel the somatization process or heighten somatic amplification.

Minimize polypharmacy. Polypharmacy may produce iatrogenic complications. Unnecessary medications should be tapered and withdrawn. This process may be long and complicated (i.e., months to several years), and it is important to take a staged approach with small, realistically achievable steps.

Provide specific therapy when indicated. A variety of specific therapies have been recommended for the somatoform disorders, which are discussed later in this chapter. Physiotherapy or massage may be helpful in diminishing musculoskeletal pain in patients with somatoform disorders.

Change social dynamics that reinforce symptoms. Many patients' lives come to revolve around their symptoms and use of the health care system. Regularly scheduled follow-up means that the patient no longer has to present a symptom as a "ticket of admission" to the physician's office. Important members of the patient's social support system may be persuaded to reward consistently nonillness-related behaviors. Social skills building, life skills training, assertiveness training, and physical reactivation programs may be indicated.

Recognize and control negative reactions or countertransference. Patients with somatization disorder evoke powerful emotional responses in physicians, which may result in less than optimal clinical care (Hahn et al. 1994; Sharpe et al. 1994). The range of emotions experienced by physicians may include guilt for failing to "help" the patient, fear that the patient will make a complaint, and anger at the patient's entitlement. The physician may be dismissive of the patient or, alternatively, may collude with the patient in excessive investigations to exclude physical disease in "a suspension of professional judgment" (Bass and Murphy 1990). The treating physician must identify something about the patient that is either likable or interesting that will help to sustain his or her involvement—in the most difficult patients, it may simply be a sense of amazement at the degree of disturbance. A physician caring for these patients must also be able to set clear limits as to his or her availability. If all else fails, it may be necessary to transfer the care of difficult patients to a colleague at least temporarily.

SOMATOFORM DISORDERS

The common feature shared by the somatoform diagnoses is "the presence of physical symptoms that suggest a general medical condition (hence, the term *somatoform*) and are not fully explained by a general medical condition, by the direct effects of a substance, or by another mental disorder (e.g., Panic Disorder) . . . the physical symptoms are not intentional (i.e., under voluntary control)" (American Psychiatric Association 1994, p. 445).

Somatization Disorder

Definition. Somatization disorder has a lengthy history and is based on Briquet's syndrome (Feighner et al. 1972). DSM-IV diagnostic criteria for somatization disorder are shown in Table 11–5.

Epidemiology. The general population lifetime prevalence of somatization disorder is estimated at 0.1%–2% (Swartz et al. 1986). Because patients with somatization disorder seek out medical help, their prevalence in medical settings is higher than in the general population and has been diagnosed in 5% of outpatient medical clinic patients (deGruy et al. 1987a) and in 9% of one sample of 213 medical and surgical inpatients (deGruy et al. 1987b). The disorder is uncommon in men (Golding et al. 1991), with recent estimates of lifetime prevalence of 0.2%–2% in women and less than 0.2% in men (American Psychiatric Association 1994). Women and men with somatization disorder have similar clinical characteristics, including comorbid psychopathology (Golding et al. 1991). By definition, the syndrome must begin before age 30, but most often symptoms begin in the teens, often with menarche, or less commonly in the early 20s. The risk for depression, alcohol abuse, and antisocial personality disorder is increased in the first-degree relatives of individuals with somatization disorder (Golding et al. 1992).

Clinical features. The classic patient with somatization disorder is a woman who began to experience medically unexplained symptoms in early adolescence and has shown a fluctuating, waxing and waning course over the years with a medical history that documents

Table 11–5. DSM-IV criteria for somatization disorder.

A history of many physical complaints beginning before age 30 years that occur over a period of several years and result in treatment being sought or significant impairment in social, occupational, or other important areas of functioning.

B. Each of the following criteria must have been met, with individual symptoms occurring at any time during the course of the disturbance:

   (1) *four pain symptoms:* a history of pain related to at least four different sites or functions (e.g., head, abdomen, back, joints, extremities, chest, rectum, during menstruation, during sexual intercourse, or during urination)

   (2) *two gastrointestinal symptoms:* a history of at least two gastrointestinal symptoms other than pain (e.g., nausea, bloating, vomiting other than during pregnancy, diarrhea, or intolerance of several different foods)

   (3) *one sexual symptom:* a history of at least one sexual or reproductive symptom other than pain (e.g., sexual indifference, erectile or ejaculatory dysfunction, irregular menses, excessive menstrual bleeding, vomiting throughout pregnancy)

   (4) *one pseudoneurological symptom:* a history of at least one symptom or deficit suggesting a neurological condition not limited to pain (conversion symptoms such as impaired coordination or balance, paralysis or localized weakness, difficulty swallowing or lump in throat, aphonia, urinary retention, hallucinations, loss of touch or pain sensation, double vision, blindness, deafness, seizures; dissociative symptoms such as amnesia; or loss of consciousness other than fainting)

C. Either (1) or (2):

   (1) after appropriate investigation, each of the symptoms in Criterion B cannot be fully explained by a known general medical condition or the direct effects of a substance (e.g., a drug of abuse, a medication)

   (2) when there is a related general medical condition, the physical complaints or resulting social or occupational impairment are in excess of what would be expected from the history, physical examination, or laboratory findings

D. The symptoms are not intentionally produced or feigned (as in factitious disorder or malingering).

repeated unexplained physical complaints. Accompanying this chronic polysymptomatic pattern is the patient's subjective assessment of herself as "sickly."

Associated features. Patients with somatization disorder have high rates of psychiatric comorbidity for both Axis I and Axis II diagnoses. As many as 75% of patients with somatization disorder have comorbid Axis I diagnoses (Katon et al. 1991; Swartz et al. 1986), of which the most common are major depression, dysthymia, panic disorder, simple phobia, and substance abuse. Patients with somatization disorder often have multiple social problems and chaotic lifestyles characterized by poor interpersonal relationships, disruptive or difficult behavior, and substance abuse (Cassem and Barsky 1991; Ford 1983) and show significant occupational and social impairment. Women with somatization disorder are more likely to have a history of sexual abuse than are women with primary mood disorders (Morrison 1989).

Clinical course and prognosis. "Somatization disorder is a chronic but fluctuating disorder that rarely remits completely. A year seldom passes without the individual seeking some medical attention prompted by unexplained somatic symptoms" (American Psychiatric Association 1994, p. 447). Patients may have iatrogenic disease or injury secondary to unnecessary medical investigations, treatments (e.g., dependence on psychoactive substances that may have initially been unwittingly prescribed for symptom control), and surgical procedures.

Differential diagnosis. The differential diagnosis of somatization disorder includes

- General medical disorders presenting with confusing or vague symptomatology or characterized by multiple symptoms in various organ systems
- Anxiety disorders—panic disorder is characterized by multiple somatic symptoms,

but the symptoms are specifically limited to the panic attack. Generalized anxiety disorder may be characterized by multiple somatic symptoms but is accompanied by unrealistic worry, which is not limited to health concerns or symptoms.

- Depressive disorders—physical complaints may be prominent during depressed mood states but are limited to these episodes.
- Schizophrenia with multiple somatic delusions—the delusions are typically bizarre.
- Other somatoform disorders—by definition, somatization disorder includes symptoms compatible with other somatoform diagnoses. If the symptoms occur exclusively during the course of somatization disorder, then additional diagnoses are not made.
- Factitious disorder with predominantly physical symptoms—intentional symptom production occurs for the purpose of assuming the sick role and obtaining medical care.
- Malingering—intentional symptom production is motivated by external incentives.

Undifferentiated Somatoform Disorder

Definition. Undifferentiated somatoform disorder is a residual category for individuals who do not meet criteria for somatization disorder or another somatoform disorder.

Clinical and associated features. DSM-IV diagnostic criteria are listed in Table 11–6. Patients with undifferentiated somatoform disorder may have one symptom or multiple symptoms.

Epidemiology. It is probable that 4%–11% of the population have multiple, medically unexplained symptoms consistent with a subsyndromal form of somatization disorder (Escobar et al. 1989).

Clinical course and prognosis. The course of this disorder varies given that it is probably quite heterogeneous.

Differential diagnosis. The differential diagnosis of undifferentiated somatoform disorder includes

- Mood and anxiety disorders—medically unexplained symptoms commonly occur in these disorders.

Table 11–6. DSM-IV diagnostic criteria for undifferentiated somatoform disorder

A. One or more physical complaints (e.g., fatigue, loss of appetite, gastrointestinal or urinary complaints).

B. Either (1) or (2):
   (1) after appropriate investigation, the symptoms cannot be fully explained by a known general medical condition or the direct effects of a substance (e.g., a drug of abuse, a medication)
   (2) when there is a related general medical condition, the physical complaints or resulting social or occupational impairment is in excess of what would be expected from the history, physical examination, or laboratory findings

C. The symptoms cause clinically significant distress or impairment in social, occupational, or other important areas of functioning.

D. The duration of the disturbance is at least 6 months.

E. The disturbance is not better accounted for by another mental disorder (e.g., another somatoform disorder, sexual dysfunction, mood disorder, anxiety disorder, sleep disorder, or psychotic disorder).

F. The symptom is not intentionally produced or feigned (as in factitious disorder or malingering).

- Factitious disorder with predominantly physical symptoms—intentional symptom production occurs for the purpose of assuming the sick role and obtaining medical care.
- Malingering—intentional symptom production is motivated by external incentives.

Hypochondriasis

Definition. Hypochondriasis is characterized by fears of having a disease or the belief that one has a serious disease based on the misinterpretation of bodily symptoms that persists despite medical reassurance (American Psychiatric Association 1994). DSM-IV criteria for hypochondriasis are shown in Table 11–7.

Epidemiology. Current prevalence rates for primary and secondary forms of hypochondriasis of 3%–13% have been reported for study samples from medical and psychiatric settings (Kellner 1986). The disorder appears to be equally common in men and women (American Psychiatric Association 1994). The disorder can begin at any age, but the most common age at onset is in early adulthood (American Psychiatric Association 1994).

Clinical features. The core feature of hypochondriasis is fear of disease or conviction that one has a disease despite normal physical examinations and investigations and physician reassurance. Bodily preoccupation (i.e., increased observation of and vigilance toward bodily sensations) is common. The preoccupation may be with a particular bodily function or experience (e.g., heartbeat), a trivial abnormal physical state (e.g., cough), which is taken as evidence of disease, a vague physical sensation, or a preoccupation with a particular disease (e.g., cancer). Patients with hypochondriasis believe that good health is a relatively symptom-free state and, in comparison to control patients, they are more likely to

Table 11–7. DSM-IV diagnostic criteria for hypochondriasis

A. Preoccupation with fears of having, or the idea that one has, a serious disease based on the person's misinterpretation of bodily symptoms.

B. The preoccupation persists despite appropriate medical evaluation and reassurance.

C. The belief in Criterion A is not of delusional intensity (as in delusional disorder, somatic type) and is not restricted to a circumscribed concern about appearance (as in body dysmorphic disorder).

D. The preoccupation causes clinically significant distress or impairment in social, occupational, or other important areas of functioning.

E. The duration of the disturbance is at least 6 months.

F. The preoccupation is not better accounted for by generalized anxiety disorder, obsessive-compulsive disorder, panic disorder, a major depressive episode, separation anxiety, or another somatoform disorder.

Specify if:
  With poor insight: if, for most of the time during the current episode, the person does not recognize that the concern about having a serious illness is excessive or unreasonable

consider symptoms to be indicative of disease (Barsky et al. 1993).

Associated features. High medical utilization is common, and the potential exists for iatrogenic damage from repeated investigations. Interpersonal relationships typically deteriorate because of the preoccupation with disease. Occupational functioning is often compromised with increased time taken off from work and decreased performance when the individual is at work because of the preoccupation with disease.

Clinical course and prognosis. Primary hypochondriasis appears to be a chronic condition, and thus, some have argued that it might be better understood in terms of a personality style or characteristic (Tyrer et al. 1990). Some forms of secondary hypochondriasis remit with resolution or treatment of the underlying condition (e.g., major life stressors, mood or anxiety disorders).

Differential diagnosis. The differential diagnosis of hypochondriasis includes

- General medical conditions—often the early stages of a variety of rheumatological, immunological, endocrine, and neurological diseases may be associated with subtle pathology that may not be detected by physical examination or laboratory investigation but may be noticeable in some way to patients. Hypochondriasis may also coexist with medical pathology (Barsky et al. 1986).
- Axis I disorders—a number of Axis I disorders may be characterized by a degree of hypochondriacal concern. These disorders include major depression, dysthymia, the anxiety disorders (including panic disorder, generalized anxiety disorder, obsessive-compulsive disorder), and somatization disorder.
- Psychotic disorders, including major depression, with psychotic features; schizophrenia; and delusional disorder, somatic type, are characterized by the fixed quality of the delusional belief in contrast to the hypochondriacal patient, who is convinced of the veracity of his or her concerns but is able to consider the possibility that the feared disease is not present.

Conversion Disorder

Definition. DSM-IV diagnostic criteria for conversion disorder are shown in Table 11–8.

Epidemiology. The prevalence of conversion disorder varies between rates of 0.3% in the general population, 1%–3% in medical outpatient settings, and 1%–4.5% in inpatient neurological and medical settings. Women outnumber men with the disorder in a ratio varying from 2:1 to 10:1 (Murphy 1990). Men are more likely to present with conversion symptoms related to military service and industrial accidents (Folks and Houck 1993). Onset is typically in adolescence or early adulthood,

Table 11–8. DSM-IV diagnostic criteria for conversion disorder

A. One or more symptoms or deficits affecting voluntary motor or sensory function that suggest a neurological or other general medical condition.

B. Psychological factors are judged to be associated with the symptom or deficit because the initiation or exacerbation of the symptom or deficit is preceded by conflicts or other stressors.

C. The symptom or deficit is not intentionally produced or feigned (as in factitious disorder or malingering).

D. The symptom or deficit cannot, after appropriate investigation, be fully explained by a general medical condition, or by the direct effects of a substance, or as a culturally sanctioned behavior or experience.

E. The symptom or deficit causes clinically significant distress or impairment in social, occupational, or other important areas of functioning or warrants medical evaluation.

F. The symptom or deficit is not limited to pain or sexual dysfunction, does not occur exclusively during the course of somatization disorder, and is not better accounted for by another mental disorder.

Specify type of symptom or deficit:
  With motor symptom or deficit
  With sensory symptom or deficit
  With seizures or convulsions
  With mixed presentation

but cases have been described in children (Shapiro and Rosenfeld 1987) as well as in later life. The need for caution about making the diagnosis comes from findings that between 13% and 35% of patients given a diagnosis of conversion disorder in earlier studies were subsequently diagnosed with a medical condition that explained the symptom (Slater and Glithero 1965; Stefansson et al. 1976).

Clinical features. Conversion symptoms are neurological in nature and affect voluntary motor or sensory functioning. Common conversion symptoms include motor symptoms (e.g., paralysis, disturbances in coordination or balance, localized weakness, akinesia, dyskinesia, aphonia, urinary retention, and difficulty swallowing), sensory symptoms (e.g., blindness, double vision, anesthesia, paresthesia, deafness), and seizures or convulsions that may have voluntary motor or sensory components. Unilateral symptoms are more likely to occur on the left side of the body as is true for somatoform pain, hyperventilation, and hypochondriasis (Toone 1990). The neurophysiological basis for the lateralization is unclear (Toone 1990). The diagnosis of conversion is "predicated on two sets of negatives: (i) signs and symptoms of physical ill health which the physician refuses to accept, and (ii) inferences (by the physician) of psychological disturbance which the patient (usually) rebuts" (Toone 1990, p. 215). Psychological mechanisms were specifically implicated in prior diagnostic definitions, but the definition according to DSM-IV only requires that psychological factors be associated with symptom onset or exacerbation. Earlier discussions of conversion focused on the etiological role of primary gain. For example, a conflict about aggression might be symbolically expressed through a paralyzed arm. Secondary gain is intrinsic to the sick role and thus is present in many general medical conditions and psychiatric disorders. Secondary gain may occur in conversion disorder patients, but it is not consciously sought. This contrasts with malingering in which symptoms are produced intentionally, motivated by external incentives, or factitious disorders in which symptoms are produced intentionally to assume the sick role.

Associated features. Little systematic study of comorbid Axis I diagnoses has been done. Protracted conversion reactions may be associated with secondary physical changes (e.g., disuse atrophy).

Clinical course and prognosis. The course of conversion disorder is unknown, but individual episodes of conversion are usually of short duration with sudden onset and resolution, although recurrence of symptoms over time is common (American Psychiatric Association 1994; Murphy 1990). In some cases, conversion symptoms may last years. Factors reported to predispose to conversion disorder are antecedent physical disorders in the individual or a close contact, which provide a model for the symptoms occurring; and severe social stressors including bereavement, rape, incest, warfare, and other forms of psychosocial trauma (Toone 1990). The prognosis of conversion disorder depends on a number of factors, including 1) acuteness of onset, 2) presence of major stressors, 3) duration of symptoms before treatment, 4) symptom pattern, 5) personality, and 6) the sociocultural context within which the illness developed (Toone 1990). Good prognosis has been linked to acute and recent onset, traumatic or stressful life event at onset, good premorbid health, and absence of other major medical or psychiatric illnesses (Lazare 1981). The majority of patients show a rapid response to treatment. Patients with pseudoseizures, tremor, and amnesia are particularly likely to have a poor outcome (Toone 1990).

Differential diagnosis. The differential diagnosis of conversion disorder includes

- General medical disorder—occult presentations of a variety of neurological, substance-induced, and general medical conditions may be mistakenly diagnosed as conversion disorder. Conversion symptoms may occur in individuals with documented medical disorders (e.g., "pseudoseizures" in individuals with epilepsy).
- Other somatoform disorders—pain disorder is diagnosed if the conversion symptom is limited to pain.
- Mood, anxiety, and psychotic disorders—conversion disorder is not diagnosed if the symptoms are better accounted for by another mental disorder.
- Dissociative disorders—share with conversion disorder symptoms that suggest neurological dysfunction. Both disorders may be diagnosed if criteria are met.
- Factitious disorder with predominantly physical symptoms—intentional symptom production occurs for the purpose of assuming the sick role and obtaining medical care.
- Malingering—intentional symptom production is motivated by external incentives.

Body Dysmorphic Disorder

Definition. The hallmark of body dysmorphic disorder (BDD) is the preoccupation with an imagined defect in appearance (if a slight physical anomaly is present, the individual's concern with it is judged to be markedly excessive) that is accompanied by significant distress or impairment in social or occupational functioning (American Psychiatric Association 1994). DSM-IV diagnostic criteria are shown in Table 11–9.

Epidemiology. The prevalence of BDD is unknown, although it is probably not rare (Hollander et al. 1992; Phillips 1991). Syndrome onset is typically in adolescence (Hollander et al. 1992; Phillips 1991; Phillips et al. 1993). Many years may pass before diagnosis

Table 11–9.   DSM-IV diagnostic criteria for body dysmorphic disorder

A. Preoccupation with an imagined defect in appearance. If a slight physical anomaly is present, the person's concern is markedly excessive.

B. The preoccupation causes clinically significant distress or impairment in social, occupational, or other important areas of functioning.

C. The preoccupation is not better accounted for by another mental disorder (e.g., dissatisfaction with body shape and size in anorexia nervosa).

because of reluctance to reveal symptoms (American Psychiatric Association 1994).

Clinical features.   Most patients with BDD have concerns about more than one body part (Hollander et al. 1992; Phillips 1991; Phillips et al. 1993). The intensity of the preoccupation with the bodily "defect" has been described as "torturing" and "tormenting," and it dominates their lives and severely limits social and occupational functioning. Many patients engage in "checking" behaviors such as observing themselves in the mirror or measuring the body part of concern. The distinction between delusional and nondelusional intensity of symptoms is often difficult to make (Hollander et al. 1992; Phillips et al. 1993).

Associated features.   Other Axis I disorders are common. Many patients with BDD also have obsessive-compulsive disorder. Psychosocial dysfunction is often profound, with social withdrawal and functioning below capacity occupationally.

Clinical course and prognosis.   BDD is usually chronic, with few symptom-free intervals, although the intensity of the symptoms may vary over time (American Psychiatric Association 1994). Patients with BDD often seek and obtain inappropriate medical and surgical treatment (Phillips et al. 1993).

Differential diagnosis.   The differential diagnosis of BDD includes

- Other Axis I disorders—A diagnosis of BDD is not made when another Axis I disorder better accounts for the behavior.
- Bodily dissatisfaction that is "normal" —concerns about appearance are common within our society, and there is a divergence of opinion as to what constitutes "normal" appearance (Murphy 1990).
- Delusional disorder, somatic type—this additional diagnosis can be made when the preoccupation reaches delusional intensity (Hollander et al. 1992; Phillips et al. 1993).

Pain Disorder

Definition.   Pain disorder in DSM-IV is the latest incarnation of somatoform pain disorder (DSM-III-R) and psychogenic pain disorder (DSM-III). DSM-IV diagnostic criteria are shown in Table 11–10. Psychological factors are judged to be important in the onset, severity, exacerbation, or maintenance of the pain, and some patients will also have a medical condition that is judged to be etiologically significant.

Epidemiology.   Pain is the most common symptom in medical settings and is associated with both physical and mental illness (Benjamin 1989). The prevalence of pain disorder is unknown. The disorder may begin at any age. First-degree biological relatives of patients with chronic pain disorder may have increased rates of depressive disorders, alcohol dependence, and chronic pain compared with the general population (American Psychiatric Association 1994).

Clinical features.   Patients with chronic pain who were diagnosed previously as having psy-

Table 11–10. DSM-IV diagnostic criteria for pain disorder.

A. Pain in one or more anatomical sites is the predominant focus of the clinical presentation and is of sufficient severity to warrant clinical attention.

B. The pain causes clinically significant distress or impairment in social, occupational, or other important areas of functioning.

C. Psychological factors are judged to have an important role in the onset, severity, exacerbation, or maintenance of the pain.

D. The symptom or deficit is not intentionally produced or feigned (as in factitious disorder or malingering).

E. The pain is not better accounted for by a mood, anxiety, or psychotic disorder and does not meet criteria for dyspareunia.

Code as follows:

307.80 Pain disorder associated with psychological factors: psychological factors are judged to have the major role in the onset, severity, exacerbation, or maintenance of the pain. (If a general medical condition is present, it does not have a major role in the onset, severity, exacerbation, or maintenance of the pain.) This type of pain disorder is not diagnosed if criteria are also met for somatization disorder.

Specify if:

   Acute: duration of less than 6 months
   Chronic: duration of 6 months or longer

307.89 Pain disorder associated with both psychological factors and a general medical condition: both psychological factors and a general medical condition are judged to have important roles in the onset, severity, exacerbation, or maintenance of the pain. The associated general medical condition or anatomical site of the pain is coded on Axis III.

Specify if:

   Acute: duration of less than 6 months
   Chronic: duration of 6 months or longer

chogenic or somatoform pain disorder were described as having "the disease of the Ds":

■ **D**isability
■ **D**isuse and degeneration of functional capacity secondary to pain behavior
■ **D**rug misuse
■ **D**octor shopping
■ **D**ependency (emotional)
■ **D**emoralization
■ **D**epression
■ **D**ramatic accounts of illness (Brena and Chapman 1983)

Associated features. Depression is diagnosed frequently in patients with chronic pain syndromes; estimates range widely between 8% and 80%, with the majority of studies finding that at least half of their chronic pain sample is depressed (Smith 1992).

Clinical course and prognosis. Iatrogenic complications include dependence on narcotic analgesics and benzodiazepines and unnecessary surgical interventions. Poor outcome has been associated with untreated pain of long duration, somatization, unemployment at the start of treatment, and receiving compensation (S. Tyrer 1992).

Differential diagnosis. For a more detailed discussion of the differential diagnosis of pain disorder, see Bouckoms, Chapter 31, in this volume.

Somatoform Disorder Not Otherwise Specified

This diagnosis is used for patients with somatoform symptoms that do not meet diagnostic criteria for any of the specific somatoform disorders.

◼ MANAGEMENT AND TREATMENT

The management of the somatoform disorders shares many features with the management of somatization outlined earlier in the chapter (see Table 11–4).

Therapeutic Role of Consultation With a Consultation-Liaison Psychiatrist

Psychiatric consultation has been shown to reduce health care expenditures in patients with somatization disorder without compromising patients' health status or satisfaction with health care. An intervention consisting of a psychiatric consultation and a letter to the referral source that described basic information about somatization disorder and outlined recommendations for management similar to those shown in Table 11–11 led to a decline of 53% in quarterly health charges, mostly accounted for by decreased hospitalization costs (Smith et al. 1986).

Approach to the Patient

In addition to the general comments made about the patient with somatic symptoms, specific approaches have been described for patients with conversion disorder, including 1) explaining to the patient that his or her conversion symptoms are not caused by a serious disease, 2) refraining from confronting the patient, and 3) providing some form of "face-saving" mechanism for symptom resolution such as physical therapy or the suggestion that the patient will improve over a specified period.

Pharmacotherapy of Somatoform Disorders

Pharmacotherapy of somatoform disorders is in its infancy. Treatments for hypochondriasis have included high-dose fluoxetine. Secondary hypochondriasis in patients with depression has been treated with amitriptyline (Kellner et al. 1986). In small series of patients

Table 11–11.   Writing a consultation report for patients with somatization disorder

Based on the study of Smith et al. (1986), the consultation report to the physician referring a patient for psychiatric assessment for multiple, medically unexplained symptoms should include the following:

1. A description of somatization disorder, including a description of its chronic relapsing course, the multiple symptoms associated with the diagnosis, its low morbidity and mortality, and the likelihood of periods when other psychiatric diagnoses may develop and be appropriate targets for treatment

2. Recommendations for regularly scheduled appointments, with frequency based on the patient's current frequency of visits and an explanation that this schedule is designed to remove the need to have symptoms present before visiting the doctor

3. Recommendations that symptoms not be taken at face value but that a physical examination be performed to assess for disease

4. Recommendations that further diagnostic procedures, hospitalizations, and surgery be avoided unless there are clear medical indications to do so

5. Recommendations that medications be kept to the minimum

6. Suggestions as to how the physician may communicate with the patient about his or her symptoms based on the consultant's understanding of the patient's psychology; such suggestions might include the recommendation that the patient not be told that the symptoms are "all in your head" but rather "the symptoms are in your body, but we have to pay attention to all of the factors that might be affecting them." The radio metaphor might be included if the patient found it helpful.

with BDD, successful pharmacotherapy has been reported with imipramine and doxepin (Brotman and Jenike 1984), clomipramine (Hollander et al. 1989), fluoxetine (Hollander et al. 1989; Phillips et al. 1993), and tranylcypromine (Jenike 1984). Studies of larger case series have suggested that some patients respond better to serotonin reuptake-blocking antidepressants (Hollander et al. 1992; Phillips et al. 1993). Analgesics have a very limited role to play in somatoform pain disorder. The use of narcotic analgesics in nonmalignant chronic pain states is controversial and is generally thought to be inappropriate (France et al. 1988). However, psychotropic medications are frequently indicated (France and Krishnan 1988). Tricyclic antidepressants decreased pain in patients with chest pain and normal angiography (Cannon et al. 1994) and in women with chronic pelvic pain (Walker et al. 1991). The mechanism(s) of action are unclear and may include visceral analgesia (Cannon et al. 1994) and improvement in sleep, which results in a reduction in the level of pain or the distress associated with it.

Physical Reactivation and Physical Therapy

Physical reactivation via a gradually escalating program of exercise (e.g., walking, swimming) often improves the quality of life in patients with a variety of somatoform disorders. It may be difficult to engage these patients in exercise, but once they become more active, they often find it pleasurable and report feelings of accomplishment, reduced stress, and greater confidence in their body. Physical therapy is invaluable in patients who have conversion disorder and may be the only treatment required (Delargy et al. 1986).

Relaxation Therapies, Meditation, and Hypnotherapy

Relaxation therapies have been used to modulate somatic sensations as part of a more comprehensive group treatment program for hypochondriasis (Barsky et al. 1988b). Relaxation therapy, biofeedback, meditation, and hypnotherapy have all been used in patients with somatoform pain (Andrasik 1986). Hypnosis has been used diagnostically and thera-

peutically in patients with conversion disorder (see review by Van Dyck and Hoogduin 1989).

Behavioral Treatment

Learning theory models have been proposed for the treatment of several somatoform disorders. Hypochondriasis has been treated with exposure and response prevention individually tailored to the patient's specific problem behaviors (Visser and Bouman 1992). Prevention of reassurance seeking was a key component of treatment because it is conceptualized as an anxiety-reducing ritual that is reinforced by the reassurance received (Warwick 1992). BDD has been successfully treated in some patients with behavioral techniques such as desensitization, live and fantasy exposure, and assertiveness training (Marks and Mishan 1988). Operant treatments of somatoform pain seek to remove positive reinforcers of pain and are more effective than other forms of treatment at increasing physical activity and reducing medication consumption (Benjamin 1989).

Cognitive Therapy

Cognitive therapy has been used in both individual and group formats for several somatoform disorders. A cognitive model directs attention to factors that maintain preoccupation with worries about health, including attentional factors, avoidant behaviors, beliefs, and misinterpretation of symptoms, signs, and medical communications (Salkovskis 1989). Cognitive therapy for somatoform pain is used to help the patient identify and replace inappropriate negative beliefs or attributions with more appropriate ideas or coping strategies (Benjamin 1989) and produces greater reduction in pain complaints than do other forms of treatment (Benjamin 1989).

Individual Psychotherapy

In general, psychoeducational and supportive techniques predominate, although insight-oriented therapy may be indicated in some patients (Ford 1983).

Group Psychotherapy

Group therapy may be particularly useful in the management of somatoform disorders. When social and affiliative needs are gratified via the group, patients' need to somatize to establish or maintain relationships may be reduced (Ford 1984).

Marital and Family Therapy

Most families will benefit from information and psychoeducational approaches (Lazare 1981). It is important to identify the family's attitude and response because they may have a conscious or unconscious interest in maintaining a symptom in a patient (Toone 1990).

◼ References

Abbey SE, Garfinkel PE: Chronic fatigue syndrome and psychiatry. Can J Psychiatry 35:625–633, 1990

American Psychiatric Association: Diagnostic and Statistical Manual of Mental Disorders, 4th Edition. Washington, DC, American Psychiatric Association, 1994

Andrasik F: Relaxation and biofeedback for chronic headaches, in Pain Management: A Handbook of Psychological Treatment Approaches. Edited by Holzman AD, Turk DC. New York, Pergamon, 1986, pp 213–239

Barsky AJ, Wyshak G, Klerman GL: Hypochondriasis: an evaluation of the DSM-III criteria in medical outpatients. Arch Gen Psychiatry 43:493–500, 1986

Barsky AJ, Goodson JD, Lane RS, et al: The amplification of somatic symptoms. Psychosom Med 50:510–519, 1988a

Barsky AJ, Geringer E, Wood CA: A cognitive-educational treatment for hypochondriasis. Gen Hosp Psychiatry 10:322–327, 1988b

Barsky AJ, Coeytaux RR, Sarnie MK, et al: Hypochondriacal patients' beliefs about good health. Am J Psychiatry 150:1085–1089, 1993

Bass C, Benjamin S: The management of chronic somatisation. Br J Psychiatry 162:472–480, 1993

Bass C, Murphy M: The chronic somatizer and the Government White Paper. J R Soc Med 83:203–205, 1990

Benjamin S: Psychological treatment of chronic pain: a selective review. J Psychosom Res 33:121–131, 1989

Brena SF, Chapman SL (eds): Management of Patients With Chronic Pain. New York, Spectrum, 1983

Brotman AW, Jenike MA: Monosymptomatic hypochondriasis treated with tricyclic antidepressants. Am J Psychiatry 141:1608–1609, 1984

Cannon RO, Quyyumi AA, Mincemoyer R, et al: Imipramine in patients with chest pain despite normal coronary angiograms. N Engl J Med 330:1411–1417, 1994

Cassem NH, Barsky AJ: Functional somatic symptoms and somatoform disorders, in Massachusetts General Hospital Handbook of General Hospital Psychiatry, 3rd Edition. Edited by Cassem NH. Boston, MA, Mosby Year Book, 1991, pp 131–157

Chambers J, Bass C: Towards a confident diagnosis of non-cardiac chest pain, in Medical Symptoms Not Explained by Organic Disease. Edited by Creed F, Mayou R, Hopkins A. London, The Royal College of Psychiatrists and The Royal College of Physicians of London, 1992, pp 17–24

Creed F, Guthrie E: Techniques for interviewing the somatising patient. Br J Psychiatry 162:467–471, 1993

deGruy F, Columbia L, Dickinson P: Somatization disorder in a family practice. J Fam Pract 25:45–51, 1987a

deGruy F, Crider J, Hashimi DK, et al: Somatization disorder in a university hospital. J Fam Pract 25(6):579–584, 1987b

Delargy MA, Peatfield RC, Burt AA: Successful rehabilitation in conversion paralysis. BMJ 292:1730–1731, 1986

Drossman DA, McKee DC, Sandler RS, et al: Psychosocial factors in the irritable bowel syndrome. Gastroenterology 95:701–708, 1988

Drossman DA, Leserman J, Nachman G, et al: Sexual and physical abuse in women with functional or organic gastrointestinal disorders. Ann Intern Med 113:828–833, 1990

Eisenberg L: Disease and illness: distinctions between professional and popular ideas of sickness. Cult Med Psychiatry 1:9–23, 1977

Eisendrath SJ: Factitious physical disorders: treatment without confrontation. Psychosomatics 30:383–387, 1989

Escobar JI, Manu P, Matthews D, et al: Medically unexplained physical symptoms, somatization disorder and abridged somatization: studies with the Diagnostic Interview Schedule. Psychiatric Developments 3:235–245, 1989

Feighner JP, Robins E, Guze SB, et al: Diagnostic criteria for use in psychiatric research. Arch Gen Psychiatry 26:57–63, 1972

Folks DG, Houck CA: Somatoform disorders, factitious disorders, and malingering, in Psychiatric Care of the Medical Patient. Edited by Stoudemire A, Fogel BS. New York, Oxford University Press, 1993, pp 267–287

Ford CV: The Somatizing Disorders: Illness as a Way of Life. New York, Elsevier, 1983

Ford CV: Somatizing disorders, in Helping Patients and Their Families Cope With Medical Problems. Edited by Roback HB. Washington, DC, Jossey-Bass, 1984, pp 39–59

France RD, Krishnan KRR: Psychotropic drugs in chronic pain, in Chronic Pain. Edited by France RD, Krishnan KRR. Washington, DC, American Psychiatric Press, 1988, pp 322–374

France RD, Krishnan KRR, Manepalli AN: Analgesics in chronic pain, in Chronic Pain. Edited by France RD, Krishnan KRR. Washington, DC, American Psychiatric Press, 1988, pp 414–444

Goldberg D, Gask L, O'Dowd T: The treatment of somatization: teaching techniques of reattribution. J Psychosom Res 33:689–695, 1989

Golding JM, Smith GR Jr, Kashner TM: Does somatization disorder occur in men? Clinical characteristics of women and men with multiple unexplained somatic symptoms. Arch Gen Psychiatry 48:231–235, 1991

Golding JM, Rost K, Kashner TM, et al: Family psychiatric history of patients with somatization disorder. Psychiatr Med 10:33–47, 1992

Guthrie E: The management of medical outpatients with non-organic disorders: the irritable bowel syndrome, in Medical Symptoms Not Explained by Organic Disease. Edited by Creed F, Mayou R, Hopkins A. London, The Royal College of Psychiatrists and The Royal College of Physicians of London, 1992, pp 60–69

Hahn SR, Thompson KS, Wills TA, et al: The difficult doctor-patient relationship: somatization, personality and psychopathology. J Clin Epidemiol 47:647–657, 1994

Hollander E, Liebowitz MR, Winchel R, et al: Treatment of body-dysmorphic disorder with serotonin reuptake blockers. Am J Psychiatry 146:768–770, 1989

Hollander E, Neville D, Frenkel M, et al: Body dysmorphic disorder: diagnostic issues and related disorders. Psychosomatics 33:156–165, 1992

Hopkins A: The management of patients with chronic headache not due to obvious structural disease, in Medical Symptoms Not Explained by Organic Disease. Edited by Creed F, Mayou R, Hopkins A. London, The Royal College of Psychiatrists and The Royal College of Physicians of London, 1992, pp 34–46

Jenike MA: A case report of successful treatment of dysmorphophobia with tranylcypromine. Am J Psychiatry 141:1463–1464, 1984

Katon W, Ries RK, Kleinman A: The prevalence of somatization in primary care. Compr Psychiatry 25:208–215, 1984

Katon W, Lin E, Von Korff M, et al: Somatization: a spectrum of severity. Am J Psychiatry 148:34–40, 1991

Kellner R: Somatization and Hypochondriasis. New York, Praeger, 1986

Kellner R: Psychosomatic Syndromes and Somatic Symptoms. Washington, DC, American Psychiatric Press, 1991

Kirmayer LJ, Robbins JM (eds): Current Concepts of Somatization: Research and Clinical Perspectives. Washington, DC, American Psychiatric Press, 1991a

Kirmayer LJ, Robbins JM: Three forms of somatization in primary care: prevalence, co-occurrence, and sociodemographic characteristics. J Nerv Ment Dis 179:647–655, 1991b

Kleinman A: Social Origins of Distress and Disease: Depression, Neurasthenia, and Pain in Modern China. New Haven, CT, Yale University Press, 1986

Kleinman A: The Illness Narratives: Suffering, Healing and the Human Condition. New York, Harper & Row, 1988

Kroenke K, Mangelsdorff D: Common symptoms in ambulatory care: incidence, evaluation, therapy and outcome. Am J Med 86:262–266, 1989

Lazare A: Current concepts in psychiatry: conversion symptoms. N Engl J Med 305:745–748, 1981

Linzer M, Varia I, Pontinen M, et al: Medically unexplained syncope: relationship to psychiatric illness. Am J Med 92 (suppl 1A):18S–25S, 1992

Lipowski ZJ: Somatization: the concept and its clinical application. Am J Psychiatry 145:1358–1368, 1988

Marks I, Mishan J: Dysmorphophobic avoidance with disturbed bodily perception: a pilot study of exposure therapy. Br J Psychiatry 152:674–678, 1988

Mayou R: Illness behavior and psychiatry. Gen Hosp Psychiatry 11:307–312, 1989

Mayou R: Somatization. Psychother Psychosom 59:69–83, 1993

McDougall J: Theaters of the Body: A Psychoanalytic Approach to Psychosomatic Illness. New York, WW Norton, 1989

Mechanic D: The concept of illness behaviour: culture, situation and personal predisposition. Psychol Med 16:1–7, 1986

Morrison J: Childhood sexual histories of women with somatization disorder. Am J Psychiatry 146:239–241, 1989

Murphy MR: Classification of the somatoform disorders, in Somatization: Physical Symptoms and Psychological Illness. Edited by Bass C. Oxford, Blackwell Scientific, 1990, pp 10–39

Pennebaker JW, Watson D: The psychology of somatic symptoms, in Current Concepts of Somatization: Research and Clinical Perspectives. Edited by Kirmayer LJ, Robbins JM. Washington, DC, American Psychiatric Press, 1991, pp 21–36

Phillips KA: Body dysmorphic disorder: the distress of imagined ugliness. Am J Psychiatry 148:1138–1149, 1991

Phillips KA, McElroy SL, Keck PE, et al: Body dysmorphic disorder: 30 cases of imagined ugliness. Am J Psychiatry 150:302–308, 1993

Pilowsky I: Abnormal illness behavior. Psychiatr Med 5:85–91, 1987

Quill TE: Somatization disorder: one of medicine's blind spots. JAMA 254:3075–3079, 1985

Rodin G: Somatization and the self: psychotherapeutic issues. Am J Psychother 38:257–263, 1984

Salkovskis PM: Somatic problems, in Cognitive Behaviour Therapy for Psychiatric Problems. Edited by Hawton K, Salkovskis PM, Kirk J, et al. Oxford, Oxford University Press, 1989, pp 235–276

Shapiro EG, Rosenfeld AA: The Somatizing Child: Diagnosis and Treatment of Conversion and Somatoform Disorders. New York, Springer-Verlag, 1987

Sharpe M, Bass C: Pathophysiological mechanisms in somatization. International Review of Psychiatry 4:81–97, 1992

Sharpe M, Peveler R, Mayou R: The psychological treatment of patients with functional somatic symptoms: a practical guide. J Psychosom Res 36:515–529, 1992

Sharpe M, Mayou R, Seagroatt V, et al: Why do doctors find some patients difficult to help? QJM 87:187–193, 1994

Shaw J, Creed F: The cost of somatization. J Psychosom Res 35:307–312, 1991

Simon GE: Somatization and psychiatric disorders, in Current Concepts of Somatization: Research and Clinical Perspectives. Edited by Kirmayer LJ, Robbins JM. Washington, DC, American Psychiatric Press, 1991, pp 37–62

Slater E, Glithero E: A follow-up of patients diagnosed of suffering from "hysteria." J Psychosom Res 9:9–14, 1965

Smith GR: The epidemiology and treatment of depression when it coexists with somatoform disorders, somatization, or pain. Gen Hosp Psychiatry 14:265–272, 1992

Smith GR, Monson RA, Ray DC: Psychiatric consultation in somatization disorder: a randomized controlled study. N Engl J Med 314:1407–1413, 1986

Stefansson JG, Messina JA, Meyerowitz S: Hysterical neurosis, conversion type: clinical and epidemiological considerations. Acta Psychiatr Scand 53:119–138, 1976

Sullivan M, Clark MR, Katon WJ, et al: Psychiatric and otologic diagnoses in patients complaining of dizziness. Arch Intern Med 153:1479–1484, 1993

Swartz M, Blazer D, George L, et al: Somatization disorder in a community population. Am J Psychiatry 143:1403–1408, 1986

Taylor GJ: Alexithymia: concept, measurement and implications for treatment. Am J Psychiatry 141:725–732, 1984

Toone BK: Disorders of hysterical conversion, in Somatization: Physical Symptoms and Psychological Illness. Edited by Bass C. Oxford, Blackwell Scientific, 1990, pp 207–234

Torgersen S: Genetics of somatoform disorders. Arch Gen Psychiatry 43:502–505, 1986

Tyrer P, Fowler-Dixon R, Ferguson B, et al: A plea for the diagnosis of hypochondriacal personality disorder. J Psychosom Res 34:637–642, 1990

Tyrer S: Psychiatric assessment of chronic pain. Br J Psychiatry 160:733–741, 1992

Van Dyck R, Hoogduin K: Hypnosis and conversion disorders. Am J Psychother 93:480–493, 1989

Visser S, Bouman TK: Cognitive-behavioural approaches in the treatment of hypochondriasis: six single case cross-over studies. Behav Res Ther 30:301–306, 1992

Walker E, Katon W, Harrop-Griffiths J, et al: Relationship of chronic pelvic pain to psychiatric diagnoses and childhood sexual abuse. Am J Psychiatry 145:75–80, 1988

Walker EA, Roy-Byrne PP, Katon WJ, et al: Psychiatric illness and irritable bowel syndrome: a comparison with inflammatory bowel disease. Am J Psychiatry 147:1656–1661, 1990

Walker EA, Roy-Byrne PP, Katon WJ, et al: An open trial of nortriptyline in women with chronic pelvic pain. Int J Psychiatry Med 21:245–252, 1991

Walker EA, Katon WJ, Jemelka RP, et al: Comorbidity of gastrointestinal complaints, depression and anxiety in the Epidemiologic Catchment Area (ECA) study. Am J Med 92 (suppl 1A):26S–30S, 1992

Warwick H: Provision of appropriate and effective reassurance. International Review of Psychiatry 4:76–80, 1992

Chapter 12

Anxiety and Panic

Eduardo A. Colón, M.D.
Michael K. Popkin, M.D., F.A.P.M.

In this chapter, we focus on anxiety and panic encountered by the consultation-liaison psychiatrist working in the hospital's medical-surgical wards. The psychiatric consultant must be able to discern 1) whether anxiety is of sufficient degree to exceed what constitutes a normative response to the challenges presented by medical illness and hospitalization, and 2) if such a threshold is crossed, to what etiological factor or factors it may be ascribed. Objective parameters are tenuous here; the decision about what is pathological is frequently facilitated by the recognition that the patient is not coping effectively with the demands of hospitalization and that symptomatology is accelerating (or that the patient is visibly struggling and losing ground). The second task involves considering several clinical factors. Is the anxiety a reactive (psychological) response to medical illness as stressor? Is the anxiety a concomitant of a preexisting or established psychiatric disorder that has been exacerbated or unmasked by the medical illness process? Is the anxiety derivative of the pathophysiology of the medical illness or a by-product (albeit untoward) of the treatment process?

DEFINITIONS/CENTRAL ELEMENTS

Anxiety is a state of fear or a subjective feeling of apprehension, dread, or foreboding. It is manifested by a wide array of physical signs and measures of autonomic activation. Regardless of etiology, anxiety "can present with disruption of practically any bodily system" (Hall 1980, p. 147). We conceptualize anxiety partly in terms of an unduly labile or overactive autonomic nervous system. Given specific internal or external challenges, some individuals respond with a degree of autonomic activation that yields overt physical symptomatology (Table 12–1). Autonomic overactivation can take either an acute or a chronic form. In the former, alarm (flight or fight) features predominate; in the latter, heightened vigilance is the predominant element of the presentations.

Table 12–1. Physical signs and symptoms of anxiety

Anorexia
"Butterflies" in stomach
Chest pain or tightness
Diaphoresis
Diarrhea
Dizziness
Dry mouth
Dyspnea
Faintness
Flushing
Hyperventilation
Light-headedness
Muscle tension
Nausea
Pallor
Palpitations
Paresthesias
Sexual dysfunction
Shortness of breath
Stomach pain
Tachycardia
Tremulousness
Urinary frequency
Vomiting

Source. Adapted from Wise MG, Taylor SE: "Anxiety and Mood Disorders in Medically Ill Patients." *Journal of Clinical Psychiatry* 51 (suppl 1):27–32, 1990. Copyright 1990, Physicians Postgraduate Press. Used with permission.

Table 12–2 lists the diagnoses found in the anxiety disorders section of DSM-IV (American Psychiatric Association 1994). Several of these diagnoses are the regular domain of the consultation psychiatrist; we review them in the following paragraphs in terms of their central elements.

Panic disorder is classified in DSM-IV as either with or without agoraphobia. These disorders entail recurrent unexpected panic attacks followed by worry, concern, and behavior changes related to the attacks. The attacks are not due to a general medical condition or the

Table 12–2. DSM-IV anxiety disorders

Panic disorder without agoraphobia
Panic disorder with agoraphobia
Posttraumatic stress disorder
Acute stress disorder
Generalized anxiety disorder
Anxiety disorder due to a general medical condition
Substance-induced anxiety disorder
Specific phobia
Agoraphobia without history of panic disorder
Social phobia
Obsessive-compulsive disorder
Anxiety disorder not otherwise specified

direct effects of a substance. Table 12–3 presents DSM-IV criteria for a panic attack.

A diagnosis of *posttraumatic stress disorder* (PTSD) requires that a trauma is "persistently reexperienced" and that there is avoidance of stimuli linked to the trauma, numbing, and persistent arousal.

Table 12–3. DSM-IV criteria for panic attack

A discrete period of intense fear or discomfort, in which four (or more) of the following symptoms developed abruptly and reached a peak within 10 minutes:

(1) palpitations, pounding heart, or accelerated heart rate
(2) sweating
(3) trembling or shaking
(4) sensations of shortness of breath or smothering
(5) feeling of choking
(6) chest pain or discomfort
(7) nausea or abdominal distress
(8) feeling dizzy, unsteady, lightheaded, or faint
(9) derealization (feelings of unreality) or depersonalization (being detached from oneself)
(10) fear of losing control or going crazy
(11) fear of dying
(12) paresthesias (numbness or tingling sensations)
(13) chills or hot flushes

Acute stress disorder involves exposure to a traumatic event plus resultant dissociative symptoms, reexperiencing of the trauma, avoidance of associated stimuli, increased arousal, significant distress, or social/occupational impairment. Symptoms must last for more than 2 days but less than 4 weeks and emerge within a month of the trauma. As in PTSD, the condition is not substance induced or the result of a general medical condition.

Generalized anxiety disorder is characterized by excessive anxiety plus "apprehensive expectation" about a number of events or activities. The worrying is difficult to control and commonly evokes restlessness, fatigue, irritability, muscle tension, and sleep dysfunction.

Anxiety disorder due to a general medical condition incorporates generalized anxiety, panic attacks, or obsessions or compulsions thought to be etiologically related to general medical conditions.

Substance-induced anxiety disorder is reserved for instances in which a clinical constellation of generalized anxiety, panic attacks, or obsessive-compulsive symptoms is linked to substance intoxication or withdrawal. The symptoms must emerge within a month of substance use or withdrawal and are not better accounted for by another anxiety disorder that is not substance induced.

Other anxiety disorders, particularly *specific phobias,* are frequently encountered by consultation-liaison psychiatrists. For example, patients who have claustrophobia often have difficulty completing a magnetic resonance imaging (MRI) scan.

EPIDEMIOLOGY: ISSUES OF COMORBIDITY AND CAUSALITY

Prevalence of Anxiety Disorders in the General and Medical-Surgical Populations

The National Institute of Mental Health (NIMH) estimated lifetime and 6-month prevalence rates of specific mental disorders in the general population by means of the Diagnostic Interview Schedule (DIS; Robins et al. 1981). Table 12–4 presents lifetime prevalence rates of anxiety disorders.

A range of studies in the ambulatory or outpatient setting have addressed the prevalence and nature of psychiatric conditions, including anxiety disorders, in primary care populations. These studies suggest that one-quarter to one-third of such patients have a formal psychiatric disorder that is often unrecognized by the primary care physician (Barrett et al. 1988; Bridges and Goldberg 1985; Hoeper et al. 1979; Schulberg et al. 1985).

Although the consultation setting has not had the benefit of epidemiological efforts on the scale of the ECA, over the years various

Table 12–4. Lifetime prevalence rates (three Epidemiologic Catchment Area sites): anxiety disorders

Disorder	New Haven, CT 1980–1981 (*N* = 3,058)	Baltimore, MD 1981–1982 (*N* = 3,481)	St. Louis, MO 1981–1982 (*N* = 3,004)
Anxiety/somatoform disorders	10.4 (0.6)	25.1 (0.8)	11.1 (0.7)
Phobia	7.8 (0.4)	23.3 (0.8)	9.4 (0.6)
Panic	1.4 (0.2)	1.4 (0.2)	1.5 (0.3)
Obsessive-compulsive	2.6 (0.3)	3.0 (0.3)	1.9 (0.3)
Somatization	0.1 (0.1)	0.1 (0.1)	0.1 (0.1)

Source. Adapted from Robins LN, Helzer JE, Weissman MM, et al: "Lifetime Prevalence of Specific Psychiatric Disorders in 3 Sites." *Archives of General Psychiatry* 41:949–958, 1984. Copyright 1984, American Medical Association. Used with permission.

consultation-liaison investigators have attempted to gauge the extent of anxiety in the general hospital inpatient areas.

Several investigators have estimated or reported the prevalence of anxiety disorders or anxiety symptoms among medical-surgical inpatients and outpatients. Such estimates have generally ranged between 10% and 30%. Using ECA data, Wells and colleagues (1988) found that patients with a chronic medical condition had a significantly higher adjusted lifetime prevalence of anxiety disorders than those without such a medical condition. They also observed that "more than eleven percent of the persons with chronic medical conditions had a recent anxiety disorder" (Wells et al. 1988, p. 979). Subsequently, Wells's group also studied the prevalence of eight chronic medical conditions in a sample of adults with anxiety disorder relative to the prevalence rates in adults without anxiety. In the second study, the authors noted that "the only psychiatric disorders uniquely associated with current active chronic medical conditions were anxiety disorders, suggesting that the association between anxiety disorders and chronic medical conditions develops *more quickly* than associations between medical conditions and other psychiatric disorders" (Wells et al. 1988, p. 980).

The prevalence rates of anxiety or symptoms of anxiety per se in medically ill patients do not distinguish between those instances in which the medical illness physiologically caused the psychiatric symptoms and those in which the anxiety is a reactive response or in which the anxiety antedates the physical disorder.

Schuckit (1983) reported that 10%–40% of medical patients with anxiety had toxic or medical etiologies for their psychiatric symptoms. Hall (1980) identified a hierarchy of medical conditions that induce anxiety. He identified that neurological and endocrine disorders accounted for the majority of "medical causes" of anxiety.

Karajgi et al. (1990) used the Structured Clinical Interview for DSM-III-R (Spitzer et al. 1990) to evaluate 50 consecutive ambulatory patients with chronic obstructive pulmonary disease (COPD). Overall prevalence of anxiety disorders was 16%; 8% had a diagnosis of panic disorder. Although the overall prevalence rate was similar to that found in the general population, the rate for panic disorder was approximately five times greater than that found in the general public. The investigators suggested that a disturbance of carbon dioxide (CO_2) response may be operative in panic disorder. Yellowlees et al. (1987) had earlier reported a 34% prevalence of anxiety disorders in a series of COPD patients; however, 27 of 50 patients in the study had been receiving corticosteroids before admission.

Frequencies of Toxic and Medical Etiologies of Anxiety Disorders

As a number of writers have emphasized, the roster of medical disorders that can directly or indirectly produce anxiety is extensive (Table 12–5). Anxiety can be caused by a gamut of endocrinological disturbances. Using the DIS, Lustman et al. (1986) found lifetime prevalence rates of 26.5% for phobic disorders and 41% for generalized anxiety disorder in type I and II diabetic patients. A second group of disorders likely to give physiological rise to anxiety are neurological diseases; these include encephalitis, multiple sclerosis, Wilson's disease, Huntington's disease, poliomyelitis, myasthenia gravis, polyneuritis, porphyria, cerebral syphilis, combined systems disease, and tumors of the central nervous system (CNS).

An example of fine work in this area is the study by Stein et al. (1990) that evaluated anxiety disorders in patients with Parkinson's disease. In an unselected sample of patients with idiopathic Parkinson's disease, Stein et al. used a range of rating scales and found that 38% of patients received a current DSM-III-R (American Psychiatric Association 1987) anxiety disorder diagnosis. These diagnoses included

Table 12–5. Medical conditions presenting with anxiety

Adrenal dysfunction/Cushing's disease

Angina

Brucellosis

Carcinoid syndrome

Cerebral arteriosclerosis

Collagen-vascular disease

Coronary insufficiency

Diabetes mellitus

Drug effects: stimulants—caffeine, cocaine, amphetamines

Drug withdrawal: antianxiety agents, caffeine, alcohol, sedatives, opiates

Hyperparathyroidism, pseudohyperparathyroidism

Hypoglycemia, hyperinsulinemia

Pancreatic tumor

Pheochromocytoma

Psychomotor epilepsy, complex partial seizures

Pulmonary emboli

Thyroid disease: hyperthyroidism, hypothyroidism, thyroiditis

Source. Adapted from Popkin 1993.

Table 12–6. Medications associated with anxiety

Anesthetics/analgesics

Antidepressants (tricyclics, SSRIs, bupropion)

Antihistamines

Antihypertensives

Antimicrobials

Bronchodilators

Caffeine preparations

Calcium-blocking agents

Cholinergic-blocking agents

Digitalis

Estrogen

Ethosuximide

Heavy metals and toxins

Hydralazine

Insulin

Levodopa

Muscle relaxants

Neuroleptics

Nonsteroidal anti-inflammatories

Procaine

Procarbazine

Sedatives

Steroids

Sympathomimetics

Theophylline

Thyroid preparations

Note. SSRIs = selective serotonin reuptake inhibitors.

generalized anxiety disorder, panic disorder, and social phobia. Notably, 29% had clinically significant social phobias. Those with anxiety disorders were no more severely disabled than the others and were not differentiated by duration or intensity of L-dopa treatment. Swedo et al. (1989) suggested that basal ganglia dysfunction was instrumental in the genesis of obsessive-compulsive symptoms in patients with Sydenham's chorea. Autoantibodies may thus have a part in the evolution of anxiety disorders.

It has long been recognized that anxiety symptoms and syndromes may be caused by medications and/or substances of abuse. The list of such causes includes aspirin intolerance, drug intoxication, caffeinism, and withdrawal from CNS depressant drugs. Many medications are capable of engendering anxiety (Table 12–6).

Levenson et al. (1992) studied the relation between psychopathology and resource use in general medical inpatients and identified 22% of a sample of 1,020 inpatients as very anxious. Seventy percent of the patients with anxiety had significant depression scores as well. Similarly, 60% of those with elevated depression scores had an anxiety score above the designated cutoff. Their data showed that high psychopathology patients had longer stays and higher costs during the index hospitalization. This finding, which was not a function of difference in severity of medical illness, applied to the anxious patients as a subcategory.

BIOLOGY OF ANXIETY

Neurotransmitters

The understanding of neurotransmitter systems, including their function and role in anxiety and other psychiatric disorders, has increased dramatically. The role of noradrenergic systems has been the focus of many panic disorder studies (Gorman et al. 1987). Locus coeruleus stimulation in animals generates behavioral responses consistent with clinical anxiety. Locus coeruleus ablation, on the other hand, decreases fearful responses (Redmond et al. 1976). Drugs that increase noradrenergic function in humans increase anxiety symptoms. Yohimbine, an α_2-receptor antagonist, increases anxiety in patients with panic disorder (Breier 1991). These studies all suggest an association between anxiety and noradrenergic systems.

Sodium lactate has become the most widely studied and accepted agent for panic induction (Pitts and McClure 1967). Other induction methods include CO_2, caffeine, and cholinomimetic agents (Gorman et al. 1987). Papp et al. (1993) studied respiratory changes in panic disorder and proposed a unifying biochemical hypothesis. These authors underscored the presence of an unstable autonomic system, with hypersensitive CO_2 chemoreceptors.

γ-Aminobutyric acid (GABA) is a major inhibitory CNS neurotransmitter that is used by up to 40% of neurons (Zorumski and Isenberg 1991). Benzodiazepine receptors are linked to GABA receptors, and their interactions result in alterations in neuronal inhibition. Activation of benzodiazepine receptors results in increased affinity of GABA to its receptors, resulting in augmentation of chloride flow into the neuron through open chloride channels. This process causes electrochemical hyperpolarization and neuronal inhibition. Antagonists that block the actions of benzodiazepines, such as flumazenil, a diazepam-binding inhibitor, and benzodiazepine inverse agonists, such as

β-carboline derivatives, cause anxiety in animals and humans (Coupland et al. 1992; Zorumski and Isenberg 1991).

It has been hypothesized that patients with panic disorder experience alterations in benzodiazepine receptor sensitivity, with their set point shifted toward an inverse agonist position (Coupland et al. 1992). Hypotheses regarding the possible alterations in the GABA-benzodiazepine receptor complex are summarized by Salzman et al. (1993). These include abnormalities in benzodiazepine receptor activity, dysregulated linkage between the subunits of the GABA-benzodiazepine complex, abnormal benzodiazepine ligands, and sensitivity to endogenous inverse agonists or to diazepam-binding inhibitor.

The successful treatment of panic disorder and generalized anxiety disorder with agents affecting serotonin function, such as tricyclic antidepressants, serotonin reuptake blockers, and serotonin agonists, suggests that serotonin has a role in anxiety disorders (Power and Cowen 1992). The effects of buspirone, an azaspirodecanedione compound, and related compounds support this hypothesis, in light of their lack of direct effect on GABA systems. Behavioral, electrophysiological, and biochemical studies suggest that buspirone acts as an agonist at presynaptic 5-HT_{1A} receptors (Tunnicliff 1991).

Anatomical Substrate

Pharmacological challenge studies, as well as electrical lesions and stimulation studies, have suggested a significant role for the locus coeruleus in modulating anxiety and panic disorder. Redmond (1987, p. 973) has described the potential role of this nucleus as an alarm system and identifies various points at which aberrations in the nucleus coeruleus may produce pathological anxiety.

It has long been postulated that the limbic system plays a central role in emotional responses. Multiple interconnections between the amygdala, the hippocampus, and other limbic structures appear to facilitate the processing of exteroceptive and interoceptive stimuli. Projections from the amygdala and hypothalamus modulate autonomic and endocrine responses involved in the regulation of anxiety (Reiman 1988). Amygdala stimulation in humans induces anxiety and fear (Chapman et al. 1954).

The potential importance of temporal-lobe structures in anxiety was recently highlighted by studies suggesting increased blood flow bilaterally during lactate-induced panic attacks. In addition, abnormal asymmetry of blood flow oxygen utilization rates was found in the parahippocampal region in patients prone to panic, and increased temporal blood flow in healthy control subjects has been demonstrated during anticipatory anxiety (Reiman et al. 1989). However, some of these changes may reflect extracranial muscle contraction during anxiety (Drevets et al. 1992).

The frontal lobes have also been implicated in the genesis and modulation of anxiety. An apparent reduction in cerebral metabolic rate of glucose in the orbitomedial region occurs in patients who undergo capsulotomy for severe anxiety disorders (Mindus et al. 1986), which suggests that the frontal-lobe system has a role in the modulation of anxiety.

■ CLINICAL CONSIDERATIONS

Anxiety Disorder Due to a General Medical Condition

First and foremost, the consultation-liaison psychiatrist who encounters significant anxiety in the medical patient must entertain the possibility that the anxiety is mediated by the medical illness. The clinician is remiss if he or she conceptualizes anxiety in the medical-surgical setting in terms of psychological response or psychogenic issues without first touching the "organic" base.

DSM-IV permits identification of specific anxiety constellations under the "general medical" rubric. Hall (1980) has suggested that secondary anxiety can be differentiated from primary anxiety by 1) onset before age 18 or after age 35 years in patients with no personal or familial psychiatric histories, 2) characteristic fluctuations in severity and duration, 3) duration of less than 2 years, 4) absence of other psychiatric symptoms (e.g., phobias, conversion disorder), and 5) absence of a recent major psychosocial stressor. Starkman et al. (1990) found that anxiety was a qualitatively different experience for a patient with pheochromocytoma and that these symptoms did not correlate with peripheral norepinephrine or epinephrine levels.

Many clinicians are inclined to rely heavily on a temporal relation to establish an organic-etiological relation. Although temporal relation is an instructive parameter, it may be misleading and subject to errors of recall. It is also apparent that psychiatric symptomatology may antedate the clinical recognition of the physical illness—that is, anxiety and depression may be the first presenting features of a medical illness. Likewise, it is by no means clear that correction of the medical illness or its treatment will result in the elimination of the psychiatric symptoms. The symptoms may develop a "life of their own."

Panic Disorder

Panic has probably received the most attention of the anxiety disorders emerging in association with medical illness. The most convincing report involved a group of patients ($n = 35$) with idiopathic cardiomyopathies awaiting cardiac transplantation (Kahn et al. 1987). Eighty-three percent of the group met criteria for at least probable panic disorder. In several other medical conditions, panic disorder was diagnosed at rates of 10%–25% (Cassem 1990). These rates far exceed those found in the general population. Rates of panic disorder have been estimated to be between 33% and 43% among patients with chest pain whose cardiac catheterizations revealed normal coronary arteries (Bass and Wade 1984; Carter et al. 1992; Cormier et al. 1988; Katon 1984; Mukerji et al. 1987; Roll and Theorell 1987). There are few current data to indicate whether panic emerging in the medical patient differs from that seen in the primary psychiatric setting. In addition, no data are available about factors such as course and onset in the medical setting.

Generalized Anxiety Disorder

This entity has traditionally been underdiagnosed by consultation-liaison psychiatrists.

Generalized anxiety disorder that is encountered in consultation-liaison psychiatry is an established condition that is often intensified or unmasked in the general hospital setting. Motor tension is typical of generalized anxiety disorder and may include trembling and twitching. In addition, autonomic hyperactivity, vigilance, and scanning are part of the overall clinical picture. Age at onset is usually during the 20s or 30s. There is some indication that symptomatology abates or is reduced with aging, particularly if the individual has achieved personal success (Uhde and Nemiah 1989). Studies of generalized anxiety disorder in the consultation setting are lacking and needed. Trepacz et al. (1988) reported a very high prevalence of generalized anxiety disorder in a series of patients with untreated Graves' disease. We reported a lifetime prevalence of 32% for generalized anxiety disorder and a 6-month prevalence of 17% in a series of patients with type I diabetes mellitus seen as candidates for pancreas transplantation (Popkin et al. 1988).

Posttraumatic Stress Disorder and Acute Stress Disorder

Consultation-liaison psychiatrists usually have little difficulty in recognizing the constellation that is still best grasped in terms of Horowitz's

model of information overload and its processing. In his seminal work on stress response, Horowitz (1976) conceptualized stress as a situation in which the individual is suddenly confronted (or assaulted) with information that is affectively overwhelming or extremely powerful. In the hospital setting, this might encompass, for example, being told that one requires radical surgery (e.g., an amputation), that one has a terminal illness or a malignancy, or that a new round of chemotherapy is needed.

Like other powerful insults, such information is likely to initially elicit a period of disbelief and/or outcry. This is generally followed by "numbing" and brief immobilization. Horowitz (1976) described that after this initial period, the individual experiences a protracted period of oscillation. In this phase of stress response, the affectively charged information alternately is repressed from consciousness and then (in pendular fashion) swings back intrusively, unsolicited into consciousness. This intrusive process may involve flashbacks or vivid imagery.

Horowitz recommended that the clinician or therapist must preclude the "pendulum" from becoming fixed at either repression or persistent awareness. Horowitz urged that treatment or therapy consist of tolerable doses of awareness in which the overwhelming affect is slowly processed or gradually incorporated. Ultimately, cognitive restructuring occurs; the new information is integrated. Its accompanying affect is addressed. In the model, the pendulum of processing then comes to rest—dead center.

Phobias

Phobias are characterized by persistent avoidance behavior "secondary to irrational fears of a specific object, activity, or situation" (Uhde and Nemiah 1989, p. 973). Intellectually, the individual usually recognizes that such fears are unreasonable, but he or she cannot dispel or surmount them. DSM-IV identifies three groupings for phobias: 1) agoraphobia without history of panic disorder, 2) specific phobia (with five categories or types), and 3) social anxiety disorder.

Agoraphobia is the fear of being in places or situations from which escape might be difficult (or embarrassing) or in which help might not be available should incapacitating symptoms arise.

Specific and social phobias tend to be shrouded by the patient and are unlikely to be identified by the primary physician unless the degree of impairment is pronounced or interferes with clinical care—for example, when a claustrophobic patient cannot tolerate an MRI procedure or when phobias involve blood, infection, or injury.

Obsessive-Compulsive Disorder

This disorder centers on recurrent obsessions or compulsions that cause marked distress, are time-consuming, or significantly interfere with functioning or relationships. These behaviors are ego-dystonic phenomena; the individual recognizes obsessions as foreign to his or her personality and compulsions as unreasonable.

ASSESSMENT AND DIFFERENTIAL DIAGNOSIS

Assessing anxiety in medically ill patients requires a comprehensive evaluation with particular focus on medical, psychological, and environmental contributors to the patient's presentation. The hospital environment itself fosters various degrees of anxiety. At first glance, anxiety symptoms may appear to be "understandable" in this context. However, even "understandable" anxiety is distressing and can complicate the course and management of medical conditions.

DSM-IV provides guidelines for diagnoses in the differential diagnosis of anxiety. However, the acute onset of anxiety may preclude diagnoses that have duration criteria, such as panic disorder, major depression, and generalized anxiety disorder. In addition, the etiological roles of toxic and medical contributors are not always clear, as required in the diagnosis of anxiety disorders due to a general medical condition. Anxiety is often the presenting symptom of a mood disorder, an impending or fully developed delirium, or a substance-induced mental disorder. In addition, anxiety symptoms in the medical setting may represent the recurrence or exacerbation of a preexisting psychiatric condition.

The patient's psychiatric history provides information and clues about biological vulnerability and whether the current symptoms are the result of a preexisting condition. Significant anxiety in a patient with no personal or family psychiatric history should heighten suspicion that toxic or medical factors might be contributing to the presenting symptoms. Similarly, a positive psychiatric history should not blind the examiner to other possible medical etiologies and contributing factors.

As discussed earlier in this chapter, a variety of medical disorders, toxic substances, and medications may cause or exacerbate anxiety (Tables 12–5 and 12–6). In addition to acute toxicity from drugs such as cocaine and amphetamines, over-the-counter preparations for the treatment of cold symptoms, weight suppression, or sleep induction may generate significant anxiety or agitation (Abramowicz 1984; R. J. Goldberg 1987). Patients withdrawing from alcohol, opiates, benzodiazepines, and barbiturates usually present with marked anxiety, delirium, or seizures. Patients frequently underreport their actual use of any of these agents or may be unable to provide this information because their medical condition is too severe. Clinicians must thoroughly review the patient's medications and substance use history to be able to assess acute anxiety in the medical setting. Families or friends can be of great assistance in this regard. They should be asked to bring in all of the patient's medications, prescribed or otherwise.

An essential aspect of treatment is to explore the patient's beliefs, fears, and overall psychological response. The experience of cognitive dysfunction in delirium, for example, presents an overwhelming psychological threat to some patients, which may be ameliorated by anticipating its likelihood, symptoms, and course (Popkin 1993). Patients may experience significant anxiety after the delirium resolves, as they attempt to integrate their recollections, discomfort, or anxiety due to the sense of lost time and as they try to integrate and understand experiences that have been particularly threatening or confusing (Mackenzie and Popkin 1980).

A variety of potential stressors in the medical setting play a significant role in patients' sense of fear and anxiety. A number of central themes may appear (Derogatis and Wise 1989a; R. J. Goldberg 1987), including a sense of alienation and separation anxiety, loss of physical control, physical damage or loss of vitality, threats to narcissistic integrity, and the threat of death. Often, patients' lack of understanding of their situation, or their personal interpretation of their conditions, will generate undue fear and apprehension.

As part of the assessment of a patient's anxiety, the psychiatric consultant must attempt to understand the patient's typical repertoire of coping strategies. This will guide the psychiatrist's interventions to help the patient utilize previously helpful and adaptive strategies or to encourage the development of new strategies.

Corroborative history is essential because access to an acutely ill patient is limited by time constraints, reduced endurance, pain, or sedation. In addition, patients may attempt to present themselves in the most favorable light, minimizing or denying relevant psychiatric history.

Diagnostic tests in the assessment of patients with anxiety include laboratory examination, electrocardiogram (ECG), brain imaging studies (CT, MRI), analysis of cerebrospinal fluid, psychiatric rating scales, and sometimes electroencephalogram (EEG). Laboratory examination should be based on suspected metabolic and electrolyte disturbances. Monitoring

of the ECG and cardiac status is essential in patients presenting with chest pain, shortness of breath, and anxiety, especially in patients at high risk for cardiac illness. Brain imaging studies will help to exclude CNS structural lesions and to establish the presence of hydrocephalus, atrophy, or demyelination. Examination of cerebrospinal fluid is essential in suspected CNS infection, subarachnoid hemorrhage, or the diagnosis of demyelinating or inflammatory processes. The EEG may be helpful when seizure activity is suspected or to establish generalized cerebral dysfunction in delirium.

A number of instruments have been developed to assist in the evaluation and monitoring of anxiety symptoms (Derogatis and Wise 1989b; Kellner and Uhlenhuth 1991). These instruments include self-rating and clinician rating scales.

Among self-rating instruments, those commonly utilized include the State-Trait Anxiety Inventory (STAI; Spielberger et al. 1970), the Symptom Checklist—90 (SCL-90-R; Derogatis 1983), Beck's Anxiety Inventory (Beck et al. 1988), and the General Health Questionnaire (GHQ; D. P. Goldberg and Hillier 1979). Clinician-based rating scales include the Hamilton Anxiety Scale (HAS; Hamilton 1959) and the Anxiety Status Inventory (ASI; Zung 1971). These instruments help to quantify and monitor the course of anxiety but vary in their length and degree of emphasis on somatic or psychological symptoms. Although many of these scales are used in medical and surgical settings, there is no gold standard. This leads to difficulties in comparing studies in this area. Direct observation by the examiner and nursing staff and reports from family, friends, or significant others are usually more helpful in the overall assessment and monitoring of clinical course than are rating scale scores alone.

TREATMENT AND MANAGEMENT

Recognition of medical or toxic causes of anxiety should lead to attempts to correct the underlying etiology or to remove any offending agents. For example, managing anxiety secondary to hyperthyroidism must target the underlying pathophysiology, with palliative treatment until the primary process resolves. Even after resolution of the acute medical process, patients may continue to experience anticipatory anxiety or become hypervigilant about changes in somatic function and may require ongoing treatment and monitoring.

Benzodiazepines, Hypnotics, and Barbiturates

The agents most commonly used to manage anxiety in the medical setting are the benzodiazepines (Table 12–7). Their rapid onset of action, ease of administration, and effectiveness when used appropriately offer several advantages. Benzodiazepines offer a wide spectrum of duration of action and can be classified as being of short-to-medium or long elimination half-life (Salzman et al. 1993). Agents with longer half-lives include diazepam, chlordiazepoxide, clorazepate, prazepam, and halazepam. Lorazepam, alprazolam, and oxazepam

have short-to-medium half-lives.

Agents with longer half-lives can be administered less frequently and may be easier to taper after prolonged use. They are more likely to accumulate in patients with impaired hepatic function and in patients taking multiple medications that undergo hepatic metabolism. Agents with shorter elimination half-lives reach steady state much more rapidly and can be eliminated in a shorter time; thus, they are reasonable options for the short-term management of anxiety (R. J. Goldberg 1987). Lorazepam and oxazepam have no active metabolites, whereas alprazolam has active metabolites of little apparent clinical significance (Rickels and Schweizer 1987). These compounds are therefore best suited for patients who have liver impairment, who are taking multiple medications, or in whom careful titration of sedative effects is required.

Midazolam has a very rapid onset and a short duration of sedative action, with profound amnestic potential (Khanderia and Pandit 1987). Therefore, it is used for anesthesia and for acute sedation during procedures

Table 12–7. Benzodiazepine characteristics

Drug	Dose equivalent (mg)	Active metabolites	Half-life (hours)
Triazolam	0.25	-	1.5–5
Midazolam		+	2–5
Oxazepam	15.0	-	5–15
Temazepam	15.0	-	9–12
Alprazolam	0.5	+	12–15
Halazepam	20.0	+	12–15
Lorazepam	1.0	-	10–20
Estazolam	0.33	+	10–24
Chlordiazepoxide	10.0	+	5–30
Clonazepam	0.5	-	18–50
Diazepam	5.0	+	20–70
Clorazepate[a]	7.5	+	30–100
Prazepam[a]	10.0	+	30–100
Flurazepam[a]	15.0	+	30–120

[a]Metabolites are active agents.

Source. Adapted from Wise MG, Taylor SE: "Anxiety and Mood Disorders in Medically Ill Patients." *Journal of Clinical Psychiatry* 51 (suppl 1):27–32, 1990. Copyright 1990, Physicians Postgraduate Press. Used with permission.

such as endoscopy. Because of the potential for acute reversal of sedation when the drug is discontinued, midazolam is sometimes used for the management of acute agitation in the intensive care unit. However, this use can often lead to prolonged administration, tolerance, dose escalation, withdrawal syndromes, and worsening of confusion (Finley and Nolan 1989).

Among these agents, only midazolam and lorazepam are reliably absorbed when administered intramuscularly (R. J. Goldberg 1987). Temazepam, triazolam, quazepam, and flurazepam are sedative-hypnotic benzodiazepines. Use of these agents over a prolonged period can lead to disturbed sleep patterns and rebound insomnia when discontinued. Hypnotic agents with a shorter duration of action and without active metabolites would be less likely to cause daytime sedation, but may be more likely to cause memory problems.

Benzodiazepine use can cause oversedation and other direct effects on CNS function, such as confusion, ataxia, decreased coordination, decreased swallowing, and diminished respiratory drive, which are all significant problems for medically ill patients (R. J. Goldberg 1987). Physiologically, benzodiazepines reduce the ventilatory response to hypoxia (Lakshminarawan et al. 1976). Patients with moderate to severe lung disease are at risk for CO_2 retention with longer-acting benzodiazepines, even at relatively low doses (Thompson and Thompson 1987). Intermediate-acting benzodiazepines without active metabolites (oxazepam and lorazepam) may be less likely than other benzodiazepines to cause hypoxia (Denaut et al. 1975). The potential for inducing cognitive changes, including amnesia, is particularly problematic when agents with a shorter duration of action are used intravenously (Healy et al. 1983; Wolkowitz et al. 1987). Monitoring patients for CNS impairment, especially in debilitated and elderly patients, is essential. Abrupt discontinuation of benzodiazepines, especially when used for prolonged periods of time, may result in rebound anxiety and withdrawal syndromes, including irritability, increased anxiety, confusion, and seizures (Petursson and Lader 1981).

Caution is mandatory when administering benzodiazepines to patients with respiratory impairment because of the potential for decreased ventilatory drive. This risk is of particular concern in patients with significant CO_2 retention, although low doses may be helpful in other patients with lung disease (Mitchells-Heggs et al. 1980). Anxiety may cause difficulties in weaning patients from ventilatory support, but oversedation will hinder weaning and should be avoided.

Neuroleptics

Although the routine use of neuroleptics for anxiety is not advocated in light of their propensity for producing side effects such as tardive dyskinesia and extrapyramidal symptoms, these agents can be utilized judiciously in specific situations. Neuroleptics are the pharmacological treatment of choice for agitation in delirium; higher-potency agents minimize the potential anticholinergic and cardiovascular side effects. Combining neuroleptics such as haloperidol with benzodiazepines such as lorazepam is increasingly popular. The clinical synergism provides additional sedation and lowers the likelihood of extrapyramidal side effects (Menza et al. 1988).

In addition, neuroleptics are particularly useful in treating anxiety and other psychiatric disorders resulting from high-dose steroids (Hall et al. 1979). Patients with severe, refractory anxiety or panic or those in whom sedation from benzodiazepine agents cannot be tolerated may benefit from a cautious trial of neuroleptics.

The treating physician must observe patients for the emergence of acute dystonia, akathisia, anticholinergic side effects, and neuroleptic malignant syndrome. Studies in the literature suggest that patients with human immunodeficiency virus (HIV) infection may be more susceptible to neuropsychiatric side effects of neuroleptics; therefore, low doses should be used initially (Edelstein and Knight 1987).

Antidepressants

Antidepressants are effective in the treatment of some anxiety syndromes, especially panic disorder (Ballenger 1991), but their effectiveness in the treatment of generalized anxiety is not as clear (Rickels and Schweizer 1987). Tricyclic antidepressants are helpful in patients with mixed anxiety and depression; however, studies addressing efficacy in the medical setting are limited, and concerns persist about decreased efficacy and heightened potential for side effects (Popkin et al. 1985). In particular, delirium and anticholinergic side effects are significant concerns. Delayed onset of therapeutic effects can present a problem when acute interventions appear necessary. Low-dose antidepressants such as trazodone are sometimes used for sedation and sleep induction, especially in situations in which benzodiazepines are not desirable. In patients with pain syndromes, antidepressants may provide additive benefits, combining sedation, decreased anxiety, and pain relief.

The use of newer antidepressants, particularly the serotonin reuptake blockers, has increased significantly in the medical setting. Side-effect profiles include lowered seizure threshold with bupropion (Johnston et al. 1991) and the potential for gastrointestinal distress, headaches, agitation, and insomnia with serotonin reuptake inhibitors (Rickels and Schweizer 1990). Potential drug interaction needs to be considered (Riesenman 1995).

β-Blockers

Because of their direct blockade of catecholaminergic effects, β-blockers are sometimes used to mitigate the peripheral manifestations of anxiety. They are particularly helpful in the treatment of conditions accompanied by increased adrenergic stimulation, such as hyperthyroidism. The effect of these agents in anxiety disorders, particularly panic disorder, however, is disappointing at best (Rickels and Schweizer 1987).

Nonbenzodiazepine Anxiolytics

Recent attention has focused on the potential use of nonbenzodiazepine anxiolytics in medical and surgical patients. Buspirone is quite attractive because of its apparent lack of abuse potential, sedative effects, and psychomotor dysfunction (Wheatley 1988). Buspirone's usefulness, however, is limited by the delay in onset of therapeutic response; demonstrable effects require 2 or more weeks. The most common side effects of buspirone include gastrointestinal distress, headaches, dizziness, and nervousness (Newton et al. 1986). Some studies have suggested that ventilatory drive might increase with buspirone administration (Garner and Eldridge 1989). Therefore, this agent may be useful in anxious patients with lung disease or who require ventilatory support (Craven and Sutherland 1991; Mendelson et al. 1991).

Psychotherapy

Supportive psychotherapy can help patients cope with the emergence of acute stressors during the hospitalization. Faced with fear and physical discomfort, the anxious patient may benefit from attempts to bolster his or her coping strategies. The effects of this complex environment require the consultation psychiatrist to assume a flexible approach, adjusting goals and interventions to the patient's changing needs. The consultation psychiatrist's tasks may include ensuring ongoing communication between the patient and care providers; providing or facilitating ongoing education about the patient's condition or treatment; and clarifying the patient's perceptions, fears, and needs. Supportive psychotherapy plays a central role in the management of anxiety in the hospitalized patient and is essential to the clinical practice of consultation-liaison psychiatry (Popkin 1993).

Brief psychodynamic psychotherapy can help a patient develop insight into the personal meaning or importance of specific events or situations. Psychodynamic psychotherapy can be accomplished, or at least begun, with attentive patients during hospitalization. Observing interaction patterns between patients and care providers (including the consultant) provides information that can help to clarify maladaptive strategies and patterns. Resistance should not generally be interpreted directly in hospitalized patients. Hospitalization tends to induce regression; anxious regressed patients need to have their current level of psychological defensive functioning supported.

Behavioral psychotherapy provides an opportunity for acute anxiety reduction, enhancement of the patient's sense of mastery, and clarification of measurable goals. Behavioral interventions commonly used in consultation-liaison psychiatry include relaxation techniques, systematic desensitization, biofeedback, meditation, hypnosis, and establishment of graded goals with simple reinforcement schedules.

Recent attention has focused on the potential efficacy of cognitive-behavior therapy in the treatment of anxiety disorders (Sokol et al. 1989; Welkowitz et al. 1991). Although several different approaches are encompassed under this heading, all approaches assume that cognitions play a central role in the patient's affect. Cognitive-behavioral psychotherapy involves active exploration, clarification, and testing of the patient's perceptions and beliefs (Turk et al. 1983).

In addition, during involvement with the anxious patient, the consultant becomes the link to the medical team caring for the patient. In a busy medical service, the escalating anxiety manifested by the patient can be perceived as based on unreasonable demands or uncooperativeness with care and may lead to further isolation of the patient. The consultant can assist nursing staff in providing structure and setting limits and in facilitating the provision of adequate medical care. In addition, medical and nursing personnel may find it helpful to discuss with the psychiatric consultant their own difficulties in managing the symptoms or behavior of particular patients.

Attention to the nature and quality of the anxious patient's social support network will facilitate the patient's symptom management on a medical ward. The effect of social support on emotional well-being and health outcomes has received significant empiric and clinical support (Rowland 1989; Wortman 1984). Lewis and Beavers (1977, p. 402) identified the family as "the most neglected component of the treatment system." The family's presence and involvement can be a source of support and reassurance, but can also heighten the patient's or the caretakers' anxiety. Attention to family members' perceptions of the patient's condition and needs, as well as their own level of anxiety and how this is communicated to the patient, may result in a significant decrease in anxiety or difficulties in management.

REFERENCES

Abramowicz M: Drugs that cause psychiatric symptoms. Med Lett Drugs Ther 26:75–78, 1984

American Psychiatric Association: Diagnostic and Statistical Manual of Mental Disorders, 3rd Edition, Revised. Washington, DC, American Psychiatric Association, 1987

American Psychiatric Association: Diagnostic and Statistical Manual of Mental Disorders, 4th Edition. Washington, DC, American Psychiatric Association, 1994

Ballenger JC: Long-term pharmacologic treatment of panic disorder. J Clin Psychiatry 52 (suppl): 18–23, 1991

Barrett JE, Barrett JA, Oxman TE, et al: The prevalence of psychiatric disorders in a primary care practice. Arch Gen Psychiatry 45:1100–1106, 1988

Bass C, Wade C: Chest pain with normal coronary arteries: a comparative study of psychiatric and social morbidity. Psychol Med 14:51–61, 1984

Beck AT, Epstein N, Brown G, et al: An inventory for measuring clinical anxiety: psychometric properties. J Consult Clin Psychol 56:893–897, 1988

Breier A: Panic disorder: clinical features, neurobiology, and pharmacotherapy. New York State Journal of Medicine 91:43S–47S, 1991

Bridges KW, Goldberg DP: Somatic presentation of DSM-III psychiatric disorders in primary care. J Psychosom Res 29:563–569, 1985

Carter C, Maddock R, Amsterdam E, et al: Panic disorder and chest pain in the coronary care unit. Psychosomatics 33:302–309, 1992

Cassem NH: Depression and anxiety secondary to medical illness. Psychiatr Clin North Am 13:597–612, 1990

Chapman WP, Scroeder HR, Geyer G, et al: Physiological evidence concerning the importance of the amygdaloid nuclear region in the integration of circulating function and emotion in man. Science 120:949–950, 1954

Cormier LE, Katon W, Russo J, et al: Chest pain with negative cardiac diagnostic studies: relationship to psychiatric illness. J Nerv Ment Dis 176:351–358, 1988

Coupland N, Glue P, Nutt D: Challenge tests: assessment of the noradrenergic and GABA systems in depression and anxiety disorders. Mol Aspects Med 13:221–247, 1992

Craven J, Sutherland A: Buspirone for anxiety disorders in patients with severe lung disease (letter). Lancet 338:249, 1991

Denaut M, Yernault J, DeCoster A: A double-blind comparison of the respiratory effects of parenteral lorazepam and diazepam in patients with COLD. Curr Med Res Opin 2:611–615, 1975

Derogatis LR: SCL-90-R Manual II. Towson, MD, Clinical Psychometric Research, 1983

Derogatis LR, Wise TN: Clinical assessment of anxiety and depression in the medical patient, in Anxiety and Depressive Disorders in the Medical Patient. Washington, DC, American Psychiatric Press, 1989a, pp 99–139

Derogatis LR, Wise TN: Screening and psychological assessment of anxiety and depression, in Anxiety and Depressive Disorders in the Medical Patient. Washington, DC, American Psychiatric Press, 1989b, pp 71–98

Drevets WC, Videen TO, Miezin FM, et al: PET images of blood flow changes during anxiety: correction. Science 256:1696, 1992

Edelstein H, Knight RT: Severe parkinsonism in two AIDS patients taking prochlorperazine (letter). Lancet 2:341–342, 1987

Finley PR, Nolan PE Jr: Precipitation of benzodiazepine withdrawal following sudden discontinuation of midazolam. DICP 23:151–152, 1989

Garner SJ, Eldridge FL: Buspirone, an anxiolytic drug that stimulates respiration. Am Rev Respir Dis 139:945–950, 1989

Goldberg DP, Hillier VF: A scaled version of the General Health Questionnaire. Psychol Med 9:139–145, 1979

Goldberg RJ: Anxiety in the medically ill, in Principles of Medical Psychiatry. Edited by Stoudemire A, Fogel BS. Orlando, FL, Grune & Stratton, 1987, pp 177–203

Gorman JM, Fyer MR, Liebowitz MR, et al: Pharmacologic provocation of panic attack, in Psychopharmacology: The Third Generation of Progress. Edited by Meltzer HY. New York, Raven, 1987, pp 985–993

Hall RCW: Anxiety, in Psychiatric Presentations of Medical Illness. New York, Spectrum, 1980, pp 180–210

Hall RCW, Popkin MK, Stickney SK, et al: Presentation of the steroid psychoses. J Nerv Ment Dis 167:229–236, 1979

Hamilton M: The assessment of anxiety states by rating. Journal of Medical Psychology 32:50–55, 1959

Healy M, Pickens R, Meisch R, et al: Effects of clorazepate, diazepam, lorazepam and placebo on human memory. J Clin Psychiatry 44:436–439, 1983

Hoeper EW, Nyczc GR, Cleary PD: Estimated prevalence of RDC mental disorder in primary care. International Journal of Mental Health 8:6–15, 1979

Horowitz M: Stress Response Syndrome. New York, Jason Aronson, 1976

Johnston JA, Lineberry CG, Ascher JA, et al: A 102-center prospective study of seizure in association with bupropion. J Clin Psychiatry 52:450–456, 1991

Kahn JP, Drusin RE, Klein DF: Idiopathic cardiomyopathy and panic disorder: clinical association in cardiac transplant candidates. Am J Psychiatry 144:1327–1330, 1987

Karajgi B, Rifkin A, Doddi S, et al: The prevalence of anxiety disorders in patients with chronic obstructive pulmonary disease. Am J Psychiatry 147:200–201, 1990

Katon W: Panic disorder and somatization: review of 55 cases. Am J Med 77:101–106, 1984

Kellner R, Uhlenhuth EH: The rating and self-rating of anxiety. Br J Psychiatry 159 (suppl 12):15–22, 1991

Khanderia U, Pandit SK: Use of midazolam hydrochloride in anesthesia. Clin Pharm 6:533–547, 1987

Lakshminarawan S, Sahn S, Hudson L: Effects of diazepam on ventilatory responses. Clin Pharmacol Ther 20:173–183, 1976

Levenson JL, Hamer RM, Rossiter C: Psychopathology and pain in medical inpatients: predict resource use during hospitalization but not rehospitalization. J Psychosom Res 36:585–592, 1992

Lewis JM, Beavers WR: The family of the patient, in Psychiatric Medicine. Edited by Usdin G. New York, Brunner/Mazel, 1977, pp 401–424

Lustman PJ, Griffith LS, Clouse RE, et al: Psychiatric illness in diabetes mellitus: relationship to symptoms and glucose control. J Nerv Ment Dis 174:736–742, 1986

Mackenzie TB, Popkin MK: Stress response syndrome occurring after delirium. Am J Psychiatry 137:1433–1435, 1980

Mendelson WB, Maczaj M, Holt J: Buspirone administration to sleep apnea patients. J Clin Psychopharmacol 11:71–72, 1991

Menza MA, Murray GB, Holmes VF, et al: Controlled study of extrapyramidal reactions in the management of delirious, medically ill patients: intravenous haloperidol versus intravenous haloperidol plus benzodiazepines. Heart Lung 17:238–241, 1988

Mindus P, Ericson K, Greitz T, et al: Regional cerebral glucose metabolism in anxiety disorders studied with positron emission tomography before and after psychosurgical intervention: a preliminary report. Acta Radiol Suppl 369:444–448, 1986

Mitchells-Heggs P, Murphy K, Minty K, et al: Diazepam in the treatment of the dyspnea in the "pink-puffer" syndrome. QJM 49:9–20, 1980

Mukerji V, Beitman BD, Alpert MA, et al: Panic disorder: a frequent occurrence in patients with chest pain and normal coronary arteries. Angiology 38:236–240, 1987

Newton RE, Marunycz JD, Alderdice MT, et al: Review of the side-effect profile of buspirone. Am J Med 80 (suppl 3B):17–21, 1986

Papp LA, Klein DF, Gorman JM: Carbon dioxide hypersensitivity, hyperventilation, and panic disorder. Am J Psychiatry 150:1149–1157, 1993

Petursson H, Lader MH: Withdrawal from long-term benzodiazepine treatment. BMJ 283:643–645, 1981

Pitts FN, McClure JN: Lactate metabolism in anxiety neurosis. N Engl J Med 227:1329–1336, 1967

Popkin MK: Consultation-liaison psychiatry, in Comprehensive Textbook of Psychiatry, 6th Edition. Edited by Kaplan HI, Sadock BJ. Baltimore, MD, Williams & Wilkins, 1993, pp 1592–1605

Popkin MK, Callies AL, Mackenzie TB: The outcome of antidepressant use in the medically ill. Arch Gen Psychiatry 42:1160–1163, 1985

Popkin MK, Callies A, Lentz RD, et al: Prevalence of major depression, simple phobia, and other psychiatric disorders in patients with longstanding type I diabetes mellitus. Arch Gen Psychiatry 45:64–68, 1988

Power AC, Cowen PJ: Neuroendocrine challenge tests: assessment of 5-HT function in anxiety and depression. Mol Aspects Med 13:205–220, 1992

Redmond DEJ: Studies of the nucleus coeruleus in monkeys and hypotheses for neuropsychopharmacology, in Psychopharmacology: The Third Generation of Progress. Edited by Meltzer HY. New York, Raven, 1987, pp 967–975

Redmond DEJ, Huang YH, Snyder DR, et al: Behavioral changes following lesions of the locus coeruleus in Macaca arctoides (abstract). Neuroscience Abstracts 1:472, 1976

Reiman E: The quest to establish the neural substrates of anxiety. Psychiatr Clin North Am 11:295–307, 1988

Reiman EM, Fusselman MJ, Fox PT, et al: Neuroanatomical correlates of lactate-induced anxiety attacks. Arch Gen Psychiatry 46:493–500, 1989

Rickels K, Schweizer EE: Current pharmacotherapy of anxiety and panic, in Psychopharmacology: The Third Generation of Progress. Edited by Melzer HY. New York, Raven, 1987, pp 1193–1203

Rickels K, Schweizer E: Clinical overview of serotonin reuptake inhibitors. J Clin Psychiatry 51 (suppl B):9–12, 1990

Riesenman C: Antidepressant drug interactions and the cytochrome P450 system: a critical appraisal. Pharmacotherapy 15:845–995, 1995

Robins LN, Helzer JE, Croughan J, et al: National Institute of Mental Health Diagnostic Interview Schedule: its history, characteristics, and validity. Arch Gen Psychiatry 38:381–389, 1981

Robins LN, Helzer JE, Weissman MM, et al: Lifetime prevalence of specific psychiatric disorders in 3 sites. Arch Gen Psychiatry 41:949–958, 1984

Roll M, Theorell T: Acute chest pain without obvious organic cause before age 40-personality and recent life events. J Psychosom Res 31:215–221, 1987

Rowland J: Interpersonal resources: social support, in Handbook of Psychooncology: Psychological Care of the Patient With Cancer. Edited by Holland JC, Rowland JH. New York, Oxford University Press, 1989, pp 58–71

Salzman C, Miyawake EK, le Bars P, et al: Neurobiologic basis of anxiety and its treatment. Harvard Review of Psychiatry 1:197–206, 1993

Schuckit M: Anxiety related to medical disease. J Clin Psychiatry 44:31–37, 1983

Schulberg HC, Saul M, McClelland M: Assessing depression in primary medical and psychiatric practices. Arch Gen Psychiatry 12:1164–1170, 1985

Sokol L, Beck AT, Greenberg RL, et al: Cognitive therapy of panic disorder: a nonpharmacological alternative. J Nerv Ment Dis 177:711–716, 1989

Spielberger CD, Gorsuch RC, Lushene RE: Manual for the State-Trait Anxiety Inventory. Palo Alto, CA, Consulting Psychologists, 1970

Spitzer RL, Williams JBW, Gibbon M, et al: User's Guide for the Structured Clinical Interview for DSM-III-R (SCID). Washington, DC, American Psychiatric Press, 1990

Starkman MN, Cameron OG, Nesse RM, et al: Peripheral catecholamine levels and the symptoms of anxiety: studies in patients with and without pheochromocytoma. Psychosom Med 52:129–142, 1990

Stein MB, Heuser IJ, Juncos JL, et al: Anxiety disorders in patients with Parkinson's disease. Am J Psychiatry 147:217–220, 1990

Swedo SE, Rappaport JL, Cheslow DL, et al: High prevalence of obsessive-compulsive symptoms in patients with Syndenham's chorea. Am J Psychiatry 146:246–249, 1989

Thompson W, Thompson T: Pulmonary disease, in Principles of Medical Psychiatry. Edited by Stoudemire A, Fogel B. Orlando, FL, Grune & Stratton, 1987, pp 553–570

Trepacz PT, McCue M, Klein I: A psychiatric and neuropsychological study of patients with untreated Graves' disease. Gen Hosp Psychiatry 10:39–55, 1988

Tunnicliff G: Molecular basis of buspirone's anxiolytic action. Pharmacol Toxicol 69:149–156, 1991

Turk DC, Meichenbaum D, Genest M: Pain and Behavioral Medicine. New York, Guilford, 1983

Uhde TW, Nemiah JC: Panic and generalized anxiety disorders, in Comprehensive Textbook of Psychiatry/V, 5th Edition. Edited by Kaplan HI, Sadock BJ. Baltimore, MD, Williams & Wilkins, 1989, pp 952–973

Welkowitz LA, Papp LA, Cloitre M, et al: Cognitive-behavior therapy for panic disorder delivered by psychopharmacologically oriented clinicians. J Nerv Ment Dis 179:472–476, 1991

Wells KB, Golding JM, Burnham MA: Psychiatric disorder in a sample of the population with and without chronic medical conditions. Am J Psychiatry 145:976–981, 1988

Wheatley D: Use of anti-anxiety drugs in the medically ill. Psychother Psychosom 49:63–80, 1988

Wolkowitz OM, Weingartner H, Thompson K, et al: Diazepam-induced amnesia: a neuropharmacological model of "organic amnestic syndrome." Am J Psychiatry 144:25–29, 1987

Wortman CB: Social support and the cancer patient: conceptual and methodologic issues. Cancer 53 (suppl 10):2339–2362, 1984

Yellowlees PM, Alpers JH, Bowden JJ, et al: Psychiatric morbidity in patients with chronic airflow obstruction. Med J Aust 146:305–307, 1987

Zorumski CF, Isenberg KE: Insights into the structure and function of GABA-benzodiazepine receptors: ion channels and psychiatry. Am J Psychiatry 148:162–173, 1991

Zung WKW: A rating instrument for anxiety disorders. Psychosomatics 12:371–379, 1971

Chapter 13

Substance-Related Disorders

John E. Franklin, Jr., M.D.
Richard J. Frances, M.D.

Substance-related disorders in the general hospital present unique challenges to consultation-liaison psychiatrists. Because of the number of consultation problems, a thorough knowledge of substance abuse, especially recognition and acute management, is essential. The hospital staff is prone to misunderstand, to neglect, and to be biased toward substance-abusing patients. In addition, the span of issues faced by the consultation-liaison psychiatrist includes drug overdose; withdrawal regimens; initial diagnosis; engaging patients in a therapeutic process; evaluating pain medication; assessing patients for liver and kidney transplantation, patients with trauma and burns (who have a high frequency of drug dependency), and pregnant substance abusers; drug abuse problems in geriatric or adolescent patients; and referral or triage to substance abuse specialists.

DSM-IV SUBSTANCE-RELATED DISORDERS

DSM-IV (American Psychiatric Association 1994) does not limit the definition of substances taken by individuals to chemicals used to alter mood or behavior. For example, over-the-counter and prescription medications (e.g., steroids, antihistamines, and anticholinergics) that have psychoactive effects are classified using an *other (or unknown) substance–related category*. Substance-related disorders are divided into *substance use disorders,* which include abuse and dependence, and *substance-induced disorders,* which include intoxication, withdrawal, delirium, dementia, amnestic, psychotic, mood, sexual dysfunction, anxiety, and sleep disorders.

DSM-IV criteria for substance dependence have not changed substantially (Table 13–1). Also, criteria related to physiological dependence (i.e., tolerance and withdrawal) are now

Table 13–1.   DSM-IV criteria for substance dependence

A maladaptive pattern of substance use, leading to clinically significant impairment or distress, as manifested by three (or more) of the following, occurring at any time in the same 12-month period:

   (1) tolerance, as defined by either of the following:

      (a) a need for markedly increased amounts of the substance to achieve intoxication or desired effect

      (b) markedly diminished effect with continued use of the same amount of the substance

   (2) withdrawal, as manifested by either of the following:

      (a) the characteristic withdrawal syndrome for the substance (refer to Criteria A and B of the criteria sets for withdrawal from the specific substances)

      (b) the same (or a closely related) substance is taken to relieve or avoid withdrawal symptoms

   (3) the substance is often taken in larger amounts or over a longer period than was intended

   (4) there is a persistent desire or unsuccessful efforts to cut down or control substance use

   (5) a great deal of time is spent in activities necessary to obtain the substance (e.g., visiting multiple doctors or driving long distances), use the substance (e.g., chain-smoking), or recover from its effects

   (6) important social, occupational, or recreational activities are given up or reduced because of substance use

   (7) the substance use is continued despite knowledge of having a persistent or recurrent physical or psychological problem that is likely to have been caused or exacerbated by the substance (e.g., current cocaine use despite recognition of cocaine-induced depression, or continued drinking despite recognition that an ulcer was made worse by alcohol consumption)

---

grouped, and the clinician must specify whether physiological dependence is part of the substance dependence.

Definitions

Withdrawal.   *Withdrawal* symptoms occur after cessation or decreased use of alcohol or medications in individuals who are physiologically dependent. Withdrawal can sometimes precipitate 1) delirium, 2) psychotic disorders, 3) mood disorders, 4) anxiety disorders, and 5) sleep disorders.

Tolerance.   *Tolerance* is an acquired decrease in the effects of a substance caused by lower blood or brain substance levels after ingestion or by increased cellular resistance. For example, Minion et al. (1989) reported a series of patients in an emergency room whose average blood alcohol concentration (BAC) was

467 mg/dL—a level known to cause coma or death in an alcohol-naive individual; 88% of these patients were oriented to time, person, and place. Tolerance is influenced by innate, acquired, or learned factors.

ALCOHOL USE DISORDERS

Several alcohol-related hospitalizations can occur before a direct connection is made between a patient's alcohol use and medical problems. Alcoholic patients tend to experience many alcohol-related problems before seeking professional help, particularly before attending Alcoholics Anonymous (AA) meetings (Bucholz and Homan 1992). Resistance to the term *alcoholism* frequently inhibits physicians from exploring the connections between abuse and biopsychosocial consequences. A hospital survey by Moore et al. (1989) found that psychiatrists positively identified alcohol abuse two-thirds of the time, whereas physicians treating gynecology patients diagnosed the disorder only 10% of the time.

Epidemiology

The Epidemiologic Catchment Area (ECA) study found that 13.6% of the general population have a lifetime prevalence of alcohol abuse or dependence (Robins et al. 1984). Follow-up data from the same ECA population reported a 1-year prevalence for alcohol disorders of 7.4%. Only 22% of these people ever used any mental health/addiction service; of these, about half were seen by specialty mental health/addiction professionals, and the other half were examined by general medical professionals (Regier et al. 1993).

Alcohol-related problems usually begin between ages 16 and 30 years. In addition, Regier et al. (1990) reported that 53% of those with an alcohol disorder or drug abuse also have a comorbid psychiatric disorder.

A conservative estimate is that 25% of general hospital inpatients and 20% of medical outpatients have alcohol-related disorders (Cleary et al. 1988; Moore et al. 1989). Unfortunately, only about 20%–50% of the general hospital population's alcohol problems are diagnosed (Moore et al. 1989).

Patients with alcoholism usually resist and avoid doctors because of denial, embarrassment, problems with authority figures, and poor self-care. Occasionally, the medical condition is the only apparent indication of alcohol abuse. Despite this, the patient must come to the same realization as other alcoholic persons: "I just can't drink anymore." Vaillant's (1983) seminal study highlights the fact that medical complications are sometimes the main reason for abstinence.

Medical and Other Complications

Common alcohol-related medical conditions include gastritis, pneumonia, liver failure, subdural hematoma, ulcer, pancreatitis, cardiomyopathy, anemia, peripheral neuropathy, fetal alcohol syndrome, Korsakoff's psychosis, and alcoholic dementia. Liver disease ranks as the ninth leading cause of death; alcoholism is a major cause of liver disease. Seventy-five percent of patients with chronic pancreatitis have alcoholism (Van Thiel et al. 1981). Alcohol use also contributes to increased rates of mouth, tongue, larynx, esophagus, stomach, liver, and pancreatic cancer (Fraumeni 1982).

The U.S. Department of Health and Human Service's Seventh Special Report to the U.S. Congress on Alcohol (1990) estimated that 200,000 deaths per year are alcohol-related. Each year, 25,000 people die and 150,000 are permanently disabled because of alcohol-related traffic accidents. There is also an association between alcohol use and violent crime, including assault, rape, child molestation, attempted murder, and murder. One study of 2,095 trauma victims found that 41% were drinking before their injury (Meyers et al. 1990). Unfortunately, these patients' alcohol problems are underrecognized and undertreated on trauma services and burn units (Bernstein et al. 1992). Burns in alcohol and drug users result in longer treatment times with more complications (Kelley and Lynch 1992).

Alcoholism, which is strongly associated with suicide, increases rates between 60 and 120 times that of the nonalcoholic population; the lifetime risk of suicide in alcoholic patients is estimated to be 2%–3.4% (Murphy and Wetzel 1990). Alcoholic patients who attempt suicide may have more severe alcohol problems and greater comorbidity than those who do not attempt suicide (Murphy et al. 1992; Roy et al. 1990).

Alcohol Intoxication

The effects of alcohol intoxication range from mild inebriation to respiratory depression, coma, and rarely, death. γ-Aminobutyric acid

(GABA)-activated neurotransmission, N-methyl-D-aspartate (NMDA) receptors, and second-messenger systems all mediate physiological effects (Franklin and Frances 1992). Alcohol activates GABA chloride ion channels, inhibits NMDA-activated ion channels, and potentiates 5-HT$_3$-activated ion channels. GABA subunits may change structurally as tolerance and dependence develop.

The body metabolizes alcohol at the rate of 100 mg/kg/hour. Approximately 1.5 hours are required to metabolize one shot of whiskey. Among individuals who have not developed tolerance, BACs of 0.03 mg% can lead to euphoria, 0.05% can cause mild coordination problems, and 0.1 mg% usually causes ataxia. Anesthesia, coma, and death are associated with BACs of greater than 0.4 mg% (Adams and Victor 1981). After tolerance develops, chronic heavy drinkers reach high blood levels with fewer of these effects. The "first-pass" metabolism of alcohol by gastric tissue is lower in women with alcoholism than in men with alcoholism. This may explain the increased bioavailability of alcohol, higher rates of liver cirrhosis, and lower thresholds for intoxication in women (Frezza et al. 1990).

Uncomplicated Alcohol Withdrawal

In individuals who have developed tolerance, alcohol withdrawal symptoms develop when a relative decline in blood alcohol levels occurs; therefore, symptoms can occur while drinking continues. A coarse, fast-frequency generalized tremor appears that increases during motor activity or stress (e.g., when the hand or the tongue is extended). The tremor typically peaks 24–48 hours after the last drink and subsides after 5–7 days of abstinence. Patients also often show signs of autonomic hyperactivity, including elevated blood pressure, heart rate greater than 100 beats/minute, sweating, malaise, nausea, vomiting, anxiety, and disturbed sleep.

History is usually difficult to obtain during

medical emergencies. A patient who is not suspected of having alcohol dependency often suddenly develops withdrawal symptoms 3 days after surgery. It is sometimes difficult to distinguish withdrawal from other postsurgical complications. Medical conditions such as infections and hypertension or treatments such as propranolol and clonidine often alter vital signs or partially conceal or confuse the clinical picture. In addition, patients frequently receive benzodiazepines for preoperative insomnia or anxiety. These as-needed doses may mask or delay autonomic symptoms of withdrawal but not eliminate the potential for serious delayed withdrawal complications. In addition, the patient is sometimes so seriously ill that the possibility of withdrawal is not considered.

Alcohol Withdrawal Seizures

Withdrawal seizures typically occur 7–38 hours after last alcohol use, with peak frequency at approximately 24 hours (Adams and Victor 1981). Ten percent of patients with chronic alcoholism experience multiple seizures (Espir and Rose 1987). Hypomagnesemia, respiratory alkalosis, hypoglycemia, increased intracellular sodium, and upregulation of NMDA receptors all potentially contribute to alcohol withdrawal seizures. One-third of patients who have withdrawal seizures develop alcohol withdrawal delirium.

Alcohol Withdrawal Delirium (Delirium Tremens)

Delirium tremens (DT) is characterized by confusion, disorientation, fluctuating or clouded consciousness, and perceptual disturbances. Typical signs and symptoms include delusions, vivid hallucinations, agitation, insomnia, mild fever, and marked autonomic arousal. Patients frequently report vivid visual hallucinations such as insects, small animals, or other perceptual distortions; these hallucinations are associated with feelings of terror and agitation. Symptoms of DT usually appear 2–3 days after cessation of heavy drinking, with peak intensity on the fourth to fifth day. Patients often show a repetitive pattern of DT each time they withdraw from alcohol (R. G. Turner et al. 1989). Withdrawal symptoms, which can wax and wane, usually subside after 3 days of adequate treatment. Untreated DT can last as long as 4–5 weeks. DT occurs more frequently and is particularly dangerous in patients who have infections, subdural hematomas, trauma, liver disease, or metabolic disorder. In the hospital, physical restraints and 24-hour sitters are sometimes needed to protect the patient and to ensure that intravenous lines are preserved.

Alcohol-Induced Psychotic Disorder

Chronic alcohol hallucinosis—alcohol-induced psychotic disorder in DSM-IV—is defined as vivid auditory hallucinations that last at least 1 week and occur shortly after the cessation or reduction of heavy alcohol ingestion. The hallucinosis presents with a clear sensorium and few autonomic signs or symptoms. The hallucinations sometimes include familiar noises or clear voices; the patient usually responds to these hallucinations with fear, anxiety, and agitation (Lishman 1978). Diagnosis is based on a history of recent heavy alcohol use and the absence of schizophrenia or mania.

Alcohol-Induced Persisting Amnestic Disorder

Alcohol-induced persisting amnestic disorder (Wernicke-Korsakoff syndrome) begins with an abrupt onset of truncal ataxia, ophthalmoplegia, and delirium (Wernicke's encephalopathy). Brew (1986) recommended that the clinician not require all three signs; the presence of two suggests a form of the disorder. The etiology of the disorder is thiamine deficiency due to dietary, medical, or genetic factors. For example, Blass and Gibson (1977) reported a familial transketolase deficiency that causes low vitamin B levels in a subgroup at risk for the syndrome. Thiamine deficiency may cause

death or, more commonly, persisting amnesia (Korsakoff's psychosis). Approximately 80% of patients with Wernicke's encephalopathy who are treated and survive develop persisting amnesia (Reuler et al. 1985). The amnesia is a severe anterograde type (i.e., memory is not transferred from immediate to long-term memory storage). Postmortem examinations show lesions in the brain stem and diencephalon (Mensing et al. 1984).

Neurological Disease

Alcohol-induced dementia is another example of a neuropsychiatric disorder found in patients with chronic alcoholism. Other nervous system disorders associated with chronic alcoholism include polyneuropathies, hepatic encephalopathy, acute or chronic subdural hematoma, and cerebellar degeneration with truncal ataxia.

Liver Disease

Alcohol has direct toxic effects on the liver (Lieber 1988). Alcohol dehydrogenase, a liver enzyme, metabolizes alcohol to toxic acetaldehyde. Aldehyde dehydrogenase completes the transformation of acetaldehyde to acetic acid; lactic acid, uric acid, and fat accumulation are by-products in this process. In addition, alcohol hepatitis can cause acute death or cirrhosis. Inflammation and liver cell destruction kill 10%–30% of patients who develop cirrhosis. The only definitive way to diagnose alcohol-induced cirrhosis is by liver biopsy.

Interaction of Alcohol and Medications

The interaction between alcohol and medications can have a wide range of effects (i.e., from lethal overdoses to undermedication; Table 13–2). Alcohol is partly metabolized through the hepatic microsomal enzyme system that metabolizes other drugs. Acutely, alcohol can slow metabolism and increase blood levels of medications, such as oral anticoagulants, diaz-

Table 13–2.   Effects of medication interactions with alcohol

Medication	Effects
Disulfiram (Antabuse)	Flushing, diaphoresis, vomiting, confusion
Anticoagulants (oral)	Increased anticoagulation effect with acute alcohol intoxication, decreased effect after chronic alcohol use
Griseofulvin	Minor Antabuse reactions
Tranquilizers, narcotics, antihistamines	Increased central nervous system depression
Diazepam	Increased absorption of diazepam
Phenytoin	Increased anticonvulsant effect with acute intoxication; after chronic alcohol abuse, alcohol intoxication or withdrawal may lower seizure threshold
Salicylates	Gastrointestinal bleeding
Chlorpromazine	Increased levels of alcohol
Monoamine oxidase inhibitors	Adverse reactions to tyramine in some alcoholic beverages

Source.   Adapted from Frances RJ, Franklin JE Jr: "Alcohol and Other Psychoactive Substance Use Disorders," in *The American Psychiatric Press Textbook of Psychiatry,* 2nd Edition. Edited by Hales RE, Yudofsky SC, Talbott JA. Washington, DC, American Psychiatric Press, 1994, p. 364. Used with permission.

epam, and phenytoin, which compete for cytochrome P450 enzymes. Chronically, because of cytochrome P450 enzyme induction, alcohol can lead to increased metabolism and decreased blood levels of these medications. Chronic alcohol intake can also lead to acetaminophen toxicity as a result of accumulation of toxic metabolites (Table 13–3).

Conversely, some medications can influence alcohol's metabolism. For example, chlorpromazine, chloral hydrate, and cimetidine increase blood alcohol levels by inhibiting alcohol dehydrogenase. Alcohol enhances diazepam absorption, which decreases its safety margin and increases the possibility of overdose. In addition, alcohol increases the potency of other central nervous system (CNS) depressants, such as narcotics and antihistamines, and has unpredictable effects when used with CNS stimulants. Mild disulfiram-like reactions can occur with oral hypoglycemics (e.g., tolbutamide, chlorpropamide), griseofulvin, metronidazole, and quinacrine. Continued use of salicylates and alcohol can lead to gastrointestinal bleeding. Because some alcoholic beverages contain tyramine, monoamine oxidase inhibitors are best avoided in the treatment of active or recovering alcoholic patients.

Table 13–3.   Alcohol effects on cytochrome P450 enzymes

Acute users
  Slows P450 metabolism; therefore, increases levels of medications dependent on system for metabolism
Chronic users
  Increases P450 metabolism; therefore, decreases the levels of medications dependent on P450 metabolism or increases toxic metabolites (e.g., increases acetaminophen toxic metabolites)

Psychiatric Consultation

The consultation-liaison psychiatrist must have an appropriate attitude and possess specific knowledge to work with patients who have substance use disorders (Table 13–4). At times, especially in critically ill patients, medical problems overshadow substance abuse issues.

Substance-abusing patients typically do not request psychiatric consultation and often are not told that a psychiatric consultation was requested. The earlier the consultation, the

Table 13–4. General consultant issues for patients with substance use disorders

Have a high suspicion for drug abuse.

Obtain urine toxicology screens whenever possible, immediately following admission.

Know general principles of detoxification (i.e., know indications for inpatient versus outpatient and pharmacological versus observational detoxification).

Realize that tailored detoxification is often needed in medically ill patients.

Be aware that, when treating polysubstance dependence, sedative detoxification occurs first.

Use challenge tests or estimate conservatively if unsure of initial detoxification dose.

Know equivalent doses of sedatives and opiates.

Recognize drug-drug interactions.

Be able to differentiate major psychopathology, metabolic and neurological conditions, and withdrawal versus intoxication.

better. A valuable window of vulnerability exists in medically ill patients while they are sick; they are often more open to treatment recommendations. Some patients are reluctant to fully disclose substance abuse or dependence because of potential legal problems (e.g., motor vehicle accidents or fear of job loss).

Acute Assessment

It is sometimes difficult during the initial consultation to differentiate the effects of alcohol intoxication, withdrawal, and chronic use from other psychiatric disorders. Spider nevi, palmar erythema, cigarette burns between the index and middle fingers, poor dental care, jaundice, enlarged liver, abdominal pain, peripheral neuropathy, and muscle weakness are clinical signs of alcoholism. When patients present as severely intoxicated, comatose, or semicomatose, head and spinal cord injuries, hypoglycemia, diabetic coma, hepatic coma, cardiac arrhythmias, myasthenia, subdural hematoma, and drug overdose can be ruled out.

Laboratory Testing

Blood γ-glutamyltransferase (GGT) is increased in more than 50% of patients who have an alcohol problem and in 80% of alcoholic patients with liver dysfunction (Trill et al. 1984); serum glutamic-oxalacetic transaminase (SGOT) is increased in 46% of patients with alcoholism. Decreased white blood cell count and increased mean corpuscular volume (MCV), uric acid, triglyceride, aspartase aminotransferase, and urea are also common in alcoholism. In patients with advanced cirrhosis, liver function is sometimes normal; however, prothrombin time is prolonged. One-third of patients with alcoholism have increased blood glucose levels. It is not uncommon for patients with inadequate calorie intake to have decreased blood glucose levels and mild hypertension (Table 13–5).

Screening Tests

Two widely used brief screening tests to detect alcoholism are the self-administered Michigan Alcoholism Screening Test (MAST) and the clinician-administered CAGE questionnaire (Ta-

Table 13–5. Laboratory findings associated with alcohol abuse

Alcohol present in blood

Positive breathalyzer test

Elevated mean corpuscular volume (MCV)

Elevated serum glutamic-oxalacetic transaminase (SGOT), serum glutamic-pyruvic transaminase (SGPT), lactate dehydrogenase (LDH)

Elevated serum γ-glutamyltransferase (SGGT) (particularly sensitive)

Decreased albumin, vitamin B_{12}, folic acid

Increased uric acid, elevated amylase, evidence of bone marrow suppression

Prolonged prothrombin time (cirrhosis)

Source. Adapted from Frances RJ, Franklin JE Jr: *Concise Guide to Treatment of Alcoholism and Addictions.* Washington, DC, American Psychiatric Press, 1989, p. 74. Used with permission.

Table 13–6. CAGE screen for diagnosis of alcoholism

Have you ever

C Thought you should CUT back on your drinking?

A Felt ANNOYED by people criticizing your drinking?

G Felt GUILTY or bad about your drinking?

E Had a morning EYE-OPENER to relieve hangover or nerves?

Note. Two or three positive responses = high index of suspicion; four positive responses = pathognomonic. The sensitivity and specificity for elderly persons for a cutoff score of 1 are 86% and 78%, respectively, and 70% and 91% for a cutoff score of 2 (Buchsbaum et al. 1992).
Source. Reprinted from Ewing JA: "Detecting Alcoholism: The CAGE Questionnaire." *Journal of the American Medical Association* 252:1905–1907, 1984. Copyright 1984, American Medical Association. Used with permission.

ble 13–6). The MAST is a 25-question form that is 90% sensitive; the CAGE is a 4-item test.

Acute Management and Treatment of Alcohol-Related Disorders

Intoxication. The behavior associated with intoxication is managed by decreasing external stimuli, interrupting alcohol ingestion, and protecting individuals from harming themselves and others until the toxic effects of alcohol disappear. In potentially fatal overdoses, hemodialysis is sometimes attempted; otherwise, careful observation is all that is needed.

Withdrawal. Usually, the choice of inpatient versus outpatient treatment for withdrawal depends on severity of symptoms, stage of withdrawal, medical and psychiatric complications, presence of polysubstance abuse, patient cooperation, ability to follow instructions, social support systems, patient history, and increasingly, insurance or managed care reimbursement policies. Consultation requests often involve patients whose withdrawal symp-

toms are only partially detoxified or patients who are not yet beyond danger of serious medical complications.

Regardless of the medications requested on the doctor's order sheet, the nurse's medication log is the only reliable source to determine which medications a patient has actually received. Full detoxification, a modified detoxification schedule, or as-needed medication is used depending on the severity of dependence, medical condition, detoxification history, vital signs, and mental status. In alcoholic patients with moderate to severe dependence or histories of moderate to severe withdrawal symptoms, full medical detoxification should proceed; as-needed medications alone should not be relied on in these patients (Table 13–7).

Although nonpharmacological inpatient treatment is sometimes employed in patients

Table 13–7. General principles of medical detoxification

Prevent complications of withdrawal, and increase patient comfort.

Select a cross-tolerant medication that has a longer half-life during taper.

Know that clonazepam is useful in hospital settings because of self-taper (Note: effective for alprazolam detoxification).

Select an intermediate-half-life benzodiazepine, such as lorazepam, for patients who are very sick, liver compromised, or elderly (i.e., do not use long half-life benzodiazepines).

Note that, if lorazepam is used to manage withdrawal, it must be tapered (i.e., it does not self-taper).

Give explicit instructions to medical staff regarding signs and symptoms of withdrawal and medication schedule.

Adjust medications based on signs and symptoms; allow some flexibility in protocol.

Avoid as-needed dosing alone when detoxification is clearly needed (e.g., in patients with chronic severe use or history of withdrawal complications).

Avoid clonidine and propranolol because they mask symptoms and signs of withdrawal.

with uncomplicated withdrawal (Hayashida et al. 1989), pharmacological treatment of withdrawal symptoms relieves discomfort and prevents complications such as seizures and DT. Some evidence suggests that repeated withdrawal may hasten cognitive decline, possibly mediated by high levels of cortisol (Linnoila 1989). Safe detoxification occurs when patients' autonomic signs and symptoms are adequately controlled. Sedation is a clinically useful indicator for adequate treatment in early withdrawal.

Benzodiazepines are recommended for the treatment and prevention of withdrawal symptoms. Benzodiazepines are safe, are easy to administer (orally, intramuscularly, or intravenously), have anticonvulsant properties, and are efficacious. Diazepam and chlordiazepoxide are commonly used. Benzodiazepines such as lorazepam or oxazepam should be used in patients with severe liver disease and elderly patients because these drugs are metabolized via conjugation versus oxidation; otherwise, no clear efficacy differences are found among benzodiazepines. Lorazepam is better absorbed intramuscularly than are other benzodiazepines.

For outpatient alcohol withdrawal treatment, 25–50 mg of chlordiazepoxide is prescribed orally four times a day on the first day, followed by a 20% decrease in dose every day for a 5-day period (Table 13–8). Standard inpatient detoxification is 25–100 mg chlordiazepoxide orally four times a day and an additional 25–50 mg every 2 hours, as needed (Table 13–8). The patient is observed for signs of agitation, tremulousness, or increased vital signs. The total amount given over 24 hours is tapered over 5–7 days; the 24-hour dose is equally divided during the day. Diazepam is recommended in patients with cross-addiction to other depressant drugs or with a history of seizures. Diazepam is also often used for standard detoxification. Diazepam is given in doses of 20 mg/hour up to 60 mg or until symptoms are controlled (Sellers et al. 1983). Because diazepam and its active metabolites have long half-lives, diazepam self-tapers when discontinued.

Nutritional deficiencies of thiamine, vitamin B_{12}, and folic acid should be corrected with oral thiamine (100 mg/day), folic acid (1 mg/day orally for 5 days), daily multivitamins, and adequate nutrition. Clinicians should administer thiamine 100–200 mg intramuscularly or intravenously for 3 days in cases of very poor nutrition; thiamine must be given before glucose because glucose infusion depletes thiamine stores. Patients with a history of alcohol withdrawal seizures should receive intramuscular magnesium sulfate, 1 g/2 mL (50% solution) four times a day for 2 days. When sweating, fever, or vomiting causes severe dehydration, attention to rehydration and electrolyte replacement is essential.

Table 13–8. Standard treatment regimen for alcohol withdrawal

Outpatient

Chlordiazepoxide 25–50 mg orally four times on first day; 20% decrease in dose each day over a 5-day period

Daily clinic visits to assess clinical symptoms and vital signs. Family members may be useful in monitoring withdrawal symptoms.

Inpatient

Chlordiazepoxide 25–100 mg or lorazepam 1–4 mg orally four times on first day; 20% decrease in dose each day over 5–7 days

In addition, chlordiazepoxide 25–100 mg or lorazepam 1–4 mg orally, every 6 hours as needed for agitation, tremors, or increased vital signs

Thiamine 100 mg orally four times daily

Folic acid 1 mg orally four times daily

One multivitamin per day

Magnesium sulfate 1 g intramuscularly every 6 hours for 2 days (if seizure risk)

Source. Adapted from Frances RJ, Franklin JE Jr: "Alcohol and Other Psychoactive Substance Use Disorders," in *The American Psychiatric Press Textbook of Psychiatry,* 2nd Edition. Edited by Hales RE, Yudofsky SC, Talbott JA. Washington, DC, American Psychiatric Press, 1994, p. 373. Used with permission.

Patients with a history of epilepsy may require additional anticonvulsant medication. However, for uncomplicated withdrawal seizures, adding anticonvulsants to benzodiazepines is not always necessary. Diazepam, 10 mg intravenously, usually inhibits status epilepticus; however, the addition of phenytoin is occasionally necessary.

Alcohol-induced psychotic disorder.   If patients develop alcohol hallucinosis during detoxification, a potent antipsychotic such as haloperidol, 2–5 mg orally twice a day, is typically needed to control agitation and hallucinations. The clinician should reassess medications shortly after cessation of symptoms because continued neuroleptics are seldom needed.

Wernicke's encephalopathy and persistent amnesia.   Wernicke's encephalopathy should be treated with parenteral thiamine, 100 mg every hour, with titration upward until ophthalmoplegia has resolved; this usually prevents progression. Ophthalmoplegia usually responds fairly quickly; truncal ataxia may persist. Thiamine is always given before glucose loading. Fluvoxamine reportedly reduces memory deficits in patients with persistent amnesia; these benefits are hypothesized to occur through its serotonergic effects (Martin et al. 1989).

Long-Term Management

In the general hospital, a number of barriers exist to detection and treatment of substance abuse disorder. Denial by the patient and the staff is usually present. Motivating factors for treatment, such as legal problems and job loss, are often absent. Patients with alcoholism sometimes admit to addiction but do not realize or deny its relation to their medical problems.

It is difficult to arrange appropriate aftercare during a short hospitalization or when financial resources are limited. Patients' insurance coverage for substance abuse treatment varies considerably. Patients with little or no coverage usually have to wait until public treatment slots are available. While waiting, patients often relapse.

Patients in recovery for substance abuse often must face the dilemma of whether to take mood-altering substances (e.g., narcotics for pain, anxiolytics for sedation). Recovery teaches people to avoid all mood-altering substances because they can lead to relapse or a substitute addiction. If the hospitalization is elective, such as for ambulatory surgery, the issue can be discussed with drug treatment staff members or AA sponsors. When the issue is discussed up front and adequate support is provided, these patients do well. The clinician should encourage AA members and sponsors to visit the patient and should discontinue mood-altering medication as soon as possible.

Patients with concomitant chronic medical illnesses that limit participation in formal substance treatment programs pose special problems. Patients may encounter difficulties with transportation (e.g., physical limitations or unreliable transportation) or difficulty sustaining the concentration necessary to take full advantage of formal rehabilitation programs. These patients often feel estranged from the "world of the well." Devising aftercare programs tailored to patients' needs is often difficult. Patients are sometimes seen individually and attend AA or professional groups as tolerated.

Disulfiram is an important treatment adjunct for many patients with alcoholism. It provides an added buffer between the impulse to drink and alcohol use. However, consultation-liaison psychiatrists rarely recommend starting disulfiram in the general hospital patient. Contraindications to disulfiram include severe liver disease, pregnancy, heart disease, and psychosis. Disulfiram also has important drug-drug interactions (e.g., it increases levels of phenytoin, isoniazid).

Frequently, a family crisis brings the patient to treatment. Evaluation and treatment of the patient's family are essential because a family system that accommodates the patient's drinking may also reinforce it. Including the family in treatment increases the chances that the patient will remain sober.

Referral Options

The two most common referral options are to a specialized substance treatment program or to AA. Most United States alcohol treatment programs emphasize a combination of psychoeducation, a 12-step program, and individual, group, and family counseling.

Regular AA attendance is associated with favorable outcome (Sheeren 1988; Vaillant 1983). A prospective study of employed alcoholic patients found that treatment plus AA was more effective than AA alone in helping employed alcohol abusers attain and continue abstinence (Walsh et al. 1991). AA officially supports the use of psychotropic medications when necessary.

Treatment Outcome

Treatment outcome studies are difficult. Thus far, the literature indicates that favorable patient factors, such as having a stable family, a stable job, less sociopathy, less psychopathology, and a negative family history for alcoholism, are better predictors of positive outcome than the type of treatment received (Frances et al. 1984). Approximately one-third of patients with alcoholism stop drinking without formal treatment intervention, one-third improve with treatment, and one-third never achieve sobriety.

SEDATIVE, HYPNOTIC, OR ANXIOLYTIC ABUSE/DEPENDENCE

Abuse rarely starts as a result of treatment for acute anxiety or insomnia in a hospitalized patient. The risk of sedative abuse in chronically medically ill outpatients is far greater.

Medical and Other Complications

As with alcohol, intoxication, withdrawal, withdrawal delirium, and amnestic disorder can occur with other sedative-hypnotics. Because the half-life of most benzodiazepines is much longer than that of alcohol, withdrawal symptoms are delayed. For example, withdrawal symptoms occur 7–10 days after abrupt cessation of diazepam. Seizures may herald withdrawal and are a potential complication of high-dose, unexpected, or poorly managed benzodiazepine withdrawal. Benzodiazepine use is associated with hip fractures in the elderly (Ray and Griffin 1989).

Prevention and Acute Management

Preventing habituation to sedative-hypnotic drugs is the best prevention of abuse and dependence. Limited prescriptions, single-source policies (i.e., obtaining all benzodiazepine prescriptions from one provider), and appropriate follow-up are necessary. Generally, benzodiazepines are used to treat specific symptoms, are used only for short periods, and are avoided in patients with alcoholism and those with a history of substance abuse. In people recovering from anxiety disorders, benzodiazepines should be tried only after behavioral and other pharmacological treatments fail. Buspirone is often helpful in such individuals. If benzodiazepines are prescribed, a single provider should closely monitor the patient, and the dosage should not escalate (Dupont and Saylor 1991).

Treatment of sedative-hypnotic withdrawal is similar to that for withdrawal from alcohol. A cross-tolerant sedative is given to prevent withdrawal symptoms, and the daily dose is gradually decreased; long-acting barbiturates or benzodiazepines are recommended. Because of potential medical complications during detoxification, especially among high-dose abusers, inpatient treatment is preferred. Clonazepam is a benzodiazepine with a moderately long half-life (23 ± 5 hours) that has shown promise in treating alprazolam withdrawal. Alprazolam is particularly difficult to taper after long-term use or high-dose abuse. It binds very tightly to the benzodiazepine-GABA receptor complex; therefore, significant rebound anxiety or withdrawal symptoms can occur with small decreases in dosage.

The most important factor in minimizing complications during benzodiazepine withdrawal is to decrease the dose by approximately 10% per day; the terminal 10% should be tapered slowly to zero over a 3- to 4-day period (Table 13–9). Generally, detoxification is accomplished within a 10- to 14-day period, but in certain individuals, longer detoxification is required. This is true particularly when patients have been taking benzodiazepines for many years or when the drug resists tapering (e.g., alprazolam and lorazepam). In such cases, tapering may take weeks or months.

OPIOID-RELATED DISORDERS

Opiate abuse presents in various ways in patients on a general medical unit (Table 13–10).

Table 13–9. Benzodiazepine detoxification

Estimate usual daily dosage by history or pentobarbital challenge test.

Convert dosage into equivalent daily dosage of diazepam; administer that dosage daily for 2 days.

Decrease diazepam dosage 10% per day thereafter.

Add diazepam 5 mg orally every 6 hours if needed for signs of increased withdrawal (increased pulse, increase in blood pressure, diaphoresis).

When the diazepam dosage approaches 10% of starting dosage, reduce dosage slowly over 3–4 days and then discontinue.

Source. Adapted from Frances RJ, Franklin JE Jr: "Alcohol and Other Psychoactive Substance Use Disorders," in *The American Psychiatric Press Textbook of Psychiatry*, 2nd Edition. Edited by Hales RE, Yudofsky SC, Talbott JA. Washington, DC, American Psychiatric Press, 1994, p. 378. Used with permission.

Consultation requests include the follow-up of patients taking methadone, patients thought or known to be dependent on prescription or illicit opiates, patients who engage in "drug-seeking" behavior, patients who require behavioral management of personality problems that interfere with medical care, and patients who overdose. Opioid-dependent patients often provoke angry reactions from the staff, such as discharging a patient too soon or underprescribing pain medications.

Polysubstance abuse is extremely common among people addicted to opiates. "Speedballing" with heroin and cocaine is one of the most frequently used combinations. Synthetic opiates, such as fentanyl, are abused by individuals who have easy access, such as nurses, physicians, and especially anesthesiologists. Contaminated needles and impure drugs can lead to endocarditis, septicemia, pul-

Table 13–10. Clinical cues to possible opiate abuse or dependence in general hospital patients

History

Exaggerated pain complaints in relation to physical findings

Drug-seeking behavior

Recent multiple outpatient medical visits for pain complaints requiring a narcotic prescription

"Allergic" to every analgesic except meperidine

Physical examination

Pupillary constriction

Withdrawal signs: hyperthermia, hypertension, tachycardia, diaphoresis, nausea, pupillary dilation

Hyperpigmentation over veins, tourniquet areas, tattoos, abscesses

Jaundice

Laboratory findings

Positive toxic screen

Increased transaminases

Decreased globulins

Hospital course

Demanding, unruly, or agitated behavior

Threats to leave against medical advice

monary emboli, pulmonary hypertension, skin infections, hepatitis, and HIV infection.

Pathophysiology

There are several subtypes of opioid receptors (i.e., mu, delta, kappa, lambda, iota, and epsilon) (Simon 1992). (Note: the sigma receptor is no longer considered an opioid receptor.) The mu receptor—the classic morphine receptor—has selective affinity for heroin, meperidine, hydromorphone, and methadone. The mu receptor is very sensitive to naloxone (opioid antagonist) and mediates analgesia, euphoria, sedation, meiosis, and respiratory depression. The 50 current endogenous opioids interact with these 5 major receptors (T. R. Kosten 1990). Certain individuals may be prone to opioid addiction because of a hypothesized lack of endogenous opioid peptides.

Neuroadaptive changes at receptor sites are hypothesized to produce dependence and tolerance, especially tolerance to respiratory depression. Once neuroadaptation occurs, removal of the opioid from receptors produces withdrawal symptoms. Neuroadaptation appears to result from modulation in the numbers or conformations of opioid receptors.

Opioid receptors are located in the locus coeruleus; chronic administration of opioids inhibits the firing rates of the locus coeruleus's norepinephrine system. In contrast, opioid withdrawal increases noradrenergic activity in the locus coeruleus, which results in withdrawal symptoms.

Comorbidity

Rounsaville et al. (1982) found that 80% of opiate-addicted patients had histories of psychiatric disorders, frequently mood disorders. During initial rehabilitation, symptoms of major depression are not as likely to remit as they are in alcoholic patients.

Intoxication and Withdrawal

Physical signs of intoxication include pupillary constriction (so-called pinpoint pupils), decreased gastrointestinal motility, marked sedation, slurred speech, and impairment in attention and memory. The onset of opioid withdrawal depends on the half-life of the opioid and the chronicity of use. For example, symptoms begin approximately 10 hours after the last dose of short-acting opioids, such as morphine and heroin.

Mild opioid withdrawal presents as a flu-like syndrome, with symptoms of anxiety, dysphoria, yawning, sweating, rhinorrhea, lacrimation, pupillary dilation, piloerection, mild hypertension, tachycardia, and disrupted sleep. Severe withdrawal symptoms include hot and cold flashes, deep muscle and joint pain, nausea, vomiting, diarrhea, abdominal pain, weight loss, fever, and gooseflesh. Subacute, protracted withdrawal symptoms can last for several weeks.

The clinician should suspect an opioid overdose in any patient who presents in a coma, especially when associated with respiratory depression, pupillary constriction, or the presence of needle marks. In any comatose patient who has overdosed on opioids, 0.4 mg naloxone is given immediately and is repeated because of naloxone's short duration of action. The clinician must remember that excessive naloxone can precipitate severe withdrawal symptoms.

Acute Management and Treatment

Two methods of treatment are available for opioid-dependent individuals in a general hospital—methadone maintenance or detoxification. Detoxification is often needed for patients who use street drugs like heroin or prescription drugs like oxycodone, meperidine, or codeine. When opioid dependence is questionable, the consultant should perform a naloxone challenge test by administering 0.4 mg naloxone intravenously. Abrupt worsening of the patient's symptoms (i.e., withdrawal occurs or worsens) strongly supports a diagnosis of opioid dependence. Table 13–11, which lists equal doses of opioids, is provided for conversion purposes during withdrawal or maintenance.

Methadone maintenance. In 1965, Dole and Nyswander first postulated that methadone would diminish drug-seeking behavior, increase personal productivity, and decrease illicit activities because wide fluctuations in opioid blood levels would cease. In "hard-core addicts" (i.e., opioid-addicted patients who use drugs two or more times per day for more than a year or are continuously involved in drug street life), methadone continues to contribute to improved health, decreased crime, increased employment, and decreased risk of HIV (Dole and Nyswander 1965).

Methadone is relatively long acting and has a half-life of 24–36 hours. The long half-life pre-

Table 13–11. Opioid potency conversion

| Drug | Equal dose (mg) | |
	Intramuscular	Oral
Morphine	10	60
Hydromorphone (Dilaudid)	1.5	7.5
Methadone (Dolophine)	10	20
Oxycodone (Percocet)	15	30
Levorphanol (Levo-Dromoran)	2	4
Oxymorphone (Numorphan)	1	10 (PR)
Heroin	5	60
Meperidine (Demerol)	75	—
Codeine	130	200

Note. PR = per rectum.
Source. Reprinted from Foley KM: "The Treatment of Cancer Pain." *New England Journal of Medicine* 313:85, 1985. Copyright 1985, Massachusetts Medical Society. Used with permission.

vents extreme fluctuation in opioid blood levels. Methadone also blunts the euphoric response to illicit heroin. Unlike heroin, which has a half-life of 8–12 hours, methadone is taken once daily orally, intramuscularly (in divided doses), or intravenously (one-third of oral maintenance dose). Once-daily administration provides a structure for rehabilitation. The addicted person no longer needs illegal activities to support a costly habit. Common side effects of methadone are sedation, mild euphoria, constipation, and reduced sweating.

A frequent mistake made by the medical staff is to base methadone dosage solely on how a patient looks, how a patient says he or she feels, or vital signs. Hospitalized patients who were taking methadone should continue to receive methadone based on their preadmission dosage, which should be verified with the methadone clinic, unless the methadone is medically contraindicated. For opioid-dependent patients hospitalized on a general medical unit who were not taking methadone, 30–40 mg/day is a reasonable starting dose. Additional doses of 5 mg twice a day are added, based on signs of withdrawal. Patients must be observed closely for oversedation or undertreatment. An average maintenance dose is 60–80 mg; 80–120 mg is occasionally needed.

Detoxification from heroin and other opiates. Detoxification from heroin, morphine, meperidine, and weak opioids (e.g., codeine and oxycodone) is generally accomplished by giving 20 mg of methadone and then decreasing the dosage by 20% each day over a 5- to 7-day period. Higher initial doses are typically needed for high-dose heroin users (i.e., habits greater than $50 per day).

In hospitalized patients who are dependent on prescribed opioids, detoxification can be accomplished by converting the daily dosage to codeine dosage, then tapering the liquid syrup codeine amount by 20% per day (Table 13–12). On an outpatient basis, detoxification is achieved by starting methadone at 20 mg and decreasing by 1 mg/day over a 20-day period. People who are dependent on synthetic narcotics, such as oxycodone or hydrocodone, can slowly taper the medication over several weeks. Outpatient detoxification of prescribed opioid drugs is seldom successful unless the patient is involved in a well-structured outpatient program.

Detoxification using clonidine. Clonidine helps to suppress opioid withdrawal symptoms because it suppresses locus coeruleus activity and reduces autonomic activity. Although clonidine suppresses autonomic signs of withdrawal, it is less effective in relieving subjective discomfort (Jasinski et al. 1985). An abrupt switch to clonidine is less disruptive if the methadone dose is first stabilized at 20 mg or less. Clonidine is given three times daily in individual doses starting at 0.1–0.3 mg, and the dosage is increased to a 2-mg/day total over an 8- to 14-day period. A Catapres TTS-1 patch is also used, with oral doses of clonidine given as necessary. Sedation and hypotension (blood pressure < 90/60 mm Hg) are common side effects and limit the use of clonidine.

Detoxification using naltrexone. Naltrexone is an opioid antagonist that blocks opioid receptors and prevents the euphoric effects of opioids. Its long-term use results in gradual extinction of drug-seeking behavior; it is a tool in abstinence-oriented treatment (Greenstein et

Table 13–12. Detoxification from prescription opiates

Taper drug itself over several weeks or convert dose to equivalent codeine dose (see Table 13–11). Use liquid form of codeine and taper 20% per day over 5–7 days.

OR

Methadone 20 mg divided into twice-daily doses will be effective for most initial symptoms from prescription medications. Taper over 5 days for inpatients; 2–3 weeks for outpatients.

al. 1984). Because naltrexone is an opioid antagonist, it will likely precipitate withdrawal symptoms in an opiate-dependent individual.

Detoxification using clonidine and naltrexone. A combination of clonidine and low-dose naltrexone is sometimes used for heroin detoxification. Naltrexone may "reset" opioid receptors. The combination may shorten the withdrawal period to 3 or 4 days, and the addition of naltrexone does not increase withdrawal symptoms. This combination has been used successfully for outpatients; however, higher doses of clonidine are often necessary (Stine and Kosten 1992).

Opiate Addiction and Pain

In all cases, pain management is directed to the primary disorder. The consultant must ensure that adequate pain medications are prescribed in cancer patients and that as-needed medication schedules are avoided. Opiate-dependent patients are more demanding and drug-seeking; expectations and behavioral limits must be established early. The medical staff must assume responsibility for adequate pain management—they must avoid excessive negotiations. Opioid-dependent patients may require up to double amounts of narcotics for acute pain control as a result of opioid tolerance. When opioids are used for analgesia, such as for postoperative pain, the opioids should be tapered at the same percentage rate in both non-opioid-dependent and opioid-dependent patients.

COCAINE-RELATED DISORDERS

Epidemiology

An estimated 79,398 emergency department visits for cocaine use were documented in the 1990 Drug Abuse Warning Network (DAWN) (National Institute on Drug Abuse 1990). According to the National Institute on Drug Abuse (1991) study, 1.9 million individuals in the

United States used cocaine during a 1-month period. Crack cocaine is used by a small subset of that population; it is popular among younger, more serious cocaine users (Smart 1991).

Pharmacology

Cocaine hydrochloride ("coke," "snow," "blow") is a white crystal powder derived from coca leaves and coca paste. It is usually diluted to 20% purity ("stepped on") by mixing it with other local anesthetics, such as lidocaine or procaine, or various sugars. Freebase cocaine is prepared from the hydrochloride salt by alkalinization and extraction with organic solvents. "Crack" or "rock" is a prepackaged freebase form of cocaine ready for smoking. "Freebasing" is smoking freebase cocaine; the onset of intense euphoria occurs within seconds. Because freebase cocaine is absorbed directly from the lungs, it goes immediately to the brain, bypassing the liver. Euphoric effects depend on blood level and on the slope to peak concentration. Most cocaine is hydrolyzed in the body to benzoylecgonine, which is detected in the urine up to 36 hours after use. High doses are detectable for up to 3 weeks. Rapid tolerance develops to cocaine's euphoric effects. Cocaine and alcohol may combine to make a toxic metabolite cocaethyline, which is potentially quite cardiotoxic.

Pathophysiology

Cocaine blocks reuptake of neuronal dopamine, serotonin, and norepinephrine. With repeated cocaine use, tolerance develops as a result of decreased reuptake inhibition and release of catecholamines and altered receptor sensitivity. Hypotheses to explain the severe craving associated with cocaine use include cortical kindling (Halikas et al. 1991), altered catecholamine receptor sensitivity (Gawin and Kleber 1986), and dopamine depletion (Dackus and Gold 1985).

Intoxication

Intoxication is characterized by euphoria, hyperalertness, grandiosity, and impaired judgment. Individuals are more gregarious or withdrawn; may have increased anxiety, restlessness, and vigilance; and exhibit stereotypical behavior. Maladaptive behavior includes fighting, psychomotor agitation, and impaired social or occupational functioning.

Paranoia occurs with high doses and chronic or binge use of cocaine; it is usually of brief duration.

Withdrawal or Abstinence

Efforts to systematically study and correlate abstinence phenomena with neurobiological findings identify three phases:

1. *Phase 1* ("the crash") consists of depression, suicidal ideation, insomnia, anxiety, irritability, and intense cocaine craving usually during the first day postwithdrawal.
2. *Phase 2* consists of cocaine craving with irritability, anxiety, and decreased capacity to experience pleasure and lasts for a few days.
3. *Phase 3* consists of milder episodic craving stimulated by conditioned environmental factors (Gawin and Kleber 1986).

Medical and Other Complications

Cocaine use is associated with acute and chronic medical ailments (e.g., chronic intranasal use leads to septal necrosis). Anesthetic properties of cocaine can lead to oral numbness and dental neglect; cocaine binges can cause malnutrition, severe weight loss, and dehydration.

Cocaine can cause acute agitation, diaphoresis, tachycardia, metabolic and respiratory acidosis, cardiac dysrhythmia, grand mal seizures, and, ultimately, respiratory arrest. Treatment of seizures and acidosis is essential. Myocardial infarctions, likely caused by tachycardia, coronary vasoconstriction, and increased platelet "stickiness," as well as subarachnoid hemorrhages and acute rhabdomyolysis are all reported with cocaine use (Lichtenfeld et al. 1986; Nadamanee et al. 1989; Roth et al. 1988; Virmani et al. 1988). Pregnant women who use cocaine are at increased risk for abruptio placentae; their babies often show decreased interactive behavior (Chasnoff et al. 1985).

Acute Management and Referral

Agitation and anxiety associated with cocaine intoxication are treated with diazepam or lorazepam. When cocaine psychosis occurs, haloperidol or chlorpromazine is usually an effective treatment.

Tricyclic antidepressants are occasionally used to treat the severe anhedonia and cocaine craving that result from β-adrenergic and dopaminergic receptor supersensitivity. Gawin et al. (1989) conducted a double-blind, random-assignment, 6-week comparison of desipramine, lithium, and placebo in cocaine-abusing outpatients. Cocaine craving and use were significantly reduced in the group given desipramine. More recent work (Fischman et al. 1990) found that desipramine did not attenuate cocaine use and was associated with irritability and cardiovascular toxicity. Two well-designed studies reported that desipramine did not control cocaine use in methadone-maintained patients (T. R. Kosten et al. 1992). Low-dose desipramine, however, was found to be useful in reducing cocaine-related panic attacks (Brystritsky et al. 1991).

Indications for inpatient treatment are 1) chronic freebase or intravenous use, 2) concurrent dependency with other addictive drugs or alcohol, 3) concurrent serious medical or psychiatric problems, 4) severe impairment in psychosocial functioning, 5) insufficient motivation for outpatient treatment, 6) lack of family and other supports, or 7) failure of outpatient treatment.

AMPHETAMINE-RELATED DISORDERS

Amphetamines ("speed") have stimulant and reinforcing properties similar to those of cocaine. Amphetamines block reuptake of dopamine, serotonin, and norepinephrine and have profound effects on dopamine storage release. The signs and symptoms of amphetamine use include tachycardia, elevated blood pressure, pupillary dilation, agitation, elation, loquacity, and hypervigilance. Amphetamine psychosis can resemble acute paranoid schizophrenia. Visual hallucinations are common. Binge episodes, called "runs," which are similar to those experienced with cocaine use, often alternate with symptoms of a severe crash.

Acute Management

Treatment of individuals who abuse amphetamines daily or intravenously requires inpatient hospitalization to treat violence, psychosis, and depression, as well as suicidal ideation during withdrawal. In an amphetamine overdose, acidifying the urine with vitamin C speeds elimination. Antipsychotic medications, such as haloperidol, should be used to treat paranoid or delusional symptoms.

PHENCYCLIDINE-RELATED DISORDERS

Phencyclidine (PCP) is an anesthetic agent that first appeared as a street drug in the 1960s; PCP abuse peaked between 1978 and 1980. Current street samples sold as PCP vary greatly in purity. Smoking marijuana cigarettes laced with PCP is the most common form of administration. Ketamine, a related compound, has gained recent popularity.

Although the mechanism of PCP's action is unclear, it may act at opiate and NMDA receptors. PCP induces several mental disorders, including intoxication, delirium, delusions, flash-backs, mood disorders, and anxiety.

Medical and Other Complications

Psychoactive effects of PCP generally begin within 5 minutes and plateau at 30 minutes after use. Volatile emotionality is the predominant behavioral presentation. Affects range from intense euphoria to anxiety, and behavior can include stereotypical repetitive activities and bizarre aggression. Distorted perceptions, numbness, and confusion are also common. Associated physical signs include high blood pressure, muscle rigidity, ataxia, and, at higher dosages, hypersalivation, hyperthermia, involuntary movements, and coma; high-dose PCP toxicity can simulate neuroleptic malignant syndrome. Rhabdomyolysis in overdoses can lead to acute renal failure. Dilated pupils and nystagmus, particularly vertical nystagmus, should alert the consultation-liaison psychiatrist to PCP use. Chronic psychotic episodes are also reported following use.

Acute Management

Acute reactions generally require pharmacological intervention. Intravenous diazepam is the drug of first choice; antipsychotics are occasionally necessary. Because supportive treatment is also necessary, management in a medical setting is preferred. Following ingestion of PCP, the urine can remain positive for 7 days; false-negative results can occur. PCP elimination is initially enhanced by ammonium chloride and subsequently by ascorbic acid or cranberry juice (Aronow et al. 1980).

◼ NICOTINE-RELATED DISORDERS

Tobacco addiction is the most preventable health problem in the United States. Approximately 60 million Americans smoke tobacco; 390,000 deaths per year are secondary to nicotine, and $24 billion per year are spent on its use (McGinnis and Foege 1993). In the United States, approximately 35% of men and 30% of women smoke cigarettes (Centers for Disease Control and Prevention 1993). Because most general hospitals are smoke-free, nicotine withdrawal should be considered in the differential diagnosis of any anxious or dysphoric patient.

Predisposition/Risk Factors and Comorbidity

Cigarette smokers generally begin smoking as teenagers; use is associated with peer tobacco use, parental tobacco use, and other substance abuse. High stress, poor social support, maladjustment, anxiety, and low self-confidence are associated with poor treatment outcome; these factors may also promote continued use. A strong association exists between alcohol and smoking, especially in women and patients with alcoholism. However, alcoholic patients quit smoking at the same rate as nonalcoholic patients. Smoking cessation may correlate with alcohol recovery.

Two separate groups examined the relation between nicotine dependence and major depression. Breslau et al. (1993), in a prospective study, suggested an association between nicotine dependence and major depression in women. Kendler et al. (1993) found a strong relation between average lifetime daily cigarette smoking and lifetime prevalence of depression.

A well-established association exists between tobacco use and chronic obstructive lung disease, lung cancer, oral cancers, and hypertension. Tobacco use also complicates prescribed medication use by increasing liver drug metabolism and decreasing drug levels. Mothers who smoke are more likely than mothers who do not smoke to have low-birth-weight babies (U.S. Department of Health and Human Services 1988). The success rate with every attempt to quit is 5%, and 50% of individuals eventually quit.

Effects

Tobacco use can produce a calming, euphoric effect in chronic users, which is more pronounced after a period of tobacco deprivation. Symptoms of acute nicotine poisoning include nausea, salivation, abdominal pain, vomiting and diarrhea, headaches, dizziness, and sweating; inability to concentrate, confusion, and tachycardia can also occur (Hughes and Hatsukami 1986). Nicotine increases activity of several neurotransmitters.

Management

Behavioral, cognitive, educational, self-help, and pharmacological approaches are all used to treat nicotine dependence. Despite this, the vast majority (95%) of individuals who stop smoking receive no formal intervention; research is needed to clarify how and why these individuals discontinued use. Tunstall et al. (1985) reviewed factors that influenced treatment outcome. All of the following factors are associated with poor long-term outcome: environmental stress, poor social support, smoking among family members, lack of educational information, female gender, poor overall adjustment, low self-confidence, poor motivation, and high pretreatment cotinine levels (a metabolite of nicotine). Fear of weight gain frequently delays quitting. Cognitive-behavioral and pharmacological strategies (e.g., serotonergic agents) are sometimes used to treat weight gain associated with cessation.

Nicotine gum is a pharmacological method used to prevent smoking while maintaining blood nicotine levels to minimize withdrawal symptoms (Raw 1985). Nicotine gum is prescribed for use every 30 minutes or as needed. Effectiveness is maximized with therapeutic contact. However, considerable relapse occurs after gum use is stopped (Hall et al. 1985). In a hospital setting, nicotine gum may not be practical. One-year postintervention effectiveness is between 25% and 40% in most intensive smoking cessation programs, which is approximately the same rate as that for other substance abuse treatment (Fiore et al. 1990).

Transdermal nicotine patch. A recent meta-analysis of published nicotine patch studies suggested that behavioral therapies may maximize the use of nicotine patches. The patch alone doubles the chance of quitting; the patch plus behavioral treatment doubles the rate of cessation compared with the patch alone (Fiore et al. 1994). We recommend short-term commercial patches for medically ill hospitalized patients who have heavy nicotine addiction because 50% will experience significant withdrawal. Nicotine patches might not be appropriate in some hospitalized medical patients (e.g., patients with gastrointestinal distress). Most general hospitals have antismoking rules, but it is unfortunate that few have adequate smoking cessation programs.

SUMMARY

Substance-related disorders are commonly found in medically ill patients. The consultation-liaison psychiatrist must know how to identify such patients quickly, treat withdrawal symptoms, and initiate appropriate referral for long-term treatment.

REFERENCES

Adams RD, Victor M: Principles of Neurology. New York, McGraw-Hill, 1981

American Psychiatric Association: Diagnostic and Statistical Manual of Mental Disorders, 4th Edition. Washington, DC, American Psychiatric Association, 1994

Aronow R, Miceli JN, Done AK: A therapeutic approach to the acutely overdosed PCP patient. J Psychoactive Drugs 12:259–267, 1980

Bernstein L, Jacobsberg L, Ashman T, et al: Detection of alcoholism among burn patients. Hosp Community Psychiatry 43:255–256, 1992

Blass JP, Gibson GE: Abnormality of a thiamine requiring enzyme in patients with Wernicke-Korsakoff syndrome. N Engl J Med 297:1367–1370, 1977

Breslau N, Kilbey M, Andreski P: Nicotine dependence and major depression: new evidence from a prospective investigation. Arch Gen Psychiatry 50:31–43, 1993

Brew BJ: Diagnosis of Wernicke's encephalopathy. Aust N Z J Med 16:676–678, 1986

Brystritsky A, Ackerman DL, Pasnau RO: Low dose desipramine treatment of cocaine-related panic attacks. J Nerv Ment Dis 179:755–758, 1991

Bucholz KK, Homan SM: When do alcoholics first discuss drinking problems? J Stud Alcohol 53:582–589, 1992

Buchsbaum DG et al: Screening for drinking disorders in the elderly using the CAGE questionnaire. J Am Geriatr Soc 40(7):662–665, 1992

Centers for Disease Control and Prevention: National Health Interview Surveys, 1965–91. Data compiled by the Office on Smoking and Health. Atlanta, GA, Centers for Disease Control and Prevention, 1993

Chasnoff IJ, Burns WJ, Scnoll SH: Cocaine use in pregnancy. N Engl J Med 313:666–669, 1985

Cleary PD, Miller M, Bush BT, et al: Prevalence and recognition of alcohol abuse in a primary care population. Am J Med 85:466–471, 1988

Dackus CA, Gold MS: New concepts in cocaine addiction: the dopamine depletion hypothesis (review). Neurosci Biobehav Rev 9:469–477, 1985

Dole VP, Nyswander ME: A medical treatment of heroin addiction. JAMA 193:646–650, 1965

Dupont RL, Saylor KE: Sedatives/hypnotics and benzodiazepines, in Textbook of Addictive Disorders. Edited by Frances RJ, Miller SI. New York, Guilford, 1991, pp 69–102

Espir ML, Rose FC: Alcohol, seizures and epilepsy. J R Soc Med 9:542–543, 1987

Fiore MC, Novotny TE, Pierce JP, et al: Methods used to quit smoking in the United States: do cessation programs help? JAMA 263:2760–2765, 1990

Fischman MU, Foltin RW, Nestadt G, et al: Effects of desipramine maintenance on cocaine self-administration by humans. J Pharmacol Exp Ther 253:760–770, 1990

Frances RJ, Bucky S, Alexopoulos GS: Outcome study of familial and nonfamilial alcoholism. Am J Psychiatry 141:1469–1471, 1984

Franklin JE Jr, Frances RJ: Alcohol-induced organic mental disorders, in The American Psychiatric Press Textbook of Neuropsychiatry, 2nd Edition. Edited by Yudofsky SC, Hales RE. Washington, DC, American Psychiatric Press, 1992, pp 563–583

Fraumeni JF: Epidemiology of cancer, in Cecil Textbook of Medicine, 16th Edition. Edited by Wyngaarden JB, Smith LH. Philadelphia, PA, WB Saunders, 1982, pp 1047–1051

Frezza M, Di Padova G, Pozzato G, et al: High blood alcohol levels in women: the role of decreased gastric alcohol dehydrogenase activity and first-pass metabolism. N Engl J Med 322:95–99, 1990

Gawin FH, Kleber HD: Abstinence symptomatology and psychiatric diagnosis in cocaine abusers. Arch Gen Psychiatry 43:107–113, 1986

Gawin FH, Kleber HD, Byck R, et al: Desipramine facilitation of initial cocaine abstinence. Arch Gen Psychiatry 46:117–121, 1989

Greenstein RA, Arndt IC, McLellan T, et al: Naltrexone: a clinical perspective. J Clin Psychiatry 45:23–37, 1984

Halikas JA, Crosby RD, Carlson GA, et al: Cocaine reduction in unmotivated crack users using carbamazepine versus placebo in a short term, double-blind crossover design. Clin Pharmacol Ther 50:81–95, 1991

Hall SM, Tunstall C, Rugg D, et al: Nicotine gum and behavioral treatment in smoking cessation. J Consult Clin Psychol 53:256–258, 1985

Hayashida M, Alterman AI, McLellan AT, et al: Comparative effectiveness and costs of inpatient and outpatient detoxification of patients with mild to moderate alcohol withdrawal syndrome. N Engl J Med 320:358–365, 1989

Hughes JR, Hatsukami D: Signs and symptoms of tobacco withdrawal. Arch Gen Psychiatry 43:289–294, 1986

Jasinski DR, Johnson RE, Kocher TR: Clonidine in morphine withdrawal. Arch Gen Psychiatry 42:1063–1066, 1985

Kelley D, Lynch JB: Burns in alcohol and drug users result in longer treatment times with more complications. J Burn Care Rehabil 13 (2 pt 1): 218–220, 1992

Kendler KS, Neale MC, MacLean CJ, et al: Smoking and major depression: a causal analysis. Arch Gen Psychiatry 50:36–43, 1993

Kosten TR: Neurobiology of abused drugs. J Nerv Ment Dis 178:217–227, 1990

Kosten TR, Morgan CM, Falcione J, et al: Pharmacotherapy for cocaine abusing methadone-maintained patients using amantadine or desipramine. Arch Gen Psychiatry 49:894–898, 1992

Lichtenfeld J, Rubin DB, Feldman RS: Subarachnoid hemorrhage precipitated by cocaine snorting. Arch Neurol 41:223–224, 1986

Lieber C: Biochemical and molecular basis of alcohol-induced injury to liver and other tissues. N Engl J Med 319:1639–1647, 1988

Linnoila M: Alcohol withdrawal syndrome and sympathetic nervous system function. Alcohol Health and Research World 13:355–357, 1989

Lishman WA: Organic Psychiatry. Philadelphia, PA, JB Lippincott, 1978

Martin PR, Adinoff B, Eckhardt MJ, et al: Effective pharmacotherapy of alcoholic amnestic disorder with fluvoxamine. Arch Gen Psychiatry 46: 617–621, 1989

McGinnis JM, Foege WH: Actual causes of death in the U.S. JAMA 270:2207–2212, 1993

Mensing JW, Hoogland PH, Sloff JL: Computed tomography in the diagnosis of Wernicke's encephalopathy: a radiological-neuropathological correlation. Ann Neurol 16:363–365, 1984

Meyers HB, Zepeda SG, Murdock MA: Alcohol and trauma: an endemic syndrome. West J Med 153:149–153, 1990

Minion GE, Slovid CM, Boutiette L: Severe alcohol intoxication: a study of 204 consecutive patients. Clinical Toxicology 27:375–384, 1989

Moore RD, Bone LR, Geller G, et al: Prevalence, detection and treatment of alcoholism in hospitalized patients. JAMA 261:403–407, 1989

Murphy GE, Wetzel RD: The lifetime risk of suicide in alcoholism. Arch Gen Psychiatry 47:383–392, 1990

Murphy GE, Wetzel RD, Robine E, et al: Multiple risk factors predict suicide in alcoholism. Arch Gen Psychiatry 49:459–463, 1992

Nadamanee K, Gorelick DA, Josephson MA: Myocardial ischemia during cocaine withdrawal. Ann Intern Med 111:876–880, 1989

National Institute on Drug Abuse: Annual data 1989: data from the Drug Abuse Warning Network. Series 1, No 9 (DHHS Publ No ADM-90-17). Rockville, MD, U.S. Department of Health and Human Services, National Institute on Drug Abuse Statistical Series, 1990

National Institute on Drug Abuse: National household survey on drug abuse: population estimates 1991 (DHHS Publ No ADM-92-1897). Rockville, MD, U.S. Department of Health and Human Services, 1991

Raw M: Does nicotine chewing gum really work? BMJ 290:1231–1232, 1985

Ray A, Griffin MR: Benzodiazepines of long and short elimination half-life and the risk of hip fracture. JAMA 262:3303–3307, 1989

Regier DA, Farmer ME, Rae DS, et al: Comorbidity of mental disorders with alcohol and other drug abuse: results from the Epidemiologic Catchment Area (ECA) study. JAMA 264:2511–2518, 1990

Regier DA, Narrow WE, Rae DS, et al: The de facto US Mental and Addictive Disorders Service System: Epidemiologic Catchment Area prospective 1-year prevalence rates of disorders and services. Arch Gen Psychiatry 50:85–94, 1993

Reuler JB, Girard DE, Cooney TG: Wernicke's encephalopathy. N Engl J Med 312:1035–1039, 1985

Robins LN, Helzer JE, Weissman MM, et al: Lifetime prevalence of specific psychiatric disorders in three sites. Arch Gen Psychiatry 41:949–958, 1984

Roth D, Alarcon FJ, Fernandez JA: Acute rhabdomyolysis associated with cocaine intoxication. N Engl J Med 319:673–677, 1988

Rounsaville BJ, Weissman MM, Kleber H, et al: The heterogenicity of psychiatric diagnoses in treated opiate addicts. Arch Gen Psychiatry 39:161–166, 1982

Roy A, Lamparski D, DeJong J, et al: Characteristics of alcoholics who attempt suicide. Am J Psychiatry 147:761–765, 1990

Sellers EM, Naranjo CA, Harrison M, et al: Diazepam loading: simplified treatment of alcohol withdrawal. Clin Pharmacol Ther 34:822–826, 1983

Sheeren M: The relationship between relapse and involvement in alcoholics anonymous. J Stud Alcohol 49:104–106, 1988

Simon EJ: Opiates: Neurobiology. Baltimore, MD, Williams & Wilkins, 1992

Smart RG: Crack cocaine use: review of prevalence and adverse effects. Am J Drug Alcohol Abuse 17:13–26, 1991

Stine SM, Kosten TR: Use of drug combinations in treatment of opioid withdrawal. J Clin Psychopharmacol 3:203–209, 1992

Trill E, Dristenson H, Fex G: Alcohol related problems in middle-aged men with elevated serum gamma glutamyltransferase: a prevention medical investigation. J Stud Alcohol 45:302–309, 1984

Tunstall CD, Ginsberg D, Hall SM: Quitting smoking. International Journal of the Addictions 20:1089–1112, 1985

Turner RG, Lichstein PR, Peden JG, et al: Alcohol withdrawal syndromes: a review of pathophysiology, clinical presentations and treatment. J Gen Intern Med 4:432–444, 1989

U.S. Department of Health and Human Services: The health consequences of smoking: nicotine addiction: a report of the Surgeon General (DHHS Publ No CDC-88-8406). Washington, DC, U.S. Department of Health and Human Services, 1988

U.S. Department of Health and Human Services: Seventh Special Report to the United States Congress on Alcohol and Health. Rockville, MD, National Institute on Alcohol Abuse and Alcoholism, 1990

Vaillant GE: Natural History of Alcoholism. Cambridge, MA, Harvard University Press, 1983

Van Thiel DH, Lipsitz HD, Porter LE, et al: Gastrointestinal and hepatic manifestations of chronic alcoholism. Gastroenterology 81:594–615, 1981

Virmani R, Robinowitz M, Smialek JE, et al: Cardiovascular effects of cocaine: an autopsy study of 40 patients. Am Heart J 115:1068–1076, 1988

Walsh DC, Ringson RW, Merrigan DM, et al: A randomized trial of treatment options for alcohol abusing workers. N Engl J Med 325:775–782, 1991

Chapter 14

Eating Disorders

Richard C. W. Hall, M.D.

Eating disorders are serious psychiatric disorders that are often encountered in a consultation-liaison setting. They are often unrecognized and produce multiple inexplicable symptoms, laboratory findings, and complications in patients admitted with other diagnoses. The reader is referred to the references marked with an asterisk at the end of this chapter for a more in-depth review of the management of eating disorders.

ANOREXIA NERVOSA

Epidemiology

The incidence and prevalence of anorexia have remained relatively constant since the beginning of this century (Hall and Beresford 1989b). In females between ages 12 and 18 years, the prevalence is between 1 in 100 and 1 in 800.

Course

The onset is insidious and the course progressive. Anorexia occurs most often in young women between ages 13 and 18 years; however, cases are reported in patients as young as 5 years and as old as 60 years (Halmi et al. 1979; Palazzali 1978).

The onset of anorexia nervosa often begins with a period of dieting. Over time, the patient develops an intense fear of becoming obese, a disturbance of body image, a progressive and significant weight loss, and a persistent refusal, despite encouragement, to maintain normal body weight.

The course of anorexia is episodic or unremitting until death. The most frequent pattern in patients who have anorexia for 3 years or more is a persistent, uncompromising maintenance of anorexic behavior. Disordered anorexic thought processes, however, may persist for months to years after return to an acceptable weight.

Predisposing factors. Predisposing factors include a history of sexual abuse (50% of these patients) or a recently stressful life situation such as a change in schools, move, divorce, death of a parent, estrangement from parents, or loss of a suitor or boyfriend. The personality profile suggests that patients with anorexia are "the best and the brightest." These patients are characteristically model children who are perfectionistic, compulsive, careful, and "peacemakers." They are often self- sacrificing and rigidly incorporate parental values. Anorexic symptoms are a call for attention and help. The individual with anorexia is unable to meet his or her needs through any means other than self-injury.

Anorexia is more commonly found in the mothers and sisters of anorexic patients. The first-degree biological relatives of anorexic patients are four times more likely to have major affective disorders (unipolar or bipolar disorder) than are control subjects, whereas alcoholism is represented four to eight times more frequently in families with anorexic members than in control families.

Outcome. Although the mortality from anorexia nervosa has diminished during the last 10 years, it is the highest of all psychiatric disorders. The death rate remains between 5% and 18%. Brotman et al. (1985) cautioned that as many as 22% of patients with persistent anorexia die as a result of the disorder. The most frequent causes of death are cardiac arrhythmias with sudden cardiac death, seizures, gastrointestinal bleeding, renal failure, and secondary infection (Sullivan 1995).

Clinical Features

Severe weight loss associated with anorexia often necessitates hospitalization to prevent death by starvation. The patients at greatest medical risk are those who have alternating episodes of anorexia and bulimia. These patients often achieve their anorexic goals through total starvation; bizarre eating patterns (e.g., only lettuce); the rumination of food (i.e., chewing, swallowing, and regurgitating food or chewing food and spitting it out), self-induced vomiting; or the use of diuretics, laxatives, emetics, enemas, and over-the-counter or prescription diet pills. They also often engage in excessive exercise. They commonly use stimulants such as caffeine, phenylpropanolamine, amphetamines, and/or cocaine to maintain energy and curb hunger.

Amenorrhea can occur before or after the onset of anorexia. Patients with anorexia, even when profoundly emaciated, report that they feel fat and often are preoccupied with particular parts of their bodies.

An important diagnostic feature is the absence of hunger. After a certain point in starvation, central peptides are released, which diminish or obviate hunger. A second physiological plateau is reached when these patients enter the phase of terminal starvation, during which cachetin is released and interferes with the cells' ability to utilize energy.

Patients with anorexia deny the severity of their illness and often come to medical attention only after a crisis. Anorexic patients' stubborn resistance to therapy and profound denial of the severity of their illness cause extreme difficulty during treatment.

Patients with anorexia can also have a variety of other psychiatric symptoms including depression, obsessive-compulsive behavior (such as hand washing, hoarding food), and organic mental syndrome with episodes of agitation, confusion, and disorientation. Organic mental syndrome often responds to low doses of a phenothiazine such as perphenazine, 2–6 mg/day. Zinc sulfate supplementation, 220 mg/day for 10 days, and oral thiamine, 100 mg/day, help to prevent this disorder.

Many patients with anorexia report that they are happy only when disabled by weight loss. They view medical sequelae as external confirmation that they are seriously ill and therefore deserve attention from close friends and family. It is not uncommon for patients with anorexia to report that they want to be close to death so that they can have the option of dying quickly if they choose (Hall and Beresford 1989a).

BULIMIA NERVOSA

In the United States, bulimia nervosa is more likely to interfere with a young person's successful completion of college than any other medical or psychiatric disorder. A review by the Eating Disorders Task Force of the American Psychiatric Association (1993) concluded that bulimia is a condition that is associated with severe and potentially fatal medical complications that warrants careful medical evaluation.

Epidemiology

The prevalence of bulimia, particularly in college women, is increasing. The prevalence of bulimia is estimated to be between 4% and 12% of college-age women and approximately 0.4% of college-age men (Hall 1996).

Course

The disorder usually begins between early to mid-adolescence and early adult life and usually has a chronic intermittent course. Bulimic behavior usually begins as an attempt to control weight but rapidly progresses to a point at which it affects all aspects of the patient's life and is no longer voluntary (Hall and Beresford 1989a, 1990; Hall et al. 1989a).

Predisposing factors. Bulimic patients often have a family history of obesity. Major affective disorders occur two to four times more often in the first-degree biological relatives of bulimic patients than in the general population.

Clinical Features

Patients with bulimia are aware that their eating pattern is abnormal but are fearful of eating normally. At some time during their lives, 50%–70% of patients with bulimia develop a full-blown major depressive episode. Attention and concentration are diminished in patients with severe bulimia. This inability to concentrate is the most likely cause of their academic difficulties.

Approximately 80% of bulimic eating

binges are planned; 20% occur as a reaction to emotional stress. Once the binge begins, attempts by friends or relatives to stop it can cause disruptive behavior and/or violence.

Patients with bulimia often exercise excessively and abuse laxatives, diuretics, ipecac, and over-the-counter and illicit stimulants (e.g., phenylpropanolamine, amphetamines, cocaine) (Varner 1995). Most bulimic patients are overweight at some time before the onset of bulimia. Most (60%–80%) are of normal weight or slightly overweight when first seen. Unlike patients with anorexia, patients with bulimia maintain libido and desire interpersonal contact.

Hall et al. (1989a) reported that, in a hospitalized population, 13% of patients with anorexia, 8% of patients with bulimia, and 25% of patients with restrictive anorexia alternating with bulimia chronically abused laxatives, compared with 8% of a control group of female patients with other psychiatric disorders. These findings are similar to those reported by Mitchell et al. (1986), who noted that laxative abusers were twice as likely to abuse diuretics, 2.5 times more likely to abuse diet pills, and 4 times more likely to experience a serious medical complication than were non-laxative-abusing patients with anorexia or bulimia.

■ MEDICAL COMPLICATIONS

Hospitalized Patients With Anorexia and Bulimia

Hall and Beresford (1990) carefully evaluated 276 anorexic and bulimic patients admitted to an eating disorders unit and compared them with 78 depressed control patients for the occurrence of medical disorders. Two hundred distinct medical diagnoses were made in the 276 patients studied. The diagnosis of previously unrecognized medical disorders in the patients with eating disorders was nearly twice that of patients in the control group (statistically significant at $P = .001$). Forty percent of the patients with bulimia had a severe medical complication that was dangerous to life or limb or, if left untreated, would likely have long-term medical sequelae. The results were highly significant because these patients were young and presented in large numbers to general hospitals. Almost 90% of the serious medical complications were previously unrecognized by the patient or his or her physician, even though the majority of these patients had ongoing medical care.

Patients who had mixed anorexia and bulimia were at greatest risk for the development of serious medical complications. Of the patients with restrictive anorexia that alternated with bulimia, 84% had a significant medical complication, whereas 71% of the patients with only restrictive anorexia had medical complications that required treatment.

Based on this study, Hall and Beresford (1990) stressed the importance of an effective laboratory evaluation for a newly hospitalized patient with a suspected eating disorder (Table 14–1).

Hypomagnesemia and hypokalemia are common problems; refractory hypokalemia is occasionally caused by a persistent unrecognized hypomagnesemia (Boyd et al. 1983; Hall et al. 1988a, 1988b; Wong et al. 1983). Profound hypomagnesemia is most likely to occur in patients with alternating anorexia and bulimia

who abuse laxatives and diuretics (Hall et al. 1990). Table 14–2 shows the medical complications found in patients during the study by Hall and Beresford (1990).

The persistent hypokalemia can result in cardiac arrhythmias, profound muscular weakness, rhabdomyolysis, and glucose intolerance. Hypoproteinemia with massive "marching" edema is an ominous sign of impending cardiac decompensation and hypovolemic shock. This condition usually occurs in patients with severe anorexia who abuse laxatives and have profoundly low serum protein levels on admission.

Patients frequently have a moderate anemia with a hematocrit between 30 and 35. Severe anemia with a hematocrit below 25 occurs in 5%–10% of hospitalized patients; bone marrow biopsies show severely reduced or absent iron stores and low red blood cell folate levels. The routine replacement of iron, folate, vitamin B_{12}, and zinc is appropriate, as is the routine replacement of thiamine (100 mg/day orally) to obviate starvation-induced mental changes.

Persistent cardiac arrhythmias occur in

Table 14–1. Laboratory evaluation for a newly hospitalized patient with a suspected eating disorder

Complete blood count with differential

SMAC-21 or equivalent, including serum electrolytes and liver function studies, blood urea nitrogen, creatinine, and serum magnesium levels

Urinalysis

Electrocardiogram

Urine toxicology

Specific pancreatic amylase (or a routine amylase and, if positive, a lipase)

Table 14–2. Medical complications frequently encountered in hospitalized patients with anorexia or bulimia

Complication	Prevalence (%)
Persistent cardiac arrhythmia	33
Hypomagnesemia	25
Peptic ulcer disease	10–16
Severe anemia	5–10
Seizures	4
Esophageal tears	3
Pancreatitis (often associated with excessive thiazide diuretic abuse)	1
Renal insufficiency	1
Hypokalemia	30
Hyponatremia	20
Hypocalcemia	15
Leukopenia	35

one-third of the hospitalized patients with anorexia and are often associated with substernal chest pain and a history of syncope. Profoundly ill patients with anorexia have difficulty maintaining body temperature and blood pressure; 60% of the severely ill patients with anorexia in Hall's study (Hall and Beresford 1989a, 1990) developed cardiac arrhythmias secondary to electrolyte disorders, particularly hypokalemia. Peptic ulcer occurs in patients hospitalized for eating disorders. Esophageal ulcerations and tears occur most frequently in patients with a history of alternating restrictive anorexia and bulimia. Cerebral cortical atrophy and ventricular dilatation occur in both anorexic and bulimic patients, particularly in patients with a history of restrictive anorexia alternating with bulimia (Nussbaum et al. 1980).

Patients With Anorexia

The most frequent signs and symptoms encountered in patients with anorexia are listed in Table 14–3. The acute medical emergencies associated with eating disorders include arrhythmias, infections, persistent syncope, delirium, grand mal seizures, acute gastric rupture, toxic megacolon, esophageal tears with bleeding, development of Barrett's esophagus with bleeding, and acute upper or lower gastrointestinal bleeding. These patients often develop osteoporosis and may present with various pathological fractures, particularly of the small bones of the feet, as well as vertebral compression fractures (Brincat et al. 1983).

A variety of deficiency states and unusual disorders are reported in patients with anorexia. These include pellagra, which may present with dermatitis, diarrhea, and dementia; thiamine deficiencies, which present with organic mental syndrome; and polyvitamin disorders, which present with stomatitis, fissuring at the corner of the mouth, and hair loss. Zinc deficiencies are common (Castillo-Duran et al. 1987; Esca et al. 1979).

The menstrual pattern of anorexic patients

Table 14–3. Signs and symptoms frequently found in patients with anorexia

Most common
Progressive weight loss to the point of emaciation and organic mental impairment
Return to prepubescent levels of development, with regression of breasts and secondary sexual characteristics
Significant orthostatic hypotension
Inability to maintain body temperature with lowered core temperature
Appearance of lanugo
Amenorrhea
Constipation
Acrocyanosis
Muscular weakness and wasting
Loss of subcutaneous fat throughout the body
Pericardial thinning
Bradycardia
Hypercarotenemia
Peripheral "marching" edema

Other
Petechiae
Ecchymoses
Tremor
Ataxia
Confusion
Auditory and/or visual hallucinations
Acute gastric dilatation with periumbilical and midepigastric tenderness or pain
Signs of "pig-bel" (acute clostridial gastritis)

Associated with bulimia
Nausea
Spontaneous (i.e., nonvolitional) reflex vomiting of any food ingested
Persistent lancinating epigastric pain
Abdominal bloating and distension
Intractable constipation
Pyrosis
Flatulence
Belching or diarrhea alternating with constipation

is affected by both their degree of starvation and their level of physical activity. Research findings suggest that increased physical activity worsens a patient's menstrual dysfunction. Studies have also found that bone density is better maintained in patients who continue to exercise (Hall and Beresford 1990).

Substance use.   Patients with anorexia and bulimia often poison themselves through the consumption of stimulants or substances to induce purging. In addition, patients with eating disorders often consume large quantities of caffeine in diet sodas, coffee, and tea. The symptoms of caffeine toxicity include profound gastrointestinal upset, heartburn, tachycardia, arrhythmia, myoclonic twitching, and transient psychotic episodes. Patients have been reported to have consumed 3–10 g/day of caffeine and died (Shaul et al. 1984).

Ipecac toxicity is also encountered in patients with anorexia and bulimia. Two toxic alkaloids of ipecac—emetine and cephaeline—accumulate because of slow excretion from the body. These substances can prolong the Q-T interval and produce atrial and ventricular arrhythmias. Laxative abuse is frequently associated with hypochloremic, metabolic acidosis and hypocalcemia, particularly in patients who abuse phosphate-containing laxatives (Oster et al. 1980).

Cardiac abnormalities.   Cardiac arrhythmias and grand mal seizures are a frequent cause of death in patients with anorexia. Most cardiac arrhythmias are precipitated by the electrolyte abnormalities described earlier in this chapter. Fohlin (1977) demonstrated that up to 87% of patients with anorexia nervosa develop cardiac abnormalities at some time during their disease.

The high-protein liquid diets that many of these patients abuse can produce profound fatigue, dehydration, hair loss, orthostatic hypotension, arrhythmias, and myocarditis (Bistrian 1981). In addition, hypomagnesemia can induce coronary artery spasm leading to acute myocardial ischemia and chest pain.

Cardiac failure can occur during the refeeding phase of treatment; refeeding is a more dangerous time than the period of gradual starvation. If refeeding is too rapid, particularly in individuals who place stress on the heart by exercise, dyspnea followed by heart failure is common. Refeeding dyspnea usually begins between the second and fifth month of refeeding and is associated with an elevated venous pressure. Gradual refeeding of severely starved anorexic patients over a 2- to 4-month period, with an average weight gain of not more than 5 pounds per week, is safest despite insurance companies' pressure for more rapid weight gain.

The electrocardiogram (ECG) changes and coronary ischemia seen on admission in anorexic patients usually improve rapidly following hydration, renourishment, and the correction of electrolyte abnormalities (Hoffman and Hall 1990). The most frequent electrocardiographic abnormalities encountered include ST segment depression, inversion of T waves, low voltage, bradycardia, and the presence of U waves associated with hypokalemia and hypomagnesemia. The most dangerous findings encountered include supraventricular arrhythmias with premature ventricular beats and ventricular tachycardia. Prolonged Q-T intervals are associated with, and may predict, the sudden development of life-threatening arrhythmias in patients with anorexia. Bradycardia occurs in up to 87% of anorexic patients; a significant diminution in myocardial mass (i.e., decrease in left-ventricular wall thickness and a reduction in cardiac chamber size) also occurs (Fohlin 1977; Thurston and Marks 1974). Hypotension, with blood pressure consistently below 90/60 mm Hg, is reported in as many as 85% of patients with anorexia (M. P. Warren and Vandewyle 1979).

In patients who have anorexia, the peripheral conversion of thyroxine (T_4) to triiodothyronine (T_3) is inhibited, and levels of T_3 are decreased as much as 50% below normal values. In addition, total T_4 levels are often lower than expected but remain in the low end of the normal range. Free T_4 is normal. The resultant metabolic downregulation produces a variety of symptoms, including cold intolerance, drying of the skin, bradycardia, carotenemia, hypercholesterolemia, and constipation. This constellation of symptoms is called euthyroid sick syndrome (Croxson and Ibbertson 1977; Miyai et al. 1975).

Renal abnormalities. Renal abnormalities occur in up to 70% of patients who have chronic anorexia nervosa. Such patients present with increased levels of blood urea nitrogen, diminished glomerular filtration rates, diminished renal concentrating capability, pitting edema, renal calculi, hypokalemic nephropathy, diabetes insipidus–like states, and a variety of electrolyte abnormalities (Brotman et al. 1986; Mira et al. 1984; Schwartz and Relman 1967; Sheinin 1989; Silber and Kass 1984; S. E. Warren and Steinberg 1979). Hypokalemic nephropathy with renal tubular vacuolization is a particularly ominous finding in patients with anorexia and bulimia who have abused diuretics and laxatives. Chronic renal failure often develops in these patients.

Electrolyte abnormalities. Mitchell et al. (1983), in a study of 168 patients with bulimia, anorexia, or atypical eating disorders, found that 49% had electrolyte abnormalities. They noted increased bicarbonate (HCO_3) concentrations in 27%, hypochloremia in 24%, hyperchloremia in 5.4%, hypokalemia in 14%, and decreased HCO_3 in 8.3%. High phosphate levels are common in patients who vomit excessively.

Edema. Peripheral edema is seen in approximately 20% of patients with severe anorexia and is more likely to occur during the refeeding period than during starvation. Two forms of edema occur: 1) plasma proteins and albumin are normal, and 2) plasma protein, particularly albumin, is profoundly decreased (this is a more serious type of edema).

Hematological abnormalities. The hematological change most frequently accompanying severe anorexia (50% of cases) is a pancytopenia; bone marrow biopsies show marrow hypoplasia (Bowers and Eckert 1978; Myers et al. 1981; Reiger et al. 1978).

Hematological changes are common in patients with bulimia and include leukopenia, relative lymphocytosis, and, in severe cases, particularly those associated with abuse of phenothaline laxatives, a hypocellular bone marrow that is filled with large amounts of gelatinous mucopolysaccharide.

Endocrine abnormalities. Patients with anorexia have many profound endocrine changes. In summary, the endocrine changes in patients with anorexia and anorexia alternating with bulimia include T_4 levels in the lower range of, or just below, clinical laboratory norms, as well as T_3 levels that are somewhat reduced. Elevated serum concentrations of triiodothyronine (reverse T_3) are often associated with diminished levels of serum T_3. Some clinical laboratory equipment does not detect reverse T_3 and may produce a false picture of hypothyroidism (euthyroid sick syndrome) (Wartofsky and Burman 1982). The administration of thyroid hormones to euthyroid starved patients is dangerous and should be avoided. If routine T_3 levels are low, the clinician should obtain a T_3 level by radioimmunoassay as well as a thyroid-stimulating hormone level before any thyroid replacement is begun.

Amenorrhea usually begins in patients who are more than 15% below median ideal body weight. Many patients do not resume menses until they gain 8–10 pounds over the weight at which menstruation ceased (Kay and Leigh 1954).

Other common endocrine changes encountered in patients with anorexia include lowered levels of follicle-stimulating hormone, luteinizing hormone, and serum estrogen. Testosterone levels are lowered in male anorexic patients. All of these changes also occur with starvation.

Patients With Bulimia

Many of the medical complications that occur in patients with bulimia are discussed in the previous section on anorexia. The most frequent serious medical complications of bulimia are electrolyte imbalances, profound dehydration, hypovolemic shock, cardiac arrhythmias, esophageal tears, gastric rupture, peptic ulcer, blood loss, anemia with syncope, seizure, and organic mental syndrome, particularly confusional states.

In addition, patients with bulimia are at risk for a variety of dental problems, such as the erosion of tooth enamel, development of gum abscesses, and obstruction or inflammation of salivary ducts, which causes parotid inflammation and enlargement ("chipmunk cheeks"). They are also more likely to develop pyorrhea of the gums, ulcerations of the oral mucosa, and a loss of tongue papillae. Characteristically, tooth size is reduced and teeth are more sensitive because of thinning enamel. Patients often have a sore throat caused by the constant irritation from gastric acid, as well as a history of intermittent recurrent mid-periumbilical abdominal pain, esophageal irritation, crushing esophageal pain, and bouts of mild hematemesis. Mallory-Weiss tears of the esophagus are common, and Boerhaave's syndrome (esophageal rupture caused by vomiting) is reported (Russell 1979; Wilbur and Washburn 1978).

Parotid enlargement occurs in 10% of bulimic patients; 50% of these patients have elevated serum amylase levels. In patients who also report abdominal pain, a serum lipase is useful to rule out pancreatitis. If lipase is elevated, the source of the elevated amylase is likely the pancreas. If lipase is within normal limits, the source is the parotid glands.

More than 60 deaths as a result of acute gastric dilatation have occurred in bulimic patients. If gastric rupture occurs, the mortality exceeds 80%. Bulimic patients are at risk for the development of peptic ulcer (as many as 16%).

Other gastrointestinal disorders associated with bulimia include pancreatitis (secondary to dehydration and the use of thiazide diuretics), nutritional hepatitis, chronic cholecystitis, gastritis, irritable colon, rectal bleeding, adynamic ileus, toxic megacolon, nocturnal fecal soiling (secondary to laxative abuse), melena, ileitis, and superior mesenteric artery syndrome (Evans 1968; Gavish et al. 1987; Jennings and Klidjian 1974; Mitchell et al. 1982).

A variety of neurological and psychiatric symptoms are associated with severe bulimia. These include the development of seizures; paresthesias; muscular weakness; changes in sensorium; delirium; dementia; headache; dizziness; gait disorders; tetany; unilateral pupillary dilation; facial weakness; auditory, visual, and tactile hallucinations; derealization; depersonalization; and depression (Rau and Green 1978; Remick et al. 1980).

TREATMENT

Anorexia

The treatment of patients with eating disorders is first directed toward stabilizing their medical condition. After initial medical stabilization, a complete blood count with differential and SMAC-21 are recommended, at least weekly during the acute stage of treatment, to monitor for surreptitious activity and abnormal physiological states. Treatment is directed toward medical management, nutritional rehabilitation, and psychoeducation, as well as family, individual, and group therapy. For patients with anorexia, an educational program taught by an experienced dietitian is valuable.

During the early stages of treatment, a weight gain of 5 pounds/week is typically established. If the patient is unable to consume reasonable quantities of solid food, supplemental feedings with Ensure, Sustacal, or Glucerna are often helpful. If serum proteins are low, Dalmark gelatin twice each day is added to the regimen. Patients are also given

220 mg/day zinc sulfate for 10 days, 100 mg/day oral thiamine, and a multivitamin with minerals. Vital signs are carefully monitored every 6 hours during the first 3–4 weeks of treatment. Patients are weighed daily in a gown. If the patient is unable to eat or if weight continues to decline, the patient is placed on strict one-to-one (i.e., nurse is with patient at all times) or bed rest. If the patient has neurological symptoms, such as weakness and headaches, the consultant should obtain a computed tomography (CT) or magnetic resonance imaging (MRI) scan. If the patient reports amenorrhea for 2 years or more or complains of bone or back pain, appropriate radiographs and a bone density scan should be ordered.

Organic confusional states are treated with low doses of appropriate neuroleptics. In my experience, patients tolerate low-dose perphenazine (i.e., 2–4 mg at bedtime) quite well. Antidepressants are less effective during severe starvation than after the patient returns to normal weight. The discharge goal weight is established on admission and is no less than 80% of the median ideal body weight; the goal is to reach median ideal body weight by the time of discharge, if possible, or within 1–3 months postdischarge. Noradrenergic antidepressants enhance central norepinephrine function and stimulate food consumption in these patients (Leibowitz 1986).

Therapy is directed toward redefining interpersonal relationships; providing control over feelings of helplessness, hopelessness, and worthlessness; increasing self-esteem; providing specific coping tools; redefining family interactions; and helping the patient to become less fearful about normal body size and eating. Considerable effort is directed toward changing the anorexic patient's attitude and cognitions about his or her body size, food consumption, and weight.

Bulimia

Much of the treatment for anorexia also applies to the patient with bulimia. Hospitalized patients usually have experienced a significant medical consequence of bulimia; thus, medical stabilization is the foremost issue. Once stabilized, either inpatient or outpatient treatment with careful monitoring and follow-up is necessary. Bulimic patients benefit from individual, group, and family therapy, as well as cognitive-behavioral restructuring techniques. Although self-help groups are a useful adjunct, they do not substitute for psychotherapy. In addition, self-help groups that are based on 12-step models are counterproductive for many patients.

Although a large number of drugs are clinically useful in the treatment of bulimia, most eating disorder specialists today treat these patients with fluoxetine, imipramine, desipramine, or doxepin—the latter is particularly useful if esophagitis, gastritis, or peptic ulcers are present. Blood level monitoring is essential for proper adjustment of these medications. Some studies suggest that fluoxetine is a particularly useful drug (Mitchell 1992).

Outcome studies suggest that patients with bulimia do best when treated with a combination of individual, group, and family psychotherapy in addition to pharmacotherapy. At the end of 2 years of intensive combined therapy, 40%–60% of patients achieve abstinence from purging behavior, and an additional 10%–30% show marked improvement (Hall 1991).

■ REFERENCES[1]

American Psychiatric Association: Practice Guideline for Eating Disorders. Washington, DC, American Psychiatric Association, 1993

Bistrian BR: The medical treatment of obesity (editorial). Arch Intern Med 141:429–430, 1981

---

[1]An asterisk (*) indicates references referred to in the first paragraph of this chapter that readers can refer to for a more in-depth review of the management of eating disorders.

Bowers T, Eckert E: Leukopenia in anorexia nervosa. Arch Intern Med 138:1520–1524, 1978

Boyd JC, Bruns DE, Wills MR: Frequency of hypomagnesemia in hypokalemic states. Clin Chem 29:178–179, 1983

Brincat M, Parsons V, Studd J: Anorexia nervosa (letter). British Journal of Medicine 287:1306, 1983

*Brotman AW, Rigotti NA, Herzog DB: Medical complications of eating disorders. Compr Psychiatry 26:258–272, 1985

*Brotman AW, Stern TA, Brotman DL: Renal disease and dysfunction in two patients with anorexia nervosa. J Clin Psychiatry 47:433–436, 1986

Castillo-Duran C, Heresi G, Fisberg M, et al: Controlled trial of zinc supplementation during recovery from malnutrition: effects on growth and immune function. Am J Clin Nutr 45:602–608, 1987

Croxson MS, Ibbertson HK: Low serum triiodothyronine (T3) and hypothyroidism in anorexia nervosa. J Clin Endocrinol Metab 44:167–174, 1977

Esca SA, Brenner W, Mach K, et al: Kwashiorkor-like zinc deficiency syndrome in anorexia nervosa. Acta Derm Venereol (Stockh) 59:361–364, 1979

Evans DS: Acute dilatation and spontaneous rupture of the stomach. Br J Surg 55:940–942, 1968

Fohlin L: Body composition, cardiovascular and renal function in adolescent patients with anorexia nervosa. Acta Paediatr Suppl 268:3–20, 1977

*Gavish D, Eisenberg S, Berry EM, et al: Bulimia: an underlying behavioral disorder in hyperlipidemic pancreatitis: a perspective-multidisciplinary approach. Arch Intern Med 147:705–708, 1987

*Hall RCW: Management of eating disorders (audiotape). Audio-Digest Psychiatry 20(14), July 19, 1991

Hall RCW: Eating disorders, in The American Psychiatric Press Textbook of Consultation-Liaison Psychiatry. Edited by Rundell JR, Wise MG. Washington, DC, American Psychiatric Press, 1996, pp 486–504

*Hall RCW, Beresford TP: Bulimia nervosa: diagnostic criteria, clinical features and discrete clinical subsyndromes. Psychiatr Med 7:13–25, 1989a

*Hall RCW, Beresford TP: Anorexia nervosa: diagnostic, prognostic and clinical features. Psychiatr Med 7:3–12, 1989b

*Hall RCW, Beresford TP: Medical complications of anorexia and bulimia, in Clinical Diagnosis and Management of Eating Disorders. Edited by Hall RCW. Longwood, FL, Ryandic Publishing, 1990, pp 165–192

*Hall RCW, Hoffman RS, Beresford TP, et al: Hypomagnesemia in patients with eating disorders. Psychosomatics 29:264–272, 1988a

*Hall RCW, Hoffman RS, Beresford TP, et al: Refractory hypokalemia secondary to hypomagnesemia in eating disorder patients. Psychosomatics 29:435–438, 1988b

Hall RCW, Hoffman RS, Beresford TP, et al: Physical illness encountered in patients with eating disorders. Psychosomatics 39:174–191, 1989a

*Hall RCW, Hoffman RS, Beresford TP, et al: Unrecognized physical illness in patients with eating disorders, in Recent Advances in Psychiatric Medicine. Edited by Hall RCW. Littleton, MA, PSG Publishing, 1989b, pp 68–80

*Hall RCW, Beresford TP, Hall AK: Hypomagnesemia in eating disorder patients: clinical signs and symptoms, in Clinical Diagnosis and Management of Eating Disorders. Edited by Hall RCW. Longwood, FL, Ryandic Publishing, 1990, pp 193–203

*Halmi KA, Casper RC, Eckert ED, et al: Unique features associated with the age of onset of anorexia nervosa. Psychiatr Res 1:209–215, 1979

Hoffman RS, Hall RCW: Reversible EKG changes in anorexia nervosa, in Clinical Diagnosis and Treatment of Eating Disorders. Edited by Hall RCW. Longwood, FL, Ryandic Publishing, 1990, pp 211–216

Jennings KP, Klidjian AN: Acute gastric dilatation in anorexia nervosa. BMJ 2:477–478, 1974

Kay DW, Leigh D: The natural history, treatment and prognosis of anorexia nervosa. Journal of Mental Science 100:411–431, 1954

Leibowitz SF: Brain monoamines and peptides: role in the control of eating behavior. Federation Proceedings 45:1396–1403, 1986

*Mira M, Stewart PM, Abraham SF: Hypokalemia and renal impairment in patients with eating disorders. Med J Aust 140:290–293, 1984

*Mitchell JE: Psychobiology of bulimia nervosa (audiotape). Audio-Digest Psychiatry 21(22), November 23, 1992

*Mitchell JE, Pyle RL, Mine RA: Gastric dilatation as a complication of bulimia. Psychosomatics 23:96–97, 1982

*Mitchell JE, Pyle RI, Eckert ED, et al: Electrolyte and other physiologic abnormalities in patients with bulimia. Psychol Med 13:273–278, 1983

*Mitchell JE, Boutacoff LI, Hatsukami D, et al: Laxative abuse as a variant of bulimia. J Nerv Ment Dis 174:174–176, 1986

Miyai K, Yamamoto T, Azukizawa M, et al: Serum thyroid hormone and thyrotropin in anorexia nervosa. J Clin Endocrinol Metab 40:334–338, 1975

Myers TJ, Perkerson MD, Witter BA, et al: Hematologic findings: anorexia nervosa. Conn Med 45:14–17, 1981

*Nussbaum M, Shenker IR, Marc J, et al: Cerebral atrophy in anorexia nervosa. J Pediatr 5:867–869, 1980

Oster JR, Masterson BPJ, Rogers AI: Laxative abuse syndrome. Am J Gastroenterol 74:451–458, 1980

Palazzali MS: Self Starvation. New York, Jason Aronson, 1978

Rau JH, Green RS: Soft neurological correlates of compulsive eaters. J Nerv Ment Dis 166:435–437, 1978

Reiger W, Brady JP, Weisberg E: Hematologic changes in anorexia nervosa. Am J Psychiatry 135:984–985, 1978

Remick RA, Jones NW, Campos PE: Postictal bulimia (letter). J Clin Psychiatry 41:256, 1980

*Russell GFM: Bulimia nervosa: an ominous variant of anorexia nervosa. Psychol Med 9:429–448, 1979

Schwartz WB, Relman AS: Effects of electrolyte disorders on renal structure and function. N Engl J Med 276:383–389, 452–458, 1967

Shaul PW, Farrell MK, Maloney MJ: Caffeine toxicity as a cause of acute psychosis in anorexia nervosa. J Pediatr 105:493–495, 1984

*Sheinin JC: Medical aspects of eating disorders. Adolesc Psychiatry 13:405–421, 1989

Silber TJ, Kass EJ: Anorexia nervosa and nephrolithiasis. J Adolesc Health Care 5:50–52, 1984

Sullivan PF: Mortality in anorexia nervosa. Am J Psychiatry 157:1073–1074, 1995

*Thurston J, Marks SP: Electrocardiographic abnormalities in patients with anorexia nervosa. Br Heart J 36:719–723, 1974

Varner LM: Dual diagnosis: patients with eating and substance- related disorders. J Am Diet Assoc 95:224–225, 1995

Warren MP, Vandewyle RI: Clinical and metabolic features of anorexia nervosa. Am J Obstet Gynecol 117:415–418, 1979

Warren SE, Steinberg SM: Acid-base and electrolyte disturbances in anorexia nervosa. Am J Psychiatry 136:415–418, 1979

Wartofsky L, Burman KD: Alterations in thyroid function in patients with systemic illness: the "euthyroid sick syndrome." Endocr Rev 3:164–217, 1982

Wilbur TL, Washburn RN: Clinical features and treatment of functional or nervous vomiting. JAMA 110:477–480, 1978

Wong ET, Rude RK, Singer FR, et al: A high prevalence of hypomagnesemia and hypermagnesemia in hospitalized patients. Am J Clin Pathol 79:348–352, 1983

Chapter 15

Sleep Disorders

Jeffrey B. Weilburg, M.D.
John W. Winkelman, M.D., Ph.D.

CLASSIFICATION OF SLEEP DISORDERS

DSM-IV (American Psychiatric Association 1994) contains a useful section on sleep disorders. In this chapter, we follow DSM-IV classification whenever possible. The other current classification schema for sleep disorders is the International Classification of Sleep Disorders (ICSD; American Sleep Disorders Association 1990). The ICSD manual provides more detailed and comprehensive information than DSM-IV, so it is also a valuable resource for consultation psychiatrists. DSM-IV includes cross-references to the ICSD.

PHYSIOLOGY OF NORMAL SLEEP

Sleep is a dynamic process that is organized on the basis of electroencephalogram (EEG), electromyographic, and electrooculographic data into rapid eye movement (REM) sleep and non-REM (NREM) sleep. NREM sleep is further divided into stages 1, 2, 3, and 4. NREM stages 3 and 4 are often considered together as delta (or slow-wave) sleep.

Sleep normally proceeds smoothly through NREM stages 1, 2, and delta, returning to stage 2 before entering the first REM period, typically 70–90 minutes after sleep onset. The rhythmic alternation of NREM and REM has a cycle length of about 90 minutes, and REM periods increase in length as the night progresses. Delta sleep occurs mostly during the early part of the night and tapers off with successive cycles.

The circadian cycling of sleep and wakefulness directly affects the regulation of a wide variety of neuroendocrine functions (e.g., the secretion of cortisol and growth hormone). Sleep disruption may therefore secondarily affect endocrine status. Body temperature also follows a circadian rhythm in healthy adults, varying between 1.0°C and 1.2°C from its peak in the late afternoon to its nadir in the early morning. Abnormalities in temperature cycling may be correlated with some forms of insomnia, and disruption of sleep cycling may affect temperature cycling.

Environmental factors such as noise and temperature affect the quality and quantity of an individual's sleep. Noise can interfere with falling asleep and can produce arousals. Noise-induced arousal thresholds are lowest in light sleep and when the noise has a significance to the sleeper (e.g., a monitor alarm will be significant to a patient who has a cardiac monitor) (Johns and Doré 1978; Jones et al. 1979). However, the influence of physical surroundings on sleep is surprisingly small. Indwelling venous and arterial catheters may disrupt sleep if they produce pain or other discomfort; however, the mere presence of these devices appears to have minimal effects on sleep architecture (Jarrett et al. 1984; Johns and Doré 1978).

When patients register complaints about disturbed sleep, the psychiatric consultant may verify that basic patient comfort has been reasonably attended to and that the nursing routine is adjusted to minimize unnecessary intrusion. However, the consultant should focus attention on identifying the specific physiological and emotional factors underlying a patient's sleep complaints, as outlined below, rather than expending too much effort on adjusting environmental factors.

Age, premorbid sleep patterns, and general health status may affect sleep. For example, compared with younger individuals, elderly people generally sleep less efficiently and less deeply and have less delta sleep and more awakenings (Reynolds et al. 1985b). Daytime sleepiness tends to be more common in elderly persons, and it is more difficult for them to adjust to changes in the sleep-wake schedule. Some patients are normally short sleepers, sleeping less than 7 hours each night without compromised daytime function. Significant weight loss—at times a consequence of chronic illness—has been associated with short, fragmented sleep. The consultant should consider these factors when evaluating the degree of sleep disruption in hospitalized patients. The consultant's goal in managing sleep disruption in such patients should be to restore sleep to a prehospitalization baseline, unless treatment of a sleep disorder itself is the reason

for admission or a clinically significant sleep disorder has been identified in the workup.

SLEEP PATTERNS IN PATIENTS IN INTENSIVE CARE UNITS

Patients in intensive care units (ICUs) tend to have several characteristic patterns in their sleep. These patterns appear in a similar fashion in patients with a variety of underlying medical and surgical problems and include decreased total sleep time (TST), disrupted day/night circadian cycles, and disrupted sleep architecture.

Decreased Total Sleep Time

Several investigators (Aurell and Elmquist 1985; Broughton and Baron 1978; Johns et al. 1974; Orr and Stahl 1977; Richards and Bairnsfather 1988) reported marked decreases in the TST of patients in ICUs. A mean TST of 2 hours was noted during the first 48 hours after noncardiac surgery (Aurell and Elmquist 1985). Investigators found that patients in ICUs typically appear to be sleeping, lying quietly with their eyes closed, but the EEG demonstrates a pattern consistent with drowsiness or stage 1 sleep interrupted frequently by brief arousals (Broughton and Baron 1978).

Disrupted Day/Night Circadian Cycles

Many patients in the ICU have periods of sleep that are brief and distributed fairly evenly throughout the 24-hour day rather than consolidated at night (Broughton and Baron 1978; Dohno et al. 1979; Johns et al. 1974; Karacan and Williams 1969; Kavey and Altshuler 1979; Richards and Bairnsfather 1988). This pattern was common to patients in ICUs despite different surgical procedures, medications, and related complications (Aurell and Elmquist 1985; Broughton and Baron 1978; Dohno et al. 1979; Johns et al. 1974; Kavey and Altshuler 1979).

Disrupted Sleep Architecture

The severity of the degree of disruption of the sleep architecture tends to vary directly with the severity of the illness (Dohno et al. 1979). When a patient remains in the ICU, sleep tends to improve over 4–7 days if the overall condition improves (Johns et al. 1974). However, if delirium or complications supervene, sleep often remains disrupted for prolonged periods.

Most authors conclude that some endogenous derangement of sleep-wake regulating systems in the central nervous system (CNS) is the basis for sleep disruption in patients in ICUs (Aurell and Elmquist 1985; Broughton and Baron 1978; Dohno et al. 1979). The specific factors producing this derangement are poorly understood, but no specific disease process or drug can be found to account for the disturbances described above. Although anxiety (stress) and nursing routine may add to the disrupted sleep seen in patients in ICUs (Yinnon et al. 1992), these factors are not the primary cause of the disruption.

Clinical Consequences of Sleep Changes

The clinical consequences, if any, of the sleep changes seen in patients in ICUs are not clear. Early studies suggested that delirium or psychosis might be produced by sleep deprivation. Sleep deprivation was thus advanced as a cause of "ICU psychosis." Subsequent work indicates that healthy subjects who undergo prolonged sleep deprivation have brief periods when sleep intrudes into waking (microsleeps), during which time unusual or confused behavior may occur. Sleep deprivation can also produce mood lability, irritability, and cognitive changes such as slow reaction time. However, sleep deprivation itself does not appear to produce psychosis or delirium (L. C. Johnson 1982; Williams et al. 1967).

Patients will occasionally be admitted to an ICU for problems directly related to a primary sleep disorder. For example, serious injuries may occur during episodes of REM sleep behavior disorder, night terrors, or sleepwalking (Schenck and Mahowald 1991). (REM sleep behavior disorder is a newly recognized condition in which patients ambulate—sometimes in an agitated fashion—while they are in REM sleep. For more information on this disorder, refer to the ICSD manual.) Pulmonary hypertension, right heart failure, and nocturnal cardiac arrest may occur secondary to severe sleep apnea. Therefore, these sleep disorders should be factored into a complete differential diagnosis, especially when more common causes of problems like those noted above have been ruled out.

■ SLEEP IN PATIENTS IN MEDICAL AND SURGICAL INPATIENT UNITS

The disturbances of sleep found in patients on the medical and surgical floors are similar to those observed in ICU patients but are not as severe and tend to resolve more readily as patients' conditions improve. Indeed, the majority of studies demonstrated that, in many patients, sleep spontaneously returns to baseline despite continued hospitalization. Therefore, the consultant should not assume that a patient's presence on the medical or surgical ward is enough in itself to produce disrupted sleep. According to Kavey and Altschuler (1979, pp. 686–687), "a hospitalized patient's summary statement of the quality of the night's sleep correlates poorly with the electrophysiological data," so "while asking how a patient slept is perhaps politic, it is unlikely to elicit a meaningful answer unless followed by a more detailed inquiry." Patients and nursing staff may make helpful observations regarding sleep-related respiration, movement, and behavior. Family members and bed partners may reveal details about the patient's sleep characteristics before hospitalization.

Transient insomnia (i.e., of a duration less than 1 week) is probably both common and underdiagnosed in medical and surgical patients. Berlin and colleagues (1984) diagnosed transient insomnia in 71% of 100 consecutive patients referred for psychiatric consultation in a general hospital. Notably, no mention of sleep disturbance was found in the medical records of 54% of patients who were found to have sleep disorders by the consulting psychiatrist.

Hypnotic agents are often routinely prescribed for general hospital patients, but the rational basis for this practice has not been established. A retrospective randomly selected chart review conducted in 1982 on 23 medical and 20 surgical patients in a general hospital showed that prescriptions for hypnotics to be administered as needed were written for 46% of those on the medical service but were actually used by only 31% (Perry and Wu 1984). Among those on the medical service who used the hypnotics, the rate of use declined with increasing length of hospital stay. In contrast, orders were written for as-needed hypnotics for 96% of the surgical patients; 88% of those on the surgical service actually used a hypnotic at least once, and the frequency of hypnotic usage increased with increasing length of hospital stay. However, no clear correlation was found between the writing of an as-needed prescription for hypnotics and the presence of sleep disturbance, perceived quality of sleep, primary diagnosis, or actual use of hypnotics. These observations suggest that consultants should use hypnotics only when treating specific sleep problems.

APPROACH TO THE PATIENT COMPLAINING OF INSOMNIA

Insomnia is generally defined as a complaint of trouble falling asleep or staying asleep or of nonrestorative sleep, with these sleep abnormalities being associated with daytime distress such as anergy, malaise, cognitive slowness, and irritability. Mild transient sleep disturbance secondary to anxiety or physical discomfort is

very common in hospitalized patients. If the sleep disruption is self-limited and is not associated with daytime compromise, there is no need to make a diagnosis of insomnia or to treat with hypnotics. More severe or persistent sleep disruption that can be linked with daytime distress may be regarded as a clinical problem worth pursuing. In such cases, insomnia might be identified as a primary clinical problem.

Several subtypes of insomnia are found in hospitalized patients. The most common is mild, transient insomnia, which, in most cases, occurs secondary to adjustment disorder in patients in whom the medical illness or the hospitalization and the related psychosocial disruption are the stressors. Insomnia secondary to anxiety or mood disorder is also seen commonly in hospitalized patients. Nocturnal panic attacks may be initially reported as insomnia, so a careful history of nocturnal events and experiences is important. Both major depression and dysthymia are common in hospitalized patients, and both frequently produce difficulty falling asleep, difficulty staying asleep, or early morning waking.

Patients with narcissistic or obsessional disorders, especially when subjected to the stress of illness and hospitalization, may become angry, frustrated, or agitated if they are unable to sleep. Such patients focus on sleep and ruminate about being deprived of the rest they believe they need and deserve.

Psychoses of any type may produce trouble falling and staying asleep, both before and during the episode of illness. Before ascribing insomnia to a patient's preexisting psychosis, however, it is important to rule out sleep disruption caused by toxic and medical factors such as delirium due to medication or direct adverse drug effects (e.g., neuroleptic-induced akathisia).

The next most common insomnia subtype found in hospitalized patients is classified in DSM-IV as sleep disorder due to a general medical condition, insomnia type. The specific nature of the medical disorder should be noted—for example, sleep disorder due to asthma, insomnia type. For this diagnosis to be made, the sleep disturbance and/or the related daytime distress must be significant in itself and sufficient to warrant being addressed as a new and distinct clinical problem, and the insomnia must be judged to be produced directly by the specific medical disorder.

In many cases, it may be difficult to determine whether a medical disorder or the medications used in treatment are causing the insomnia. For example, both Parkinson's disease and carbidopa can produce insomnia. If it appears that the insomnia is more a function of the drug than of the medical problem, a diagnosis of substance-induced sleep disorder, insomnia type, may be made instead. Patients who have been dependent on alcohol, caffeine, nicotine, or stimulants may experience withdrawal in the hospital and may experience insomnia as a withdrawal symptom. Patients with chronic alcoholism may have significantly disturbed sleep even after months of abstinence. Such patients may also be diagnosed with substance abuse-related insomnia. A careful history, with an interview of those who know the patient, may be required to make this diagnosis.

Patients who learn to associate sleep with frustration or dysphoria may develop conditioned, or psychophysiological, insomnia. Such patients may have only anxious or depressive traits rather than formal Axis II or adjustment disorders, but, when stressed by illness or hospitalization, they may have significant insomnia. A careful history will reveal long-standing intermittent insomnia, which is sometimes better when the patient is in a novel environment such as a hotel. For practical purposes, the consultant may manage such patients in a manner similar to how patients with anxiety disorders are managed (see section, "Treatment of Insomnia," later in this chapter). The possibility should be considered that insomnia is being caused by medication-induced periodic leg movements of sleep

(PLMS). Table 15–1 lists medications that can cause insomnia. In our experience, medication-induced insomnia is much more commonly seen among outpatients than among hospitalized patients.

Delirium may be a subtle and transient problem in some patients. Nocturnal agitation with resultant insomnia may be the initial, and in some cases the major, presenting feature of delirium. The consultant should always have a high index of suspicion for delirium as a cause of insomnia in hospitalized medically ill patients. Nurses may be instructed to perform careful mental status examinations at night, which can assist in proper diagnosis.

Table 15–1. Insomnia secondary to drugs or medications: substance-induced sleep disorder, insomnia type

Alcohol (withdrawal, long-term abuse)

Antiasthmatics, decongestants (β_2-agonists, pseudoephedrine, phenylephrine)

Antidepressants: phenelzine, tranylcypromine, protriptyline, desipramine, imipramine, amoxapine, fluoxetine and other selective serotonin reuptake inhibitors (by direct stimulant properties and, in some, by induction of PLMS), tricyclic withdrawal

Antihypertensives, methyldopa, diuretics, reserpine, clonidine (nightmares, PLMS)

Cimetidine

Heavy metal toxicity: arsenic, mercury, lead, copper

L-Dopa, baclofen, methysergide

Neuroleptics: phenothiazines, butyrophenones (can induce PLMS)

Sedative-hypnotics (rebound insomnia following withdrawal after long-term abuse): barbiturates, benzodiazepines, narcotics

Stimulants: amphetamines; methylphenidate; pemoline; cocaine; caffeine and stimulant xanthines in coffee, tea, cola, chocolate

Tetracycline (nightmares)

Thyroxine, steroids, birth control pills

Tobacco (direct stimulation, withdrawal, conditioned awakening to smoke)

Note. PLMS = periodic leg movements of sleep.

Most patients with sleep apnea complain of excessive daytime sleepiness, but some also complain of insomnia. Because sleep apnea is both potentially fatal if misdiagnosed or mismanaged and potentially correctable if discovered, and because sleep apnea may be present yet underrecognized in elderly patients or in those with pulmonary, cardiac, neurological, or other illness, the consultant should always consider it in the differential diagnosis of insomnia (see section, "Sleep Apnea," later in this chapter for further discussion).

TREATMENT OF INSOMNIA

For patients with insomnia secondary to medical or psychiatric disorders, optimized treatment of the underlying disorder is the first step. Behavioral management techniques, such as progressive muscle relaxation, hypnosis, or guided imagery, along with attention to the rules of sleep hygiene, may help some patients who have insomnia secondary to psychiatric disorders, particularly adjustment and anxiety disorders (Turner and Ascher 1979). Caffeine appears to increase insomnia in hospitalized patients (Victor et al. 1981), so simply removing coffee, tea, and cola beverages from the diets of patients complaining of insomnia may be of practical utility. Patients with anxiety disorders may be sensitive to the stimulant side effects of antidepressants used to treat mood or anxiety disorders and, as a result, may experience insomnia during the early phase of treatment. Trazodone, 25–100 mg, may be added to moderate the insomnia-producing effects of potentially stimulating antidepressants such as fluoxetine (Nierenberg et al. 1994).

Benzodiazepine hypnotics have been and remain a mainstay of drug treatment for insomnia secondary to psychiatric and medical disorders in hospitalized patients. Benzodiazepines may be used when insomnia symptoms persist despite treatment of the primary cause of insomnia, such as pain, depression, or conges-

tive heart failure (CHF). Because they may induce significant nocturnal respiratory compromise, benzodiazepines should be used with caution when patients have significant chronic obstructive pulmonary disease (COPD), obesity- or cardiac-related hypoventilation, or CHF (Guilleminault 1990). Benzodiazepines can impair ventilation in patients with sleep apnea and thus should be used with caution in such patients. Elderly patients are particularly sensitive to the cognitive compromise produced by benzodiazepines, and falls can result from impaired cognition or motor coordination. Therefore, in elderly patients, benzodiazepines should be used cautiously and in reduced dosages.

Benzodiazepines should be used at the lowest effective dose and only while the insomnia complaint remains acute. It has yet to be established whether the newer benzodiazepine hypnotics—quazepam, estazolam, and zolpidem—offer clear advantages over older agents for hospitalized patients with medical and surgical problems (Salazar-Gruesco et al. 1988). In general, drugs with a rapid onset of action (such as diazepam, triazolam, and zolpidem) are the agents of choice to help those who have trouble falling asleep, whereas drugs with a somewhat delayed onset of action (such as clonazepam, temazepam, and quazepam) are useful for those who have sleep interruption. Withdrawal problems (rebound anxiety or insomnia) may occur when short-acting benzodiazepines such as triazolam or alprazolam are used to treat daytime anxiety. In our experience, patients with insomnia secondary to anxiety disorders may be particularly sensitive to withdrawal and rebound phenomena. Longer-acting benzodiazepines such as clonazepam may improve both daytime anxiety and insomnia for such patients. Diazepam and clonazepam may be useful for patients with insomnia produced by leg cramps or PLMS.

Chloral hydrate, paraldehyde, and barbiturates should be used rarely, if at all, because these drugs have a greater tendency to depress respiration and are generally less effective than benzodiazepines. Clinical lore suggests that sedating antihistamines such as diphenhydramine and hydroxyzine may be useful in some patients, but their efficacy for the treatment of insomnia is not well established, and the possibility of their causing antihistamine-induced delirium in some patients makes these agents of questionable value (Nicholson et al. 1985; Rickels et al. 1983).

Neuroleptics should be used in hospitalized patients to control insomnia secondary to psychosis, psychotic depression, and acute mania. Neuroleptics may also be extremely helpful in controlling disturbed sleep secondary to delirium in elderly individuals and in ICU patients. This use is especially important if concomitant agitation and irritability pose a risk to a patient who is already compromised by medical illness or whose postsurgical status requires compliance with restrictions posed by drains, intravenous drug administration, and dressings. Neuroleptics may also be used to control mania secondary to steroids or other medications. Low to moderate doses of benzodiazepines such as lorazepam may be used adjunctively with neuroleptics to induce sleep and to manage nocturnal delirium or agitation.

In depressed patients with insomnia, sedating antidepressants (e.g., doxepin or trazodone) may be given. Tricyclic antidepressants may induce or worsen preexisting sleep-related movement disorders and thus may precipitate or worsen insomnia in some patients. Likewise, some antidepressants such as fluoxetine, imipramine, desipramine, protriptyline, and the monoamine oxidase inhibitors (MAOIs) may be stimulating and may produce insomnia (see Table 15–1). Lithium may disrupt sleep continuity if polyuria supervenes. Many consultation-liaison psychiatrists use low- to moderate-dose trazodone in combination with morning doses of selective serotonin reuptake inhibitors (SSRIs) for initial management of insomnia.

■ APPROACH TO THE PATIENT COMPLAINING OF EXCESSIVE DAYTIME SOMNOLENCE

Evaluating a patient who complains of excessive daytime somnolence (EDS) requires a careful history and, occasionally, objective measures of sleepiness. Multiple etiologies of EDS exist, and the most common is inadequate TST; however, EDS that is caused by a primary sleep disorder is the result of an inability to obtain restorative sleep and therefore will not be relieved simply by the patient's achieving more sleep.

As with insomnia, the approach to the management of the patient with EDS begins with clarification of the nature of the complaint. EDS is characterized by falling asleep inappropriately during the day. Many patients fail to report the extent of their somnolence because of inattention, cognitive decline, and memory disturbance. On the other hand, fatigue, lethargy, depression, delirium, boredom, obtundation, and abulia are often described by patients as "sleepiness"; however, these patients may not have inappropriate episodes of sleep during the day. The sleepiness associated with psychiatric disorders is likely to be related to impaired attention, energy, or motivation. Other conditions, such as depression, can lead to sleeping excessive lengths of time or to spending excessive time awake in bed, but objective measures do not support the conclusion that the patient has EDS. These patients, if kept to a "normal" sleep schedule, will not have inappropriate levels of daytime somnolence (Nofzinger et al. 1991).

The hospital setting is a poor environment in which to assess EDS because hospitalized patients frequently sleep during the day for a variety of reasons that are no cause for concern. Interviews with family members or housemates can help define the extent and duration of sleep problems. Bed partners can describe snoring or abnormal behaviors during sleep. A history of job loss, injury, or motor vehicle accidents may reflect dysfunctions associated with EDS.

In addition to a careful history, objective measures are sometimes indicated. The gold standard for EDS evaluation is the Multiple Sleep Latency Test (MSLT), which determines latency to EEG-defined sleep averaged over five naps during the day (Carskadon 1986). Mean sleep latencies of less than 5 minutes are pathological. Once the presence of EDS is clearly established—on the basis of the history and, if necessary, evaluation with the MSLT—the differential diagnosis of the underlying cause of EDS can be considered.

◼ SLEEP APNEA

Sleep-disordered breathing is identified by means of polysomnographic evaluation in a sleep laboratory in which the EEG, electrooculogram, electromyogram, respiratory effort, oxygen saturation, and air flow from the nares and mouth are recorded. Two types of apnea are recognized, although they commonly coexist in the same patient: 1) obstructive, in which air flow is compromised despite respiratory effort; and 2) central, in which little, if any, respiratory effort is made. Whereas hypopnea is a minimum of a one-third reduction in air flow, apnea is defined as a complete elimination of air flow, lasting for a minimum of 10 seconds, that causes a reduction in oxyhemoglobin saturation. These episodes are usually followed by a brief arousal. Sleep apnea is defined as more than five apnea or hypopnea episodes per hour of sleep. The severity of sleep apnea is determined by the respiratory index (number of hypopnea or apnea episodes per hour), the extent of the oxygen desaturation (oxygen nadir and number of desaturations below 85%), the sleep fragmentation caused by respiratory events, and any associated cardiac arrhythmia.

Symptoms of sleep apnea are due to sleep fragmentation and cardiopulmonary stress associated with obstructed respiration (see Table 15–2). Reduced air flow produces oxyhemoglobin desaturation, and obstruction in the upper airway leads to compensatory increases in respiratory effort. Repetitive brief arousals produce daytime somnolence. Hypoxia and high intrathoracic pressures lead to increases in pulmonary artery pressure, which have been shown to produce right heart failure, systemic hypertension, and stroke, although the confounding variable of obesity limits conclusions of such studies (Millman 1985; Partinen and Palomaki 1985). Studies have indicated that one-quarter to one-third of patients with a diagnosis of moderate to severe apnea do not survive beyond 8–10 years (He et al. 1988; Partinen and Guilleminault 1990). Finally, the severity of apnea and subsequent hypoxemia during the early morning might explain currently available population studies suggesting higher mortality rates (Mitler et al. 1987).

Table 15–2.   Signs and symptoms of obstructive sleep apnea syndrome

Central nervous system
 Excessive daytime somnolence
 Nocturnal restlessness
 Depression
 Cognitive deterioration
 Morning headache
 Loss of sexual drive

Respiratory
 Snoring
 Dry mouth/sore throat

Cardiac
 Hypertension
 Right heart failure
 Arrhythmias

Gastrointestinal
 Gastroesophageal reflux

Autonomic nervous system
 Nocturnal diaphoresis

Renal
 Nocturia and nocturnal enuresis

Hematological
 Polycythemia

The pathophysiology of central sleep apnea differs from that of the obstructive form. Rather than an obstruction in the upper airway, the abnormality in central sleep apnea is in the central drive for respiration. Central sleep apnea usually produces less oxyhemoglobin desaturation and does not produce the high intrathoracic pressures of obstructive apnea. Most patients with pure central sleep apnea describe insomnia and not excessive daytime somnolence (Roehrs et al. 1985).

Treatment of sleep apnea is multifaceted. The first step is an investigation of the potential underlying medical and anatomical etiologies (see Table 15–3). Minimum evaluation includes thyroid indices and direct or endoscopic evaluation of the upper airway. If the patient is overweight, a referral to a nutritionist is essential. Patients should eliminate nocturnal alcohol or sedatives because these reduce activity of the upper airway musculature and extend the duration of apneas.

The mainstay of treatment for both obstructive and central sleep apnea is nasal continuous positive airway pressure (CPAP). Positive pressure is delivered via a plastic mask over the nose; the pressure is adjusted in the sleep laboratory to eliminate sleep-related obstructive events, including snoring.

Resection of nasal polyps or hypertrophied adenoids and tonsils can reduce obstructive events and may enhance CPAP compliance. More aggressive surgical management—that is, uvulopalatopharyngoplasty—is reserved for CPAP treatment failures because of unpredictable efficacy of such procedures (the chance of a successful outcome is 50% in the hands of even a highly skilled surgeon).

■ NARCOLEPSY

Narcolepsy is a disorder characterized by both excessive daytime sleepiness and the associated REM symptoms of cataplexy, sleep paralysis, and hypnagogic hallucinations. The preva-

Table 15–3. Risk factors for obstructive sleep apnea

General
  Obesity
  Increasing age
  Male gender
  Postmenopausal status (women)
  Nocturnal alcohol or sedative-hypnotic use

Reduction in upper airway patency
  Hypertrophic tonsils or adenoids
  Nasal septum deviation
  Nasal polyps
  Neoplasms
  Storage diseases (e.g., amyloidosis)
  Craniofacial abnormalities (e.g., Pierre Robin syndrome, Treacher Collins syndrome)
  Retrognathia
  Micrognathia
  Macroglossia (e.g., Down's syndrome)

Metabolic abnormalities
  Hypothyroidism
  Acromegaly
  Prader-Willi syndrome

Neurological disorders
  Parkinson's disease
  Syringomyelia
  Shy-Drager syndrome
  Mitochondrial encephalomyopathy

lence is approximately 0.05% in the general population.

There is no cure for narcolepsy, so treatment is directed toward relief of daytime sleepiness and REM-related phenomena. Dextroamphetamine (up to 60 mg/day) or methylphenidate (up to 60 mg/day) restores alertness to an average of 70% of normal (Mitler and Hajdukovic 1991). Both medications are available in sustained-release formulations; these are usually administered in twice-daily doses of 30 mg each. Prophylactic naps, when feasible, can reduce the total daily dose of stimulants required. Because of their potent REM suppression effects, antidepressants are the treatment of choice for patients with cataplexy, sleep paralysis, and hypnagogic hallucinations. Tricyclic antidepressants, MAOIs, and serotonergic uptake inhibitors are all effective, although the greatest clinical experience has been amassed with protriptyline and clomipramine.

RESTLESS LEGS SYNDROME AND PERIODIC LEG MOVEMENTS OF SLEEP

Restless legs syndrome (RLS) is a movement disorder characterized by both sensory and motor components. Patients commonly describe an achy or "crawling" paresthesia, usually in the legs. Frequently, the sensory and motor aspects of the disorder are worse at night when immobility is necessary, so the presenting complaint of this movement disorder is sleep disturbance.

Many patients with RLS also manifest the associated movement disorder, PLMS, in which involuntary movements of the affected limbs occur episodically during sleep, approximately every 20–40 seconds. Such movements are brief (0.5–5 seconds) and are most common in the dorsiflexors of the foot and flexors of the lower leg. However, the movements can be quite disruptive of sleep continuity, producing nocturnal arousals or actual awakenings.

RLS occurs in association with a number of medical problems, such as renal failure, diabetes, chronic anemia, and peripheral nerve injuries. It may appear during otherwise uncomplicated pregnancy, with aging, or as an apparently idiopathic problem in its own right. RLS and PLMS may also be induced by various medications.

Treatment of the underlying causes of RLS and PLMS (removal of offending medications, correction of electrolyte disturbance or anemia) can at times eliminate the disturbance, but generally, only symptomatic relief is possible. The primary therapeutic agents are benzodiazepines, dopamine agonists, and narcotics.

SLEEP IN PATIENTS WITH SELECTED MEDICAL CONDITIONS AND DISORDERS

Characteristic changes in the clinical and polysomnographic features of sleep are associated with some medical illnesses.

Cardiac Disease

Dysrhythmias. Patients with ventricular arrhythmias may have a decreased rate of arrhythmias during sleep, but some—especially those with sleep apnea, alveolary hypoventilation, or COPD—can develop significant worsening of arrhythmias during either REM or NREM sleep (Bond et al. 1973; Lown et al. 1973; Nevins 1972; Smith et al. 1972). Atrial arrhythmias may worsen during sleep (Bond et al. 1973; Lown et al. 1973).

Conduction system abnormalities, especially in patients with comorbid nocturnal hypoxia, can worsen during sleep (Miller 1982). Benzodiazepines may precipitate or worsen hypoxia, so consultants should use these drugs with caution in patients with conduction system abnormalities.

Patients with sleep apnea can develop bradycardia at the beginning of an apneic spell, which may progress to asystole in severe cases. Dramatic increases in heart rate can occur as respiration resumes.

Coronary artery disease. Cardiac ischemia frequently occurs during sleep in patients with coronary artery disease (CAD). The ischemia may produce anginal pain, which awakens the patient, or the episode may be silent (e.g., signified only by ST segment depression on cardiac monitoring).

There is a relation between nocturnal angina and REM sleep in some patients (Broughton and Baron 1978; Cassano et al. 1981; Nowlin et al. 1965). Variant (spasm) angina can occur during REM, sometimes in association with frightening dreams (King et al. 1973).

Chronic Obstructive Pulmonary Disease

Patients with COPD have frequent arousals during sleep, decreased sleep efficiency, and significant sleep-related oxygen desaturations (especially during REM) of uncertain etiology

(Klink and Quan 1987; Perez-Padilla et al. 1985). The role of nasal oxygen as a treatment for these sleep-related desaturations is controversial. Benzodiazepines or other sedatives can precipitate clinically significant sleep apnea in patients with COPD and must be used with caution (Cohn et al. 1992; Guilleminault 1990). Whether neuroleptics induce respiratory compromise in patients with COPD has not, to our knowledge, been studied, but no evidence of such compromise has been noted in our experience with neuroleptics in patients in ICUs.

Endocrine Disease

Hyperthyroidism typically increases and hypothyroidism decreases delta sleep, but the clinical significance of these effects is uncertain. Goiter, diabetes, and use of exogenous androgen can predispose to sleep apnea (Guilleminault et al. 1981; M. W. Johnson et al. 1984; Millman 1985; Young et al. 1986).

Pregnancy

Sleep changes, probably related to hormonal alterations, may occur in some women during pregnancy (Errante 1985). Increased sleep time and daytime sleepiness appear in the first trimester; after this time, sleep patterns normalize, and then in the third trimester, a shift toward decreased TST occurs. Stage 4 sleep may decrease as term approaches, but this sleep change resolves postpartum. REM sleep may also decline before term and resolve in the first 2 weeks postpartum.

Neurological Disease

Epilepsy.   In generalized epilepsy, convulsive seizures appear equally distributed during waking and sleep in the majority of patients with epilepsy. Convulsive seizures occur exclusively during sleep in about 8% of patients (morpheic epilepsy) (Fisch and Pedley 1987). Patients with only nocturnal seizures may have normal daytime EEGs. Most patients with partial epilepsy have daytime seizures exclusively, with exclusive nocturnal seizures occurring in 11% of this population (Baldy-Moulinier 1982). Patients with partial epilepsy appear to have lighter, more unstable sleep; a higher frequency of complaints of EDS; and subjectively unsatisfying sleep compared with subjects without epilepsy or patients with generalized epilepsy.

Headache.   Vascular headaches often appear during sleep, either at night or during an afternoon nap. An association between REM and the onset of some migrainous headaches has been reported. Both cluster headache and chronic paroxysmal hemicrania also often have REM-related onset. Patients with vascular and mixed vascular/tension headaches often complain of insomnia and sometimes show frequent awakening, abnormal sleep architecture, and overall decreases in REM sleep (Dexter 1986). Patients with vascular headaches have an incidence of somnambulism, enuresis, and night terrors higher than that found in the general population (Pradalier et al. 1987).

Stroke.   Strokes often begin during nocturnal sleep, and there is a high incidence of stroke among patients with snoring and sleep apnea. Strokes that affect medullary and pontine areas may produce sleep apnea or aggravate preexisting mild apnea. Strokes in a variety of locations can produce alterations in the sleep-wake cycle, decreased sleep efficiency, decreased time, and drowsiness and, in rare cases, can induce narcolepsy (Aldrich and Naylor 1989; Kapen et al. 1990).

Degenerative diseases.   Degenerative CNS diseases such as Huntington's disease, progressive supranuclear palsy, spinocerebellar degeneration, olivopontocerebellar degeneration, and torsion dystonia often produce insomnia, EDS, circadian cycle disturbances, and parasomnias (Hansotia et al. 1985; Jankel et al. 1983; Katayama et al. 1985; Lavigne et al. 1991).

Patients with Tourette's syndrome may experience nocturnal tics, insomnia, and parasomnias, which remit or worsen as a function of the severity of the syndrome itself (Erenberg 1985). These problems tend to become less common as patients enter adulthood.

Senile dementia of the Alzheimer's type, multi-infarct dementia, alcoholic dementia, Pick's disease and other frontal degenerative processes, Creutzfeldt-Jakob disease, and obstructive hydrocephalus can all produce sleep problems secondary to nocturnal delirium (sundowning). The likelihood of sundowning increases as the dementing illness worsens or comorbid medical problems supervene (Evans 1987).

Sleep apnea exacerbates cognitive decline. There may be a direct correlation between apnea and dementia among women, beyond the increased incidence of both disorders that are present at baseline with advancing age (Bliwise 1993; Reynolds et al. 1985a).

Patients with dementia typically have fragmented nocturnal sleep. They have increased awake time at night and nap frequently during the day. This disruption of the normal circadian sleep-wake cycle, and a decrease in total delta sleep, tends to worsen with the progression of the dementia (Prinz et al. 1982).

Parkinson's disease and related conditions (Shy-Drager syndrome, striatonigral degeneration, Parkinson's–amyotrophic lateral sclerosis–dementia complex) frequently produce insomnia characterized by frequent nocturnal awakenings and excessive daytime napping (Mouret 1975). Disordered breathing secondary to interference with the operation of the muscles of respiration may add to sleep fragmentation. Sleep disruption may also occur because of the inability to move normally in bed, painful leg cramps, nightmares, and PLMS. Dementia, which occurs in approximately

one-third of patients with Parkinson's disease, may further complicate matters. One of the most common sources of sleep disturbance among patients with Parkinson's disease and related conditions is the antiparkinsonian medications themselves. L-Dopa and bromocriptine can induce parasomnias (somnambulism, pavor nocturnus), PLMS, nightmares, visual hallucinations, dystonias, and choreiform movements.

Parkinsonian-related sleep changes tend to worsen as the disease progresses and as the duration of treatment lengthens. Careful timing of L-dopa compound administrations (earlier in the day), use of multiple classes of drugs (selegiline, amantadine, anticholinergic agents) concomitantly, and careful, short-term use of benzodiazepine hypnotics with short or intermediate duration of action may be helpful (Nausieda et al. 1982).

Other neurological conditions. Sleep apnea can occur during postpolio syndrome, years after the disease itself has resolved (Cosgrove et al. 1987; Guilleminault and Motta 1978). In a similar fashion, apnea and Kleine-Levin syndrome have been reported as late complications of encephalitis (Merriam 1986). Narcoleptic sleep attacks and cataplexy have been reported in some patients with multiple sclerosis (Poirier et al. 1987). Lesions involving brain stem respiratory centers may, in rare instances, produce "sleep-related neurogenic tachypnea" (a proposed diagnosis in the ICSD), which is characterized by an increase in respiratory rate during sleep of at least 20% over the rate in the waking state. Sleep fragmentation with a complaint of EDS may appear with this condition.

Gastrointestinal Disease

Peptic ulcer disease, hiatal hernia, gastroesophageal reflux, or colitis may produce insomnia, often related to nocturnal pain (Orr 1989). Patients with hepatic failure often have insomnia; the insomnia worsens as the hepatic failure progresses. Even mild hepatic encephalopathy may produce insomnia, so supporting full compliance with protein restrictions may be clinically useful. Benzodiazepines such as lorazepam and oxazepam that do not require metabolism by the hepatic microsymal system are the preferred agents in treating insomniac patients with hepatic failure or in the elderly with hepatic compromise.

Gastroesophageal reflux is a very common problem and causes awakenings during sleep (Lavigne et al. 1991). *Peptic ulcer disease* also can produce pain-related awakenings during sleep (Orr 1989). There is a circadian rhythm to gastric acid secretion, with a maximum reached between 9:00 P.M. and midnight. Gastric acid secretion may be increased as a function of *rebound from antacid use,* and *sedatives* may inhibit esophageal acid clearance, so the alteration in the timing of administration of these agents may improve sleep in some patients.

Musculoskeletal Disease

Patients with *fibromyalgia syndrome* frequently complain of insomnia (Moldofsky 1989). Such patients may have sleep interruption from muscle and joint pain and may show the intrusion of alpha EEG activity into delta sleep (called *alpha-delta sleep*), which may interfere with the restorative quality of their sleep. Patients with arthritis of various types and with related connective tissue disease may also have pain-related insomnia complaints.

Cancer

Insomnia appears to be a common complaint of patients with a wide variety of malignancies; the mechanisms remain obscure (Derogatis et al. 1979; Silberfarb et al. 1993).

Other Diseases and Conditions

Obstructive sleep apnea from tonsillar enlargement is a potential complication of *amyloidosis* (Carbone et al. 1985). Patients with *uremic renal failure* may demonstrate decreased amounts of delta sleep and have a relatively high incidence of PLMS, producing complaints of insomnia or EDS that are generally related to the severity of the uremia (Karacan et al. 1972). The incidence of sleep apnea also appears to be significantly increased in patients with renal failure (Kimmel et al. 1989).

Summary

Psychiatric consultants should perform a formal assessment of sleep and related issues on each patient they see. A high index of suspicion for delirium as the cause of nocturnal agitation and related sleep complaints should be maintained, especially for patients in ICUs, elderly individuals, and patients on multiple medications. An attempt to discover a particular etiology for a sleep or related problem—be it medical, drug related, or psychiatric—should be made, and treatment should be focused as specifically as possible on this etiology. Sedative-hypnotics should not be prescribed until this attempt is made and factors such as sleep-related respiratory status have been considered.

References

Aldrich MS, Naylor MW: Narcolepsy associated with lesions of the diencephalon. Neurology 18:1505–1508, 1989

American Psychiatric Association: Diagnostic and Statistical Manual of Mental Disorders, 4th Edition. Washington, DC, American Psychiatric Association, 1994

American Sleep Disorders Association: International Classification of Sleep Disorders: ICSD Diagnostic and Coding Manual. Rochester, MN, American Sleep Disorders Association, 1990

Aurell J, Elmquist D: Sleep in the surgical intensive care unit: continuous polygraphic recording of sleep in nine patients receiving postoperative care. BMJ 2290:1029–1032, 1985

Baldy-Moulinier M: Temporal lobe epilepsy and sleep organization, in Sleep and Epilepsy. Edited by Sterman MB, Shouse MN, Passouant P. New York, Academic Press, 1982, pp 347–359

Berlin RM, Litovitz GL, Diaz MA, et al: Sleep disorders on a psychiatric consultation service. Am J Psychiatry 141:582–584, 1984

Bliwise DL: Sleep in normal aging and dementia. Sleep 16:40–81, 1993

Bond WC, Bohs C, Ebey J, et al: Rhythmic heart rate variability related to stages of sleep. Conditional Reflex 8:98–107, 1973

Broughton R, Baron R: Sleep patterns in the intensive care unit and on the ward after acute myocardial infarction. Electroencephalogr Clin Neurophysiol 45:348–360, 1978

Carbone JE, Barker D, Stauffer JL, et al: Sleep apnea in amyloidosis. Chest 87:401–403, 1985

Carskadon MA: Guidelines for the Multiple Sleep Latency Test (MSLT): a standard measure of sleepiness. Sleep 9:519–524, 1986

Cassano GB, Maggini C, Guazzelli M, et al: Nocturnal angina and sleep. Prog Neuropsychopharmacol Biol Psychiatry 5:99–104, 1981

Cohn MA, Morris DD, Juan D, et al: Effects of estazolam and flurazepam on cardiopulmonary function in patients with chronic obstructive pulmonary disease. Drug Saf 7:152–158, 1992

Cosgrove JL, Alexander MA, Kitts EL, et al: Late effects of poliomyelitis. Arch Phys Med Rehabil 68:4–7, 1987

Derogatis LR, Feldstein M, Morrow G, et al: A survey of psychotropic drug prescriptions in an oncology population. Cancer 44:1919–1929, 1979

Dexter J: The relationship between disorders of arousal from sleep and migraine (abstract). Headache 26:322, 1986

Dohno S, Paskewitz D, Lynch JJ, et al: Some aspects of sleep disturbance in coronary patients. Percept Mot Skills 18:199–205, 1979

Erenberg G: Sleep disorders in Gilles de la Tourette's syndrome (letter). Neurology 35:1397, 1985

Errante J: Sleep deprivation or postpartum blues? Topics in Clinical Nursing 6(4):9–18, 1985

Evans K: Sundown syndrome in institutionalized elderly. J Am Geriatr Soc 35:101–108, 1987

Fisch BJ, Pedley TA: Generalized tonic-clonic epilepsies, in Epilepsy: Electro-Clinical Syndromes. Edited by Luders H, Lesser RP. New York, Springer-Verlag, 1987, pp 151–185

Guilleminault C: Benzodiazepines, breathing, and sleep. Am J Med 88 (suppl 3A):25–28, 1990

Guilleminault C, Motta J: Sleep apnea syndrome as a long term sequela of poliomyelitis, in Sleep Apnea Syndromes. Edited by Guilleminault C. New York, Alan R Liss, 1978, pp 309–315

Guilleminault C, Briskin JG, Greenfield MS, et al: The impact of autonomic nervous system dysfunction on breathing during sleep. Sleep 4:263–278, 1981

Hansotia P, Wall R, Berendes J, et al: Sleep disturbance and severity of Huntington's disease. Neurology 35:1672–1674, 1985

He J, Kryger MH, Zorick FJ, et al: Mortality and apnea index in obstructive sleep apnea. Chest 94:9–14, 1988

Jankel WR, Allen RP, Niedermeyer E, et al: Polysomnographic findings in dystonic musculorum. Sleep 6:281–285, 1983

Jarrett DG, Greenhouse JB, Thompson SB, et al: Effect of nocturnal intravenous cannulation on sleep EEG measures. Biol Psychiatry 19:1537–1550, 1984

Johns MW, Doré C: Sleep at home and in the sleep laboratory. Ergonomics 21:325–330, 1978

Johns MW, Large AA, Masterson JP, et al: Sleep and delirium after open heart surgery. Br J Surg 61:377–381, 1974

Johnson LC: Sleep deprivation and performance, in Biological Rhythms, Sleep and Performance. Edited by Webb WB. New York, Wiley, 1982, pp 111–142

Johnson MW, Anch AM, Remmers JE, et al: Induction of the obstructive sleep apnea syndrome in a woman by exogenous androgen administration. Am Rev Respir Dis 128:1023–1025, 1984

Jones J, Hoggart B, Withey J, et al: What the patients say: a study of reactions to an intensive care unit. Intensive Care Med 5:89–92, 1979

Kapen S, Maas C, Nichols C, et al: Obstructive sleep apnea is a major risk factor for stroke. Neurology 40 (suppl 1):136, 1990

Karacan I, Williams RL: Sleep characteristics of patients with angina pectoris. Psychosomatics 10:280–284, 1969

Karacan I, Williams RL, Bose J, et al: Insomnia in hemodialytic and kidney transplant patients (abstract). Abstracts of paper presented to the 11th annual meeting of the Association for the Psychophysiological Study of Sleep. Psychophysiology 9:137, 1972

Katayama S, Yokoyana S, Hiramo Y, et al: TRH and Sleep Abnormalities in Spinocerebellar Degeneration. Amsterdam, Elsevier, 1985, pp 227–230

Kavey NB, Altshuler KZ: Sleep in herniorrhaphy patients. Am J Surg 138:682–687, 1979

Kimmel PW, Miller G, Mendelson WB, et al: Clinical studies: sleep apnea syndrome in chronic renal disease. Am J Med 86:308–314, 1989

King M, Zir L, Kaltman AJ, et al: All-night polygraphic studies of nocturnal angina pectoris. Am J Med Sci 265:419–422, 1973

Klink M, Quan SF: Prevalence of reported sleep disturbances in a general adult population and their relationship to obstructive airway diseases. Chest 91:540–546, 1987

Lavigne GJ, Velley-Miguel AM, Montplaisir J, et al: Muscle pain, dyskinesia, and sleep. Can J Physiol Pharmacol 69:678–682, 1991

Lown B, Tykoscinski M, Garfein A, et al: Sleep and ventricular premature beats. Circulation 48:691–701, 1973

Merriam AE: Kleine-Levin syndrome following acute viral encephalitis. Biol Psychiatry 21:1301–1304, 1986

Miller WP: Cardiac arrhythmias and conduction disturbances in the sleep apnea syndrome. Am J Med 73:317–321, 1982

Millman RP: Sleep apnea in hemodialysis patients: the lack of testosterone effect. Nephron 40:401–410, 1985

Mitler M, Hajdukovic R: Relative efficacy of drugs for the treatment of sleepiness in narcolepsy. Sleep 14:218–220, 1991

Mitler MM, Hajdukovic RM, Shafor R, et al: When people die: cause of death versus time of death. Am J Med 82:266–274, 1987

Moldofsky H: Nonrestorative sleep and symptoms after a febrile illness in patients with fibrositis and chronic fatigue syndromes. J Rheumatol 16 (suppl 19):150–153, 1989

Mouret J: Difference in sleep in patients with Parkinson's disease. Electroencephalogr Clin Neurophysiol 38:563–567, 1975

Nausieda P, Weiner W, Kaplan LR, et al: Sleep disruption in the course of chronic levodopa therapy: an early feature of the levodopa-induced psychosis. Clin Neuropharmacol 5:183–194, 1982

Nevins DB: First and second degree AV heart block with rapid eye movement sleep. Ann Intern Med 76:981–983, 1972

Nicholson AN, Pascoe PA, Stone BM, et al: Histaminergic systems and sleep. Neuropharmacology 24:245–250, 1985

Nierenberg A, Adler L, Peselow E, et al: Trazodone for antidepressant-associated insomnia. Am J Psychiatry 151:1069–1072, 1994

Nofzinger E, Thase M, Reynolds CF, et al: Hypersomnia in bipolar depression: a comparison with narcolepsy using the multiple sleep latency test. Am J Psychiatry 148:1177–1181, 1991

Nowlin J, Troyer W, Collins WS, et al: The association of nocturnal angina pectoris with dreaming. Ann Intern Med 631:1040–1046, 1965

Orr WC: Gastrointestinal disorders, in Principles and Practice of Sleep Medicine. Edited by Kryger MH, Roth T, Dement WC. Philadelphia, PA, WB Saunders, 1989, pp 622–629

Orr WC, Stahl ML: Sleep disturbance after open heart surgery. Am J Cardiol 39:196–201, 1977

Partinen M, Guilleminault C: Daytime sleepiness and vascular morbidity at seven-year follow up in obstructive sleep apnea patients. Chest 97:27–32, 1990

Partinen M, Palomaki H: Snoring and cerebral infarction. Lancet 2:1325–1326, 1985

Perez-Padilla R, West P, Lertzman M, et al: Breathing during sleep in patients with interstitial lung disease. Am Rev Respir Dis 132:224–229, 1985

Perry SW, Wu A: Rationale for the use of hypnotic agents in a general hospital. Ann Intern Med 100:441–446, 1984

Poirier G, Montplaisir J, Dumont M, et al: Clinical and sleep laboratory study of narcoleptic symptoms in multiple sclerosis. Neurology 37:693–695, 1987

Pradalier A, Giroud M, Dry J, et al: Somnambulism, migraine and propranolol. Headache 27:143–145, 1987

Prinz PN, Vitaliano P, Vitiello MV, et al: Sleep EEG and mental function changes in senile dementia of the Alzheimer's type. Neurobiol Aging 3:361–370, 1982

Reynolds CF, Kupfer DJ, Taska LS, et al: EEG sleep in elderly depressed, demented and healthy subjects. Biol Psychiatry 20:431–442, 1985a

Reynolds CF, Kupfer DJ, Taska LS, et al: Sleep of healthy seniors: a revisit. Sleep 8:20–29, 1985b

Richards KC, Bairnsfather L: A description of night sleep patterns in the critical care unit. Heart Lung 17:35–42, 1988

Rickels K, Morris RJ, Newman H, et al: Diphenhydramine in insomniac family practice patients: a double-blind study. J Clin Pharmacol 23:235–242, 1983

Roehrs T, Conway W, Wittig R, et al: Sleep complaints in patients with sleep-related respiratory disturbances. Am Rev Respir Dis 132:520–523, 1985

Salazar-Gruesco EF, Rosenberg RS, Roos RP, et al: Sleep apnea in olivopontocerebellar degeneration: treatment with trazodone. Ann Neurol 123:399–401, 1988

Schenck CH, Mahowald MW: Injurious sleep behavior disorders (parasomnias) affecting patients on intensive care units. Intensive Care Med 17:219–224, 1991

Silberfarb P, Hauri PJ, Oxman TE, et al: Assessment of sleep in patients with lung cancer and breast cancer. J Clin Oncol 11:997–1004, 1993

Smith R, Johnson L, Rothfeld D, et al: Sleep and cardiac arrhythmias. Arch Intern Med 130:751–753, 1972

Turner RM, Ascher M: Controlled comparison of progressive relaxation, stimulus control and paradoxical intention therapies for insomnia. J Consult Clin Psychol 47:500–508, 1979

Victor BS, Lubetsky M, Greden JF, et al: Somatic manifestations of caffeinism. J Clin Psychiatry 42:185–188, 1981

Williams R, Agnew H, Webb WB: Effects of prolonged stage four and 1-REM sleep deprivation: EEG, task performance, and psychologic responses (Report No SAM-TR-67-59). United States Air Force School of Aerospace Medicine, Brooks Air Force Base, Texas, 1967

Yinnon AM, Ilan Y, Tadmor B, et al: Quality of sleep in the medical department. Br J Clin Pract 46:88–91, 1992

Young R, Waldron J, Baer S, et al: Obstructive sleep apnea in association with retrosternal goiter and acromegaly. J Laryngol Otol 100:861–863, 1986

Chapter 16

Factitious Disorders and Malingering

Charles V. Ford, M.D.
Marc D. Feldman, M.D.

Factitious disorders are among the Axis I diagnoses in DSM-IV (American Psychiatric Association 1994), whereas malingering is assigned a V code. However, these two entities differ only in whether there are clear-cut external benefits accruing from the symptom production (malingering) or whether the symptoms are produced or feigned for the sole purpose of assuming the sick role (factitious disorders). When perceived incentives are used as a diagnostic criterion, imprecision in diagnosis is bound to arise; indeed, behavior is often motivated by a variety of conscious and unconscious objectives, and a person may feign illness in order to achieve different goals at different times (see Figure 16–1). Although the medical literature contains numerous bizarre examples of simulated illness, these cases merely represent one end on a continuum of illness portrayals. On the other end are normal illness behaviors that are somewhat common, such as the use of physical symptoms to avoid undesired social obligations (e.g., a "tummy-ache" to avoid going to school).

FACTITIOUS DISORDERS

Patients who have factitious disorders intentionally feign or self-induce diseases or symptoms. These patients are conscious of their behaviors, although their underlying motivations may be unconscious. By convention, a diagnosis of factitious disorder does not apply to individuals who readily acknowledge that they have produced their own medical signs and symptoms (e.g., patients who self-mutilate).

In chronic factitious disorder, or Munchausen syndrome, self-induction of dramatic illness allows the patient to achieve the goal of multiple hospitalizations. More recent recognition of factitious disorder by proxy (or Munchausen syndrome by proxy), in which signs and symptoms are created in another per-

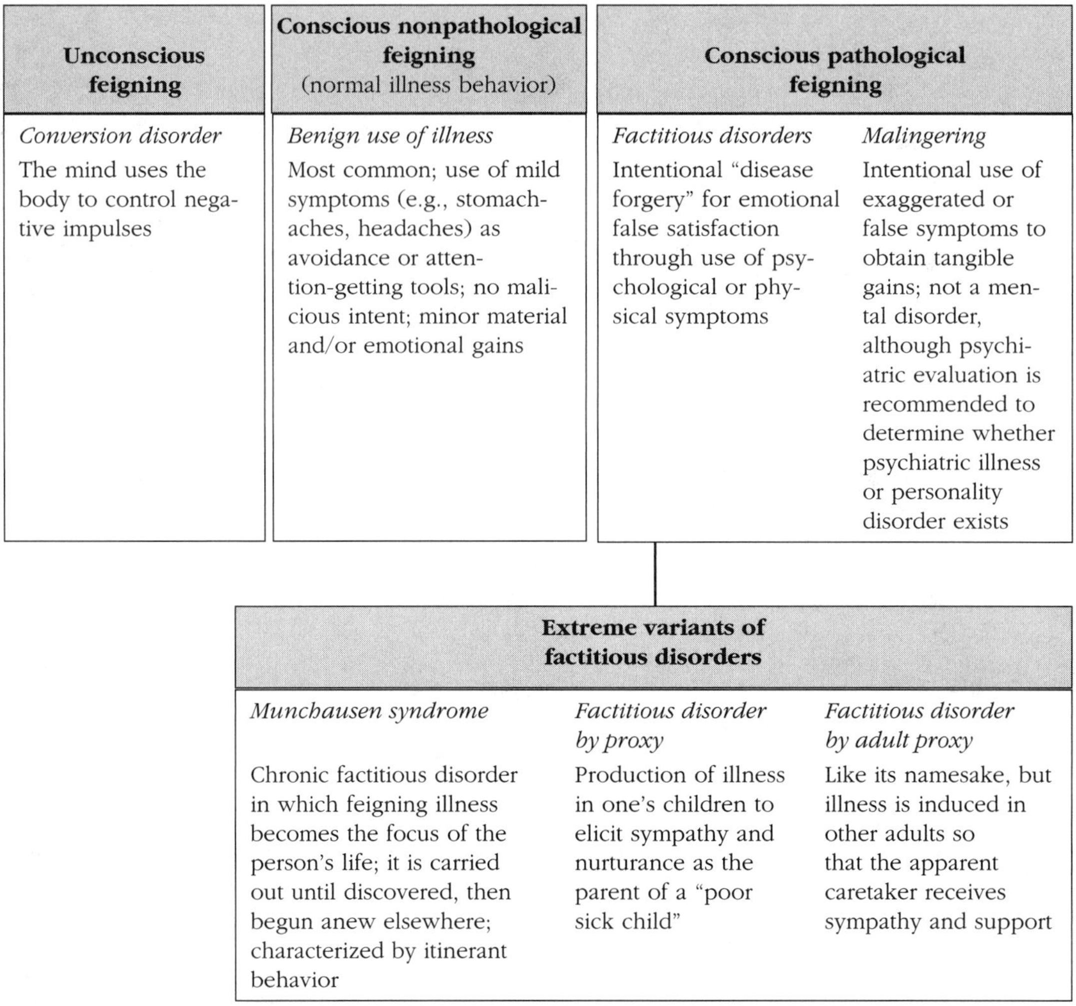

Unconscious feigning	Conscious nonpathological feigning (normal illness behavior)	Conscious pathological feigning	
Conversion disorder The mind uses the body to control negative impulses	*Benign use of illness* Most common; use of mild symptoms (e.g., stomachaches, headaches) as avoidance or attention-getting tools; no malicious intent; minor material and/or emotional gains	*Factitious disorders* Intentional "disease forgery" for emotional false satisfaction through use of psychological or physical symptoms	*Malingering* Intentional use of exaggerated or false symptoms to obtain tangible gains; not a mental disorder, although psychiatric evaluation is recommended to determine whether psychiatric illness or personality disorder exists

Extreme variants of factitious disorders		
Munchausen syndrome Chronic factitious disorder in which feigning illness becomes the focus of the person's life; it is carried out until discovered, then begun anew elsewhere; characterized by itinerant behavior	*Factitious disorder by proxy* Production of illness in one's children to elicit sympathy and nurturance as the parent of a "poor sick child"	*Factitious disorder by adult proxy* Like its namesake, but illness is induced in other adults so that the apparent caretaker receives sympathy and support

Figure 16–1. Simulation of disease.

son, has resulted in insights about children whose recurrent illnesses had previously seemed inexplicable.

Epidemiology

Information about incidence, prevalence, and demographic features must be inferred from single-case studies, a few reported series, and referral patterns. For example, Sutherland and Rodin (1990) noted that 10 of 1,288 inpatients (or 0.8%) at a large teaching hospital in Toronto who were referred consecutively for psychiatric consultation had a diagnosis of factitious disorder.

Factitious disorder by proxy currently accounts for fewer than 1,000 of the more than 2.5 million cases of child abuse reported each year in the United States, but recognition of these cases is increasing worldwide.

Demographic analyses of patients with factitious disorder suggest two general patterns. Factitious disorder patients with Munchausen syndrome tend to be middle-aged men, usually unmarried, and estranged from their families. The remaining patients with factitious disorders are usually women, ages 20–40 years, who work in medical occupations such as nursing or medical technology (Carney and Brown 1983; Ford 1983). Patients with factitious disorder by proxy are the mothers in almost all reported cases, although fathers or other caretakers are sometimes reported (Makar and Squier 1990). The victim is generally a preverbal child, but some victims are older.

Clinical Features

Factitious disorder with predominantly physical symptoms.
Essentially, every known disease has been fabricated, including esoteric maladies unfamiliar to most physicians (Feldman and Escalona 1991; Zuger and O'Dowd 1992). A partial list of diseases simulated by factitious disorder patients is provided in Table 16–1. Modern interest in factitious disorders was stimulated by Asher's (1951) whimsical article describing and naming Munchausen syndrome. Despite frequent criticism of the term, the Munchausen eponym persists when references are made to cases of chronic factitious disorder. Other features that are typically encountered in patients with Munchausen syndrome are included in Table 16–2.

Patients with Munchausen syndrome frequently present to the emergency room of large teaching hospitals during the evening hours or on the weekend, presumably because insurance offices are closed and more inexperienced members of the house staff are on duty. Dramatic signs and symptoms, such as gross bleeding, incapacitating chest pain, or apparent seizures or coma, may divert attention from other patients. Alternatively, the patient may provide a history typical of an unusual and intriguing disease, such as porphyria or Mediterranean fever. After admission to the hospital, the patient becomes widely known, sometimes offering claims such as being a former major league baseball player, an awardee of a Congressional Medal of Honor, or a foreign dignitary. Despite their reputed prominence, however, these patients infrequently receive visitors, and the physicians rarely receive telephone calls from concerned family members or friends. The patient is usually surprisingly will-

Table 16–1. Some signs, symptoms, and diseases simulated in or caused by factitious behavior

More common	Less common
Cancer	Acquired immunodeficiency syndrome (AIDS)
Chronic diarrhea	
Epilepsy	
Fever of unknown origin	Anaplastic anemia
	Cushing's disease
Hematuria	Diabetes mellitus
Hypoglycemia	Goodpasture's syndrome
Intestinal bleeding	Hemiplegia
Iron-deficiency anemia	Hypersomnia
Kidney stones	Hypertension
	Hyperthyroidism
	Hypotension
	Myocardial infarction
	Pheochromocytoma
	Pupillary dysfunction
	Reflex sympathetic dystrophy
	Septic arthritis
	Thrombocytopenia
	Torsion dystonia
	Uterine bleeding
	Ventricular tachycardia

Table 16–2. Characteristic features of Munchausen syndrome

Simulation or production of signs and symptoms that are plausible but unusual or dramatic

Pseudologia phantastica, which is engaging (but pathological) lying (e.g., the patient may falsely present himself or herself as a college president)

Peregrination, or widespread travel associated with numerous hospitalizations (more than 500 admissions have been reported for a single patient) (von Maur et al. 1973)

ing to undergo invasive tests and procedures. Ultimately, inconsistencies in the personal history or medical findings create suspicions among the staff. When caregivers become more confrontational, the patient responds with irritation, renewed physical complaints, or disruptive behavior. The patient may belligerently demand discharge against medical advice, threaten to file a lawsuit, or simply disappear.

With the more common form of factitious disorder, the features of peregrination and pseudologia phantastica are typically less pronounced or absent. Whereas referrals for consultation to major diagnostic centers are common, the individual seeks medical care within one community for symptoms that do not remit with usual treatments. Among the symptoms and signs frequently reported within this group of patients are hypoglycemic episodes (Grunberger et al. 1988), fevers of unknown etiology (Aduan et al. 1979), recurrent infections or abscesses (Reich and Gottfried 1983), and blood dyscrasias (Abram and Hollender 1974).

Factitious disorder with predominantly psychological symptoms. Factitious psychological symptoms are most often seen by clinicians in conjunction with physical complaints (authentic or fabricated). As a result, psychiatrists are more likely to encounter patients with factitious psychological symptoms on medical-surgical wards or in the emergency room than to see such patients on psychiatric units.

The symptoms most commonly reported —including depression and suicidal thinking—are frequently tied to claims of bereavement (Phillips et al. 1983; Snowden et al. 1978). The patient purports that his or her emotional distress is the result of the death of someone close to him or her, such as a parent or child. The distress appears genuine, is often accompanied by tears, and elicits sympathy from medical personnel. Later, the staff members discover that the mourned person is still very much alive, that the loss did occur but many years earlier, or that the circumstances of the

death were much less dramatic than the patient claims. Case reports also describe feigned multiple personality disorder, substance dependence, dissociative and conversion reactions, memory loss, and posttraumatic stress disorder. A variant of factitious disorder with predominantly psychological symptoms is Ganser's syndrome, which is characterized by the provision of approximate answers, or "vorbeireden," to questions (e.g., the examiner asks, "What is the color of snow?" and the patient answers "Green"). Amnesia, disorientation, and perceptual disturbances are generally present as well.

Factitious disorder with combined physical and psychological symptoms. When the patient presents with both physical and psychological factitious symptoms and neither predominate, the appropriate diagnosis is factitious disorder with combined physical and psychological symptoms.

Factitious disorder not otherwise specified. Meadow (1977) coined the term *Munchausen by proxy* (introduced as "factitious disorder by proxy" in DSM-IV) to refer to a form of child abuse in which an individual surreptitiously produces signs of disease in a child and then seeks medical care for that child. Associated with this invidious behavior are the risks associated with not only the original ailment but also the resultant procedures and medication trials.

Typically, a child is admitted to the hospital with symptoms such as seizures, bleeding, diarrhea, or respiratory/apneic difficulties. The mother accompanies the child and appears to be especially concerned, involved, and medically knowledgeable. She characteristically assists the nurses and readily consents to any invasive diagnostic procedures proposed for the child. Discovery of her role in the production of the child's symptoms may occur accidentally, such as finding her smothering the child with a pillow or introducing a toxic substance into the child's mouth or intravenous tubing. Suspicions may also arise if symptoms occur only when the mother is present in the hospital, if another child in the family has unexplained illnesses, or if the child's medical problems do not respond to appropriate treatment.

Of ominous note is the fact that 9% of these children die if they are not taken out of the home (Rosenberg 1987). In addition, severe psychological morbidity, such as hyperactivity and personal adoption of Munchausen syndrome behavior, are reported in children who are subjected to factitious disorder by proxy (McGuire and Feldman 1989).

Etiology

Most authors have emphasized psychodynamic factors as initiating and perpetuating factitious behavior. Some of the proposed psychodynamic explanations for factitious disorders are shown in Table 16–3.

Some recent explanations for Munchausen syndrome emphasize the possible role of underlying brain dysfunction. Approximately 20%–25% of patients with Munchausen syndrome have some suggestion of brain dysfunction (Ford et al. 1988; King and Ford 1988).

Differential Diagnosis and Diagnosis

The diagnosis of factitious disorders is generally established by one of four routes (Table

Table 16–3. Psychodynamic explanations for factitious disorders

Longing for nurturance and the use of illness to place demands on others to provide care

Reaction to loss; an attempt to deal with feelings of abandonment and helplessness

Use of deceit to create a feeling of power and superiority ("duping delight")

Use of deceit as a form of angry "acting out" toward physicians, who may also be serving as transference objects

Source. Babe et al. 1992; Cramer et al. 1971; Feldman and Escalona 1991; Ford 1983.

Table 16–4. Four methods to establish the diagnosis of factitious disorder

1. The patient is fortuitously discovered while engaging in factitious illness behavior (e.g., self-injecting air to create subcutaneous emphysema) (Karnik et al. 1990).

2. Incriminating paraphernalia, such as syringes and medications, are noted among the patient's belongings.

3. Laboratory findings suggest a factitious etiology (e.g., inappropriately high insulin levels and low C-peptide levels in a hypoglycemic individual surreptitiously injecting insulin) (Horwitz 1989).

4. The diagnosis is made by exclusion because there is no known disease that could explain the findings.

16–4). The consultation-liaison psychiatrist is usually asked for help either when suspicions are raised or after the diagnosis of factitious disorder is already established. When the diagnosis is not yet confirmed, the psychiatric consultant may assist the medical team by providing ethical and legal guidelines for further investigations (see subsection, "Ethical and Legal Issues," which follows). The consultant should also evaluate the patient for characteristics such as pseudologia phantastica and a concurrent personality disorder.

In order to develop a sound management plan, determination of both physical and psychiatric comorbidity in patients with factitious disorder is essential. Patients with factitious disorder may also have legitimate physical findings, the presence of which mislead their physicians. Patients with genuine diabetes may manipulate hypoglycemic agents to create symptoms (Grunberger et al. 1988).

Management

Ethical and legal issues. Patients with factitious disorders often are approached with little attention to their personal rights. This cavalier attitude developed, in part, from a belief by health care practitioners that the patients falsified their histories and physical examinations; therefore, practitioners believed there was little danger of malpractice suits. Recent changes in medical practice in the United States have emphasized patients' rights and informed consent. As a result, it is now apparent that many practices, such as clandestine searches of personal articles, are not ethically or legally acceptable (Feldman and Ford 1994). An individual suspected of factitious behavior must be accorded the same rights as other patients; among these rights are 1) personal privacy, including that of one's belongings; 2) confidentiality; and 3) informed consent, which mandates that caregivers provide information about the nature of proposed diagnostic procedures, including those aimed solely at detecting factitious behavior (Ford and Abernethy 1981; Kass 1985; Meropol et al. 1985).

Patients with factitious disorder can and do sue (*Ford v. United States of America* 1987; Lipsitt 1986). Thus, when a patient is suspected of factitious disorder, it is prudent to take the steps outlined in Table 16–5. When evaluating a patient suspected of factitious disorder, it is generally best to communicate one's concerns to the patient early in the diagnostic process. Physicians must keep in mind that they are healers and not amateur sleuths.

Factitious disorder by proxy presents a

Table 16–5. Steps to take when factitious disorders are suspected

1. Involve the hospital administration from the start.
2. Seek legal advice from the hospital's risk management department and/or the physician's own attorney.
3. Consult with the hospital ethics committee early on.
4. Maintain confidentiality to the extent specified by law. The "blacklists" of Munchausen patients advocated by some authors (Mohammed et al. 1985) are not legally acceptable in the United States (Kass 1985).

unique medicolegal challenge because it is a form of child abuse. In cases of possible factitious disorder by proxy, physicians in the United States must, by law, share their suspicions with the proper civil authorities. It must also be kept in mind that the child is at risk and helpless to protect himself or herself; therefore, more aggressive investigative approaches are justified (Samuels et al. 1992). For example, one may consider hidden video surveillance of a hospitalized child (Epstein et al. 1987).

Confrontation. Recognition is the first step in treating any disorder. The second step might be a consultation-liaison psychiatrist's discussion of factitious illness with the team. Confrontation of the patient is best accomplished by having the primary physician and consulting psychiatrist approach the patient in a noncondemning but firm manner (Hollender and Hersh 1970). The patient is told that he or she is contributing to the illness and that this behavior must reflect a high degree of emotional distress as well as difficulty in directly communicating needs. Therapeutic assistance is then offered by the psychiatrist. The patient often reacts with emphatic denial, anger, threats of lawsuit, or apparent bewilderment. A small minority of patients will accept treatment, which preferably will initially occur on an inpatient psychiatric unit. A period of inpatient treatment has the potential to facilitate a therapeutic alliance and subsequent outpatient psychotherapy. Comorbid psychiatric diagnoses, such as major depression, should be vigorously treated with the appropriate modalities (Earle and Folks 1986). A similar approach is taken with factitious disorder by proxy perpetrators, although the denial in these cases is typically tenacious and is often buttressed by spouses or other physicians. The child generally must be removed from the home regardless of whether the perpetrator acknowledges the abusive behavior.

Techniques proposed for the psychotherapy of factitious disorders have ranged from vigorous, persistent confrontation (Stone 1977) to a supportive approach incorporating face-saving measures (Eisendrath 1989). The latter approach is in wider favor among clinicians because of the emotional fragility of these patients. In view of these patients' severe underlying personality disorders, therapeutic gains are customarily very modest. Ideally, the therapist's consistency in providing support reduces the patient's need for acting-out behaviors. The primary care physician's regularly scheduled examinations of the patient serve the same purpose.

Prognosis

Factitious disorders are not benign conditions. They are associated with considerable morbidity and even mortality (Grunberger et al. 1988; Nichols et al. 1990; Sutherland and Rodin 1990). Relatively few patients accept referral for psychiatric treatment, and of these, even fewer are "cured" of their factitious behavior (Grunberger et al. 1988; Sutherland and Rodin 1990).

■ MALINGERING

By definition, individuals who exhibit malingering are motivated by specific, recognizable external incentives to produce or simulate physical or psychological illness (American Psychiatric Association 1994; Gorman 1982). Examples of these incentives are deferment from military service, avoidance of hazardous work assignments, receipt of financial rewards such as disability payments, escape from incarceration (e.g., not guilty by reason of insanity), or procurement of controlled substances. As we explore the psychological aspects of malingering, we must also keep in mind the admonition of Szasz (1956) that malingering is not a psychiatric diagnosis but an accusation.

Epidemiology

The percentage of individuals who malinger or embellish potentially compensable injuries is unknown, but it is believed to be significant. This behavior adds considerably to the cost of insurance coverage. There is no known demographic pattern for people who engage in malingering; this behavior is likely determined more by setting than by personal characteristics (Gorman 1982).

Clinical Features

Malingered symptoms fall into three major categories (Table 16–6). The deliberate embellishment of previous or concurrent illness is probably the form of malingering most frequently encountered by consultation-liaison psychiatrists. The symptoms reported are usually difficult to quantify objectively. They include pain (particularly back pain), dizziness, weakness, seizures or "spells," and features of posttraumatic stress disorder (Sparr and Pancratz 1983). Patients may intensify their complaints when they are asked directly about their symptoms or when they think that they are being observed. When distracted by television or visitors, however, they become visibly more relaxed and are able to engage in physical activities incompatible with their symptom reports.

Diagnosis

To identify malingering, the consultation-liaison psychiatrist must verify an external mo-

Table 16–6. Categories of malingered symptoms

Production or simulation of an illness (e.g., the use of thyroxine to mimic hyperthyroidism)

Exacerbation of a previous illness (e.g., deliberate infection of a surgical wound)

Exaggeration of symptoms of a previous or concurrent illness (e.g., embellished complaints of pain)

tivation and demonstrate that there is limited or no objective evidence for the patient's symptoms. One must also consider the possibility of somatoform disorders (conversion, hypochondriasis, somatization disorder, somatoform pain disorder, body dysmorphic disorder) and factitious disorders. These clinical syndromes have indistinct boundaries, so a person may meet the criteria for different disorders at different times (Ford 1992; Jonas and Pope 1985; Nadelson 1985).

Conversion disorder and malingering are on a continuum, representing opposite poles of purely unconscious and purely conscious motivation. It is difficult for the diagnostician to know the patient's location on the continuum at any moment. Patients with unconsciously determined somatoform disorders (e.g., conversion) are usually consistent in their symptom presentation, irrespective of their audience; as noted, malingerers may display markedly different behaviors when they believe that they are being observed.

Psychological testing is often helpful in identifying malingering patients. The Minnesota Multiphasic Personality Inventory—2 (MMPI-2; Hathaway and McKinley 1989) is a useful test for patients who distort their presentations (Lees-Haley and Fox 1990; McCaffrey and Bellamy-Campbell 1989; Wetzler and Marlowe 1990). Discrepancies between the validity scales, as well as between obvious and subtle clinical subscales, help to identify patients who are exaggerating their symptoms.

Management

Malingering is basically a legal rather than a medical issue. With this fact in mind, the primary physician and consultation-liaison psychiatrist must be circumspect in their approach to the patient. Every note must be written with the understanding that it will likely become a courtroom exhibit. Malingering is often listed among the diagnostic possibilities but is rarely proved conclusively in medical settings.

The patient who is suspected of malingering should not be confronted with a direct accusation. Instead, subtle communication indicates that the physician is "onto the game" (Kramer et al. 1979). One technique is to mention, almost in passing, that diagnostic tests indicate no "organic" basis for the symptoms. The malingerer may feel freer to discard the symptoms if the physician suggests that patients with similar problems usually recover after a certain procedure is performed or a particular length of time has passed. Such suggestions are often followed by perceptible improvement, if not recovery. Some patients however, in an effort to prove the existence of their disease, may vastly intensify their symptoms. In doing so, they may create such caricatures of the illness that the effort to malinger becomes obvious to all.

REFERENCES

Abram HS, Hollender MH: Factitious blood disease. South Med J 67:691–696, 1974

Aduan RP, Fauci AS, Dale DC, et al: Factitious fever and self-induced infection: a report of 32 cases and review of the literature. Ann Intern Med 90:230–242, 1979

American Psychiatric Association: Diagnostic and Statistical Manual of Mental Disorders, 4th Edition. Washington, DC, American Psychiatric Association, 1994

Asher R: Munchausen syndrome. Lancet 1:339–341, 1951

Babe KS Jr, Peterson AM, Loosen PT, et al: The pathogenesis of Munchausen syndrome: a review and case report. Gen Hosp Psychiatry 14:273–276, 1992

Carney MWP, Brown JP: Clinical features and motives among 42 artifactual illness patients. Br J Med Psychol 56:57–66, 1983

Cramer B, Gershberg MR, Stern M: Munchausen syndrome: its relationship to malingering, hysteria and the doctor-patient relationship. Arch Gen Psychiatry 24:573–578, 1971

Earle JR Jr, Folks DG: Factitious disorder and coexisting depression: a report of a successful psychiatric consultation and case management. Gen Hosp Psychiatry 8:448–450, 1986

Eisendrath SJ: Factitious physical disorders: treatment without confrontation. Psychosomatics 30:383–387, 1989

Epstein MA, Markowitz RL, Gallo DM, et al: Munchausen syndrome by proxy: considerations in diagnosis and confirmation by video surveillance. Pediatrics 80:220–224, 1987

Feldman MD, Escalona R: The longing for nurturance: a case of factitious cancer. Psychosomatics 32:226–228, 1991

Feldman MD, Ford CV: Patients or Pretenders?: The Strange World of Factitious Disorders. New York, Wiley, 1994

Ford CV: The Somatizing Disorders: Illness as a Way of Life. New York, Elsevier, 1983

Ford CV: Illness as a lifestyle: the role of somatization in medical practice. Spine 17:S338–S343, 1992

Ford CV, Abernethy V: Factitious Illness: a multidisciplinary consideration of ethical issues. Gen Hosp Psychiatry 3:329–336, 1981

Ford CV, King BH, Hollender MH: Lies and liars: psychiatric aspects of prevarication. Am J Psychiatry 145:554–562, 1988

Ford v United States of America, Civil Action No. 84–1013, U.S. Dist. (Penn.), 1987

Gorman WF: Defining malingering. J Forensic Sci 27:401–407, 1982

Grunberger G, Weiner SL, Silverman R, et al: Factitious hypoglycemia due to surreptitious administration of insulin: diagnosis, treatment and long term follow-up. Ann Intern Med 108: 252–257, 1988

Hathaway SR, McKinley JC: Minnesota Multiphasic Personality Inventory—2. Minneapolis, MN, University of Minnesota, 1989

Hollender MH, Hersh SP: Impossible consultation made possible. Arch Gen Psychiatry 23:343–345, 1970

Horwitz DL: Factitious and artifactual hypoglycemia. Endocrinol Metab Clin North Am 18:203–210, 1989

Jonas JM, Pope HG: The dissimulating disorders: a single diagnostic entity? Compr Psychiatry 26:58–62, 1985

Karnik AM, Farah S, Khadadah M, et al: A unique case of Munchausen's syndrome. Br J Clin Pract 44:699–701, 1990

Kass FC: Identification of persons with Munchausen's syndrome: ethical problems. Gen Hosp Psychiatry 7:195–200, 1985

King BH, Ford CV: Pseudologia fantastica. Acta Psychiatr Scand 77:1–6, 1988

Kramer KK, LaPiana FG, Appleton B: Ocular malingering and hysteria: diagnosis and management. Surv Ophthalmol 24:89–96, 1979

Lees-Haley PR, Fox DD: MMPI subtle-obvious scales and malingering-clinical vs simulated scores. Psychol Rep 66:907–911, 1990

Lipsitt DR: The factitious patient who sues (letter). Am J Psychiatry 143:1482, 1986

Makar AF, Squier PJ: Munchausen syndrome by proxy: father as a perpetrator. Pediatrics 85: 370–373, 1990

McCaffrey RJ, Bellamy-Campbell R: Psychometric detection of fabricated symptoms of combat-related posttraumatic stress disorder: a systematic replication. J Clin Psychol 45:76–79, 1989

McGuire TL, Feldman KW: Psychologic morbidity of children subjected to Munchausen syndrome by proxy. Pediatrics 83:289–292, 1989

Meadow R: Munchausen syndrome by proxy: the hinterland of child abuse. Lancet 2:343–345, 1977

Meropol N, Ford C, Zaner R: Factitious illness: an exploration in ethics. Perspect Biol Med 28: 269–281, 1985

Mohammed R, Goy JA, Walpole BG, et al: Munchausen's Syndrome: a study of the casualty "Black books" of Melbourne. Med J Aust 143: 561–563, 1985

Nadelson T: False patients/real patients: a spectrum of disease presentation. Psychother Psychosom 44:175–184, 1985

Nichols GR II, Davis GJ, Corey TS: In the shadow of the Baron: sudden death due to Munchausen syndrome. Am J Emerg Med 8:216–219, 1990

Phillips MR, Ward NG, Ries RK: Factitious mourning: painless patienthood. Am J Psychiatry 140:420–425, 1983

Reich P, Gottfried LA: Factitious disorders in a training hospital. Ann Intern Med 99:240–247, 1983

Rosenberg DA: Web of deceit: a literature review of Munchausen syndrome by proxy. Child Abuse Negl 11:547–563, 1987

Samuels MP, McClaughlin W, Jacobson RR, et al: Fourteen cases of imposed upper airway obstruction. Arch Dis Child 67:162–170, 1992

Snowden J, Solomons R, Druce H: Feigned bereavement: twelve cases. Br J Psychiatry 133: 15–19, 1978

Sparr L, Pancratz LD: Factitious posttraumatic stress disorder. Am J Psychiatry 140:1016–1019, 1983

Stone MH: Factitious illness: psychological findings and treatment recommendations. Bull Menninger Clin 41:239–254, 1977

Sutherland AJ, Rodin GM: Factitious disorders in a general hospital setting: clinical features and a review of the literature. Psychosomatics 31: 392–399, 1990

Szasz TS: Malingering: "diagnosis" or social condemnation? Arch Neurol Psychiatry 76:432–443, 1956

von Maur K, Wasson KR, DeFord JW, et al: Munchausen's syndrome: a thirty year history of peregrination par excellence. South Med J 66: 629–632, 1973

Wetzler S, Marlowe D: "Faking bad" on the MMPI, MMPI-2 and Millon-II. Psychol Rep 67:1117–1118, 1990

Zuger A, O'Dowd MA: The baron has AIDS: a case of factitious human immunodeficiency virus infection and review. Clin Infect Dis 14:211–216, 1992

Section III

Clinical Consultation-Liaison Settings

Chapter 17

Internal Medicine and Medical Subspecialties

Chapter Editor: Donna B. Greenberg, M.D.

In this chapter, we discuss psychiatric aspects of heart, lung, gastrointestinal (GI), and renal disease. We then review psychiatric symptoms associated with endocrine disorder, systemic lupus erythematosus, cobalamin deficiency, and the differential diagnosis of chronic fatigue.

Heart Disease

Peter Halperin, M.D.

To provide effective consultations, the consultation-liaison psychiatrist must be well-grounded in heart disease and its treatment but also must be keenly aware of the interrelation between psychosocial state and cardiac illness. Limbic-hypothalamic emotional-behavioral responses—triggered by the sympathoadrenal and other neuroendocrine systems—affect cardiac illness (Folkow 1987; Henry and Stephens 1977).

Mammals have evolved the fight-or-flight response—a powerful set of physiological reflexes that prepare the body for intense physical activity in anticipation of an event. For example, the smell or sound of a lion will instantly induce its prey to prepare for flight, a distinct evolutionary advantage. Mediated by norepinephrine and epinephrine, such signals increase heart rate, increase myocardial contractility, increase blood pressure, and regulate arterial tone so that blood goes preferentially to exercising skeletal muscle. Lipids are released from storage sites into the bloodstream to be used as a source of energy for the impending exercise. Norepinephrine also reduces the threshold for platelet aggregation, thus making clotting more likely.

These are all great advantages in the environments in which they evolved; however, the actions of norepinephrine and epinephrine have counterparts that relate to cardiovascular disease. For instance, a physiological increase in heart rate can lead to pathological arrhythmias in vulnerable individuals, normal arterial tone changes can produce coronary artery spasm, appropriate changes in blood pressure can foster sustained hypertension, increased lipid release can contribute to hyperlipidemias and other dyslipidemias (Pauletto et al. 1991), and the potentially helpful increase in clot formation can be a factor in coronary artery thrombosis and myocardial infarction (MI) (S. O. Levine et al. 1985; Markovitz and Matthews 1991).

CARDIAC PATHOLOGY AND THE NERVOUS SYSTEM

Ventricular Arrhythmias and Sudden Cardiac Death

Animal studies have demonstrated that intense emotional arousal predisposes to ventricular arrhythmias (Lown et al. 1973; Matta et al. 1976). In animal models, direct electrode stimulation of limbic structures, the hypothalamus, anterior temporal lobe, insula, and cingulate gyrus, as well as the frontal, orbital, motor, and premotor cortical areas, produces ventricular arrhythmias. Pretreatment with β-adrenergic blockers and physical ablation of peripheral sympathetic structures such as the stellate ganglion prevent the arrhythmias caused by cortical stimulation as well as arrhythmias caused by psychological stressors in animal models.

Because major depression is associated with cardiac morbidity, the interactions among the serotonin system, depression, and the heart hold great interest. In animal models (Blatt et al. 1979; Rabinowitz and Lown 1978), pharmacological maneuvers to increase central nervous system (CNS) serotonin raise the threshold for induction of ventricular arrhythmias. Increased CNS serotonin is also associated with decreased sympathetic neural activity (Antonaccio and Robson 1973). The use of newer selective serotonin reuptake inhibitors (SSRIs) may have a specific role in the care of patients with cardiac disease who have depression.

In patients with cardiac pathology, even minor psychological stress can induce arrhythmias, whereas no amount of psychological stress causes such arrhythmias in patients without myocardial impairment (Lown 1979; Reich et al. 1979). Public speaking, recall of emotionally charged events, automobile driving, and other common stressors can produce ventricular arrhythmias in susceptible patients (Lown et al. 1980; Sigler 1967; Taggart et al. 1969, 1973). In one series of such patients, stressors—from mental arithmetic to the more potent interview discussing illness and death—were much more reliable inducers of arrhythmias than physical maneuvers such as carotid sinus massage, posture changes on a tilt table, the Valsalva maneuver, hyperventilation, breath holding, and dive reflex activation (DeSilva and Lown 1978; Lown and DeSilva 1978).

Lown and Graboys (1977) suggested a role for psychiatric treatment by showing that psychological management of particular triggers can reduce the frequency of life-threatening arrhythmias. Furthermore, patients who have had a cardiac arrest are at risk for depression and posttreatment cognitive deficits (Roine et al. 1993).

Stress and Hypertension

In one well-known animal model, forced crowding, exposure to threat by cats, development in isolation, and then exposure to established mouse societies caused sustained hypertension (Henry et al. 1967). Human studies suggest that stable, safer, and rural societies have fewer hypertensive individuals than do urban societies with a higher crime rate and unstable social structures (Harburg et al. 1973; Henry and Cassel 1969; Stamler et al. 1967).

Some hypertensive patients have a more prolonged vasoconstrictive response to psychological stress than normotensive patients (Brod 1970; Brod et al. 1959). Similar responses in normotensive offspring of hypertensive parents suggest genetic transmission of a vulnerability in stress responsiveness (Ditto and Miller 1989). Behavioral studies of hypertensive patients show the most consistent correlations between hypertension and expressed or internalized hostility, especially in challenging situations that produce active, hostile coping responses (Esler et al. 1977; Light et al. 1987; Manuck et al. 1987).

Stress-Induced Ischemia

The mental stress of ordinary life is the most common precipitant of myocardial ischemia in patients with coronary artery disease (CAD) (Rozanski et al. 1988). In studies using ambulatory electrocardiograms (ECGs), investigators examined the incidence of ischemia in daily life (as defined by ST depression) in patients with angina; they found that angina is more likely to occur when patients are mentally rather than physically stressed and that most ischemic episodes are painlessly silent (Deanfield et al. 1983).

Stress and the Pathogenesis of Coronary Artery Disease

Type A behavior. Dunbar (1943) described a typical patient with heart disease compulsively working long hours without taking vacations, without delegating responsibility, without taking care of his or her health, and without acknowledging a tendency to depression. The tendency to experience internal anger while controlling its expression was another cornerstone in the psychoanalytic understanding of patients with CAD.

Sympathetic arousal and anger are evident in Friedman and Rosenman's (1974) type A behavior pattern hypothesis, which came to dominate this line of research from the 1960s to the

1980s. The type A pattern is an action-emotion complex characterized by expression of two underlying traits: hostility and "time urgency" or "hurry sickness."

Researchers in the Western Collaborative Group Study (WCGS) (Rosenman et al. 1975) found that, over an 8-year period, type A men developed CAD between 1.7 and 4.1 times more frequently than type B men when other risk factors were controlled. The data from the Framingham study supported the significance of type A behavior in men (Friedman et al. 1986). There were no comparable studies in women.

However, the Multiple Risk Factor Intervention Trial (MRFIT) study did not demonstrate a connection between type A behavior and subsequent CAD (Shekelle et al. 1983). Furthermore, a study of the WCGS cohort 20 years later did not show those who were originally designated as type A continuing to have a worsened prognosis (Miller et al. 1991; Ragland and Brand 1988). More recent prospective studies also seriously challenge the hypothesized type A link to CAD.

Compared with type B subjects, type A subjects respond with an exaggerated sympathomimetic response to laboratory challenges and stressors such as harassment during competition and work- or goal-related tasks, including exercise (DeQuattro et al. 1985; Friedman et al. 1975; Glass et al. 1980; Seraganian et al. 1985; Simpson et al. 1974; Williams et al. 1982). That β-adrenergic blockade lowers both type A behavior scores and cardiovascular responsivity also suggests the existence of a type A–sympathoadrenal connection (Krantz et al. 1982). Two studies of global type A scores did not demonstrate a correlation with severity of angiographic findings (Dimsdale et al. 1979; Sherwitz et al. 1983). However, hostility and anger measures alone have been correlated with severity of CAD on angiogram (Dembrowski et al. 1985; MacDougall et al. 1985).

The most important study to emerge from the type A literature was an extensive treatment study, the Recurrent Coronary Prevention Project (RCPP), which demonstrated that group psychotherapy that reduced type A behavior and other behavioral risks substantially lowered the incidence of recurrent MI and cardiac death in patients with a previous MI (Friedman et al. 1986).

In addition to type A behavior, other important psychosocial factors that were addressed in treatment in the RCPP may contribute information about practical behaviors that can avert an MI. First, denial of symptoms and delay in seeking medical attention were major foci of the therapy (J. J. Gill and M. Friedman, personal communication, May 1994). In the first year, patients tended to change their behavior toward increased acceptance of the meaning of symptoms, better communication with cardiologists, and less delay from pain onset before reaching the emergency room. The researchers also documented significant decreases in depression, significant increases in self-efficacy, and marginal increases in social support (Mendes de Leon et al. 1991).

For further discussion on type A behavior specifically and behavioral medicine in general, see Littman and Ketterer, Chapter 34, in this volume.

Social support. In a classic article, Ruberman and colleagues (1984) demonstrated that patients with MI who were more socially isolated and who had higher life stress and less education had more than four times the risk of death than their counterparts who had low levels of stress and isolation. More recent studies have demonstrated that social isolation (living alone) is associated with greater risk for a recurrent cardiac event (Case et al. 1992) and that patients with cardiac disease who have less social and economic resources have significantly poorer outcomes (Williams et al. 1992).

Denial. Of all the psychological and emotional conditions that affect cardiac disease, perhaps none is as clinically important as de-

nial. Patients ignore or misattribute cardiac symptoms to a more benign problem, such as heartburn, despite intellectual awareness of the symptoms of MI. Studies have disclosed a median delay time of 2.9–5.1 hours between the onset of symptoms and arrival at the emergency room (Hackett and Cassem 1969; Moss and Goldstein 1970; Simon et al. 1972). This issue is critical because 55%–80% of deaths from MI occur within 4 hours of the onset of symptoms (Wallace and Yu 1975). Techniques such as thrombolytic therapy are available in most emergency rooms and can minimize damage from an evolving infarct. The most likely explanation for patients not attributing their symptoms to their heart is fear of an MI (Hackett and Rosenbaum 1984).

However, denial may not always be detrimental to patients with cardiac disease. Hackett and co-workers (1968) demonstrated that once a patient is in the coronary care unit (CCU) in the postinfarct stage, denial of the degree of danger in his or her situation is associated with a better in-hospital clinical course. Given the greatly heightened risk of ischemia and arrhythmias in the immediate postinfarct period, the lower anxiety resulting from denial presumably decreases risk by decreasing catecholamine release.

Depression. Because depression has long been associated with increased risk of death from cardiac causes, major depression should be diagnosed and treated. Cardiac patients have a high prevalence of major depression, which modern studies using Research Diagnostic Criteria (RDC) or DSM-III (American Psychiatric Association 1980) criteria place at about 18% (Carney et al. 1988; Schleifer et al. 1989). Carney et al. (1988) determined that depression was an independent risk factor for coronary events—stronger than gender, hypertension, ventricular arrhythmias, or diabetes.

Avery and Winokur (1976) examined mortality in depressed patients who were adequately treated with medication or electroconvulsive therapy (ECT) versus inadequately treated depressed patients. They found that the rate of MI was significantly higher in the inadequately treated group over a 3-year observation period. In a more recent study of 222 hospitalized patients with MI, Lesperance and Frasure-Smith (1993) found that patients with severe depression were five times more likely to die within 6 months after discharge than were their nondepressed counterparts.

Explanations for this consistent correlation between depression and cardiovascular risk include the increased peripheral catecholamine activity found in patients with depression (Esler et al. 1982) and the correlation between lower CNS serotonin and ventricular arrhythmias. Decreased compliance with medical and lifestyle prescriptions may also contribute (Blumenthal et al. 1982).

Panic disorder.   Panic disorder, characterized by heightened sympathetic nervous system discharge and sensitivity and also perhaps by locus coeruleus dysregulation, has been associated with cardiac risk (Coryell et al. 1982) and cardiac disease (Goldberg et al. 1990). Panic disorder and myocardial ischemia can produce the same symptoms. Catecholamine-induced spasm of the coronary arterioles or microvascular angina in patients with panic disorder can be overlooked on cardiac catheterization (Cannon 1988). In one study, Chignon et al. (1993) examined the rate of panic disorder in a group of patients who were referred for ambulatory ECG testing to identify CAD. The prevalence rate of panic disorder was approximately 15% in 200 consecutively referred patients. Panic was just as prevalent among those with ECG changes. The psychiatric consultant, who may be asked whether chest pains are "real," should treat the panic disorder but should not rule out coronary disease prematurely. Coronary disease and panic disorder may occur together, and the risk of overlooking coronary disease must always be considered.

TREATMENT OF PATIENTS WITH CARDIAC DISEASE

Psychological Treatment

Three studies support the notion that psychotherapeutic and educational approaches improve the condition of hospitalized patients who have had an MI. Gruen (1975) examined the effect of individual supportive psychotherapy on such patients and found decreases in length of total hospitalization, time in intensive care, occurrence of congestive heart failure (CHF), and self-reported anxiety, as well as a faster return to normal activities 4 months after discharge. Oldenburg and co-workers (1985) compared therapy and education with routine care for hospitalized patients post-MI and found that the treated group had fewer symptoms of CAD and better psychological measures after 1 year. Frasure-Smith (1991) showed that a modest treatment protocol to evaluate and lower stress in patients after MI significantly decreased morbidity and mortality over the subsequent 5 years.

Simple meditation and muscle relaxation exercises can be quickly taught at the bedside. Patients not only reduce sympathetic discharge directly from the exercise but also secondarily gain a sense of autonomy and control in the passive environment of the hospital bed. In one study, patients who received in-hospital stress management and relaxation training after their MI improved at 6 months in both vocational and psychological status (Langosch et al. 1982). Other studies point toward an amelioration of ventricular arrhythmias among patients who practice meditation (Benson et al. 1975). The Lown group (1980) reported the case of one patient whose ventricular tachycardia terminated during meditation.

A cardiac rehabilitation team can contribute to behavioral treatment. Patients benefit from witnessing or participating in monitored exercise. Rehabilitation programs also represent a unique opportunity to bring psychosocial treatment, such as group psychotherapy, into the regimen of behavioral treatment (exercise, dietary changes, smoking cessation). (For further discussion, see Lipsitt, Chapter 33, and Chapter 34 in this volume.)

Somatic Treatment

Depression

When to begin somatic treatment of depression in patients with cardiac disease has always been a difficult judgment call. In severely depressed patients post-MI, the benefits of early somatic treatment on psychiatric and cardiological outcome may well outweigh the risks. If the depression is moderate, it may take 2–4 weeks after an MI to judge whether the mood is persistent. The precautions detailed below should be observed.

Tricyclic antidepressants. In clinical practice, tricyclic antidepressant side effects result in a high rate of discontinuation in 14%–60% of patients with cardiac disease (Roose et al. 1991b). Roose and Dalack (1992) detail the major concerns in such patients.

■ *Orthostatic hypotension:* Orthostatic blood pressure measurements should be obtained before and after treatment in any patient with cardiac disease who is given a tricyclic antidepressant. Pretreatment changes in orthostatic blood pressure predict both posttreatment hypotension and, ironically, a positive antidepressant response to tricyclic agents (Jarvik et al. 1983; Schneider et al. 1986). Not everyone with postural signs feels dizzy on rising, and the dizziness may improve even when the standing blood pressure does not. Patients with CHF are especially vulnerable to such drug-induced postural changes in blood pressure (Roose et al. 1986, 1987).

■ *Anticholinergic side effects:* Because tachycardia—typically 5 beats/minute over baseline—increases cardiac work and demand, the tricyclic antidepressants with the least anticholinergic activity (such as nortriptyline and desipramine) should be used.

■ *Conduction system effects:* At therapeutic levels, tricyclic antidepressants prolong conduction in the HV portion of the His bundle. In patients with partial bundle-branch block, tricyclic drug–induced slowing of HV time can cause complete heart block.

A Q-Tc greater than 440 msec is associated with increased risk for sudden death (Schwartz and Wolf 1978). In patients with cardiac disease, a baseline ECG should be obtained and repeated when the drug dosage has achieved therapeutic levels and at least yearly to evaluate P-R, QRS, Q-Tc duration, and the absence of bundle-branch block or complete atrioventricular (AV) block (Bigger et al. 1977, 1978; Burckhardt et al. 1987; Burrows et al. 1976, 1977; Giardina et al. 1979, 1981; Kantor et al. 1975, 1978; Luchins 1983; Raskind et al. 1982; Sigg et al. 1963; Thase and Perel 1982; Veith et al. 1982a).

■ *Myocardial contractility:* Several studies have demonstrated that tricyclic antidepressants do not adversely affect left ventricular function, even in patients with low ejection fraction (Giardina et al. 1981; Veith et al. 1982b), so this is not a concern in patients with CHF.

Bupropion. Bupropion had a low rate of orthostatic hypotension, few significant conduction disturbances, and no exacerbation of ventricular arrhythmias in 36 cardiac patients who were studied (Roose et al. 1991a); however, bupropion did cause a mild increase in supine blood pressure. Hypertension worsened in 2 of 5 patients who could not tolerate the drug.

Trazodone. The main risk of trazodone to those with cardiac disease is related to α-adrenergic blockade and postural hypotension (Himmelhoch et al. 1984). Ventricular irritability has rarely been reported (Vitullo et al. 1990).

Psychostimulants. Cardiac side effects are relatively rare from the psychostimulants methylphenidate and dextroamphetamine, and these agents are probably underutilized in patients with cardiac disease (Ballard et al. 1976; Katon and Raskind 1980; Kaufman et al. 1982; Woods et al. 1986). Reported side effects, including hypertension, tachycardia, and arrhythmias, are rare in medically ill, elderly patients. Psychostimulants have the advantages of little sedation, rapid onset (often within days), and relief of mood-related anorexia. Patients who do not tolerate tricyclic antidepressants have been shown to tolerate psychostimulants. In profoundly depressed, hospitalized patients with cardiac disease in whom depression will affect medical recovery, psychostimulants can be rapidly effective; however, blood pressure and heart rate should be monitored.

Selective serotonin reuptake inhibitors. The SSRIs, including fluoxetine, sertraline, and paroxetine, hold promise as being relatively safe for use in patients with cardiac disease. Notably, the SSRIs are devoid of anticholinergic and α-adrenergic activity. In nondepressed subjects, fluoxetine's effect on the ECG was a small decrease in resting heart rate with no change in conduction, P-R and Q-T interval, or QRS (Fisch 1985; Upward et al. 1988). Likewise, in a large sample of depressed patients, sertraline had essentially no effect on the ECG (Upward et al. 1988). However, bradycardia has been reported in two patients (Ellison et al. 1990), and atrial fibrillation was reported in one patient with heart disease who was treated with fluoxetine (Buff et al. 1991). SSRIs are much safer for the heart in overdose situations than are other classes of antidepressants. SSRIs may displace other protein-bound medications

such as digoxin and warfarin, thereby raising blood levels. Because of the narrow therapeutic window of those drugs, serum levels in patients taking digoxin and prothrombin time in patients taking warfarin should be closely monitored when SSRIs are added. Because of inhibition of liver enzymes, levels of antiarrhythmics, metoprolol, and other β-adrenergic antagonists may be higher than expected (Gram 1994).

Lithium carbonate. Lithium carbonate is generally considered safe for bipolar disorder in patients with cardiac disease, but requires careful monitoring. At therapeutic levels, conduction abnormalities have been noted even in patients without cardiac disease, especially elderly individuals (Jaffe 1977; Mitchell and MacKenzie 1982; Roose et al. 1979a, 1979b; Tangedahl and Gau 1972; Wellens et al. 1975; J. Wilson et al. 1976). The most common abnormalities are sinus node dysfunction, AV block, and (rarely at therapeutic levels) ventricular ectopy. Benign T-wave flattening or inversion is also common. Any patients taking lithium who have cardiac disease or who are older than 65 should have baseline and follow-up ECGs every 6–12 months to rule out conduction disturbances.

Electroconvulsive therapy. Zielinski and colleagues (1993) compared ECT in 40 depressed patients with and 40 patients without serious cardiac disease. Minor transitory arrhythmias or ST–T-wave changes during or immediately after treatment that resolved within minutes accounted for all complications in the subjects without heart disease and for 66% of complications in the patients with cardiac disease. One-fifth of patients with cardiac disease ($n = 8$) developed persistent ECG changes lasting hours to days, accompanied by chest pain, asystole, or arrhythmia. No deaths occurred. Preexisting ischemic heart disease predicted ischemic events as preexisting arrhythmias predicted arrhythmias. In summary, ECT with appropriate monitoring is relatively safe, even in patients with severe cardiac disease. (See Beale and Kellner, Chapter 32, in this volume for further discussion of ECT.)

Delirium

Neuroleptic medications, particularly intravenous haloperidol or droperidol, are commonly used to treat patients with agitated delirium. The risk of hypotension is related to the degree of α-adrenergic blockade of the tranquilizer. Haloperidol has less of a hypotensive effect than does droperidol. At very high doses of haloperidol given intravenously, torsades de pointes is a risk; the Q-T interval should be monitored carefully (Kriwisky et al. 1990).

Acute Anxiety

Benzodiazepines. Anxiety can have lethal complications in those with ventricular arrhythmia or in those who are awaiting electrophysiological testing, surgery, or intraabdominal defibrillator placement. Because of the risk of sympathetic arousal, benzodiazepines have become routine in CCUs and cardiac surgical units (Jefferson 1989). Benzodiazepines also reduce stress-induced catecholamine levels and platelet activation (Baer and Cagen 1987; Vogel et al. 1984). These drugs have negligible cardiovascular effects but can contribute to respiratory depression, oversedation, or delirium. Recognition of patient dependence on benzodiazepines before hospitalization is also important. Withdrawal symptoms of generalized arousal or seizures are certainly undesirable when a patient's cardiac status is compromised.

Buspirone. Buspirone lacks anticholinergic or α-adrenergic effects. It is less likely to cause respiratory depression, and, therefore, it is safer to use than diazepam in patients with respiratory illness (Rapoport et al. 1991). Buspirone may also be preferable for patients with cardiac disease who are on respirators,

but its onset of action is slow. Benzodiazepines or haloperidol may be started simultaneously with buspirone and then tapered after several weeks when buspirone begins to have an effect.

Lung Disease

Donna B. Greenberg, M.D.
Richard L. Kradin, M.D.

Chronic hypoxia compromises cognitive function and mood (Heaton et al. 1983; Prigatano et al. 1983). Changes in partial pressure of carbon dioxide (pCO_2) and acid-base balance have profound effects on cerebral blood flow and neuronal function. Acute elevations in pCO_2 compromise consciousness and mental facility. Chronic hypercapnea leads to headache and dull, unmotivated, unproductive states (Burns and Howell 1969; Neff and Petty 1972). Hypocapnea also decreases ability to rehearse or recall (Posner 1972).

The patient's assessment of the severity of dyspnea affects his or her quality of life and functional status (Moody et al. 1990). The perception of severity correlates with mood, the tendency to hyperventilate, catastrophic cognition, fear of dyspnea, and the intrapsychic meaning of the symptom (Carr et al. 1992; Demers et al. 1990; Kellner et al. 1987, 1992; D. F. Klein 1993; Morgan et al. 1983; Porzelius et al. 1992; Yellowlees et al. 1987).

■ RESPIRATION IN CLINICAL PSYCHIATRIC SYNDROMES

Respiration in Clinical Depression

Patients with clinical depression often display blunted ventilatory responses to inhaled CO_2.

Depressed and grieving patients manifest lower respiratory rates, lower resting end tidal volumes, and elevated levels of pCO_2 (Damas-Mora et al. 1976, 1982). The lung and blood levels of CO_2 are normally tightly regulated by the minute ventilation, the product of the rate and volume of air exchanged each minute. Patients who experience depression or grief do not increase the minute ventilation appropriately when they breathe a mixture of gas with high pCO_2 or low partial oxygen pressure (pO_2) (Jellinek et al. 1985; Shershow et al. 1973, 1976). Patients with depression who experience sleep disturbance are more vulnerable to CO_2 retention, so patients who have both depression and lung disease are at increased risk for complications of respiratory depression (White et al. 1983).

Respiration in Anxiety Disorders

Increased respiratory rate and changes in tidal volume are key aspects of Selye's fight-or-flight response (Selye 1956). Anxious patients have faster respiratory rates, smaller tidal volumes, and shorter breath-holding times than do control subjects (Tobin et al. 1983).

Anxious patients complain of the inability to get enough air and feelings of suffocation or oppression (Christie 1935). Anxiety-driven hyperventilation can lead to diminished cerebral blood flow, light-headedness, and feelings of depersonalization. Gasping, sighing, and air hunger are clues to the presence of panic attacks. Phobic symptoms, which are often associated with panic attacks, are another clue to the presence of anxiety disorder in patients with pulmonary disease.

D. F. Klein (1993) and co-workers recently suggested that the primary abnormality in patients with panic disorder is an enhanced central chemosensitivity to elevated levels of pCO_2. M. E. Cohen and White (1951) showed that breathing up to 4% CO_2 induced anxiety attacks in patients with anxiety neurosis.

Although most panic research has focused on the central dysregulation of breathing in response to CO_2, we have hypothesized that this dysregulation may reflect a primary or acquired instability in both central and peripheral cholinergic pathways. Indeed, preliminary results from our laboratory suggest that a subset of patients with panic disorder also show abnormally increased bronchial motor responses to the inhaled cholinergic agent methacholine (R. L. Kradin, personal communication, December 1994).

The patient with panic disorder may interpret the interoceptive sensation of dysphoria and breathlessness as catastrophic, impending suffocation; to alleviate symptoms, this cognition can be reinterpreted by behavioral and cognitive interventions (D. F. Klein 1993).

PSYCHIATRIC ASPECTS OF RESPIRATORY SYNDROMES

Chronic Obstructive Pulmonary Disease

In patients with chronic obstructive pulmonary disease (COPD), chronic hypoxia can compromise thinking and mood, which produces delirium, mood lability, and restrictions in daily activities. Patients with COPD have impaired abstracting ability and complex perceptual motor integration. These are impaired more than motor speed, strength, or gross coordination. Continuous oxygen treatment improves quality of life, neuropsychiatric function, and longevity better than nocturnal-only treatment. No change in mood has been documented (Grant et al. 1982, 1987; Heaton et al. 1983; Nocturnal Oxygen Therapy Trial Group 1980; Prigatano et al. 1983; Series and Cormier 1990).

However, the benefits of supplemental oxygen have a psychological cost. Supplemental oxygen use is a social embarrassment. Some patients feel that home oxygen marks the beginning of terminal illness, and they may withdraw socially. Others become psychologically dependent on the oxygen supply (Marchionno et al.

1985). Patients may limit their emotional expressiveness in order not to exceed lung capacity.

Borson and McDonald (1989) suggested that clues to the diagnosis of major depressive disorder in patients with COPD include the perception of activity as effortful, pervasive pessimism, diurnal mood variation with morning worsening, and early morning awakening. The prevalence of depression in individuals with COPD is 12%–15%, and panic symptoms are often linked to depression (Light et al. 1987).

The prevalence of panic symptoms may be high. A history of panic attacks has been reported in 38% of patients with COPD (Porzelius et al. 1992; Yellowlees et al. 1987). Because a significant subset of patients with COPD are predisposed to CO_2 retention, the possibility that CO_2 sensitivity generates panic cannot be excluded. Furthermore, common and possibly genetically determined elements may link the tendency to smoke and the predisposition to panic disorder (Pohl et al. 1992).

We have noted that γ-aminobutyric acid (GABA)–ergic agents suppress the respiratory pacemaker. To treat panic, benzodiazepines are used conservatively for fear of respiratory depression, but the benefits for relief of panic, anticipatory anxiety, and phobia must be weighed against the risk of CO_2 retention in any individual patient. Newer SSRIs may be useful therapeutically in this setting. To diminish fear and agitation without risking respiratory suppression, neuroleptic medications can also be beneficial in low doses. When respiratory drive is marginal, any sedative must be used cautiously.

Because of recent emphasis on treatment of inflammation in both chronic lung disease and asthma, patients with respiratory compromise commonly receive high-dose steroids. Because the psychiatric side effects of steroids are dose related, agitation and mania may be underestimated in the acute setting, and the subsequent labile or depressed states may contribute to morbidity. Steroid side effects may respond acutely to low-dose neuroleptics.

Smoking and Smoking Cessation

Nicotine, which increases heart rate and blood pressure, acts as an acute stimulus for breathing (Stolerman and Shoaib 1991). Nicotine increases dopamine release in the prefrontal cortex and nucleus accumbens (Mifsud et al. 1989). Other addictive agents such as opiates, amphetamines, and cocaine also release dopamine (DiChiara and Imperato 1988).

Alcoholism (Covey et al. 1993), generalized anxiety disorder, and panic disorder all show an increased association with cigarette smoking (Carvajal et al. 1989; Glassman 1993). Most anxious smokers report that cigarette smoking allays anxiety, despite experimental models that do not support this observation (Frederick et al. 1988).

The association between smoking and depression remains even when the variables of anxiety and alcoholism are controlled. Glassman (1993) pointed out that, even though depression was not listed as a criterion for nicotine withdrawal in DSM-III-R (American Psychiatric Association 1987), 75% of heavy cigarette smokers who attempt to quit will experience depressive symptoms. In some patients with severe psychiatric disease in remission, attempts at smoking cessation have led to severe exacerbations of symptoms that remitted with a return to smoking (Glassman 1993).

The effects of nicotine on adrenergic, serotonergic, and dopaminergic pathways modulate dysphoric symptoms. Nicotine-induced firing of dopaminergic neurons that project to prefrontal areas may also antagonize the negative symptoms in patients with schizophrenia and could help to explain the inordinately high prevalence of cigarette smoking in this population (Tung et al. 1990).

Asthma

Asthma is one of the classic psychosomatic diseases. Emotional arousal (anxiety, fear, and anger) and suggestion can cause changes in airway tone. Airway reactivity to emotion may be mediated by the vagus nerve (methacholine-induced bronchoconstriction may be blocked by methacholine) (Isenberg et al. 1992). Suggestion and emotion may preferentially affect the larger, upper airways (Lehrer et al. 1986), which are innervated by cholinergic neurons.

The challenge for patients with asthma is to lead a full life despite the tendency to wheeze. Psychoeducation, relaxation, biofeedback, and family therapy have each had a role in the care of asthma patients (Ewer and Stewart 1986; Lehrer et al. 1992). Appropriate management of prophylactic and as-needed medications is a critical aspect of education. The side effects of antiasthmatic drugs are jitteriness, palpitations, and insomnia. Those who become phobic about dyspnea may overuse bronchodilator inhalers.

Weiss (1994) described a sensible behavioral management program. He used a problem checklist to assess asthma medications, early signs of wheezing, triggers of an attack, individual behavior and behavior of other people during an attack, and the effects of asthma on social development, school, and the family (Creer 1979). A patient diary of attacks is an added resource. Weiss looks for core psychological issues that may prevent the patient from attending to early warning signals or from taking medication appropriately (e.g., fear of appearing inadequate, fear of rejection, and drive to excel athletically, such that there is a premium on keeping vulnerability secret). Weiss's advice to his patients is to know the facts and fallacies about asthma, the emotional and physical factors that precipitate and aggravate an attack, the early warning signs and what to do about them, and how to relax and breathe abdominally.

Sleep Apnea

During normal sleep, oxygenation falls and pCO_2 rises. In stage 4 sleep, breathing is regu-

lar (Fishman 1972; Hedgel and Cherniack 1988). During rapid eye movement (REM) and stages 1 and 2 non-REM sleep, irregular breathing and apnea—either obstructive, central, or both—occur. Daytime sleepiness, morning headache, restless sleep, snoring, and thrashing in bed should raise the suspicion of sleep apnea in those who complain of depression or memory loss, especially obese men. (For further information on the management of sleep apnea, see Weilburg and Winkelman, Chapter 15, in this volume.)

Gastrointestinal Disorders

Kevin W. Olden, M.D., F.A.C.P.
R. Bruce Lydiard, M.D., Ph.D.

EPIDEMIOLOGY

Functional GI disorders are extremely common. Among individuals living in households in the United States, 69% reported that in the 3 months before participation in the survey, they experienced symptoms that met the criteria for at least 1 of 25 distinct GI disorders. Symptoms consistent with functional disorders of the large bowel were reported by 44% of the sample, of the esophagus by 42%, of the gastroduodenal region by 26%, and of the anorectal area by 26% (Drossman et al. 1993).

In North America, the GI disorders that are more common in women than in men are globus, functional dysphagia, irritable bowel syndrome (IBS), constipation, abdominal pain, and functional biliary pain. Men, however, more commonly experience aerophagia and postprandial bloating (Drossman et al. 1993).

Patients with abdominal pain without diagnosis tend to have a higher number of stressful life changes, particularly the breakup of close relationships, than patients whose pain leads to appendectomy (Creed et al. 1988). A significantly higher rate of physical or sexual abuse in childhood or adulthood has been found in patients with functional GI disorders. These patients have also had more lifetime surgeries and were more likely to develop chronic or recurrent abdominal pain with multiple somatic complaints (Drossman et al. 1990b). A substantial body of literature documents a high prevalence of psychiatric disorders compared with the general population in patients with functional bowel disorders (Blanchard et al. 1990; Clouse and Alpers 1986; Esler and Goulston 1973; G. Fava and Pavan 1976; Fielding 1977; Ford et al. 1987; Hislop 1971; Langeluddecke 1985; Latimer 1983; Latimer et al. 1981; Lydiard et al. 1993; Richter et al. 1986; Talley 1993; Walker et al. 1990a, 1990b; Wender and Kalm 1983; Young et al. 1976).

The psychological and psychosocial factors that lead patients to seek health care are critical to the understanding of these patients (Drossman et al. 1988; Sandler et al. 1984; Whitehead and Schuster 1985). Consultation for bowel symptoms is often sought when symptoms are amplified by depression, anxiety, pain, and recent negative life events.

GLOBUS SENSATION

Globus is defined as a fullness, lump, or tickle in the throat at the level of the cricopharyngeal cartilage that is present for at least 3 months. It is not related to swallowing. There is no true dysphagia—that is, the patient has no difficulty swallowing solids or liquids. Any lifetime history of globus is common in healthy control subjects (46% in one study), and it occurs more commonly in women than in men (Thompson 1982). Although globus has been classically associated with emotional distress, many patients with globus demonstrate anatomical pathology (Moser et al. 1991). The differential diagnosis

includes achalasia; diffuse esophageal spasm; anatomical lesions of the tonsils, pharynx, or esophagus; cervical spondylolisthesis; gastroesophageal reflux disease; hypothyroidism; and neuromuscular dysfunction of cranial nerve IX, X, or XII (Freeland et al. 1974; Greenberg et al. 1988). Although globus has classically been called hystericus, it occurs with anatomical findings, grief, conversion disorder, panic attacks, and depression (Greenberg et al. 1988; Lehtinen and Puhakka 1976).

Globus has a strong tendency to abate on its own. Biofeedback and behavior therapy have been used with reasonable success (Hayes 1976), but no large-scale controlled trials have demonstrated the effectiveness of these interventions.

The responsible consultation psychiatrist should first consider the possibility of an organic diagnosis. Then a focused psychosocial history to identify any acute life stressors and a mental status examination should follow. Particular attention should be paid to the diagnosis of anxiety and mood disorders. Most patients respond to a brief course of supportive psychotherapy. Anxiolytics and/or antidepressants should be considered for patients with diagnosed anxiety or mood disorder.

ESOPHAGEAL DYSFUNCTION

Five patterns of esophageal dysmotility have been described: achalasia, hypertensive lower esophageal sphincter, diffuse esophageal spasm, nutcracker esophagus, and nonspecific esophageal motility disorders (NSEMD). Of these, the last three are most often associated with psychiatric comorbidity. The diagnosis of esophageal dysmotility can only be made by esophageal motility testing—that is, by passing a pressure-sensitive motility catheter through the nose into the esophagus. The use of tiny profusion catheters in combination with computer recorders has eliminated much of the technical difficulty of previous methods of motility testing, making the procedure much more comfortable for patients (Castell and Richter 1987).

The majority of patients with documented esophageal motility disorders have an Axis I psychiatric diagnosis. Clouse and Lustman (1983) found a prevalence of 84%, compared with 31% of a group of control subjects. Patients with esophageal motility disorders were likely to have major depression (52%), generalized anxiety disorder (36%), somatization disorder (20%), substance abuse disorders (20%), panic disorder (4%), and social phobia (4%).

Esophageal dysmotility is a common cause of noncardiac chest pain (Castell and Richter 1987). Panic disorder is also frequently seen in patients with chest pain and angiographically normal coronary arteries. It is likely that both esophageal dysmotility and panic attacks contribute to the complaints of chest pain in many of these patients. Beitman et al. (1987a, 1987b) showed that psychiatric treatment could reduce chest pain complaints in these patients.

Because calcium channel blockers are potent smooth muscle relaxants, it was expected that use of these drugs would result in a decrease in abnormal esophageal motility patterns and, in turn, a decrease in GI complaints. In a study of nifedipine (10–30 mg tid) compared with placebo, the esophageal motility tracings improved in the treated group, but the patients' level of psychological distress and esophageal complaints did not (Richter et al. 1987). This study would suggest that therapy targeted at the patient's emotional distress is much more efficacious in resolving symptoms than therapy targeted at the specific motility disorder.

IRRITABLE BOWEL SYNDROME

IBS is a common and sometimes debilitating disorder that affects 8%–17% of the general population (Connell et al. 1965; Drossman et al. 1982; Thompson and Heaton 1980). It ranks

second only to the common cold as a cause for absenteeism from work. IBS commonly occurs in early adulthood and affects women approximately twice as often as men (Fielding 1977; Hislop 1971). The diagnostic criteria for IBS (Connell et al. 1965; Drossman et al. 1982, 1990a; Manning et al. 1978; Thompson and Heaton 1980) are shown in Table 17–1.

Most clinicians prefer nonpharmacological modalities to treat patients with mild forms of IBS. These include education, dietary discretion, stress management techniques, and use of bulk-fiber products. In general, physicians request psychiatric consultation for patients whose conditions are refractory to such modalities.

Drossman and Thompson (1992) have suggested that for patients with IBS, clinicians should 1) schedule regular appointments with the patient to indicate that the treating clinician is committed to the patient for the long term; 2) let the patient know that IBS is often a

Table 17–1. Symptom criteria for irritable bowel syndrome

Continuous or recurrent symptoms over at least 3 months of

1. Abdominal pain, relieved with defecation or associated with a change in frequency or consistency of stool; *and/or*
2. Disturbed defecation (three or more of the following at least 25% of the time)

- Altered stool frequency
- Altered stool form (hard or loose/watery)
- Altered stool passage (straining or urgency, feeling of incomplete evacuation)
- Passage of mucus
- Bloating or feeling of abdominal distension

If above symptom criteria are met, appropriate laboratory investigations, including complete blood count and erythrocyte sedimentation rate, and sigmoidoscopy or fiberoptic examination should be conducted. Additional investigations are determined clinically (Drossman et al. 1990a).

Source. Drossman et al. 1990a.

chronic condition that requires long-term management; 3) make a positive diagnosis of IBS to reassure patients that they do not have a more serious illness such as cancer; and 4) identify reasonable treatment goals, such as better functioning, rather than complete relief from all symptoms. Psychotherapy may be indicated for some patients who have severe psychosocial stressors.

Psychiatric Morbidity in Patients With Irritable Bowel Syndrome

Treatment-seeking patients with IBS exhibit high rates of psychiatric disorders. Lydiard et al. (1993) evaluated psychiatric disorders in treatment-resistant patients with IBS who were referred to a university-based gastroenterology practice and found that 94% of the patients had a lifetime history of a major psychiatric illness. More than 80% were currently psychiatrically ill, primarily with anxiety and mood disorders. Many patients were unaware of their psychiatric diagnosis. Of the 27% of the IBS patients in the study who had panic disorder, nearly all had agoraphobia based on fear of loss of bowel control. Obsessive-compulsive disorder (OCD) has also been associated with IBS (Olden 1994); in that study, 42% of patients with OCD met diagnostic criteria for IBS, compared with 29% of control subjects who did not have OCD.

Those with significant anxiety or mood symptoms achieve only partial relief from first-line treatment modalities. Several studies have shown the benefit of psychopharmacological medications, including tricyclic antidepressants and benzodiazepines, for patients with IBS, but these studies are seriously flawed (K. B. Klein 1988). Little attention was paid to psychiatric diagnoses. Even so, the limited data available suggest that pharmacological treatment of the psychiatric disorder in patients with IBS leads to reduction in both GI and psychiatric symptoms (Lydiard et al. 1991; Noyes et al. 1990; Tollefson et al. 1991).

◼ INFLAMMATORY BOWEL DISEASE

Patients with inflammatory bowel disease (IBD), Crohn's disease, or ulcerative colitis can develop marked abnormalities of fluid and electrolyte balance as a result of their diarrhea. Chronic hematochezia and malabsorption of nutrients can lead to significant anemia (Ginsberg and Albert 1989; Gitnick 1990). Patients with IBD, independent of metabolic abnormalities, tend to have significant psychological impairment and disturbed social functioning (Drossman 1989).

When compared with patients who have other chronic medical illnesses, patients with IBD do not have any significant increase in diagnosable psychiatric disorders. Also, no relation has been found between severity of IBD and presence or absence of a psychiatric diagnosis (Helzer et al. 1984). Investigators did find a suggestion of elevated "obsessional thinking" in patients with ulcerative colitis. In addition, patients with ulcerative colitis who had undergone colectomy were more likely to have a diagnosable psychiatric disorder.

Psychiatric consultation for patients with IBD involves more than establishing the presence or absence of a diagnosable psychiatric disorder. It includes assessing the patient's quality of life: his or her ability to perform activities of daily living, to achieve sexual satisfaction, and to ambulate freely (Bergner et al. 1981; Drossman 1989; Meyers et al. 1980). A psychiatric consultant must work with all the members of the multidisciplinary team, including ostomy nurses, surgeons, and gastroenterologists, to formulate treatment strategies. In addition to psychotherapy and psychopharmacological intervention, patients can seek help from patient advocacy groups such as the Crohn's and Colitis Foundation. The support that patients receive can greatly enhance their ability to cope. The goal is to maximize the patient's total quality of life rather than merely to reduce physical symptoms.

Renal Disease

Lewis M. Cohen, M.D.

RENAL TRANSPLANTATION

Renal transplantation and the various types of dialysis have transformed the fate of people with end-stage renal disease (ESRD) and have made it possible for consultation-liaison psychiatrists to attend to the psychiatric aspects of their new lives.

Many individuals have survived more than 20 years with a kidney transplant, and we are beginning to see long-term reports in the literature—for example, from Gorlen et al. (1993) in Norway, who examined the quality of life of 33 patients who had received kidney transplantation an average of 15.6 years previously. Almost the entire sample reported a good quality of life, and three-quarters (76%) were fully rehabilitated and engaged in full-time work. Renal transplants are now the standard of comparison for research involving other organs, such as allogeneic bone marrow transplantation (Andrykowski et al. 1990).

Psychiatrists and social workers are members of most transplant teams and provide screening and support of potential kidney transplant recipients and donors (Fricchione 1989). (For further discussion regarding the issues involved in organ transplantation, see Strouse et al., Chapter 19, in this volume.)

DIALYSIS

Sexual Function

Harry Abrams (Abrams et al. 1975) found that 75% of his sample of men with ESRD reported reduced potency. Reduced potency was operationally defined as a decrease in the frequency of sexual intercourse by at least 50%. A more recent questionnaire study has again underscored the problems with sexual dysfunction and infertility and demonstrated partial improvement following transplantation (Schover et al. 1990). Further amelioration of problems with potency may follow administration of testosterone or reduction of the corticosteroid or antihypertensive dosage (Dubovsky and Penn 1980). Insertion of a penile prosthesis has also become an option (Gulledge et al. 1983). However, sexual problems continue to be largely ignored in most dialysis programs.

Quality of Life

The majority of psychosocial studies of ESRD have led investigators to conclude that the quality of life is best for successful transplant patients (Bentdal et al. 1991; Piehlmeier et al. 1991; Simmons et al. 1984), similarly good for home peritoneal dialysis patients (Bremer et al. 1989), and considerably worse for patients who receive hemodialysis (Barrett et al. 1990; Evans et al. 1985). Researchers involved in three prospective studies have concluded that, in comparison with a dialysis-treated population, people who receive kidney transplants experience improved physical and emotional outcomes (Parfrey et al. 1989; Russell et al. 1992; Simmons et al. 1981). A psychiatric history is a useful predictor of psychiatric symptomatology following transplantation (Sensky 1989).

Clinicians should not believe that transplantation is a panacea. Individuals who stay with hemodialysis may be more isolated and more receptive to the psychological and social benefits that come from structured dialysis programs.

Diminished quality of life and depression are particularly pronounced in people who have had failed transplants and are now receiving dialysis (Bremer et al. 1989). This subgroup of dialysis patients must cope with the added disappointment of staff and family. Often, they poignantly struggle with guilt over the "sacrificed" or "wasted" kidney.

Ethical Issues and Discontinuation of Dialysis

Currently, 50% of patients who begin dialysis therapy in the United States are age 60 years or older (Kutner and Brogan 1990). As the population increasingly includes patients with diabetes and dementia, as well as geriatric patients, nephrologists have begun to accept that dialysis is a type of life-support treatment that may be electively discontinued (Chazan 1990; Epstein 1979; Neumann 1992).

Although in some dialysis programs discontinuing treatment is opposed (Fisher et al. 1986), 90% of surveyed nephrologists consider treatment cessation to be an option (P. A. Singer 1992). Kjellstrand and associates (Kjellstrand and Dossetor 1992; Neu and Kjellstrand 1986) reported that dialysis termination was the second leading cause of mortality in their sample, occurring in 23% of patient deaths. Data from the ESRD Network of New England indicate that approximately 20% of the patient population die each year, and about 10% of deaths are preceded by a decision to discontinue dialysis (ESRD Network of New England 1990).

The large majority of people with ESRD do not articulate terminal care wishes, do not speak directly to their families about death, do not discuss this subject with medical staff, and do not complete the legal options available to them (L. M. Cohen et al. 1991; Holley et al. 1993; Husebye et al. 1987; Reilly 1990). People who receive dialysis are preoccupied not with death but instead with the ordinary activities of life (Norton 1969).

In our prospective study of 19 patients and families who decided to terminate dialysis, none of the patients who were able to participate in making the decision were suicidal, irrational, or had major psychiatric disorders. These patients had decided that progressive physical deterioration left them unable to enjoy life further and that dialysis was prolonging suffering rather than prolonging life (L. M. Cohen et al. 1993; McKegney and Lange 1971).

Neuropsychiatric Syndromes

Chronic renal failure causes subtle and subclinical abnormalities in concentration, problem solving, and calculation ability. Advanced uremia causes impaired mentation, lethargy, asterixis, multifocal myoclonus, and other neurobehavioral disturbances. Although these abnormalities may be reversible with dialysis, subtle deficits remain in even well-dialyzed patients (Osberg et al. 1982). Adequacy of dialysis has an effect on these subtle abnormalities in the individual patient. As a whole, better dialyzed patients have fewer electroencephalogram (EEG) abnormalities and improved concentration and sleep function (Teschan et al. 1983).

A deterioration in total intelligence as measured by the Wechsler Adult Intelligence Scale —Revised (Wechsler 1981) has also been found in chronic renal failure patients on dialysis. This decline is partly due to slowness in performing tests. Verbal skills are maintained to the original levels, but performance IQ deteriorates. Memory function, particularly working memory, is more severely affected. Many patients complain of problems in concentration, which increase demonstrably during the intervals between dialysis treatments (West 1978).

The differential diagnosis of neuropsychiatric syndromes in the patient with chronic renal failure includes hypercalcemia, hypophosphatemia, hypoglycemia, hyperglycemia, hyponatremia, hypernatremia, drug intoxication, hypertensive encephalopathy, cerebrovascular disease, subdural hematomas, meningitis, encephalitis, and normal pressure hydrocephalus. In a susceptible person, HIV encephalopathy should also be considered.

Dialysis dementia is a specific syndrome that was first reported in the early 1970s and is characterized by progressive encephalopathy, stuttering, dysarthria, dysphasia, impaired memory, depression, paranoia, myoclonic jerking, and seizures. In the course of approximately a year, the syndrome may progress to global dementia and death. This syndrome was found to correlate with high concentrations of aluminum in the brain tissue of patients and was clearly associated with outbreaks in dialysis units in which the water supply was contaminated with excess aluminum concentrations. Because water treatment in the United States now removes aluminum from dialysate water, the incidence of dialysis dementia has markedly diminished.

Psychotropic Medications

Antidepressants. Clinicians have always been alert to the possible occurrence of depression in this patient population, and the tricyclic antidepressants have been used extensively. Unfortunately, patients maintained with dialysis seemed by anecdote to be more sensitive to the side effects associated with these medications (Stoudemire et al. 1990). The explanation is unclear but may be related to an elevation of the hydroxylated tricyclic metabolites (Dawling et al. 1982). Anecdotal evidence also suggests that patients are better able to tolerate the new serotonin reuptake inhibitors as well as medications such as bupropion. A pharmacokinetic study of depressed patients with severe renal dysfunction maintained with hemodialysis showed that fluoxetine plasma concentrations were unaffected at the normal adult dosage (Bergstrom et al. 1993).

Antianxiety agents. It is probably best to avoid benzodiazepines that have pharmacologically active metabolites, such as diazepam (Levy 1985). Most clinicians rely on lorazepam, clonazepam, oxazepam, and temazepam. Dosages are usually in a range of one-half to two-thirds of that used in patients with normal renal function (Levy 1985).

Antipsychotics. Theoretically, one would imagine that patients are at greater risk for neuroleptic malignant syndrome because of the marked fluid shifts and dehydration associated with treatment (Stoudemire et al. 1991).

Likewise, neuroleptic medications may lower the seizure threshold. Nevertheless, these medications are commonly employed, often at somewhat lower starting dosages than usual. The high-potency agents, in particular, appear to be well tolerated (Levy 1985).

Mood stabilizers. Patients maintained on dialysis do not eliminate lithium and, therefore, do not require daily lithium supplementation between treatments Stoudemire et al. (1991). The protocol requires determining an appropriate dose (usually 300–600 mg), which is administered after the dialysis. Serum lithium levels are checked 2–3 hours later. Some of the alternatives to lithium, such as valproate or verapamil, may also prove to be of value for these patients.

CONCLUSION

Most patients in dialysis programs are psychologically healthy people who are suddenly faced with incredible new stresses and demands. Life on hemodialysis includes perhaps 17 different daily medications, enormous pharmaceutical and medical bills, intermittent pain and fatigue, uncertainty as to the future, long waits on a transplant list, a rigid diet, dependency on others for basic care, and exposure to peers whose conditions deteriorate or who die.

It is a pleasure and a challenge for psychiatrists to work with patients who have ESRD and with the staff that care for them.

Endocrine Disorders

Roger Kathol, M.D.

It is important to recognize which endocrine disorders are associated with high frequencies of specific psychiatric syndromes (see Table 17–2) because these might contribute to the symptoms of a patient first seen in psychiatric consultation. When the symptoms and/or signs suggest that an endocrine abnormality might be present, or when the patient presents with a psychiatric syndrome in an atypical fashion for the primary psychiatric disorder (outside the age at risk, unusual symptoms, limited family history, nonresponse to usual treatment, etc.), further investigation with laboratory tests is warranted. Endocrine tests in the absence of signs or symptoms of a specific endocrine disease, including thyroid disease (Bauer et al. 1991), are generally not indicated. This, of course, necessitates that the psychiatrist perform at least focal physical examinations for endocrine signs when endocrine disorders are seriously considered in the differential diagnosis.

DIABETES MELLITUS

The most frequent psychiatric conditions associated with diabetes mellitus include anxiety and depression (Table 17–2). Because diabetes is controlled with treatment but not cured, those patients experiencing persistent psychiatric symptoms who receive psychiatric intervention may have less disease morbidity (Table 17–3). At present, the most appropriate forms of intervention include syndrome-specific medication or cognitive-behavior psychotherapy.

HYPOTHYROIDISM

Although depression and anxiety are seen with great frequency in patients with hypothyroidism, the greatest concern is the cognitive deficits that can occur as a result of the changes in metabolic activity in the CNS. For this reason, cognition should be assessed and lifestyle adjustments made until adequate treatment has been achieved. Later assessment is important because follow-up studies of dementia

(Clarfield 1988) suggest that treatment of hypothyroidism does not necessarily reverse memory deficits.

In most patients who have either depression or anxiety with hypothyroid state, replacement of the thyroid deficiency with thyroxine will reverse psychiatric symptoms. If, however, these symptoms do not improve after adequate replacement for 1 month to 6 weeks, the clinician should consider alternative forms of direct psychiatric intervention (Table 17–3). Certainly, if a patient has life-threatening or highly debilitating symptoms of depression or anxiety, a short course of psychotropic medications could be tried while waiting for the effects of hormone replacement to occur.

HYPERTHYROIDISM

As in patients with hypothyroidism, depression and anxiety are common in patients with hyperthyroidism. In most situations, it is not difficult to identify hyperthyroid patients because of the signs and symptoms of that disease. In more than 90% of people demonstrating symptoms of depression and anxiety associated with hyperthyroidism who do not have a preexisting psychiatric condition, their symptoms will resolve during the course of treatment for the hyperthyroidism alone (Kathol and Delahunt 1986). For this reason, no other psychiatric intervention is required until an adequate trial of antithyroid medication, radioactive iodine, or thyroid surgery has been completed. As might be expected, symptoms of anxiety will disappear in direct relation with the reduction in thyroid hormone levels. Depressive symptoms are not as linearly related to thyroxine levels.

HYPERPARATHYROIDISM

Mood symptoms are commonly seen in patients with this disorder. Several case series suggest that the severity of symptoms intensi-

Table 17–2. Prevalence of psychiatric disorders among patients with endocrine disease from studies with prospective systematic evaluations

Endocrine disorder	Anxiety disorder	Major depression	Cognitive impairment	Substance abuse	Psychosis/ delirium	Any disorder
Diabetes mellitus	0%–45%[a,b,c]	7%–33%[a,b,c]	0%[c]	1%–14%[a,b,c]	0%–1%[a,b,c]	33%–71%[a,b,c]
Hypothyroidism	20%–33%[d]	33%–43%[d]	29%[e]	—	5%[e]	—
Hyperthyroidism	53%–69%[f,g]	30%–70%[f,g]	0%[f]	0%–8%[f]	0%[f,g]	53%–100%[f,g]
Hyperparathyroidism	12%[h]	11%–43%[h,i,j]	3%–39%[h,i,j]	—	3%–9%[h,j]	23%–67%[h,j]
Cushing's syndrome	18%[k]	35%–86%[k,l,m,n]	—	3%–6%[k,m]	0%[k,l,m]	80%[k,m]
Addison's disease	—	48%[o]	—	—	4%[o]	—
Pheochromocytoma	12%*–29%[†p]	12%*–18%[†p]	—	—	—	—
Acromegaly	—	2.5%[q]	—	—	—	—

Note. *Definite; †Probable plus definite.
Source. Popkin et al. 1988;[a] Wilkinson et al. 1988;[b] Lustman et al. 1986;[c] Jain 1972;[d] Nickel and Frame 1958;[e] Trzepacz et al. 1988;[f] Kathol and Delahunt 1986;[g] Joborn et al. 1986;[h] Brown et al. 1987;[i] Petersen 1968;[j] Hudson et al. 1987;[k] S. I. Cohen 1980;[l] Haskett 1985;[m] Jeffcoate et al. 1979;[n] Cleghorn 1951;[o] Starkman et al. 1985;[p] Abed et al. 1987.[q]

fies as the level of hypercalcemia increases. Delirium, psychosis, and cognitive impairment are more commonly seen in patients who have calcium levels above 15 or 16 mg/dL. Depressive symptoms but not cognitive symptoms tend to resolve with treatment (Brown et al. 1987). Cognitive symptoms may improve; however, residual symptoms usually remain.

CUSHING'S SYNDROME

Most studies indicate that 50%–80% of patients with Cushing's syndrome will also experience mild to severe depressive symptoms (see Table 17–2). It is also well documented that the depressive symptoms will be moderate to severe in up to 50% of such patients. Many will experience psychotic features, which is an unusual presentation for depression associated with medical illness. For this reason, it is critical that clinicians assess mood in individuals with Cushing's syndrome as part of the medical evaluation.

In patients who demonstrate depression, it may be necessary to institute therapy for the depression itself while awaiting the eventual resolution of both the physical and the psychiatric manifestations of Cushing's syndrome by surgical and/or medical therapy directed at the cause of hypercortisolemia. Such intervention may include medications or ECT in the more severely ill patients. Less severely ill patients can be followed through the course of treatment with either supportive counseling or cognitive-behavior therapy. Ultimately, in all patients who have a mood syndrome related to Cushing's syndrome, the depression will resolve with control of the cortisol excess alone.

It is difficult to distinguish patients with Cushing's syndrome from those with hypothalamic-pituitary-adrenal axis hyperactivity related to primary depression. To differentiate these two conditions, the patient should be treated for his or her depressive symptoms, and as the depression resolves, it should be deter-

Table 17–3. Important clinical factors among patients with endocrine disorders and psychiatric symptoms

Endocrine disease	Effect of psychiatric disorder on illness	Effect of treatment of endocrine disorder on psychiatric symptoms	When to treat psychiatric symptoms with psychiatric medications	Comments
Diabetes mellitus	Worse HbA$_1$[a] No differences in rate of diabetic complications[b]	Depression persists[b]	Early after identification	Stressful situation does not affect glucose control[c]
Hypothyroidism	May lead to misdiagnosis Need to do physical examination and medical history	Anxiety and depression resolve[d] Cognitive function stabilizes but problems persist[e] A short period of mania may occur[f]	If symptoms are life-threatening or persist >1 month after treatment with thyroid replacement	Psychiatric symptoms less severe now than before thyroid replacement; use caution when reading old literature Thyroid laboratory tests unnecessary unless signs of thyroid disease are present on examination, the patient is an elderly female,[g] or presentation is atypical If mania occurs during treatment, continue replacement; the mania will typically subside
Hyperthyroidism	May lead to misdiagnosis Need to do physical examination and medical history	Anxiety and depression resolve[h]	If symptoms are life-threatening or persist >1 month after thyrotoxicosis is treated	Same as for hypothyroidism Anxiety symptoms correlate with free T$_4$[h]
Hyperparathyroidism	Psychiatric symptoms may be first sign of hypercalcemia	Depression, but not cognitive problems,[i] resolves	If symptoms are life-threatening or persist >1 month after calcium has normalized	Calcium level should be obtained in newly diagnosed major depression, in patients with atypical presentations, or in patients with other symptoms of hypercalcemia Calcium level correlates with degree of psychiatric symptoms[j]
Pheochromocytoma	May lead to misdiagnosis if good history is not obtained and criteria for anxiety disorders are not used	Symptoms usually resolve with treatment	If symptoms are disabling or life-threatening	Anxiety disorder frequency less common than originally suspected[k]

Cushing's syndrome	Mood symptoms may be severe, with increased suicide risk[l] May lead to misdiagnosis, particularly because HPA abnormalities also occur in primary depression Physical examination is necessary	Delayed (1–3 months), but eventual resolution[m,n]	If symptoms are disabling or life-threatening If symptoms persist >2 months of glucocorticoid control	Resolution of HPA abnormalities with depression treatment and blunted ACTH after CRF or insulin-induced hypoglycemia differentiate primary depression from Cushing's syndrome in patients without physical signs[n] Family history of mood disorder less likely than among primary mood disorder patients[o]

Note. ACTH = adrenocorticotropic hormone; CRF = corticotropin-releasing factor; HPA = hypothalamic-pituitary-adrenal; T_4 = thyroxine.
Source. [a]Lustman et al. 1986; [b]Lustman et al. 1988; [c]Kemmer et al. 1986; [d]Jain 1972; [e]Haggerty et al. 1993; [f]Josephson and MacKenzie 1980; [g]Bauer et al. 1991; [h]Kathol and Delahunt 1986; [i]Brown et al. 1987; [j]Petersen 1968; [k]Starkman et al. 1985; [l]Haskett 1985; [m]Kelly et al. 1983; [n]Jeffcoate et al. 1979; [o]Hudson et al. 1987.

mined whether hypercortisolemia persists. If it does, this is suggestive evidence that Cushing's syndrome could be the cause of the patient's depression. Alternatively, the patient could be subjected to a corticotropin-releasing factor (CRF) infusion test. Patients with Cushing's syndrome will have an augmented adrenocorticotropic hormone (ACTH) response to CRF infusion, whereas patients with primary depression will have a blunted response.

ADDISON'S DISEASE

Few studies have investigated psychiatric symptoms in patients with Addison's disease since the mid-1950s. For this reason, it is impossible to determine whether psychiatric symptomatology is present with increased frequency in these patients or whether what was documented as psychiatric symptomatology was merely the apathy, fatigue, and lethargy associated with the underlying endocrine state.

CONCLUSION

Several endocrine diseases are associated with a high frequency of psychiatric symptoms or syndromes. In most instances, these symptoms resolve with adequate treatment of the endocrine disorder. If psychiatric manifestations are recognized, the patient can be informed about the course of symptoms with treatment of the endocrine disorder and the likelihood of his or her requiring other psychiatric care.

Systemic Lupus Erythematosus

Donna B. Greenberg, M.D.

Delirium, mood syndromes, generalized seizures, and signs of diffuse involvement of CNS disease are common features of systemic lupus erythematosus (SLE)

(J. Singer and Denburg 1990). The most common psychiatric presentations of active disease are brief reactive or atypical psychosis, delirium, primary generalized seizures, complex partial seizures, transverse myelitis, and global cognitive dysfunction (dementia) (Yagnik and Cohen 1988). Autoantibodies to neuronal membranes may account for most deficits. These autoantibodies reach the brain through breaks in the blood-brain barrier created by immunological vasculitis (Bluestein 1987). Autoimmune hematological abnormalities are more common in lupus patients with neuropsychiatric symptoms. Elevated cerebrospinal fluid (CSF) protein and pleocytosis are noted in patients with aseptic meningitis and focal neurological syndromes. Neuroimaging reveals perisulcal atrophy (Bresnihan 1982). Some neurological damage is associated with small vessel inflammatory vasculitis, usually with focal injury.

Mood syndromes may be the most common psychiatric presentation of patients with lupus (Baker 1973; Grigor et al. 1978), but mood change is not always due to lupus involvement in the brain. Patients with SLE are often treated with steroids, which raises the risk of steroid-related mood syndromes and psychosis. Metabolic derangement (e.g., resulting from kidney impairment) may increase the likelihood of seizures and delirium. In practice, treatment options for CNS lupus include increasing steroid medications, adding anticonvulsants and antidepressants, and, for severe depression, ECT (Allen and Pitts 1978; Douglas and Schwartz 1982; Guze 1967).

Cobalamin Deficiency

Donna B. Greenberg, M.D.

The minimal daily requirement of cobalamin is small, so deficiency is unlikely to occur in the patient with normal absorption. Deficiency occurs in patients with pernicious anemia (autoimmune loss of intrinsic factor and atrophic gastritis) and in patients with complete gastrectomy or bowel repairs that allow bacterial overgrowth in blind intestinal loops. Malabsorption from atrophic gastritis, ileal disease, and a strict vegetarian diet are additional predisposing conditions. Vitamin B_{12} deficiency is also frequent among patients with acquired immunodeficiency syndrome (AIDS) (Mantero-Atienza et al. 1991).

The sooner the treatment, the better. The ability to correct cerebral damage due to B_{12} deficiency depends on how long the condition has been present. Reversal of long-term dementia due to cobalamin deficiency may be difficult, but a clinician's alertness to clues may make this dementia a preventable condition. Other than an elevated mean corpuscular volume (MCV), the clue to vitamin B_{12} deficiency may be peripheral neurological deficits: symmetrical and progressive lower limb vibratory loss, paresthesias, and a deficit in postural sensation that causes patients to walk with a weak, unsteady, and awkward gait.

Treatment requires replacement of vitamin B_{12}, with frequent intramuscular injections over the first month, and then monthly vitamin B_{12} injections for maintenance. Studies have suggested that an oral regimen of 1 mg of B_{12} orally each day may be sufficient maintenance for many patients (Hitchcock and Toendle 1991; Lederle 1991).

Fatigue

Donna B. Greenberg, M.D.

Fatigue is one of the most common complaints heard in the doctor's office (National Ambulatory Medical Care Survey 1978). The physician's task is to find serious and treatable explanations from the history, physical examination, and common blood tests. Three syndromes—fibromyalgia, chronic fatigue syndrome (CFS), and postviral fatigue syndrome—are all contemporary diagnoses given to patients who continue to complain of fatigue without evidence of another specific medical diagnosis. In all three syndromes, psychiatric diagnoses—particularly anxiety and mood disorders—occur more often than in the general population.

FIBROMYALGIA

Fibromyalgia is a syndrome of generalized muscle pain in which sleep dysfunction and fatigue are prominent but no sign of collagen vascular disease can be documented by rheumatologists. Nonrestorative sleep, associated with EEG findings of persistent alpha waves during REM and non-REM sleep, has been thought to be a key feature (Moldofsky and Lue 1980). Among patients with fibromyalgia, fatigue occurs in 81%, sleep disturbance in 75%, and anxiety in 45%–55% (Wolfe et al. 1990). Two treatments have shown benefit in controlled studies: 25 mg amitriptyline, with and without naproxen (Carette et al. 1986; Goldenberg et al. 1986); and cyclobenzaprine plus another tricyclic (Bennett et al. 1988). In a more recent double-blind, placebo-controlled study of 208 patients who met 1990 criteria, the benefit of 50 mg amitriptyline or 30 mg cyclobenzaprine was not sustained over 6 months compared with placebo (Carette et al. 1994).

The American College of Rheumatology has recently redefined fibromyalgia as a condition of generalized pain and specific tender points, but fatigue is not a criterion because this symptom is so common in patients with comparison diagnoses such as rheumatoid arthritis (Wolfe et al. 1990). The criteria for fibromyalgia include a history of widespread pain—left and right, above and below the waist, and in the axial-cervical spine, chest, or low back. Pain must be noted in 11 of 18 tender point sites on digital palpation—the examiner must use a force of

4 kg, acknowledged to be painful by the patient. Although the elimination of fatigue as a criterion places the focus on the muscle condition, patients who appear in rheumatology offices by referral will have high rates of fatigue complaints and psychiatric comorbidity.

CHRONIC FATIGUE SYNDROME

Researchers have continued to search for the causes of other conditions of persistent fatigue. Recent studies have not supported the hypothesis that chronic or recrudescent Epstein-Barr virus (EBV) accounts for chronic fatigue symptoms. The working criteria were defined by consensus in 1988 (Holmes et al. 1988) and 1994 (Fukada et al. 1994) (Figure 17–1).

Patients with CFS often meet criteria for psychiatric illness: major depression (35%–75%), panic disorder (5%), dysthymia (5%), and somatization disorder (10%–15%) (Abbey and Garfinkel 1990). CFS is extremely heterogeneous. Katon and Russo (1992) reported that patients with a large number of medically unexplained physical symptoms, like those who meet CFS criteria, have a high prevalence of lifetime psychiatric diagnoses, the tendency to amplify symptoms, and greater-than-expected degrees of disability.

There are no specific treatments for CFS (Dawson and Sabin 1993). Gantz (1993) suggested nonsteroidal anti-inflammatory agents for myalgias and arthralgias, nonsedating antihistamines for allergies, and antidepressant medications for depressive symptoms, anxiety, and insomnia. He avoids exotic, unproved remedies. Occult diagnoses of substance abuse, primary sleep disorder, or depression with hypomania (bipolar II) should be considered. The treatment, like that for somatoform pain disorder, requires attention to emotional attributions, functional necessity, cognitive retraining, and graded increases in aerobic function. These patients often feel belittled if their physical symptoms are presumed to be

I. Clinically evaluate cases of prolonged or chronic fatigue by

   A. History and physical examination

   B. Mental status examination (abnormalities require appropriate psychiatric, psychological, or neurological examination)

   C. Tests (abnormal results that strongly suggest an exclusionary condition must be resolved)

     1. Screening laboratory tests: CBC, ESR, ALT, total protein, albumin, globulin, alkaline phosphatase, Ca, PO_4, glucose, BUN, electrolytes, creatinine, TSH, and UA

     2. Additional tests as clinically indicated to exclude other diagnoses

Exclude case if another cause for chronic fatigue is found

II. Classify case as either chronic fatigue syndrome or idiopathic chronic fatigue if fatigue persists or relapses for ≥6 months.

A. Classify as chronic fatigue syndrome if

   1. Criteria for severity of fatigue are met

   2. Four or more of the following symptoms are concurrently present for ≥6 months: (1) impaired memory or concentration, (2) sore throat, (3) tender cervical or axillary lymph nodes, (4) muscle pain, (5) multijoint pain, (6) new headaches, (7) unrefreshing sleep, (8) postexertion malaise

B. Classify as idiopathic chronic fatigue if fatigue severity or symptom criteria for chronic fatigue syndrome are not met.

III. Subgroup research cases by the presence or absence of the following essential parameters:

   A. Comorbid conditions (psychiatric conditions must be documented by use of an instrument)
   B. Current level of fatigue (measured by a scale)
   C. Duration of fatigue
   D. Current level of physical function (measured by an instrument)

Subgroup research cases further as needed by optional parameters such as epidemiological or laboratory features of interest.

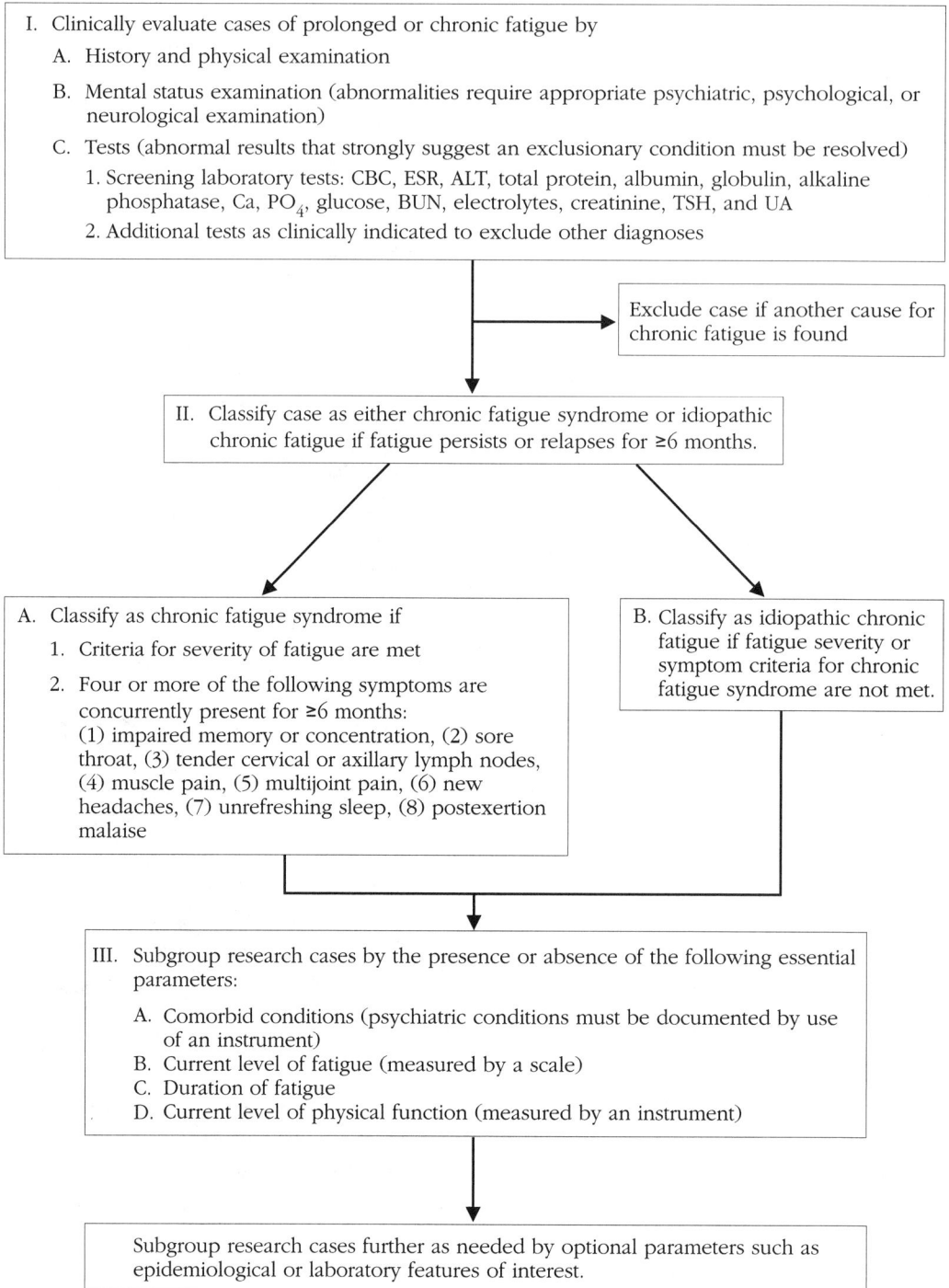

Figure 17–1. Evaluation and classification of unexplained chronic fatigue. ALT = alanine aminotransferase; BUN = blood urea nitrogen; CBC = complete blood count; ESR = erythrocyte sedimentation rate; PO_4 = phosphorus; TSH = thyroid-stimulating hormone; UA = urinalysis. *Source.* Adapted from Fukada K, Straus SE, Hickie I, et al: "The Chronic Fatigue Syndrome: A Comprehensive Approach to Its Definition and Study." *Annals of Internal Medicine* 121:953–959, 1994. Used with permission.

psychological. Acknowledging the validity of their suffering is critical.

The new criteria have excluded major depression with psychotic or melancholic features, bipolar disorder, schizophrenia, dementia, anorexia nervosa, or bulimia nervosa. Substance abuse in the last 2 years excludes patients, but anxiety disorder or nonmelancholic depression does not (Fukada et al. 1994).

Factors most important in predicting persistent illness at 2.5 years are more than eight unexplained medical symptoms, lifetime history of dysthymia, more than 1.5 years' duration of the syndrome, less education, and older age. No initial physical examination or immunological or viral measures predict persistent symptoms (Clark et al. 1995).

■ POSTINFECTION SYNDROMES POTENTIALLY ASSOCIATED WITH CHRONIC FATIGUE SYNDROME

Postviral Syndrome

Certainly, acute viral malaise is a low-energy state associated with sleepiness and elevated cytokines, but no single virus has been implicated in CFS. Patients with chronic fatigue, like much of the population, have serologies confirming exposure to a variety of viruses (Levine et al. 1992).

On the premise that viruses could be reactivated or persist when the immune system is stressed, scientists have looked for evidence of immune deficiency among patients with CFS. A prospective study among 1,200 primary care patients showed evidence that episodes of common infections were related to the onset of chronic fatigue. The strongest indicators of postinfectious fatigue were psychological distress and fatigue before infection (Wesseley et al. 1995).

Epstein-Barr Virus Infection (Mononucleosis)

The fatigue of acute mononucleosis may occur as a 3-week prodrome of malaise before exudative pharyngitis, lymphadenopathy, hepatosplenomegaly, hepatitis, or encephalitis develop; heterophile tests become positive only after several weeks. Atypical lymphocytes may be noted. The best indicator of acute infection is the presence of antibodies to viral capsid antigen immunoglobulin M (IgM), which persists for 4–8 weeks. Most patients return to work in 3 weeks, but some remain tired for months. Depression and anxiety syndromes have often been reported during the recovery phase. Recrudescent disease, with very high antibody titers, is associated with interstitial pneumonitis in immunocompromised hosts.

Lyme Disease

Lyme disease is caused by a spirochete, *Borrelia burgdorferi,* which, like neurosyphilis, has late neurotoxic features. The diagnosis of Lyme disease is clinical and relies on classical physical signs. Knowledge of a tick bite gives a clue to the diagnosis. An early sign of the disease is the appearance of erythema migrans, a red papule evolving peripherally and clearing in the center. The lesion and associated nodes fade in 1 month. Over a period of 6 months after infection, 15%–20% of patients develop lymphocytic meningitis, radicular pains, and cranial and peripheral neuropathies. Somnolence, emotionality, memory deficits, and depression are common. Other patients have facial palsy, meningitis, radiculoneuritis, chorea, cerebellar ataxia, seizures, dementia, hemiplegia, transverse myelitis, encephalomyelitis, or leukoencephalitis. Examination of CSF obtained on spinal tap shows lymphocytic pleocytosis, immunoglobulin G (IgG) and IgM, and Lyme antibodies; 80% of patients with Lyme disease also have arthritis or arthralgias. An asymmetric sensory and motor peripheral neuropathy is also seen.

Late disease is characterized by knee, hip, or shoulder arthritis, which gradually improves. Progressive encephalomyelitis is a late consequence, appearing as late as 7 years after diagnosis and characterized by encephalopathy, seizures, dementia, hemiplegia, dysphasia, hemianopsia, paresis, cranial nerve palsies, and radiculoneuropathy. CSF examination reveals lymphocytosis, high protein, IgG, and specific Lyme antibody. Magnetic resonance imaging (MRI) studies show infarct patterns, white matter disease, and hydrocephalus. Late neurological disease is treated with intravenous antibiotics, but patients respond slowly to therapy.

For a definitive diagnosis of Lyme disease, a positive enzyme-linked immunosorbent assay (ELISA) must be confirmed by a Western immunoblot. Serology may be negative because of laboratory variability or because testing is done early in the course of the disease. ELISA antibody screens may not become positive for the first 6 weeks after infection. Fear of Lyme disease is common, and because no Lyme disease test is perfect, proving that the patient's symptoms are not due to Lyme disease is a problem (Steere et al. 1993).

CONCLUSION

Axis III, the medical axis of DSM, is the focus of this chapter. The consultation-liaison psychiatrist is in the best position to combine medical knowledge with Axis I (psychiatric syndromes) and Axis II (traits and disorders) to diagnose and treat medically ill patients with respect and technical understanding.

REFERENCES

Abbey SE, Garfinkel PE: Chronic fatigue syndrome and the psychiatrist. Can J Psychiatry 35:625–633, 1990

Abed RT, Clark J, Elbadawy HF, et al: Psychiatric morbidity in acromegaly. Acta Psychiatr Scand 75:635–639, 1987

Abrams HS, Hester LR, Sheridan WF, et al: Sexual functioning in patients with chronic renal failure. J Nerv Ment Dis 160:220–226, 1975

Allen RE, Pitts FN: ECT for depressed patients with lupus erythematosus. Am J Psychiatry 135:367–368, 1978

American Psychiatric Association: Diagnostic and Statistical Manual of Mental Disorders, 3rd Edition. Washington, DC, American Psychiatric Association, 1980

American Psychiatric Association: Diagnostic and Statistical Manual of Mental Disorders, 3rd Edition, Revised. Washington, DC, American Psychiatric Association, 1987

Andrykowski MA, Altmaier EM, Barnett RL, et al: The quality of life in adult survivors of allogeneic bone marrow transplantation. Transplantation 50:399–406, 1990

Antonaccio MJ, Robson RD: Centrally mediated cardiovascular effects of 5-hydroxy-tryptophan in anesthetized dogs. J Pharm Pharmacol 25:495–497, 1973

Avery D, Winokur G: Mortality in depressed patients treated with electroconvulsive therapy and antidepressants. Arch Gen Psychiatry 33:1029–1037, 1976

Baer PG, Cagen LM: Platelet activating factor vasoconstriction of dog kidney: inhibition by alprazolam. Hypertension 9:253–260, 1987

Baker M: Psychopathology in SLE: psychiatric observations. Semin Arthritis Rheum 3:95–110, 1973

Ballard JE, Boileau RA, Sleator EK, et al: Cardiovascular responses of hyperactive children to methylphenidate. JAMA 236:2870–2874, 1976

Barrett BJ, Vavasour HM, Major A, et al: Clinical and psychological correlates of somatic symptoms in patients on dialysis. Nephron 55:10–15, 1990

Bauer MS, Halpern L, Schriger D: Screening Ambulatory Depressives for Causative Medical Illnesses: The Example of Thyroid Function Screening. A Report for the Agency for Health Care Policy and Research. Washington, DC, Agency for Health Care Policy and Research, 1991, pp 1–24

Beitman BD, Basha I, Flaker G, et al: Atypical or nonanginal chest pain: panic disorder or coronary artery disease? Arch Intern Med 147:1548–1552, 1987a

Beitman BD, Lamberti JW, Mukerji V, et al: Panic disorder in patients with angiographically normal coronary arteries: a pilot study. Psychosomatics 28:480–484, 1987b

Bennett RM, Gatter RA, Campbell SM, et al: A comparison of cyclobenzaprine and placebo in the management of fibrositis: a double blind controlled study. Arthritis Rheum 31:1535–1542, 1988

Benson H, Alexander S, Feldman CL: Decreased premature ventricular contractions through the use of the relaxation response in patients with stable ischemic heart disease. Lancet 2:380–382, 1975

Bentdal OH, Fauchald P, Brekke IB, et al: Rehabilitation and quality of life in diabetic patients after successful pancreas-kidney transplantation. Diabetologia 34 (suppl 1):S158–S159, 1991

Bergner M, Bobbitt RA, Carter WB, et al: The Sickness Impact Profile: development and final revision of a health status measure. Med Care 19:787–805, 1981

Bergstrom RF, Beasley CM Jr, Levy NB, et al: The effects of renal and hepatic disease on the pharmacokinetics, renal tolerance, and risk-benefit profile of fluoxetine. Int Clin Psychopharmacol 8:261–266, 1993

Bigger JT, Giardina E-GV, Perel JM, et al: Cardiac antiarrhythmic effects of imipramine hydrochloride. N Engl J Med 296:206–208, 1977

Bigger JT, Kantor SJ, Glassman AH, et al: Cardiovascular effects of tricyclic antidepressant drugs, in Psychopharmacology: A Generation of Progress. Edited by Lipton MA. New York, Raven, 1978, pp 1033–1046

Blanchard EB, Scharff L, Schwarz SP, et al: The role of anxiety and depression in the irritable bowel syndrome. Behav Res Ther 28:401–405, 1990

Blatt CM, Rabinowitz SH, Lown B: Central serotonergic agents raise the repetitive extrasystole threshold of the vulnerable period of the canine ventricular myocardium. Circ Res 44:723–730, 1979

Bluestein HG: Neuropsychiatric manifestations of systemic lupus erythematosus. N Engl J Med 317:309–310, 1987

Blumenthal JA, Williams RS, Wallace AG et al: Physiological and psychological variables predict compliance to prescribed exercise therapy in patients recovering from myocardial infarction. Psychosom Med 44:519–527, 1982

Borson S, McDonald GJ: Depression and chronic obstructive pulmonary disease, in Depression and Coexisting Disease. Edited by Robinson RG, Rabins PV. New York, Igaku-Shoin, 1989, pp 40–60

Bremer BA, McCauley CR, Wrona RM, et al: Quality of life in end-stage renal disease: a reexamination. Am J Kidney Dis 13:202–209, 1989

Bresnihan B: CNS lupus. Clinical Rheumatic Disease 8:183–185, 1982

Brod J: Hemodynamics and emotional stress. Bibl Psychiatr 144:13–16, 1970

Brod J, Fencl V, Jirka J: Circulatory changes underlying blood pressure elevation during acute emotional stress (mental arithmetic) in normotensive and hypertensive subjects. Clin Sci 18:269–278, 1959

Brown GG, Preisman RC, Kleerekoper M: Neurobehavioral symptoms in mild primary hyperparathyroidism: related to hypercalcemia but not improved by parathyroidectomy. Henry Ford Hosp Med J 35:211–215, 1987

Buff DD, Brenner R, Kirtane SS, et al: Dysrhythmia associated with fluoxetine treatment in an elderly patient with cardiac disease. J Clin Psychiatry 52:174–176, 1991

Burckhardt D, Raedler E, Muller V, et al: Cardiovascular effects of tricyclic and tetracyclic antidepressants. JAMA 239:213–216, 1987

Burns BH, Howell JBL: Disproportionately severe breathlessness in chronic bronchitis. QJM 38:277–294, 1969

Burrows GD, Vohra J, Hunt D, et al: Cardiac effects of different tricyclic antidepressant drugs. Br J Psychiatry 129:335–341, 1976

Burrows GD, Vohra J, Dumovic P, et al: Tricyclic antidepressant drugs in cardiac conduction. Progress in Neuropharmacology 1:329–334, 1977

Cannon RO: Causes of chest pain in patients with normal coronary angiograms: the eye of the beholder. Am J Cardiol 62:306–308, 1988

Carette S, McCain GA, Bell DA, et al: Evaluation of amitriptyline in primary fibrositis: a double-blind, placebo-controlled study. Arthritis Rheum 29:655–659, 1986

Carette S, Bell MJ, Reynolds J, et al: Comparison of amitriptyline, cyclobenzaprine, and placebo in the treatment of fibromyalgia: a randomized double-blind clinical trial. Arthritis Rheum 37:32–40, 1994

Carney RM, Rich MW, Freedland KE, et al: Major depressive disorder predicts cardiac events in patients with coronary artery disease. Psychosom Med 50:627–633, 1988

Carr RE, Lehrer PM, Hochron SM: Panic symptoms in asthma and panic disorder: a preliminary test of the dyspnea-fear theory. Behav Res Ther 30:251–261, 1992

Carvajal C, Passig C, San Martin E, et al: Prevalencia del consumo de cigarillos en pacientes psiquiatricos. Acta Psiquiatr Psicol Am Lat 35:145–151, 1989

Case RB, Moss AJ, Case N, et al: Living alone after myocardial infarction: impact on prognosis. JAMA 267:515–519, 1992

Castell DO, Richter JE: Edrophonium testing for esophageal pain: concurrence and discord. Dig Dis Sci 32:897–899, 1987

Chazan JA: Elective withdrawal from dialysis: an important cause of death among patients with chronic renal failure. Dialysis and Transplantation 19:530–538, 1990

Chignon JM, Lepine JP, Ades J: Panic disorder in cardiac outpatients. Am J Psychiatry 150:780–785, 1993

Christie RV: Some types of respiration in the neuroses. QJM 16:427–434, 1935

Clarfield AM: The reversible dementias: do they reverse? Ann Intern Med 109:476–486, 1988

Clark MR, Katon W, Russo J: Chronic fatigue, risk factors for symptom persistence in a two and a half year followup study. Am J Med 98:187–195, 1995

Cleghorn RA: Adrenal cortical insufficiency: psychological and neurological observations. Can Med Assoc J 65:449–454, 1951

Clouse RE, Alpers DH: The Relationship of Psychiatric Disorder to Gastrointestinal Illness. Annu Rev Med 37:283–295, 1986

Clouse RE, Lustman PJ: Psychiatric illness and contraction abnormalities of the esophagus. N Engl J Med 309:1337–1342, 1983

Cohen LM, Woods A, McCue J: The challenge of advance directives and ESRD. Dialysis and Transplantation 20:593–594, 1991

Cohen LM, Germain M, Woods A, et al: Patient attitudes and psychological considerations in dialysis discontinuation. Psychosomatics 34:395–401, 1993

Cohen ME, White PD: Life situations, emotions and neurocirculatory asthenia. Res Publ Assoc Res Nerv Ment Dis 12:335–357, 1951

Cohen SI: Cushing's syndrome: a psychiatric study of 29 patients. Br J Psychiatry 136:120–124, 1980

Connell AM, Hilton C, Irvine G, et al: Variation of bowel habits in two population samples. BMJ 5470:1095–1099, 1965

Coryell W, Noyes R, Clancy J: Excess mortality in panic disorder: a comparison with unipolar depression. Arch Gen Psychiatry 139:1079–1082, 1982

Covey LS, Glassman AH, Stetner F, et al: Effect of history of alcoholism or major depression on smoking cessation. Am J Psychiatry 150:1546–1547, 1993

Creed F, Craig T, Farmer R: Functional abdominal pain, psychiatric illness, and life events. Gut 29:235–242, 1988

Creer T: Asthma Therapy: A Behavioral Health Care System for Respiratory Disorders. New York, Springer, 1979

Damas-Mora J, Grant R, Kenyon P, et al: Respiratory ventilation and carbon dioxide levels in syndromes of depression. Br J Psychiatry 129:457–464, 1976

Damas-Mora J, Suster L, Jenne A: Diminished hypercapnic drive in endogenous or severe depression. J Psychosom Res 26:237–245, 1982

Dawling S, Lynn K, Rosser R, et al: Nortriptyline metabolism in chronic renal failure: metabolic elimination. Clin Pharmacol Ther 32:322–329, 1982

Dawson DM, Sabin TD: Summary and perspective, in Chronic Fatigue Syndrome. Edited by Dawson DM, Sabin TD. Boston, MA, Little, Brown, 1993, pp 195–211

Deanfield JE, Maseri A, Selwyn AP, et al: Myocardial ischemia during daily life in patients with stable angina: its relation to symptoms and heart rate changes. Lancet 2:753–758, 1983

Dembrowski TM, MacDougall JM, Williams RB, et al: Components of type A, hostility and anger in relationship to angiographic findings. Psychosom Med 47:219–226, 1985

Demers RY, Fischetti LR, Neale AV: Incongruence between self-reported symptoms and objective evidence of respiratory disease among construction workers. Soc Sci Med 30:805–810, 1990

DeQuattro V, Loo R, Foti A: Sympathoadrenal responses to stress: the linking of Type A behavior pattern to ischemic heart disease. Clin Exp Hypertens 7:469–481, 1985

DeSilva RA, Lown B: Ventricular premature beats, stress and sudden death. Psychosomatics 19:639–659, 1978

DiChiara G, Imperato A: Drugs abused by humans preferentially increase synaptic dopamine concentrations in the mesolimbic system of freely moving rats. Proc Natl Acad Sci U S A 85:5274–5278, 1988

Dimsdale JE, Hackett TP, Hutter AM, et al: Type A behavior and angiographic findings. J Psychosom Res 23:273–276, 1979

Ditto B, Miller SB: Forearm blood flow responses of offspring of hypertensives to an extended stress task. Hypertension 13:181–187, 1989

Douglas CJ, Schwartz HI: ECT for depression caused by lupus cerebritis: a case report. Am J Psychiatry 139:1631–1632, 1982

Drossman DA: Irritable bowel syndrome. Am Fam Physician 39:159–164, 1989

Drossman DA, Thompson WG: The irritable bowel syndrome: review and a graduated multicomponent treatment approach. Ann Intern Med 116:1009–1016, 1992

Drossman DA, Sandler RS, McKee DC, et al: Bowel patterns among subjects not seeking health care. Gastroenterology 83:529–534, 1982

Drossman DA, McKee DC, Sandler RS, et al: Psychosocial factors in the irritable bowel syndrome: a multivariate study of patients and nonpatients with irritable bowel syndrome. Gastroenterology 95:701–708, 1988

Drossman DA, Thompson WG, Talley NJ, et al: Identification of subgroups of functional gastrointestinal disorders. Gastroenterology International 3:159–172, 1990a

Drossman DA, Leserman J, Nachman G, et al: Sexual and physical abuse in women with functional or organic gastrointestinal disorders. Ann Intern Med 113:828–833, 1990b

Drossman DA, Li Z, Andruzzi E, et al: US householder survey of functional gastrointestinal disorders: prevalence sociodemography, and health impact. Dig Dis Sci 38:1569–1580, 1993

Dubovsky S, Penn I: Psychiatric consideration in renal transplant surgery. Psychosomatics 21:481–491, 1980

Dunbar F: Psychosomatic Diagnosis. New York, Paul B Hoeber, 1943

Ellison JM, Milofski JE, Ely E: Fluoxetine-induced bradycardia and syncope in two patients. J Clin Psychiatry 51:385–386, 1990

Epstein FH: Responsibility of the physician in the preservation of life. Arch Intern Med 139:919–920, 1979

Esler MD, Goulston KJ: Levels of anxiety in colonic disorders. N Engl J Med 288:16–20, 1973

Esler MD, Julius S, Zweifler A, et al: Mild high-renin hypertension: neurogenic human hypertension? N Engl J Med 296:405–411, 1977

Esler M, Turbott J, Schwartz R, et al: The peripheral kinetics of norepinephrine in depressive illness. Arch Gen Psychiatry 39:285–300, 1982

ESRD Network of New England. Paper presented at Medical Review Board Annual Meeting, Boston, MA, September 25, 1990

Evans RW, Manninen DL, Garrison LP, et al: The quality of life in patients with end-stage renal disease. N Engl J Med 312:553–559, 1985

Ewer TC, Stewart DE: Improvement in bronchial hyper-responsiveness in patients with moderate asthma after treatment with a hypnotic technique: a randomised controlled trial. BMJ 293:1129–1132, 1986

Fava G, Pavan L: Large bowel disorders, II: psychopathology and alexithymia. Psychother Psychosom 27:100–105, 1976

Fielding JF: The irritable bowel syndrome. Clinical Gastroenterology 6:607–622, 1977

Fisch C: Effects of fluoxetine on the electrocardiogram. J Clin Psychiatry 46:42–44, 1985

Fisher SH, Curry E, Batuman V: Stopping long-term dialysis (letter). N Engl J Med 314:1449, 1986

Fishman R: REM sleep inhibition. Exp Neurol 36:166–172, 1972

Folkow B: Psychosocial and central nervous influences in primary hypertension. Circulation 76 (suppl I):10–19, 1987

Ford J, Miller PM, Eastwood J, et al: Life events, psychiatric illness in the irritable bowel syndrome. Gut 28:50–55, 1987

Frasure-Smith N: In-hospital symptoms of psychological stress as predictors of long-term outcome after acute myocardial infarction in men. Am J Cardiol 67:121–127, 1991

Frederick T, Frerichs RR, Clark VA: Personal health habits and symptoms of depression at the community level. Prev Med 17:173–182, 1988

Freeland AP, Ardran GM, Emrys-Roberts E: Globus hystericus and reflux esophagitis. J Laryngol Otol 88:1024–1031, 1974

Fricchione GL: Psychiatric aspects of renal transplantation. Aust N Z J Psychiatry 23:407–417, 1989

Friedman M, Rosenman RH: Type A Behavior and Your Heart. New York, Knopf, 1974

Friedman M, Byers SO, Diamant RH, et al: Plasma catecholamine response of coronary-prone subjects (type A) to a specific challenge. Metabolism 24:205–210, 1975

Friedman M, Thoresen CE, Gill JJ, et al: Alteration of type A behavior and its effect on cardiac recurrences in post myocardial infarction patients: summary results of the recurrent coronary prevention project. Am Heart J 112:653–665, 1986

Fukada K, Straus SE, Hickie I, et al: The chronic fatigue syndrome: a comprehensive approach to its definition and study. Ann Intern Med 121:953–959, 1994

Gantz N: Management of a patient with chronic fatigue syndrome, in Chronic Fatigue Syndrome. Edited by Dawson DM, Sabin TD. Boston, MA, Little, Brown, 1993, pp 185–194

Giardina E-GV, Bigger JT, Glassman AH, et al: The electrocardiographic and antiarrhythmic effects of imipramine hydrochloride at therapeutic plasma concentrations. Circulation 60:1045–1052, 1979

Giardina E-GV, Bigger JT, Johnson LL: The effect of imipramine and nortriptyline on ventricular premature depolarizations and left ventricular function. Circulation 64 (suppl IV):316–320, 1981

Ginsberg AL, Albert MB: Treatment of patients with severe steroid-dependent Crohn's disease with nonelemental formula diet: identification of possible etiologic dietary factor. Dig Dis Sci 34:1624–1628, 1989

Gitnick G: Etiology of inflammatory bowel diseases: where have we been? Where are we going? Scand J Gastroenterol Suppl 175:93–96, 1990

Glass DC, Krakoff LR, Contrada R, et al: Effect of harassment and competition upon the cardiovascular and plasma catecholamine responses in type A and type B individuals. Psychophysiology 17:453–463, 1980

Glassman AH: Cigarette smoking: implications for psychiatric illness. Am J Psychiatry 150:546–553, 1993

Goldberg R, Morris P, Christian F, et al: Panic disorder in cardiac outpatients. Psychosomatics 31:168–173, 1990

Goldenberg DL, Felson DT, Dinerman H: A randomized controlled trial of amitriptyline and naproxen in the treatment of patients with fibromyalgia. Arthritis Rheum 29:1371–1377, 1986

Gorlen T, Ekeberg O, Abdelnoor M, et al: Quality of life after kidney transplantation: a 10–20 years follow-up. Scand J Urol Nephrol 27:89–92, 1993

Gram LF: Fluoxetine. N Engl J Med 20:1354–1361, 1994

Grant I, Heaton RK, McSweeny AJ, et al: Neuropsychologic findings in hypoxemic chronic obstructive pulmonary disease. Arch Intern Med 142:1470–1476, 1982

Grant I, Prigatano GP, Heaton RK, et al: Progressive neuropsychologic impairment and hypoxemia. Arch Gen Psychiatry 44:999–1006, 1987

Greenberg DB, Stern TA, Weilberg JB: The fear of choking: three successfully treated cases. Psychosomatics 29:126–129, 1988

Grigor R, Edmonds J, Lewkonia R, et al: Systemic lupus erythematosus: a prospective analysis. Ann Rheum Dis 37:121–128, 1978

Gruen W: Effects of brief psychotherapy during the hospitalization period on the recovery process in heart attacks. J Consult Clin Psychol 43:274–290, 1975

Gulledge AD, Buszta C, Montague D: Psychological aspects of renal transplantation. Urol Clin North Am 10:327–335, 1983

Guze SB: The occurrence of psychiatric illness in systemic lupus erythematosus. Am J Psychiatry 123:1562–1570, 1967

Hackett TP, Cassem NH: Factors contributing to delay in responding to the signs and symptoms of acute myocardial infarction. Am J Cardiol 24:651–658, 1969

Hackett TP, Rosenbaum JF: Emotion, psychiatric disorders, and the heart, in Heart Disease. Edited by Braunwald E. Philadelphia, PA, WB Saunders, 1984, pp 1826–1946

Hackett TP, Cassem NH, Wishnie HA: The coronary care unit: an appraisal of its psychological hazards. N Engl J Med 279:1365–1370, 1968

Haggerty JJ, Stern RA, Mason GA, et al: Subclinical hypothyroidism: a modifiable risk factor for depression? Am J Psychiatry 150:508–510, 1993

Harburg E, Erfurt JC, Hauenstein LS, et al: Socio-ecological stress, suppressed hostility, skin color, and black-white male blood pressure: Detroit. Psychosom Med 35:276–296, 1973

Haskett RF: Diagnostic categorization of psychiatric disturbance in Cushing's syndrome. Am J Psychiatry 142:911–916, 1985

Hayes LA: The use of group contingencies for behavioral control: a review. Psychol Bull 83:628–648, 1976

Heaton RK, Grant I, McSweeny AJ, et al: Psychological effects of continuous and nocturnal oxygen therapy in hypoxemic COPD. Arch Intern Med 143:1941–1947, 1983

Hedgel DW, Cherniack NS: Sleeping and breathing, in Update: Pulmonary Diseases and Disorders. Edited by Fishman AP. New York, McGraw-Hill, 1988, pp 249–261

Helzer JE, Chammas S, Norland CC, et al: A study of the association between Crohn's disease and psychiatric illness. Gastroenterology 86:324–330, 1984

Henry JP, Cassel JC: Psychological factors in essential hypertension: recent epidemiological and animal experimental evidence. Am J Epidemiol 90:171–200, 1969

Henry JP, Stephens PM: Stress, Health, and the Social Environment: A Sociobiological Approach to Medicine. New York, Springer-Verlag New York, 1977

Henry JP, Meehan JP, Stephens PM: The use of psychosocial stimuli to induce prolonged systolic hypertension in mice. Psychosom Med 29:408–432, 1967

Himmelhoch JM, Schechtman K, Auchenbach R: The role of trazodone in the treatment of depressed cardiac patients. Psychopathology 17 (suppl 2):51–63, 1984

Hislop IG: Psychological significance of the irritable colon syndrome. Gut 12:452–457, 1971

Hitchcock JN, Toendle GJ: Oral cobalamin for treatment of pernicious anemia. JAMA 265:96–97, 1991

Holley JL, Nespor S, Rault R: Chronic in-center hemodialysis patients' attitudes, knowledge, and behavior towards advance directives. J Am Soc Nephrol 3:1405–1408, 1993

Holmes GP, Kaplan JE, Gantz NM, et al: Chronic fatigue syndrome: a working case definition. Ann Intern Med 108:387–389, 1988

Hudson JI, Hudson MS, Griffing GT, et al: Phenomenology and family history of affective disorder in Cushing's disease. Am J Psychiatry 144:951–953, 1987

Husebye DG, Westlie L, Styrovoky TJ, et al: Psychological, social, and somatic prognostic indicators in old patients undergoing long-term dialysis. Arch Intern Med 147:1921–1924, 1987

Isenberg SA, Lehrer PM, Hochron S: The effects of suggestion and emotional arousal on pulmonary function in asthma: a review of a hypothesis regarding vagal mediation. Psychosom Med 54:192–216, 1992

Jaffe CM: First-degree atrioventricular block during lithium carbonate treatment. Am J Psychiatry 134:88–89, 1977

Jain VK: A psychiatric study of hypothyroidism. Psychiatrie Clin (Basel) 5:121–130, 1972

Jarvik LF, Read SL, Mintz J, et al: Pretreatment orthostatic hypotension in geriatric depression: predictor of response to imipramine and doxepin. J Clin Psychopharmacol 3:368–372, 1983

Jeffcoate WJ, Silverstone JT, Edwards CRW, et al: Psychiatric manifestations of Cushing's syndrome: response to lowering of plasma cortisol. QJM 191:465–472, 1979

Jefferson JW: Cardiovascular effects and toxicity of anxiolytics and antidepressants. J Clin Psychiatry 50:368–378, 1989

Jellinek MS, Goldenheim PD, Jenicke MA: The impact of grief on ventilatory control. Am J Psychiatry 142:121–123, 1985

Joborn C, Hetta J, Palmer M, et al: Psychiatric symptomatology in patients with primary hyperparathyroidism. Ups J Med Sci 91:77–87, 1986

Josephson AM, MacKenzie TB: Thyroid-induced mania in hypothyroid patients. Br J Psychiatry 137:222–238, 1980

Kantor SJ, Bigger JT, Glassman AH, et al: Imipramine-induced heart block. JAMA 231:1364–1366, 1975

Kantor SJ, Glassman AH, Bigger JT, et al: The cardiac effect of therapeutic plasma concentrations of imipramine. Am J Psychiatry 135:534–538, 1978

Kathol RG, Delahunt JW: The relationship of anxiety and depression to symptoms of hyperthyroidism using operational criteria. Gen Hosp Psychiatry 8:23–28, 1986

Katon W, Raskind M: Treatment of depression in the medically ill elderly with methylphenidate. Am J Psychiatry 30:106–108, 1980

Katon W, Russo JS: Chronic fatigue syndrome criteria. Arch Intern Med 152:1604–1609, 1992

Kaufman MW, Murray GB, Cassem NH: Use of psychostimulants in medically ill depressed patients. Psychosomatics 23:817–819, 1982

Kellner R, Samet JM, Pathak D: Hypochondriacal concerns and somatic symptoms in patients with chronic airflow obstruction. J Psychosom Res 31:575–582, 1987

Kellner R, Samet JM, Pathak D: Dyspnea, anxiety, and depression in chronic respiratory impairment. Gen Hosp Psychiatry 14:20–28, 1992

Kelly WF, Checkley SA, Bender DA, et al: Cushing's syndrome and depression—a prospective study of 26 patients. Br J Psychiatry 142:16–19, 1983

Kemmer FW, Bisping R, Steingruber HJ, et al: Psychological stress and metabolic control in patients with type I diabetes mellitus. N Engl J Med 314:1078–1084, 1986

Kjellstrand CM, Dossetor JB: Ethical Problems in Dialysis and Transplantation. Dordrecht, The Netherlands, Kluwer Academic Publishers, 1992

Klein DF: False suffocation alarms, spontaneous panics, and related conditions. Arch Gen Psychiatry 50:306–317, 1993

Klein KB: Controlled treatment trials in irritable bowel syndrome: a critique. Gastroenterology 95:233–241, 1988

Krantz DS, Durel LA, David JE, et al: Propranolol medication among coronary patients: relationship to type A behavior and cardiovascular response. Journal of Human Stress 8:4–12, 1982

Kriwisky M, Perry GY, Tarchitsky D, et al: Haloperidol-induced torsades de pointes. Chest 98:482–484, 1990

Kutner NG, Brogan D: Expectations and psychological needs of elderly patients. Int J Aging Hum Dev 31:239–259, 1990

Langeluddecke PM: Psychological aspects of irritable bowel syndrome. Aust N Z J Psychiatry 19:218–226, 1985

Langosch W, Seer P, Brodner G, et al: Behavior therapy with coronary heart disease patients: results of a comparative study. J Psychosom Res 26:475–484, 1982

Latimer P: Irritable bowel syndrome. Psychosomatics 24:215–218, 1983

Latimer P, Sarana S, Campbell D, et al: Colonic motor and myoelectric activity: a comparative study of normal subjects, psychoneurotic patients and patients with irritable bowel syndrome. Gastroenterology 80:893–901, 1981

Lederle FA: Oral cobalamin for pernicious anemia, medicine's best kept secret. JAMA 265:94–95, 1991

Lehrer PM, Hochron SM, McCann B, et al: Relaxation decreases large airway but not small airway asthma. J Psychosom Res 30:13–25, 1986

Lehrer PM, Sargunaraj D, Hochron S: Psychological approaches to the treatment of asthma. J Consult Clin Psychol 60:639–643, 1992

Lehtinen V, Puhakka H: A psychosomatic approach to the globus hystericus syndrome. Acta Psychiatr Scand 53:21–28, 1976

Lesperance F, Frasure-Smith N: Depression and death post-myocardial infarction (NR457), in New Research Program and Abstracts: American Psychiatric Association, 149th Annual Meeting, San Francisco, CA, 1993, p 175

Levine PH, Jacobson S, Pocinki AG, et al: Clinical, epidemiologic, and virologic studies in four clusters of the chronic fatigue syndrome. Arch Intern Med 152:1611–1616, 1992

Levine SO, Towell BL, Suarez AM, et al: Platelet aggregation and secretion associated with emotional stress. Circulation 71:1129–1134, 1985

Levy NB: Use of psychotropics in patients with kidney failure. Psychosomatics 26:699–709, 1985

Light RW, Merrill EJ, Despars JA, et al: Prevalence of depression and anxiety in patients with COPD: relationship to functional capacity. Chest 87:35–38, 1987

Lown B: Sudden cardiac death: the major challenge confronting contemporary cardiology. Am J Cardiol 43:313–328, 1979

Lown B, DeSilva RA: Roles of psychological stress and the autonomic nervous system changes in provocation of ventricular premature complexes. Am J Cardiol 41:979–985, 1978

Lown B, Graboys TB: Management of patients with malignant ventricular arrhythmias. Am J Cardiol 39:910–918, 1977

Lown B, Verrier RL, Corbalan R: Psychologic stress and the threshold for repetitive ventricular response. Science 132:834–836, 1973

Lown B, DeSilva RA, Reich P, et al: Psychophysiologic factors in sudden cardiac death. Am J Psychiatry 137:1325–1335, 1980

Luchins DJ: Review of clinical and animal studies comparing the cardiovascular effects of doxepin and other tricyclic antidepressants. Am J Psychiatry 140:1006–1009, 1983

Lustman PJ, Griffith LS, Clouse RE, et al: Psychiatric illness in diabetes mellitus: relationship to symptoms and glucose control. J Nerv Ment Dis 174:736–742, 1986

Lustman PJ, Griffith LS, Clouse RE: Depression in adults with diabetes. Diabetes Care 11:605–612, 1988

Lydiard RB, Fossey MD, Ballenger JC: Irritable bowel syndrome in patients with panic disorder (letter). Am J Psychiatry 148:1614, 1991

Lydiard RB, Fossey MD, Marsh W, et al: Prevalence of psychiatric disorders in patients with irritable bowel syndrome. Psychosomatics 34:229–234, 1993

MacDougall JM, Dembrowski TM, Dimsdale JE, et al: Components of type A, hostility and anger: further relationships to angiographic findings. Health Psychol 4:137–145, 1985

Manning AP, Thompson WG, Heaton KW, et al: Towards positive diagnosis of the irritable bowel. BMJ 2:653–654, 1978

Mantero-Atienza E, Baum MK, Morgan R, et al: Vitamin B12 in early human immunodeficiency virus-1 infection (letter). Arch Intern Med 151:1019–1020, 1991

Manuck SB, Morrison RL, Bellack AS, et al: Behavioral factors in hypertension: cardiovascular responsivity, anger, and social competence, in Anger and Hostility in Cardiovascular and Behavioral Disorders. Edited by Chesney MA, Rosenman RH. New York, Hemisphere/McGraw-Hill, 1987, pp 149–172

Marchionno PM, Kirilloff LH, Openbrier DR, et al: Effects of continuous oxygen therapy on body image and lifestyle in patients with COPD (abstract). Am Rev Respir Dis 13 (pt 2):A163, 1985

Markovitz JH, Matthews KA: Platelets and coronary heart disease: potential psychophysiologic mechanisms. Psychosom Med 53:643–668, 1991

Matta RJ, Lawler JE, Lown B: Ventricular electrical instability in the conscious dog: effects of psychologic stress and beta-adrenergic blockade. Am J Cardiol 34:594–598, 1976

McKegney FP, Lange P: The decision to no longer live on chronic hemodialysis. Am J Psychiatry 128:47–53, 1971

Mendes de Leon CF, Powell LH, Kaplan BH: Change in coronary-prone behaviors in the Recurrent Coronary Prevention Project. Psychosom Med 53:407–419, 1991

Meyers S, Walfish JS, Sachar DB, et al: Quality of life after surgery for Crohn's disease: a psychosocial survey. Gastroenterology 78:1–6, 1980

Mifsud JC, Hernandez L, Hoebel BG: Nicotine infused into the nucleus accumbens increases synaptic dopamine as measured by in vivo microdialysis. Brain Res 478:365–367, 1989

Miller TQ, Turner CW, Tindale RS, et al: Reasons for the trend toward null findings in research on type A behavior. Psychol Bull 110:469–485, 1991

Mitchell JE, MacKenzie TB: Cardiac effects of lithium in man: a review. J Clin Psychiatry 43:47–51, 1982

Moldofsky H, Lue FA: The relationship of alpha and delta EEG frequencies to pain and mood in "fibrositis" patients treated with chlorpromazine and L-tryptophan. Electroencephalogr Clin Neurophysiol 50:71–80, 1980

Moody L, McCormick K, Williams A: Disease and symptom severity, functional status, and quality of life. J Behav Med 13:297–306, 1990

Morgan AD, Peck DF, Buchanan D, et al: Psychological factors contributing to disproportionate disability in chronic bronchitis. J Psychosom Res 27:259–263, 1983

Moser G, Vacariugranser GV, Schneider C, et al: High incidence of esophageal motor disorders in consecutive patients with globus sensation. Gastroenterology 101:1512–1521, 1991

Moss AJ, Goldstein S: The pre-hospital phase of acute myocardial infarction. Circulation 41:737–742, 1970

National Ambulatory Medical Care Survey: 1975 Summary. Hyattsville, MD, National Center for Health Statistics, 1978, pp 22–26

Neff TA, Petty TL: Tolerance and survival in severe chronic hypercapnea. Arch Intern Med 129:591–596, 1972

Neu S, Kjellstrand CM: Stopping long-term dialysis: an empirical study of withdrawal of life-supporting treatment. N Engl J Med 314:14–20, 1986

Neumann ME: As dialysis becomes an extension of life, its use gains greater scrutiny (editorial). Nephrology News Issues, 1992, p 5

Nickel SN, Frame B: Neurologic manifestations of myxedema. Neurology 8:511–517, 1958

Nocturnal Oxygen Therapy Trial Group (NOTTG): Continuous or nocturnal oxygen therapy in hypoxemic chronic obstructive lung disease. Ann Intern Med 93:391–398, 1980

Norton CE: Attitudes toward living and dying in patients on chronic hemodialysis. Ann N Y Acad Sci 164:720–732, 1969

Noyes R Jr, Cook B, Garvey M, et al: Reduction of gastrointestinal symptoms with treatment for panic disorder. Psychosomatics 31:75–79, 1990

Olden KW: Brain-gut interactions. West J Med 160:55, 1994

Oldenburg B, Perkins RJ, Andrews G: Controlled trial of psychological intervention in myocardial infarction. J Consult Clin Psychol 53:852–859, 1985

Osberg JW, Mears GL, McKee DC, et al: Intellectual functioning in renal failure and chronic dialysis. Journal of Chronic Disease 35:445–447, 1982

Parfrey PS, Vavasour HM, Gault MH: A prospective study of health status in dialysis and transplant patients. Transplant Proc 20:1231–1232, 1989

Pauletto P, Scannaoieco G, Pessina AC: Sympathetic drive and vascular damage in hypertension and atherosclerosis. Hypertension 17 (suppl 4):75–81, 1991

Petersen P: Psychiatric disorders in primary hyperparathyroidism. J Clin Endocrinol Metab 28:1491–1495, 1968

Piehlmeier W, Bullinger M, Nusser J, et al: Quality of life in Type 1 (insulin-dependent) diabetic patients prior to and after pancreas and kidney transplantation in relation to organ function. Diabetologia 34 (suppl 1):S150–S157, 1991

Pohl RB, Yeragani VK, Balon R, et al: Smoking in panic disorder patients, in CME Syllabus and Scientific Proceedings in Summary Form. 145th Annual Meeting of the American Psychiatric Association. Washington, DC, American Psychiatric Association, 1992, p 84

Popkin MK, Callies AL, Lentz RD, et al: Prevalence of major depression, simple phobia and other psychiatric disorders in patients with longstanding type I diabetes mellitus. Arch Gen Psychiatry 45:64–68, 1988

Porzelius J, Vest M, Nochomovitz M: Respiratory function, cognitions, and panic in chronic obstructive pulmonary patients. Behav Res Ther 30:75–77, 1992

Posner JB: Newer techniques of cerebral blood flow measurement. Stroke 3:227–237, 1972

Prigatano GP, Parsons O, Wright E, et al: Neuropsychological test performance in mildly hypoxemic patients with chronic obstructive pulmonary disease. J Consult Clin Psychol 51:108–116, 1983

Rabinowitz SH, Lown B: Central neurochemical factors related to serotonin metabolism and cardiac ventricular vulnerability for repetitive electrical activity. Am J Cardiol 41:516–522, 1978

Ragland DR, Brand RJ: Type A behavior and mortality from coronary heart disease. N Engl J Med 318:65–69, 1988

Rapoport DM, Greenberg HE, Goldring RM: Differing effects of the anxiolytic agents buspirone and diazepam on control of breathing. Clin Pharmacol Ther 49:394–401, 1991

Raskind M, Veith RC, Barnes R, et al: Cardiovascular and antidepressant effects of imipramine in the treatment of secondary depression in patients with ischemic heart disease. Am J Psychiatry 139:1114–1117, 1982

Reich P, Murawski BJ, DeSilva RA, et al: Psychologic studies of patients with ventricular arrhythmias. Psychosom Med 41:74–79, 1979

Reilly GS: A questionnaire for dialysis patients on treatment cessation issues. Dialysis and Transplantation 19:533–545, 1990

Richter JE, Obrecht WF, Bradley LA, et al: Psychological comparison of patients with nutcracker esophagus and irritable bowel syndrome. Dig Dis Sci 31:131–138, 1986

Richter JE, Dalton CB, Bradley LA, et al: Oral nifedipine in the treatment of noncardiac chest pain in patients with the nutcracker esophagus. Gastroenterology 93:21–28, 1987

Roine RO, Kajaste S, Kaste M: Neuropsychological sequelae of cardiac arrest. JAMA 269:237–242, 1993

Roose SP, Dalack GW: Treating the depressed patient with cardiovascular problems. J Clin Psychiatry 53(suppl):25–31, 1992

Roose SP, Nurnberger JI, Dunner DL, et al: Cardiac sinus node dysfunction during lithium treatment. Am J Psychiatry 136:804–806, 1979a

Roose SP, Bone S, Haidorfer C, et al: Lithium treatment in older patients. Am J Psychiatry 136:843–844, 1979b

Roose SP, Glassman AH, Giardina E-GV, et al: Nortriptyline in depressed patients with left ventricular impairment. JAMA 256:3253–3257, 1986

Roose SP, Glassman AH, Giardina E-GV, et al: Tricyclic antidepressants in depressed patients with cardiac conduction disease. Arch Gen Psychiatry 44:273–275, 1987

Roose SP, Dalack GW, Woodring S: Death, depression and heart disease. J Clin Psychiatry 52 (no 6, suppl):34–39, 1991a

Roose SP, Dalack GW, Woodring S, et al: Cardiovascular effects of bupropion in depressed patients with heart disease. Am J Psychiatry 148:512–516, 1991b

Rosenman RH, Brand RJ, Jenkins CD, et al: Coronary heart disease in the Western Collaborative Group Study: final follow-up experience of 8-1/2 years. JAMA 233:872–877, 1975

Rozanski A, Bairey CN, Krantz DS, et al: Mental stress and the induction of silent myocardial ischemia in patients with coronary artery disease. N Engl J Med 318:1005–1011, 1988

Ruberman W, Weinblatt AB, Goldberg JD, et al: Psychosocial influences on mortality after myocardial infarction. N Engl J Med 311:552–559, 1984

Russell JD, Beecroft ML, Ludwin D, et al: The quality of life in renal transplantation—a prospective study. Transplantation 54:656–660, 1992

Sandler RS, Drossman DA, Nathan HP, et al: Symptom complaints and health care seeking behavior in subjects with bowel dysfunction. Gastroenterology 87:314–318, 1984

Schleifer SJ, Macari-Hinson MM, Coyle DA, et al: The nature and course of depression following myocardial infarction. Arch Intern Med 149:1785–1789, 1989

Schneider LS, Sloane RB, Stapes FR, et al: Pretreatment orthostatic hypotension as a predictor of response to nortriptyline in geriatric depression. J Clin Psychopharmacol 6:172–176, 1986

Schover LR, Novick AC, Steinmuller DR, et al: Sexuality, fertility, and renal transplantation: a survey of survivors. J Sex Marital Ther 16:3–13, 1990

Schwartz PJ, Wolf S: QT interval prolongation as predictor of sudden death in patients with myocardial infarction. Circulation 57:1074–1077, 1978

Selye H: The Stress of Life. New York, McGraw-Hill, 1956

Sensky T: Psychiatric morbidity in renal transplantation. Psychother Psychosom 52:41–46, 1989

Seraganian P, Hanley JA, Hollander E, et al: Exaggerated psychophysiological reactivity: issues in quantification and reliability. J Psychosom Res 29:393–405, 1985

Series F, Cormier Y: Effects of protriptyline on diurnal and nocturnal oxygenation in patients with COPD. Ann Intern Med 113:507–511, 1990

Shekelle RB, Julley SB, Neaton J, et al: Type A behavior pattern and risk of coronary death in MRFIT. Am Heart Assoc Cardiovasc Dis Epidemiol Newsletter 33:34–35, 1983

Shershow JC, King A, Robinson S: Carbon dioxide sensitivity and personality. Psychosom Med 35:155–160, 1973

Shershow JC, Kanarek DJ, Kazemi H: Ventilatory response to carbon dioxide inhalation in depression. Psychosom Med 38:282–287, 1976

Sherwitz L, McKelvain R, Laman C, et al: Type A behavior, self-involvement and coronary atherosclerosis. Psychosom Med 45:47–57, 1983

Sigg EG, Osborne M, Porol B: Cardiovascular effects of imipramine. J Pharmacol Exp Ther 141:237–243, 1963

Sigler LH: Emotion and atherosclerotic heart disease, I: electrocardiovascular changes observed on the recall of past emotional disturbances. Br J Med Psychol 40:55–64, 1967

Simmons RG, Kamstra-Hennen L, Thompson CR: Psychosocial adjustment five to nine years post transplant. Transplant Proc 13:40–43, 1981

Simmons RG, Anderson C, Kamstra L: Comparison of quality of life of patients on continuous ambulatory peritoneal dialysis, hemodialysis, and after transplantation. Am J Kidney Dis 3:253–255, 1984

Simon AB, Feinleib M, Thompson HK: Components of delay in the pre-hospital phase of acute myocardial infarction. Am J Cardiol 30:476–482, 1972

Simpson MT, Olewine DE, Jenkins CD, et al: Exercise induced catecholamines and platelet aggregation in the coronary-prone behavior pattern. Psychosom Med 36:467–487, 1974

Singer J, Denburg JA: Diagnostic criteria for neuropsychiatric systemic lupus erythematosus: the results of a consensus meeting. J Rheumatol 17:1397–1402, 1990

Singer PA: Nephrologists' experience with and attitudes towards decisions to forego dialysis. J Am Soc Nephrol 2:1235–1240, 1992

Stamler J, Stamler R, Pullman T: The Epidemiology of Essential Hypertension. New York, Grune & Stratton, 1967

Starkman MN, Zelnik TC, Nesse RM, et al: Anxiety in patients with pheochromocytomas. Arch Intern Med 145:248–252, 1985

Steere AC, Taylor E, McHugh GL, et al: The overdiagnosis of Lyme disease. JAMA 269:1812–1816, 1993

Stolerman IP, Shoaib M: The neurobiology of tobacco addiction. Trends Pharmacol Sci 12:467–473, 1991

Stoudemire A, Moran MG, Fogel BS: Psychotropic drug use in the medically ill: part I. Psychosomatics 31:377–391, 1990

Stoudemire A, Moran MG, Fogel BS: Psychotropic drug use in the medically ill: part II. Psychosomatics 32:34–46, 1991

Taggart P, Gibbons D, Somerville W: Some effects of motor car driving on the normal and abnormal heart. BMJ 4:130–134, 1969

Taggart P, Carruthers M, Somerville W: Electrocardiogram, plasma catecholamines and lipids and their modification by oxprenolol when speaking before an audience. Lancet 2:341–346, 1973

Talley NJ: Nonulcer dyspepsia: current approaches to diagnosis and management. Am Fam Physician 47:1407–1416, 1993

Tangedahl TN, Gau GT: Myocardial irritability associated with lithium carbonate therapy. N Engl J Med 287:867–868, 1972

Teschan PE, Bourne JR, Reed RB, et al: Electro-physiologic and neurobehavioral responses to therapy: the National Corroborative Dialysis Study. Kidney Int 23 (suppl 13):S58–S65, 1983

Thase ME, Perel JM: Antiarrhythmic effects of tricyclic antidepressants (letter). JAMA 248:429, 1982

Thompson WG: Sexual problems in chronic respiratory disease: achieving and maintaining intimacy. Postgrad Med 79:41–44, 47, 50–52, 1982

Thompson WG, Heaton KW: Functional bowel disorders in apparently healthy people. Gastroenterology 79:283–288, 1980

Tobin MJ, Chadha TS, Jenouri G, et al: Breathing patterns: disease subjects. Chest 84:286–294, 1983

Tollefson GD, Luxenberg M, Valentine R, et al: An open label trial of alprazolam in comorbid irritable bowel syndrome and generalized anxiety disorder. J Clin Psychiatry 52:502–508, 1991

Trzepacz PT, McCue M, Klein I, et al: A psychiatric and neuropsychological study of patients with untreated Graves' disease. Gen Hosp Psychiatry 10:49–55, 1988

Tung CS, Grenhoff J, Svensson TH: Nicotine counteracts midbrain dopamine cell dysfunction induced by prefrontal cortex inactivation. Acta Physiol Scand 138:427–428, 1990

Upward JW, Edwards JG, Goldie A, et al: Comparative effects of fluoxetine and amitriptyline on cardiac function. Br J Clin Pharmacol 26:399–402, 1988

Veith RC, Raskind MA, Caldwell JH, et al: Cardiovascular effects of tricyclic antidepressants in depressed patients with chronic heart disease. N Engl J Med 306:954–959, 1982a

Veith RC, Bloom V, Bielski R, et al: ECG effects of comparable plasma concentrations of desipramine and amitriptyline. J Clin Psychopharmacol 2:394–398, 1982b

Vitullo RN, Wharton JM, Allen NB, et al: Trazodone related exercise induced nonsustained ventricular tachycardia. Chest 98:247–248, 1990

Vogel WH, Miller J, DeTurck KH, et al: Effects of psychoactive drugs on plasma catecholamines during stress in rats. Neuropsychopharmacol 23:1105–1108, 1984

Walker EA, Roy-Byrne PP, Katon WJ: Irritable bowel syndrome and psychiatric illness. Am J Psychiatry 147:565–572, 1990a

Walker EA, Roy-Byrne PP, Katon WJ, et al: Psychiatric illness in irritable bowel syndrome: a comparison with inflammatory bowel disease. Am J Psychiatry 147:1656–1661, 1990b

Wallace WA, Yu PA: Sudden death and the prehospital phase of acute myocardial infarction. Annu Rev Med 26:1–7, 1975

Wechsler D: Wechsler Adult Intelligence Scale—Revised. San Antonio, TX, Psychological Corporation, 1981

Weiss JH: Behavioral management of asthma, in Behavioral Approaches to Breathing Disorders. Edited by Tenemon BH, Ley R. New York, Plenum, 1994, pp 205–219

Wellens H, Cats B, Durren D: Symptomatic sinus node abnormalities following lithium carbonate therapy. Am J Med 59:285–287, 1975

Wender PH, Kalm M: Prevalence of attention deficit disorder, a residual type, and other psychiatric disorders in patients with irritable colon syndrome. Am J Psychiatry 140:1579–1582, 1983

Wesseley S, Chalder T, Hirsch S, et al: Postinfectious fatigue: prospective cohort study in primary care. Lancet 345:1333–1138, 1995

West TPJ: A comparison: pre dialysis, post dialysis cognitive abilities. Dialysis and Transplantation 7:809–821, 1978

White DP, Douglas NJ, Pickett CK, et al: Sleep deprivation and the control of ventilation. Am Rev Respir Dis 128:984–986, 1983

Whitehead WE, Schuster MM: Gastrointestinal Disorders: Behavioral and Physiological Basis for Treatment. New York, Academic Press, 1985

Wilkinson G, Borsey DQ, Leslie P, et al: Psychiatric morbidity and social problems in patients with insulin-dependent diabetes mellitus. Br J Psychiatry 153:38–43, 1988

Williams RB, Lane JD, Kuhn CM, et al: Type A behavior and elevated physiological and neuroendocrine responses to cognitive tasks. Science 218:483–485, 1982

Williams RB, Barefoot JC, Califf RM, et al: Prognostic importance of social and economic resources among medically treated patients with angiographically documented coronary artery disease. JAMA 267:520–524, 1992

Wilson J, Kraus E, Bailas M, et al: Reversible sinus node abnormalities due to lithium carbonate therapy. N Engl J Med 294:1223–1224, 1976

Wolfe F, Smythe HA, Yunus MB, et al: The American College of Rheumatology 1990 criteria for classification of fibromyalgia: report of the multicenter criteria committee. Arthritis Rheum 33:160–172, 1990

Woods SW, Tesar GE, Murray GB, et al: Psychostimulant treatment of depressive disorders secondary to medical illness. J Clin Psychiatry 47:12–15, 1986

Yagnik PM, Cohen MM: Nervous system involvement, in Diagnosis and Management of Rheumatic Diseases, 2nd Edition. Edited by Katz WA. Philadelphia, PA, JB Lippincott, 1988, pp 220–223

Yellowlees PM, Alpers JH, Bowden JJ, et al: Psychiatric morbidity in patients with chronic airflow obstruction. Med J Aust 146:305–307, 1987

Young SJ, Alpers DH, Norland CC, et al: Psychiatric illness in irritable bowel syndrome: practical implications for the primary physician. Gastroenterology 70:162–166, 1976

Zielinski RJ, Roose SP, Devanand DP, et al: Cardiovascular complications of ECT in depressed patients with cardiac disease. Am J Psychiatry 150:904–909, 1993

Chapter 18

Surgery and Surgical Subspecialties

Robert O. Pasnau, M.D.
Fawzy I. Fawzy, M.D.
Christine E. Skotzko, M.D.
Thomas B. Strouse, M.D.
David K. Wellisch, Ph.D.
Alisa K. Hoffman, Ph.D.

In recent years, economic forces and changes in surgical technology have radically altered the hospital practice of general surgery. Examples include trends toward same-day admissions for planned surgical procedures, shortened hospitalization with management of complex medical regimens at home, and reliance on visiting nurses and home health care to replace hospital-based care. Technical advances, such as endoscopic procedures in lieu of open procedures, have shortened stays and reduced surgical morbidity (Phillips et al. 1993).

The effect of these changes on the patient's psychological experience of surgery is unknown. It is notable that these changes are occurring while the population grows older and is more likely to have medical diseases, two factors that independently strongly predict a vulnerability to a number of postsurgical psychiatric disorders (Lipowski 1992; Schor et al. 1992; Zisselman 1993).

In his definitive chapter on the surgical patient, Surman discussed the varied psychological problems of the surgical patient. He noted the important role that surgeons play in a patient's life:

> Two aspects of surgery speak to the reality and the excess meaning of the experience: 1. Surgery represents a decisive approach to the relief of pain and suffering. 2. Surgery involves a transference relationship with the patient in a role of heightened dependency and expectation. (Surman 1987, p. 69)

The purpose of psychiatric consultation and liaison in the management of surgical patients is to relieve emotional problems that either interfere with the impending operation or hamper convalescence. Psychiatric management is articulated with surgical treatment in order to help the patient through an otherwise difficult hospital stay. Because the aims of both surgeon and psychiatrist coincide, there should be no basic disagreement in patient management, yet without good communication and agreement of these goals, misunderstandings may occur.

General Principles

Preoperative Issues

Context of consultation. Jacobsen and Holland (1989) reported that presurgical psychiatric consultation is most commonly requested in three major areas:

1. When patients experience preoperative panic or are refusing surgery
2. When questions arise about perioperative management of patients who are taking psychotropic drugs
3. When concern exists about a patient's capacity to give informed consent or refusal

Preoperative anxiety and transient treatment refusal. The dynamic origins of preoperative anxiety include the importance of a person's history of trauma, expectations of loss versus gain at outcome of surgery, and identification with others who may have undergone similar procedures. Additionally, an array of psychological stressors are inherent in the surgical situation and affect most patients; these stressors include basic threats to bodily and psychic integrity, fears of the unknown, loss of identity and control, and fear of pain and death (Johnston 1980).

Preoperative panic or surgery refusal is estimated to occur in 5% of general surgery patients (Strain 1985). Frequently, these problems occur in patients with preexisting anxiety disorders or new-onset anxiety in the context of

serious illness. Management is directed at education, coordination of care, involvement of anesthesia personnel, and autonomy-enhancing behavioral techniques (such as self-guided relaxation exercises, effective pharmacological interventions, and efforts to introduce familiar persons into the medical setting).

Psychotropic medications. Several reviews emphasized the need for open and careful discussion between patient, surgeon, anesthesiologist, and psychiatrist of the risks and benefits of presurgical continuation or cessation of psychotropic drugs (Sedgwick et al. 1990). The appreciable psychiatric risks of discontinuing psychotropics in seriously ill patients are increasingly recognized. Therefore, many psychiatric patients should continue taking their psychotropic drugs until the time of surgery and should be carefully observed after surgery for medication interactions and emergent psychiatric symptoms. Abrupt discontinuation of maintenance psychotropic drugs can have adverse medical consequences, including malignant arrhythmias in vulnerable patients (Van Sweden 1988), withdrawal seizures (Shader and Greenblatt 1993), and a syndrome of cholinergic rebound (Dilsaver et al. 1983; Lawrence 1985).

Competency and informed consent. Few issues evoke more confusion among medical and surgical staff than a patient who refuses an apparently needed and reasonable procedure. In such a situation, a psychiatric consultation may represent the treating physician's wish to have the patient declared "incompetent," thus authorizing medical-surgical treatment over a patient's protests. Despite the general misunderstanding of the legal authority of psychiatrists in a medical setting in which the capacity to consent to or refuse treatment is at issue, the psychiatric consultant's role is extremely important in patient assessment and in facilitating good outcomes for patients and their caregivers.

True emergencies in which treatment refusal or competency is an issue are resolved de facto by Good Samaritan standards (e.g., emergency room resuscitation), by patients becoming too ill to protest, or when authorized surrogates intervene (such as individuals who possess a Durable Power of Attorney for Health Care).

In other circumstances in which a duly authorized surrogate decision maker is absent, the capacity to provide informed consent or refusal is a judicially determined issue. The psychiatrist must assess the entire situation, including the patient's current mental status and health beliefs. Following assessment, the consultant is usually able to offer valuable observations about the nature of the impasse and can help to resolve it without legal recourse or mutual dismissal of each other by patient and primary physician. Preservation of the possibility of appropriate medical treatment is an important goal.

When the surgeon and psychiatrist concur that it is appropriate to pursue judicial review of the patient's competency to consent to or to refuse a procedure or treatment, the psychiatrist must have already documented the patient's mental status examination focusing on the ingredients of capacity:

■ The consistent ability to communicate a choice
■ The capacity to demonstrate an understanding of relevant medical information, including risks and benefits
■ The capacity to appreciate the current situation and its consequences
■ The ability to manipulate information in a rational manner (Appelbaum and Grisso 1989; Hall and Ellman 1990)

A detailed description of how the patient demonstrates or fails to demonstrate these elements, with examples, should appear in the consultation report. A concise differential psychiatric diagnosis and the actual or expected

results of psychiatric treatment, when relevant, are also critical. The psychiatrist's report is expert testimony that is commonly used in the judicial review. Sufficient detail and clarity in the consultation can obviate a personal court appearance by the psychiatrist.

Psychiatric Morbidity in Postsurgical Patients

Mental disorders secondary to medical treatment or substances of abuse. Medical and substance-induced mental disorders are commonly diagnosed postoperatively in surgical patients. Most frequent among these is delirium, with a prevalence in prospectively studied surgical patients ranging from 7% to 15% (Golinger 1989; Lipowski 1992; Schor et al. 1992; Seymour and Vaz 1989; Zisselman 1993). Withdrawal from alcohol and other substances is also commonly present and underdiagnosed. Immediate preoperative patient self-medication with alcohol was documented in approximately 11% of patients in a German series (Neukam et al. 1992). Nicotine withdrawal is also common (Fiore et al. 1992).

Other psychiatric disorders. A variety of other problems can also occur, including disruptive ward behavior (acting out), new-onset or recurrent depression, mania, anxiety symptoms, brief psychoses, intoxication with iatrogenic agents, acute posttraumatic stress disorder (PTSD), and others (Porter and Rosenthal 1993; Strain 1985; Surman 1987; Vieta et al. 1993). Several studies convincingly demonstrated lengthened stays, increased costs, and excess morbidity in general hospital patients with undiagnosed or inadequately treated psychiatric disorders (Lyons et al. 1986; Thomas et al. 1988; Verboskey et al. 1993).

Treatment Considerations

Formal psychotherapy on the surgical service is often difficult to engage in because of noise, interruptions, the postoperative medical regimen, lack of recognition among the staff of the importance of psychological concerns, and other factors. Nonetheless, even brief, focused meetings are valuable and are sometimes of crucial importance in the postsurgical management of patients with borderline and other primitive personality disorders. Behavioral interventions such as treatment contracts, relaxation techniques, and guided imagery are also valuable. The principles of interpersonal therapy, with a focus on the management of critical relationships (medical staff, visiting family) and boundaries, are sometimes useful.

Psychopharmacological interventions in postoperative patients are complicated by factors such as orders to give nothing by mouth, absent or compromised gastrointestinal (GI) absorption, emerging medical problems (e.g., perioperative myocardial infarction or stroke), or drug interactions that may compromise previous effective treatments. Therefore, the psychiatrist must perform a complete assessment of the patient's postoperative physical and mental status before recommending psychopharmacological intervention and then communicate recommendations in a clear and understandable way to surgical and nursing staff. This often requires education of colleagues about the nature, course, and contemporary strategies of treatment of psychiatric disorders. Antidepressants are the only psychotropic drugs that are not clearly safe and effective when administered via parenteral routes. (Psychopharmacology is discussed in detail in Jachna et al., Chapter 30, in this volume.)

Electroconvulsive therapy (ECT) is sometimes the only viable treatment for patients on the surgical service who have major affective disorders. Such patients may have permanent GI malabsorption or other problems that make effective oral antidepressant therapy impossible. Although amitriptyline is occasionally administered intravenously, it is logistically awkward, requires cardiac monitoring, and has unproven effectiveness (Enowitch 1984;

Krebs-Roubicek et al. 1981). Sublingual methylphenidate is sometimes useful as a temporizing measure; however, it is not a definitive long-term treatment for patients with major depression. Promising nonpharmacological somatic treatments, such as therapeutic sleep deprivation and phototherapy, have not been studied in medically ill populations and are impractical in the general hospital. (ECT is discussed in detail in Beale and Kellner, Chapter 32, in this volume.)

Psychiatric consultants are sometimes asked to play a role in acute pain management, particularly when the patient is dissatisfied with previous pain management efforts, has an identified or suspected psychiatric history, is a suspected substance abuser, or is responding "atypically" to pain management (Carr et al. 1992). Because pain is a subjective somatosensory experience, staff doubtfulness about the patient's self-report carries the risk of significant undertreatment and unnecessary suffering. In such situations, the psychiatrist has multiple tasks: to form an alliance that helps to restore the patient's credibility with the treatment team; to make an intelligible psychiatric diagnosis; to comment on the potential interplay between psychiatric factors and the patient's pain experience; and to help minimize acting out among all involved parties. Of value are rational pharmacotherapy (France and Krishnan 1988), relaxation techniques, appropriate education about the psychiatric diagnosis, autonomy-enhancing interventions such as patient-controlled analgesia (the PCA pump) (Chapman 1992; Gil et al. 1990; Voulgari et al. 1991), and assiduous attention to improve communication between the patient and the treatment team. These issues are particularly relevant to the management of burn victims and patients hospitalized for head and neck surgery (both patient populations are discussed later in this chapter). (See Bouckoms, Chapter 31 in this volume, for a more extensive discussion of pain management.)

CARDIOTHORACIC SURGERY

The patient who faces cardiovascular surgery usually has a life-threatening illness, and the surgery itself carries a risk of death or morbidity. Technology such as the intra-aortic balloon pump (IABP) permits medical support of patients through illnesses that were once fatal. These factors create a setting in which prompt, focused consultation can dramatically affect outcome and reduce costs (Lazarus and Hagens 1968; Mumford et al. 1982; Surman et al. 1974).

Preoperative Issues

Competency and compliance. Consultation on competency to consent is usually related to preexisting psychiatric disorders or to secondary conditions such as delirium. (The factors that are relevant to competency are discussed in detail in Simon, Chapter 6, in this volume.) It is important to remember that statutes and procedures vary from state to state. When faced with the possibility of the death of a very ill patient, physicians will often look to family members for consent. In dire circumstances in an unresponsive patient, in which immediate surgical intervention is required and/or in which death may be imminent, consent will often be presumed.

Another common consultation question, relative to both inpatients and outpatients, is whether a patient's future compliance with medications can be predicted. Valve replacement surgery and organ transplantation are areas in which concerns about patient compliance with treatment and medication regimens are especially important. Noncompliance may result in graft failure and death. If postoperative noncompliance is likely, the psychiatrist can communicate this to the surgeon, so that the surgeon can place a valvular prosthesis that does not require the patient to take anticoagulants postoperatively; this reduces such a patient's risk of future stroke or death.

Preoperative anxiety. Contemplating impending cardiac surgery can cause significant anxiety for an individual or family. The symbolic importance of the heart and concerns when it is "broken" may foster additional discomfort.

The agitated patient. During the assessment of an agitated patient, it is important to ascertain whether a worsening medical condition is causing delirium or another disorder. Often, the underlying cardiothoracic process impairs circulation or oxygenation, putting other organs at risk for dysfunction and increasing the risk for delirium. It is important for the psychiatric consultant to determine whether a psychiatric disorder, a central nervous system (CNS) disorder, or personality traits are contributing to the clinical picture. Interventions include altering the treatment environment, eliminating toxic drugs, and maximizing patient comfort (Tesar and Stern 1986).

Another potential cause of agitation is antiemetic medication. Akathisia and other extrapyramidal side effects are often unrecognized as being caused by antiemetics such as metoclopramide, prochlorperazine, and droperidol.

Inadequate pain control is another potential cause of agitation. This is sometimes related to the patient's reluctance to inform the staff of increasing discomfort, problems in communication when a patient is on a ventilator, or inadequate dosing; in general, physicians underestimate analgesic requirements and overestimate the duration of analgesic action. Pain is most effectively treated with regular rather than as-needed dosing of analgesics.

Fear of impending surgery or uncertainty regarding outcome must also be considered in the agitated patient. If discussion does not alleviate the patient's distress, benzodiazepines may be helpful. When panic is evident, a low dose of a high-potency neuroleptic is recommended.

Cardiac assist devices. Cardiac assist devices are generally used for individuals with cardiogenic shock to support circulation to the body and prevent irreparable harm to other organ systems and the heart. These devices are used until a corrective procedure is performed or until the heart regains sufficient function. These devices include the IABP, left-ventricular assist device (LVAD), right-ventricular assist device (RVAD), extracorporeal membrane oxygenation (ECMO) device, and total artificial heart (TAH). The nature of an assist device requires that patients lie quietly, because interruption of blood flow or loosening of an attachment may result in extensive bleeding and death. For this reason, with the exception of the IABP, patients are kept heavily sedated and paralyzed. Numerous risks are associated with use of any assist devices, including infection, bleeding, and embolization.

After the initial healing period, patients with TAH and certain ventricular assist devices are allowed to awaken and actually may become ambulatory (Hravnak and George 1989; Ruzevich et al. 1990). Psychiatric assessment and support are often helpful during this period. Delirium, as expected, is common in this group, as is subtle neuropsychological and neurological impairment.

In assessing an agitated patient who has an IABP, it is necessary to ascertain whether the underlying difficulty is related to pain, to delirium, to frustration, or to other factors. Individuals may require intubation to maintain oxygenation, which makes assessment and communication even more difficult. Complaints of pain are quite common and are often attributed to position. Extension of the leg in which the device is inserted is imperative for adequate hemodynamic function. Prior back injuries and degenerative disk disease may be sources of excruciating discomfort. The incidence of delirium is reportedly as high as 34% for individuals on an IABP (Sanders et al. 1992). High-dose intravenous haloperidol is reportedly safe in the treatment of patients with agitated delirium (Tesar and Stern 1988) and is reportedly efficacious in combination with benzodiazepines in managing patients on an IABP (Sanders et al. 1992). In individuals with a history of dilated cardiomyopathy and alcohol abuse, haloperidol may present a risk of arrhythmia (Metzger and Friedman 1993) and must therefore be used with care in this population. Because most acutely ill cardiac patients occupy a monitored bed, following conduction intervals on routine electrocardiograms is recommended (Rosenbaum 1980).

Perioperative Issues

Confusion and agitation. In the immediate postoperative period, the majority of patients who have had cardiothoracic surgery are placed in an intensive care unit for close observation of vital signs and continuing assessment for blood loss. During the recovery process, anesthesia gradually wears off and members of the staff observe the patient for evidence of alertness. Depending on the surgery and the patient's condition, extubation is usually performed within a relatively short time after surgery. It is during this perioperative period that postanesthesia confusion may develop. In patients who have undergone major cardiac procedures, this state may persist to and may extend beyond the third postoperative day and may progress to postcardiotomy delirium (PCD).

Dubin and colleagues (1979, p. 586) concluded that "cardiac status, the severity of physical illness, the complexity of the surgical procedure, and preoperative organic brain disease are the determining factors in PCD." These same factors guide assessment today.

Delirium is reported in up to 70% of postcardiotomy patients (Hazan 1966; Mravinac 1991). As expected, the risk for delirium is increased in elderly patients undergoing valve replacement (Heller et al. 1970). Breuer et al. (1983) reported that postoperative IABP and pressor agents were significantly associated with prolonged PCD.

When assessing any patient for PCD, all clinical parameters should be examined: the patient, vital signs, laboratory data (preoperative and postoperative), and medications received. Medications such as midazolam and morphine—often given in the intensive care unit to quiet restless patients—can perpetuate and exacerbate the delirium. As noted above, high-potency neuroleptics are safe and effective to use in controlling agitation and do not contribute to the confusion (Sos and Cassem 1980; Tesar and Stern 1986, 1988). As for any patient in the intensive care unit, reorientation, reassurance, and explanation of procedures sometimes help to limit behavioral problems in patients who have undergone cardiotomy (Sadler 1981). These measures may also limit the need for pharmacotherapy.

Substance withdrawal. Observation during the perioperative period for substance withdrawal is imperative. Withdrawal from substances of abuse such as alcohol, benzodiazepines, narcotics, and barbiturates can cause hyperthermia, hypertension or hypotension, seizures, hallucinations, changes in respiratory rate, and delirium. These symptoms are sometimes misdiagnosed as surgical complications, and their occurrence may increase morbidity (e.g., when a confused patient pulls out an IABP). Prompt recognition and treatment of substance withdrawal can prevent unnecessary and expensive tests and harm or death.

Pain control. Analgesia must be individually tailored because patients do not respond uniformly to pain medication. It is imperative to assess the patient's underlying mental state because delirium with associated agitation in an intubated patient is sometimes mistaken for pain and treated incorrectly. Similarly, anxiety should be treated with appropriate reassurance and anxiolytics.

Ventilator weaning. Weaning causes dyspnea, which may result in anxiety, fear, helplessness, loss of vitality, and preoccupation with shortness of breath (DeVito 1990). Air hunger, either on or off the ventilator, is exacerbated by anxiety and fear. The outward manifestations of fear can lead to overmedication with sedatives and narcotics, contributing to difficulty maintaining an airway and preventing adequate oxygenation. Assessment for anxiety and delirium and recommendations for appropriate pharmacotherapy are of invaluable help in these cases.

For the patient who is having difficulty weaning, there are several prerequisites for success. Respiratory factors include adequate respiratory muscle strength, oxygenation, ventilatory demand, and work of breathing. Other important factors include adequate cardiac function, oxygen transport capacity, metabolic parameters, fluid balance, nutritional status, mental state, and psychological readiness (Henneman 1991; Knebel 1991). Psychological readiness involves fears and concerns that result from weaning trials (such as when a patient tires during a trial and, as a consequence, cannot complete the weaning process).

There are a variety of pharmacological approaches to decreasing anxiety during weaning. These include low-dose benzodiazepines and neuroleptics (Cassem and Hackett 1978). Progressive relaxation and focused biofeedback (Acosta 1988; Holliday and Hyers 1990) and hypnosis (Bowen 1989) provide alternatives. Often neglected during evaluation is inquiry into sleep hygiene. Disturbed sleep can leave the patient exhausted and ill-equipped to handle the physical and emotional challenge of weaning.

Successful weaning in some individuals requires a significant amount of time and patience. These commodities are sometimes in short supply in the fast-paced world of the cardiothoracic intensive care unit. Reassurance to staff and patient, as well as tracking performance using behavioral techniques such as a wall chart, can demonstrate daily progress for both patient and staff.

Postoperative Issues

Neuropsychological changes. Possible neurological complications during the postoperative period range from a catastrophic cerebrovascular accident to subtle cognitive changes. Risk factors for impairment are similar to those for PCD and include a patient's baseline condition, intraoperative factors, and rate of recovery. Some patients report preoperative cognitive disturbances. These may result from microemboli caused by a diseased valve or chronic atrial fibrillation (Kimball 1972; Middlekauff et al. 1991). Long-standing cardiac dysfunction such as arrhythmia, hypotension, congestive failure, and asystolic arrest may also cause subtle CNS dysfunction.

Depression and return to function. The prevalence of depression in patients who have had coronary artery bypass grafts (CABGs) averages around 25%. Major cardiac surgery often causes a significant disruption in an individual's view of self and the future. The need to make dietary and lifestyle changes may be additional perturbing factors. When one considers the prevalence of subtle cognitive impairment postoperatively and the evidence of electroencephalographic changes postoperatively—changes that seem lateralized to the left hemisphere—postcardiotomy depression is likely attributable to subtle brain injury in a susceptible individual (Witoszka et al. 1973; Zeitlhoffer et al. 1988).

Predictors for return to work after cardiotomy have been identified. An individual's expectations are strong predictors of "return to work" rates. Educational level and family income were stronger predictors than occupation or level of physical exertion required (Stanton et al. 1983).

Valve replacement. Chief among the complaints of individuals who have undergone me-

chanical valve replacement is the noise. Mechanical valves reportedly cause annoyance, disrupt sleep of both the patient and the partner, disrupt concentration, and are a source of social embarrassment for some individuals (Limb et al. 1992). These difficulties are described as more troublesome for younger individuals and women. One group of researchers found that these complaints are related to the audibility of the measured sounds from the valves (Moritz et al. 1992). Other individuals described a feeling of comfort or soothing from the regular monotonous tones but acknowledged alarm when skipped beats or an accelerated heart rate occurred.

Automatic implantable cardiac defibrillation. Individuals with sustained ventricular tachycardia unresponsive to medication or ablation are often advised to undergo implantation of an automatic implantable cardiac defibrillator (AICD). This device contains a computer that senses the heart rate and delivers an electrical shock when the heart rate reaches a preset level. The device is intended to prevent sudden death by providing immediate defibrillation—before extensive damage is done to the myocardium by the abnormal rhythm. The frequency and number of shocks delivered depend on the individual.

Implantation of these devices is associated with generalized anxiety disorder and sexual dysfunction. In addition, during a shock, the current is conducted through physical contact to another individual. Studies are under way to assess the effect of these devices on quality of life.

ORTHOPEDIC SURGERY

Psychiatric consultation for hospitalized orthopedic patients has positive effects. Following consultation, patients report improvement in their sense of well-being, the quality of their medical care, and their physical outcome. It has also been demonstrated that psychiatric consultation helps to reduce medical costs.

Delirium

Postoperative delirium has been identified as a significant problem in elderly patients undergoing total hip replacement, with the prevalence reaching 25% of these patients (Millar 1981; Sheppeard et al. 1980; Titchener et al. 1958). Multiple etiologies for postoperative delirium have been postulated, including age, preoperative cognitive deficit, magnitude of the surgery, anesthesia, sleep deprivation, and sensory deprivation. A number of preoperative and postoperative interventions—consisting of short therapeutic sessions, education/information about what could be expected to happen, relaxation exercises, and even discussion of possible postoperative delirium—seemed to decrease the incidence or at least the effect of the delirium (Rogers and Reich 1986).

Borderline Personality Disorder

Psychiatric consultants who deal with patients with borderline personality disorder should actively promote a behavioral management program that includes 1) clear communication with the patient and among the staff; 2) understanding the patient's need for the constant attention of personnel; 3) dealing with the patient's entitlement without confronting the patient's needed defenses; and 4) setting firm limits on the patient's dependency, manipulative behavior, rage, and self-destructive behaviors. The consultant should also assist the staff in diminishing the patient's fearfulness, feelings of helplessness, and any other complications that might impair the treatment team relationship (Groves 1975).

Chronic Pain

Narcotic analgesics are often included in standard treatment regimens, and a consultant should determine whether the patient has any history of substance abuse or other addictive behavior before such drugs are given. Alternative pain management methods should be considered for all patients with pain but may be especially important for the patient with chronic orthopedic pain who abuses substances. Such alternative methods are frequently quite effective and may be used in combination with each other and with pain medication. Manual or electrical massage and transcutaneous electronic nerve stimulation (TENS) may be used to stimulate mechanoreceptors, which release a synaptic transmitter (an endorphin). These techniques may produce pain relief for up to 6 hours. Massage may also increase blood flow, relax muscles, and improve muscle tone (Paterson and Burn 1985). Other alternative methods include applications of moist or dry heat, cold applications, injection of lidocaine at trigger points, injection of steroids in some joints, supports and/or braces, acupuncture, traction, physical therapy, and corrective surgery. Behavioral techniques include relaxation exercises, guided imagery, hypnosis, and biofeedback. These techniques may also serve to give patients some sense of control over their situation, thereby further decreasing levels of depression and anxiety, which again may decrease their perception of pain.

Substance Abuse

Orthopedic patients found to have substance abuse problems need careful evaluation to determine etiological factors. Did the substance abuse predate the orthopedic injury, or did it result from a chronic pain syndrome? Preexisting conditions should be dealt with in the same manner used with any other substance abusing patient. Patients with chronic pain conditions require a more aggressive approach to pain management, utilizing alternative pain control methods (e.g., relaxation, hypnosis, acupuncture, nerve blocks), as noted above. However, significant attention must be paid to rehabilitation in regard to the substance abuse.

OPHTHALMOLOGY

Usually there is no hesitation in referring to the psychiatric consultant patients who have an obvious disturbance, such as psychotic episodes and delirium (sometimes agitated by sensory deprivation or the "black patch psychosis") or when loss of vision occurs in the absence of a recognizable organic disease. However, the ophthalmologist may not know when to refer a patient who has sustained acute, partial, or total loss of vision.

Vision Loss in Children

Children who experience vision loss manifest two common responses. The first is a neurobehavioral reaction that is best interpreted as a behavioral adaptation to poor vision. The second response affects personality development by limiting social and cognitive growth. The neurobehavioral reaction is often misinterpreted by adults as a conscious attempt to misbehave. However, it is important to note that many behaviors are specific to disease states and can be addressed as such. Developmental disturbances such as delayed mobility and confusion of "I" and "you" pronouns have been noted in vision-impaired children. Often, children experience a combination of symptoms. For example, patients whose vision loss accompanies hearing loss require special rehabilitation and attention. A grieving process will sometimes continue for a long time as the child and parents compare abilities with those of children with normal sight through the many developmental stages of life.

Acute Vision Loss in Adults

Acute vision loss often results in a full grieving process. Long-standing or permanent blindness may result in depression and social isolation. A patient may experience personality changes, low motivation (in an otherwise highly motivated person), and communication problems (with the patient having lost the ability to note the emotional facial expressions of others). Good (1993) suggested that immediate interventions can minimize the impact of vision loss—for example, the provision of reading machines, guide dogs, low-vision aids, Braille instruction, and/or companionship. Introducing these aids as soon as possible reduces the amount of social isolation, desperation, and depression felt by these patients.

Visual hallucinations, although they are more common in visually impaired patients, should be carefully monitored in any patient with an ophthalmological problem because such hallucinations could be signs of a mental illness or of an organic brain disease. Perceptual disorders (such as a distortion of size and shape) or palinopsia (a visual hallucination that is characterized by the persistence of an image after its removal) may occur.

Lifestyle changes almost always accompany loss of vision; these changes, which may include loss of work and social activities, can be quite devastating for patients, and in fact may be of more importance than the disease process itself. Generally, children cope better than adults with lifestyle changes because they are more open to learning compensatory strategies.

So much of human communication involves eye contact that its loss has a great psychological effect on both the patient and the caregiver. Compared with other types of wounds, eye injuries often cause countertransference and transference reactions in people (patient, caregiver, attending physician), with the characteristics of these responses determined by the specific personalities involved.

Neuropsychiatric Aspects of Blindness

The neuropsychiatric (functional) form of vision loss is usually diagnosed when sight failure occurs in the absence of a physical explanation. Psychiatric examples include sociopathy or malingering, depression, tunnel vision among conversion disorder patients, hysteria, possible child abuse, or other affective disturbances.

Trauma to the eye can also alert an ophthalmologist to the need for a psychiatric consultation. Childhood situations such as poorly supervised play, abuse, sports-related injuries, and low socioeconomic status are considered risk factors for eye trauma. More dramatic examples include suicide attempts (such as gunshot wounds), when precautions and psychiatric care become paramount, and the "shaken baby syndrome," which may cause retinal blood vessels to rupture. Autoenucleation, or the attempted removal of one's own eye, is almost always associated with schizophrenia or severe psychiatric disorders and must be addressed as carefully as the eye injury (Good 1993).

Various topical ophthalmic medications, when absorbed systemically, may cause psychiatric problems. For instance, β-blockers used to treat glaucoma may cause depression (with symptoms ranging from mild dysphoria to anergia to suicidal ideation), hallucinations, lethargy, confusion, and impotence. Topical anticholinergics, used to provide surgical exposure and visibility, can result in diminished salivation, increased heart rate, GI disturbances, and changes in activity levels (ranging from drowsiness to transient attention deficit with hyperactivity); transient delirium may even occur. These reactions are more likely to occur in children, yet in this population they are also more likely to be missed or ignored because children may not vocalize complaints of experiencing these symptoms.

The psychiatrist must be aware of ophthalmic complications of various psychotropic medications. Some drugs with anticholinergic effects, such as tricyclic antidepressants and neuroleptics, may produce acute-angle closure glaucoma. An ophthalmic consultation is required in any psychiatric patient with a glaucoma history who is a candidate for these medications.

Blindness can occur in patients who take thioridazine at doses greater than 800 mg/day. Doses at this level should be avoided, and patients who receive 600 mg/day should have eye examinations every 6 months. Chlorpromazine can cause anterior cataracts. Lithium toxicity can cause gaze-evoked nystagmus and occasionally downbeat nystagmus, fast eye movements, oculogyric crisis, and opsoclonia. Neuroleptic drugs may also cause oculogyric crisis, which can be treated with anticholinergic medications; however, the anticholinergics may in turn result in blurred vision.

Some potential drug interactions should be noted. Ophthalmic β-blockers (such as timolol and betaxolol) may react with phenothiazines. The simultaneous use of propranolol and chlorpromazine or thioridazine results in serum elevations of the β-blocker and the neuroleptic. When calcium channel blockers are used with topical β-blockers, conduction defects, heart failure, and hypotension may result.

BURN UNITS

The role of the consultation psychiatrist on the burn unit and after hospitalization can be linked to three important phases in the care and management of the patient who has sustained burns: 1) the acute phase, 2) the reconstructive phase, and 3) the long-term adjustment phase (Welch 1987).

Acute Phase

During the first 24–72 hours after the burn occurs, the patient experiences a period of initial lucidity. This period offers the psychiatric consultant an opportunity to assess the patient's history, personality dynamics, and coping patterns. A high percentage of burn patients have important predisposing factors for burn injuries, such as alcoholism, cognitive degeneration or dementia in elderly patients, chronic mental illness, family dysfunction, or, in the case of burned children, frank neglect. In one study, MacArthur and Moore (1975) showed that 59% of men and 38% of women with burn injuries have a combination of such factors.

After the initial phase of lucidity, between 30% and 70% of burn patients develop delirium, presumably caused by stress and burn-induced metabolic disturbances (Andreasen et al. 1977). Both chlorpromazine and haloperidol have been recommended to treat burn patients with delirium. Haloperidol is usually administered in doses from 1 to 5 mg iv as a bolus, with a total dose as high as 185 mg over a 24-hour period (Cassem and Sos 1980). Chlorpromazine is also given intravenously, with 100 mg given in 100 cc of normal saline infused over 15–30 minutes. With either drug, the initial loading dose should be given at 30-minute intervals until sedation is achieved. To maintain sedation, half the total induction dose is given every 12 hours (Welch 1987).

Pain management is a crucial area of intervention for the consultation psychiatrist. Although pain is a chronic issue for the patient with a burn injury, it becomes most acute during dressing changes and debridement. The most commonly used intravenous analgesics include morphine, meperidine, methadone, and fentanyl. Each of these agents has advantages and disadvantages; dosages are highly variable from patient to patient. Because of its fast onset and short duration of action, fentanyl is recommended before dressing changes and debridement (Welch 1987).

Two major psychological issues must be addressed during this period: denial and education. Psychiatrists who are experienced in burn unit work attest to the rapid alteration between a patient's request for more information and profound denial. This rapid shifting between the two poles often confuses the family and confounds the staff. Experience has shown that it is not wise, if not unkind, to attempt to dispel denial, especially early on. On the other hand, direct questions should be answered kindly but directly. This includes the answer to

the question "Will I die?", even if the patient is in extremis.

Reconstructive Phase

The reconstructive phase extends from the end of acute surgical intervention and delirium up to discharge from the unit. Thus, this period may last for weeks or months, depending on the extent of the burn and the pace of the recovery. Because the patient is now able to face the implications of the event with clear cognitive acuity, this phase is the most psychologically difficult. However, the patient's physical problems also continue, including the pain associated with physical therapy and dressing changes. During this phase, the psychiatrist must be prepared to deal with grief, facilitate affective expression, and intervene in the management of regression.

Long-Term Adjustment Phase

Despite significant emotional distress in this phase, patients often experience difficulty engaging in psychotherapy or communicating with their families. The psychological goal is to encourage good coping.

Based on the work of Weisman and Sobel (1979), we suggest that clinicians use the following approach for patients with burn injuries:

1. Identify the primary feelings about the burn experience without making this the exclusive focus of the therapy.
2. Define a hierarchy of problems facing the patient.
3. Define a hierarchy of desired goals and solutions using a problem-solving/cognitive approach.
4. Continue to work with flexibility on the above goals while addressing other issues that worry or concern the patient.

We believe that this active-confrontational, problem-solving approach is an active ingredient in prevention of depression.

HEAD AND NECK SURGERY

Psychiatric Contraindications to Surgery

Unlike for transplant operations, the indications or contraindications for disfiguring surgeries are primarily based on medical considerations. Most head and neck cancer patients adjust to and cope very well with severely disfiguring surgeries in the service of saving their lives. However, a recent study showed that 18% of the patients reported that the disadvantages outweighed the advantages (Gamba et al. 1992). These patients responded with statements such as "I no longer recognize myself" and "I look like a monster" (Gamba et al. 1992, p. 220). For this group, survival from the cancer was less important than having a certain appearance. This finding led the authors to propose that the best way to help a patient prepare for surgery is through education. This should include discussion about how daily life functions—such as swallowing, tasting, hearing, smelling, seeing, and eating—may be altered. In addition, information about expected energy level and psychological reactions, such as depression and anxiety, should be included. Finally, presurgery education should include preparing the patient for the possibility of a psychosis or delirium.

It is very helpful for the patient to meet a person who is well adjusted after going through a similar operation. This makes the important point that people can adjust well to the procedure; in fact, one study showed that more than 86% of the head and neck patients adjusted functionally to their disfigurement. One-third of these patients had visible disfigurement as a result of surgical treatment (West 1977). A crucial ingredient in preventing untoward emotional reactions is the support that patients receive from the family and treatment team, both preoperatively and postsurgically.

Psychiatric Disorders

A patient who has previously had a psychiatric disorder is at increased risk of developing a psychiatric illness after disfiguring surgery. Psychopathology also affects the patient's ability to cope with surgery. Breitbart and Holland (1988) noted that a preexisting anxiety disorder constituted a major impediment to treatment and rehabilitation for patients with head and neck cancer.

It is not unusual for patients to experience mild depression and/or anxiety; however, a major depression or an anxiety disorder may develop. Diagnosing depression is complicated when a patient already has difficulty with sleep and appetite; these are key vegetative signs of depression. Other signs to look for, specifically with patients who will or who have had surgery for head and neck cancer, include

- Excessive dependency
- Anger
- Social withdrawal (demonstrated, for example, by very little eye contact, avoiding family gatherings)
- Feelings of hopelessness and helplessness
- Excessive pain complaints
- Noncompliance with treatment

The psychiatrist should also look for subtle, nonverbal cues revealed in gestures and expressions to detect the patient's mood following disfiguring surgical procedures.

Anxiety is also a very significant problem in patients who are disfigured. Many factors contribute to anxiety in patients who are adjusting to disfigurement. If patients were involved in an accident, an anxiety reaction to that specific trauma usually occurs, as well as anxiety about their appearance.

Many symptoms are associated with anxiety besides feeling anxious or as if one were "falling apart." Anxiety can lead to distortion of body change and body image. Patients can perceive disfigurement as much worse than it is, which can cause further isolation, depression, and anxiety.

There are several helpful interventions for anxiety. Early interventions in the postoperative period include relaxation training, guided imagery, and desensitization. A combination of imagery plus desensitization can help the patient to master fears and to learn how to relax. Cognitive restructuring is another way to reduce anxiety. With this intervention, patients measure their cognitions to determine whether they are accurate and, if not, restructure them to become less stress-inducing. Pharmacological interventions are helpful for patients who are too anxious to engage in these exercises, or for patients who are sleepless and unable to concentrate because of their anxiety symptoms.

An altered mental status is a common postoperative occurrence in patients who have had head and neck surgery. Mild disorientation, confusion, illusions, or hallucinations may represent conditions caused by sensory overload, sensory deprivation, sleep deprivation, or the shock of extremely threatening events. Adams et al. (1984), using bedside testing, found that a high percentage of patients who had been labeled as "depressed" by surgeons had substantial neuropsychological deficits.

Pain Control

Inadequate pain control contributes to increased levels of depression, pain, and anxiety, which, in turn, lead to even more increased pain. As is true with patients with burn injuries, as previously described in this chapter, we recommend that orders for pain medications be written with the provision that a "patient may decline (or defer) doses" rather than being written for as-needed dosing. This gives the patient some control, helps to provide comfort, and minimizes desperation (Shapiro and Kornfeld 1987).

Reactions to Loss and Body Image Problems

Patients who undergo disfiguring surgery experience multiple losses. There are losses of function and abilities and of specific body parts, but most important, such patients experience losses of identity and self-image. The face is crucial to an individual's identity and self-image, and so a disfiguring surgery to the facial area carries the greatest risk of emotional devastation and subsequent depression. The fear of social reaction to a facial disfigurement may lead, at times, to social isolation, which further perpetuates depression. Shame underlies such self-isolation, which also worsens depression.

Sexuality is also seriously affected by alterations in body image. Although not specifically addressing persons with head and neck cancer, Grinker (1976) stated that the "dread of exposing oneself to one's spouse as crippled, damaged, incomplete or dying may cause sexual inhibition or abstinence" (p. 131). Intimacy and sexual bodily functions are also affected by shame and embarrassment (Grinker 1976). Open communication with the treatment team about sexuality, both before and after surgery, is usually helpful.

One of the main factors that influences patients' adjustment to changes in body is how accepted they feel. Perceived absence of social support undermines recovery. Orr et al. (1989) found that patients who perceived more social support (friends more than family) had a more positive body image, greater self-esteem, and less depression than those who had less social support. The first "social exposure" that the patient has following surgery or trauma is to the treatment team. Thus, social support and communication about sensitive patient issues, such as sexuality or shame related to body image, begin in the hospital milieu. Patient acceptance begins with staff members' ability to comfortably and effectively communicate within the staff-patient relationship.

Substance Withdrawal

Populations of patients with head and neck cancer have high rates of alcoholism and drug abuse (Shapiro and Kornfeld 1987). When alcohol intake is abruptly interrupted by trauma or surgery, withdrawal often occurs.

Staff Issues

A difficult aspect of working with disfigured patients is the reactions of the hospital staff. These patients can look grotesque, exude secretions constantly, and smell repulsive and are sometimes difficult to understand because of extensive facial bandaging. It is often difficult for staff members to remember that behind the tubes, the appearance, and the excretions lies a human being (Bronheim et al. 1991). Thus, it is all too easy to reduce contact and communication with such patients, setting up a cycle of avoidance. The psychiatric consultant is not immune to these feelings. More frequent therapeutic interviews of shorter duration help to prevent therapist burnout. Human contact is of vital importance to disfigured patients because they need to express and process feelings and to be reassured that they are not abandoned because of their disfigurement.

CONCLUSION

One of the psychiatrist's major tasks in working with surgical patients is establishing a relationship with the referring surgeon, who may or may not be knowledgeable about psychiatric issues. Surgeons vary considerably, as do all human beings, in their sensitivity to these factors. Some, who have written extensively in the surgical literature, are exquisitely aware of the psychological dimensions of patient care. Others, often at the beginning of their careers, are less likely to regard these issues as sufficiently important to take up valuable time. Thus, the first rule of consultation to surgery is "Know your surgeon."

REFERENCES

Acosta F: Biofeedback and progressive relaxation in weaning the anxious patient from the ventilator: a brief report. Heart Lung 17:299–301, 1988

Adams F, Larson DL, Goeptert H: Does the diagnosis in head and neck cancer mask organic brain disease? Otolaryngol Head Neck Surg 92:618–624, 1984

Andreasen NJ, Hartford CE, Knott JR, et al: EEG changes associated with burn delirium. Diseases of the Nervous System 38:27–31, 1977

Appelbaum PS, Grisso T: Assessing patients' capacities to consent to treatment. N Engl J Med 319:1635–1638, 1989

Bowen DE: Ventilator weaning through hypnosis. Psychosomatics 30:449–450, 1989

Breitbart W, Holland J: Psychosocial aspects of head and neck cancer. Semin Oncol 15:61–69, 1988

Breuer AC, Furlan AJ, Hanson MR, et al: Central nervous system complications of coronary artery bypass graft surgery: prospective analysis of 421 patients. Stroke 14:682–687, 1983

Bronheim H, Strain JA, Biller HF: Psychiatric aspects of head and neck surgery, part II: body image and psychiatric intervention. Gen Hosp Psychiatry 13:225–232, 1991

Carr DB, Jacox AK, Chapman CR, et al (Agency for Health Care Policy and Research Consensus Panel): Acute pain management: operative or medical procedures and trauma, part 2. Clin Pharmacokinet 11:391–412, 1992

Cassem NH, Hackett TP: The setting of intensive care, in Massachusetts General Hospital Handbook of General Hospital Psychiatry. Edited by Hackett TP, Cassem NH. St Louis, MO, CV Mosby, 1978, pp 319–341

Cassem NH, Sos J: The intravenous use of haloperidol for acute delirium in intensive care settings, in Psychic and Neurologic Dysfunctions After Open Heart Surgery. Edited by Speidel H, Rodewald G. Stuttgart, Germany, Georg Theive Verlag, 1980, pp 196–199

Chapman CR: Psychological aspects of postoperative pain control. Acta Anaesthiol Belg 43: 41–52, 1992

DeVito AJ: Dyspnea during hospitalizations for acute phase of illness as recalled by patients with chronic obstructive airway disease. Heart Lung 19:186–191, 1990

Dilsaver SC, Kronfol Z, Sackelaves JC: Antidepressant withdrawal syndrome: evidence supporting the cholinergic over-drive hypothesis. J Clin Psychopharmacol 3:157–164, 1983

Dubin WR, Field HL, Gastfriend DR: Postcardiotomy delirium: a critical review. J Thorac Cardiovasc Surg 77:586–594, 1979

Enowitch BI: The treatment of depression: update 1984. Conn Med 48:703–706, 1984

Fiore MC, Jorenby DE, Baker TB, et al: Tobacco dependence and the nicotine patch: clinical guidelines for effective use. JAMA 268:2687–2694, 1992

France RD, Krishnan KRR: Psychotropic drugs in chronic pain, in Chronic Pain. Edited by France RD, Krishnan KRR. Washington, DC, American Psychiatric Association, 1988

Gamba A, Romano M, Grosso IM, et al: Psychosocial adjustment of patients surgically treated for head and neck cancer. Head Neck Surg 14:218–223, 1992

Gil KM, Ginsburg B, Muir M, et al: Patient-controlled analgesia in postoperative pain: the relation of psychological factors to pain and analgesic use. Clinical Journal of Pain 6:137–142, 1990

Golinger RC: Delirium in the surgical patient. Am Surg 55:549–551, 1989

Good WV: Ophthalmology, in Surgical Subspecialties and Trauma. Edited by Stoudemire A. New York, Oxford University Press, 1993, pp 829–838

Grinker RR: Sex and cancer. Medical Aspects of Human Sexuality 10:130–139, 1976

Groves JE: Management of the borderline patient on a medical or surgical ward: the psychiatric consultant's role. Int J Psychiatry Med 6:337–347, 1975

Hall MA, Ellman IM: The patient lacking decision-making capacity, in Health Care Law and Ethics. Edited by Hall MA, Ellman IM. Minneapolis, MN, West Publishing, 1990, pp 236–311

Hazan SJ: Psychiatric complications following cardiac surgery. J Thorac Cardiovasc Surg 51:307–319, 1966

Heller SS, Frank KA, Malm JR, et al: Psychiatric complications of open-heart surgery. N Engl J Med 283:1015–1020, 1970

Henneman EA: The art and science of weaning from mechanical ventilation. Focus on Critical Care 18:490–501, 1991

Holliday JE, Hyers TM: The reduction of weaning time from mechanical ventilation using tidal volume and relaxation biofeedback. Am Rev Respir Dis 141:1214–1220, 1990

Hravnak M, George E: Nursing considerations for the patient with a total artificial heart. Critical Care Nursing Clinics of North America 1:495–513, 1989

Jacobsen P, Holland JC: Psychological reactions to surgery, in Handbook of Psychooncology. Edited by Holland JC, Rowland JH. New York, Oxford University Press, 1989, pp 117–133

Johnston M: Anxiety in surgical patients. Psychol Med 10:145–152, 1980

Kimball CP: The experience of open heart surgery. Arch Gen Psychiatry 27:57–63, 1972

Knebel AR: Weaning from mechanical ventilation: current controversies. Heart Lung 20:321–334, 1991

Krebs-Roubicek E, Koebl J, Poeldinger W: Treatment of anxious depression with intravenous infusions of a combination of drugs. Agressologie 22:25–26, 1981

Lawrence JM: Reactions of withdrawal of antidepressants, antiparkinsonian drugs, and lithium. Psychosomatics 47:544–546, 1985

Lazarus HR, Hagens JH: Prevention of psychosis following open-heart surgery. Am J Psychiatry 124:1190–1195, 1968

Limb D, Kay PH, Murday AJ: Problems associated with mechanical heart valves. Eur J Cardiothorac Surg 6:618–620, 1992

Lipowski ZJ: Update on delirium. Psychiatr Clin North Am 15:335–346, 1992

Lyons JS, Hammer JS, Strain JJ, et al: The timing of psychiatric consultation in the general hospital and length of hospital stay. Gen Hosp Psychiatry 8:159–162, 1986

MacArthur JD, Moore FD: Epidemiology of burns. JAMA 231:259–263, 1975

Metzger E, Friedman R: Prolongation of the corrected QT and torsades de pointes cardiac arrhythmia associated with intravenous haloperidol in the medically ill. J Clin Psychopharmacol 13:128–132, 1993

Middlekauff HR, Stevenson WG, Stevenson WL: Prognostic significance of atrial fibrillation in advanced heart failure. Circulation 84:40–48, 1991

Millar HR: Psychiatric morbidity in elderly surgical patients. Br J Psychiatry 138:17–20, 1981

Moritz A, Steinseifer U, Kobinia G, et al: Closing sounds and related complaints after heart valve replacement with St Jude Medical, Duromedics Edwards, Bjork-Shiley Monostrut, and Carbomedics prosthesis. Br Heart J 67:460–465, 1992

Mravinac CM: Neurologic dysfunctions following cardiac surgery. Critical Care Nursing Clinics of North America 3:691–698, 1991

Mumford E, Schlesinger HJ, Glass GV: The effects of psychological intervention on recovery from surgery and heart attacks: an analysis of the literature. Am J Public Health 72:141–151, 1982

Neukam FW, Strauss J, Schliephake H, et al: Preoperative blood alcohol levels in patients hospitalized for prolonged surgical procedures. Klinik und Poliklinik fur Mund-, Kiefer- und Gesichtschirurgie Medizinische Hochschule Hannover 47:53–55, 1992

Orr DA, Reznikoff M, Smith GM: Body image, self-esteem, and depression in burn-injured adolescents and young adults. J Burn Care Rehabil 10:454–461, 1989

Paterson JK, Burn L: General considerations, in An Introduction to Medical Manipulation. Edited by Paterson JK, Burn L. Boston, MA, MTP Press Limited, 1985, pp 1–7

Phillips EH, Carroll BJ, Fallas MJ: Laparoscopically guided cholecystectomy: a detailed report of the first 453 cases performed by one surgical team. Am Surg 59:235–242, 1993

Porter KA, Rosenthal SH: Postoperative mania: a case report and review of the literature. Psychosomatics 34:171–173, 1993

Rogers M, Reich P: Psychological intervention with surgical patients: evaluation outcome. Adv Psychosom Med 15:23–50, 1986

Rosenbaum JF: Psychotropic drugs and the cardiac patient. Drug Ther 10:111–121, 1980

Ruzevich SA, Swartz MT, Reedy JE, et al: Retrospective analysis of the psychologic effects of mechanical circulatory support. J Heart Transplant 9:209–212, 1990

Sadler PD: Incidence, degree, and duration of post cardiotomy delirium. Heart Lung 10:1084–1092, 1981

Sanders KM, Stern TA, O'Gara PT, et al: Delirium during intra-aortic balloon pump therapy: incidence and management. Psychosomatics 33:35–44, 1992

Schor JD, Levkoff SE, Lipsitz LAZ, et al: Risk factors for delirium in hospitalized elderly. JAMA 267:827–831, 1992

Sedgwick JV, Lewis IH, Linter SP: Anesthesia and mental illness. Int J Psychiatry Med 20:209–225, 1990

Seymour DG, Vaz FG: A prospective study of elderly general surgical patients, II: postoperative complications. Age Ageing 18:316–326, 1989

Shader RJ, Greenblatt DJ: Use of benzodiazepines in anxiety disorders. N Engl J Med 328:1398–1405, 1993

Shapiro PA, Kornfeld DS: Psychiatric aspects of head and neck cancer surgery. Psychiatr Clin North Am 10:87–100, 1987

Sheppeard H, Cleak DK, Ward DJ, et al: A review of early mortality and morbidity in elderly patients following Charnley total hip replacement. Arch Orthop Trauma Surg 97:243–248, 1980

Sos J, Cassem NH: Managing post-operative agitation. Drug Ther 10:103–106, 1980

Stanton BA, Jenkins CD, Denlinger P, et al: Predictors of employment status after cardiac surgery. JAMA 249:907–911, 1983

Strain JJ: The surgical patient, in Psychiatry, Vol 2. Edited by Michels R, Cazenar JO. Philadelphia, PA, JB Lippincott, 1985, pp 1–11

Surman OS: The surgical patient, in Massachusetts General Hospital Handbook of General Hospital Psychiatry, 2nd Edition. Edited by Hackett TP, Cassem NH. Littleton, MA, PSG Publishing, 1987, pp 69–83

Surman OS, Hackett TP, Silverberg EL, et al: Usefulness of psychiatric intervention in patients undergoing cardiac surgery. Arch Gen Psychiatry 30:830–835, 1974

Tesar GE, Stern TA: Evaluation and treatment of agitation in the intensive care unit. J Intensive Care Med 1:137–148, 1986

Tesar GE, Stern TA: Rapid tranquilization of the agitated intensive care unit patient. J Intensive Care Med 3:195–201, 1988

Thomas RI, Cameron DJ, Fahs MC: A prospective study of delirium and prolonged hospital stay: exploratory study. Arch Gen Psychiatry 45:937–940, 1988

Titchener J, Zwerling I, Gottschalk L, et al: Psychological reactions of the aged in surgery. Archives of Neurological Psychiatry 79:63–73, 1958

Van Sweden B: Rebound antidepressant cardiac arrhythmia. Biol Psychiatry 24:360–369, 1988

Verbosky LA, Franco KN, Zrull JP: The relationship between depression and length of stay in the general hospital patient. J Clin Psychiatry 54:177–181, 1993

Vieta E, De Pablo J, Cirera E, et al: Rapidly cycling bipolar II disorder following liver transplantation. Gen Hosp Psychiatry 15:129–131, 1993

Voulgari A, Lykouras L, Papnikolaou M, et al: Influence of psychological and clinical factors on postoperative pain and narcotic consumption. Psychother Psychosom 55:191–196, 1991

Weisman AD, Sobel HJ: Coping with cancer through self instruction: a hypothesis. Human Stress 5:3–8, 1979

Welch CA: Psychiatric care of the burn victim, in Massachusetts General Hospital Handbook of General Hospital Psychiatry, 2nd Edition. Edited by Hackett TP, Cassem NH. Littleton, MA, PSG Publishing, 1987, pp 438–447

West DW: Social adaptation patterns among cancer patients with facial disfigurements resulting from surgery. Arch Phys Med Rehabil 58:473–479, 1977

Witoszka MM, Tamura H, Ideglia R, et al: Electroencephalographic changes and complications in open heart surgery. J Thorac Cardiovasc Surg 66:855–864, 1973

Zeitlhoffer J, Saletu B, Anderer P, et al: Topographic brain mapping of EEG before and after open-heart surgery. Neuropsychobiology 20:51–56, 1988

Zisselman MH: Recognition and management of delirium in medical-surgical patients. New Dir Ment Health Serv 57:29–37, 1993

Chapter 19

Transplantation

Thomas B. Strouse, M.D.
Deane L. Wolcott, M.D.
Christine E. Skotzko, M.D.

The development of bone marrow and solid organ transplantation is one of the true triumphs of twentieth-century medicine. Clinically successful and widely utilized bone marrow and solid organ transplantation was developed during the 1970s and 1980s. Future biomedical developments will likely extend the clinically useful role of transplantation to organs for which transplantation is still experimental or rarely used (e.g., small bowel transplantation, multiple organ transplantation).

In the early 1990s, the potential limits to the role of organ transplantation in the health care system in the United States were increasingly clear. Although innovative and strenuous efforts are being made to increase the donor organ pool (e.g., living-related partial organ donation to children and even adults), it appears that donor organ availability will remain limited for the foreseeable future. In addition, the competition between organ transplantation and other health care services for financial re-

sources may restrict the growth of organ transplantation.

Organ transplant psychiatry (OTP) is a rapidly growing area of consultation-liaison clinical activity and research (Freeman et al. 1995). Clinically, the OTP specialist functions both as a provider of patient care and as a transplant team member. An OTP specialist now needs specific knowledge and skills even beyond those of the general consultation-liaison psychiatrist in order to optimally fulfill the clinical and transplant team membership roles.

The critical patient care roles of the OTP clinician include the diagnosis and treatment of psychiatric disorders in organ transplant candidates and recipients. OTP specialists are also commonly called on to participate in the transplant candidate evaluation and selection process, which raises multiple ethical, legal, scientific, and public policy concerns. OTP specialists are also often called on to assess past, current, and predicted future transplant candidate medical treatment regimen compliance and to help manage other interpersonal and social behaviors that may interfere with optimal patient-transplant team relationships. The psychiatric assessment and management of patients with dysfunctional personality traits or formal personality disorders, patients with substance abuse histories or ongoing patterns of substance abuse, and patients with acute liver failure after drug overdose (usually with acetaminophen) are common challenges faced by the OTP specialist.

The OTP specialist is called on also to fulfill many formal or informal functions as a member of the organ transplant team. The degree to which the psychiatrist is accepted as a member of the transplant team depends on the following factors: 1) his or her ability to communicate effectively and succinctly with other team members; 2) the extent to which his or her clinical judgment is trusted; 3) his or her ability to effectively defuse adverse reactions of transplant team members to patients—conflicts that can interfere with optimal team decision making and patient care; 4) his or her ability to work collaboratively and effectively with any other psychosocial services team members (e.g., medical social workers, psychologists); and 5) his or her effectiveness in providing a listening ear and informal support to distressed transplant team members.

BIOPSYCHOSOCIAL ASSESSMENT OF TRANSPLANT CANDIDATES AND LIVING RELATED DONORS

Team Concept

The complexity of solid organ transplantation requires that a multidisciplinary team participate in caring for transplant applicants, candidates, and recipients as well as for living donors. In the assessment phase, persons with life-threatening illnesses are screened for entrance into the transplant candidate pool.

The composition of the transplant selec-

tion team varies among centers. Almost all programs include internists and surgeons with specialization in the relevant organ system(s). Members of this group typically serve as gatekeepers, controlling the flow of patients into the evaluation phase.

Psychosocial data are important and are generally reviewed before the acceptance of an individual as a transplant candidate (Wolcott 1991) or living related donor. Interest in the use of psychosocial screening criteria has existed since the inception of organ transplantation with renal cadaveric and living donor transplantation (Eisendrath et al. 1969; Fellner 1971; Vidt 1971).

Consultation-liaison psychiatrists are exceptionally well suited to lead the clinical psychosocial assessment of applicants. Among the reasons for medical psychiatrists to coordinate psychosocial assessment is the potential for somatic symptoms of chronic illness to mimic symptoms of psychiatric illness (Mai 1987). Among the skills required of a team psychiatrist are competency in the assessment of substance abuse (including abstinence and relapse risk), character disorder, and the potential for unacceptable or undesirable psychosocial outcomes as well as skill in the diagnosis and treatment of primary versus secondary ("organic") psychiatric disorders.

Transplant centers commonly rely heavily on nursing coordinators to facilitate the patient's entry into the formal assessment phase. Coordinators ensure that all of the necessary screenings and assessments are performed. In addition, coordinators are involved in patient teaching, and they provide support to patients and family members.

Social work assessment of the patient's home environment, support system, disposition, and housing needs is common to most programs (Levenson and Olbrisch 1993b). Stability of marital relationship, availability of involved others, and financial and geographic resources are important factors to be considered.

TRANSPLANTATION ISSUES THAT FREQUENTLY LEAD TO PSYCHIATRIC CONSULTATION

Ethical Considerations

Despite annual increases in the numbers of organ transplants performed in the United States, potential recipients still outnumber donors (Surman 1989). Transplant selection committees provide local gatekeeping for the precious resource of donor organs and are thus inherently involved in a selection process based on ethical, psychosocial, and biomedical factors (Freeman et al. 1992; Jonsen 1989).

Both clinicians and observers of the transplant field are increasingly aware of the intertwining nature of medical, psychiatric, psychosocial, and ethical issues in the assessment of organ transplant candidates (Craven and Rodin 1992; Fox and Swazey 1992). This observation is not surprising because the tasks of psychosocial assessment require careful judgments about a patient's coping style, illness behavior, ability to form an alliance with the medical team, needs for emotional support, and financial and other material resources (Freeman et al. 1992; see Table 19–1). Beyond these tasks, psychosocial teams are called on to make complex predictions about posttransplant quality of life, the adequacy of family support systems, the impact of transplantation on preexisting psychiatric illness, and future compliance. It is generally agreed that psychosocial assessment should promote fairness, equal access, and the avoidance of harm to the patient (Lowy and Martin 1992). Frequently, however, mental health clinicians are aware of conflicts between the apparent wishes or best interests of the patient (e.g., life extension, receiving transplant) and the reasonable needs of the transplant program (e.g., for compliance, solid sobriety, or enthusiastic participation by the patient in treatment) (Gellman 1989; Murray 1989).

Are there ethical remedies to these inherent problems? Most authors conclude that psychosocial selection processes should include at minimum "informed consent" for patients—that is, a clear accounting of the purpose and use by the selection committee of psychosocial data (Lowy and Martin 1992). Surman and Purtillo (1992) and Wolcott (1990) stress the importance of developing scientifically valid, data-based criteria for exclusion. Loewy (1987) argues that committees should take care to avoid "social worth" considerations. Based in part on the Americans With Disabilities Act, Merrikin and Overcast (1987) discourage disqualification of patients because of mental conditions.

Evaluating Living Donors

Whole or partial organs donated by living relatives are an increasingly important source of

Table 19–1. Psychosocial screening criteria for solid organ transplantation

Absolute contraindications

Active substance abuse

Psychosis significantly limiting informed consent or compliance

Refusal of transplant and/or active suicidal ideation

Factitious disorder with physical symptoms

Relative contraindications

Dementia or other persistent cerebral dysfunction, if

- Adequate psychosocial resources to supervise compliance cannot be arranged OR
- Of a type known to correlate with high risk of adverse posttransplant neuropsychiatric outcome (e.g., alcohol dementia, frontal-lobe syndromes)

Treatment-refractory psychiatric illness, such as intractable, life-threatening mood disorder, schizophrenia, eating disorder, character disorder

Noncompliance with the transplant system, unwillingness to participate in necessary psychoeducational/psychiatric treatment tissue grafts. Living donors now account for about 20% of kidneys transplanted in the United States. The donation of partial organ segments, from both paired and single organ systems (lung, liver)—primarily by parents to children—is a growing transplant practice (Broelsch et al. 1990; Goldman 1993).

There are no standardized criteria for the assessment of potential living related organ donors. Nevertheless, many transplant centers involve psychiatrists in prospective patient screening. Potential donors should be assessed for the same standard ingredients of informed consent that apply in any other presurgical situation. However, in assessing potential donors, a variety of other areas are also important, including

- Family dynamics and the potential for coercion of a particular member into donating
- The implied obligation of the recipient of the "gift"
- Evolving family relationships and the potential for the donor to have magical beliefs that long-standing interpersonal problems will be healed by his or her donation
- Personal, cultural, or religious concerns about organ donation
- The potential for underlying psychopathology to be exacerbated by the psychobiological stress of donation

In the only available study of psychiatric outcomes in donors of partial liver segments, Goldman (1993) described 20 patients from the University of Chicago. Psychological outcomes appeared to parallel findings from the literature on kidney donors.

Rating Scales in Candidate Assessment

Two rating scales are available for the clinical assessment of psychosocial factors in transplant candidates: the Psychosocial Assessment of Candidates for Transplant (PACT), developed by Olbrisch and co-workers (1989), and the Transplantation Evaluation Rating Scale (TERS), developed by Twillman et al. (1993). Both scales include weighted ratings for psychiatric diagnoses, substance abuse, health behaviors, compliance, social support, prior coping, and disease-specific coping. The TERS also rates affective and mental states.

PSYCHIATRIC DISORDERS IN CANDIDATES FOR TRANSPLANTS

Patients With Cardiac Disease

Anxiety symptoms are often directly related to a patient's cardiac status. Kahn et al. (1987) reported that 83% of individuals with idiopathic cardiomyopathy had probable panic disorder versus 16% of individuals with postinfarction heart failure, rheumatic heart disease, or congenital heart disease. Wells et al. (1989) discovered a significantly greater degree of lifetime and recent anxiety disorders in persons with heart disease compared with a group of individuals with no chronic medical condition.

Freeman and colleagues (1988b) reported adjustment disorders in 25% of individuals who were seen before heart transplantation. Dysthymic disorder and organic mental disorder accounted for 4% of disorders in this population. Kuhn et al. (1990) reported adjustment disorders in 19% of candidates and neuropsychiatric syndromes in 12%. Despite the relatively low rate of frank delirium reported, other investigators have found evidence of cognitive impairment in a great percentage of candidates for heart transplant (Schall et al. 1989).

Patients With Pulmonary Disease

Patients who are candidates for single or double lung transplantation have serious limitations in daily functioning that are directly related to their underlying disease. Wells et al. (1989) examined the recent and lifetime prevalence of psychiatric disorders in a group of individuals with self-reported chronic lung disease and found that their lifetime risk for mood disorder, substance-related disorders, and anxiety disorder was significantly higher than that of a control group with no chronic medical condition. Kellner and co-workers (1992) found that the degree of dyspnea in patients with chronic pulmonary conditions was positively correlated with the degree of depression and anxiety.

Not surprisingly, when Craven (1990b) examined a consecutive series of applicants for lung transplantation, he found that 50% reported a history of psychiatric disorder. These disorders included organic brain syndrome (19%), major depression (16%), panic or anxiety disorder not otherwise specified (11%), and alcohol or other substance abuse (11%).

Patients With Liver Disease

Delirium, including hepatic encephalopathy, is the most common psychiatric disorder found in patients with liver disease both before and after transplantation. Trzepacz et al. (1989) found rates of hepatic encephalopathy approaching 20% in prospectively studied candidates for liver transplant at the University of Pittsburgh. "Subclinical" encephalopathy probably occurs at much higher rates (Trzepacz et al. 1988), although large-scale prospective studies that would document the incidence are not available. During the posttransplant period, the prevalence of delirium is also high. Although it is widely accepted that liver transplantation is associated with improvement in neuropsychological (Tarter et al. 1992) and neuropsychiatric functioning, secondary neuropsychiatric syndromes are diagnosed postoperatively in up to 33% of liver recipients (DeGroen and Craven 1992; DeGroen et al. 1987; Tollemar et al. 1988). Some patients have prolonged delirium that progresses to syndromes resembling dementia (DeGroen and Craven 1992).

Several primary psychiatric disorders have been reported in candidates for liver transplant. In the series described above, Trzepacz et al. (1989) found that 20% of candidates had current adjustment disorders, 4.5% had major depression, 9% met the criteria for alcohol abuse or alcohol dependence, and 2% met criteria for abuse of other substances.

Patients With Renal Disease

Major depression, as diagnosed with the Diagnostic Interview Schedule (Robins et al. 1981), was found in 8.1% of an unselected sample of 99 patients undergoing renal dialysis. Of these depressed patients, 50% had a history of major depression (Rodin and Voshart 1987); another 12% of patients met the criteria for past major depression only. Major depression has been described in as few as 5% (Smith et al. 1985) and as many as 22% (Lowry 1979) of patients undergoing dialysis. Cognitive problems and syndromes resembling dementia have been reported to be associated with chronic renal disease and dialysis (Alter et al. 1989; Nissenson et al. 1987). These disorders may reverse after renal transplant.

PSYCHIATRIC DISORDERS, THEIR RELATION TO SELECTION CRITERIA, AND PREDICTION OF OUTCOME

Table 19–1 shows proposed absolute and relative biopsychosocial contraindications for organ transplantation. In this table, we combined current standards of practice, to the extent that they are readily available, with provisionally data-based predictors of poor outcomes in the domains of graft survival, perioperative medical and psychological morbidity, and quality of life (House and Thompson 1988; Kuhn et al. 1988a, 1988b, 1988c; Levenson and Olbrisch 1987, 1993a; Surman 1992; Wolcott 1990).

Although surveys (Levenson and Olbrisch 1993b; Olbrisch and Levenson 1991) have documented that 100% of responding liver transplant programs—and high percentages of other organ transplant programs—use psychosocial assessments in candidate selection, consensus is lacking about absolute or relative psychosocial contraindications to transplant, with the prominent exception of active substance abuse or florid, nondelirious psychosis. Ethicists, legal scholars, and clinicians, however, have worried about the potential for prejudicial application of selection standards (Lowy and Martin 1992; Merrikin and Overcast 1987), particularly to underserved, psychiatrically ill patients.

Most transplant psychiatrists embrace the view that psychosocial factors should not be taken as immutable or as definitively precluding candidacy, a priori (Surman 1989, 1992). Instead, factors once rigidly considered as absolute contraindications to transplant are best viewed as risk factors and as targets for aggressive intervention. Treatable psychiatric illness remains frequently unrecognized and undertreated in the United States (Regier et al. 1993) and is probably more prevalent among potential recipients of transplants.

Substance-Related Disorders

Alcohol causes major health problems in the United States, and its abuse accounts for approximately one-third of patients with end-stage liver disease who present for transplant evaluation and one-half of all patients with end-stage liver disease (Loewy 1987). Additionally, alcohol-related cardiomyopathy is a common reason for heart transplantation, accounting for a significant—although unknown—measure of the 30% of patients with "idiopathic" cardiomyopathy who are evaluated for transplants (Burdine et al. 1990). Lucey and colleagues (1990; Lucey and Beresford 1992) pioneered an approach to the assessment of alcoholic patients for organ transplantation based in part on the seminal work of George Vaillant (1983). The Beresford algorithm emphasizes careful diagnosis, the impor-

tance of recognition by the patient and family of alcoholism as a disease, assessment of social stability factors, and evaluation for the attainment of commonly accepted predictors of long-term abstinence from alcohol.

Abuse of substances other than alcohol receives much less attention in the transplant literature. Gastfriend et al. (1989) convincingly demonstrated that substance abuse in transplant recipients is highly correlated with noncompliance and graft loss. Additionally, immunocompromised transplant recipients are vulnerable to fungal, bacterial, and viral infections, lung injury, and multiple other medical complications of exposure to inhaled, injected, and orally administered recreational drugs.

Psychotic Illness

A limited amount of literature exists about transplantation performed in patients with schizophrenia or other chronic psychotic illnesses. DiMartini and Twillman (1994) recently described successful liver and bone marrow transplants in two schizophrenic men. Sills and Popkin (1992) reported on a case of elective removal of a transplanted kidney from a patient who demonstrated recurrent organic psychosis, noncompliance, antisocial behavior, and alcohol abuse after his transplant.

Kidney transplantation provides a unique alternative to the life-sustaining technology of chronic dialysis; other transplanted organs sustain life, whereas technologies cannot. With its attendant freedom from the logistical difficulties of chronic dialysis, Surman (1989) suggests that kidney transplant is almost always a better alternative for psychiatrically ill patients.

Suicidal Ideation and/or Transplant Refusal

It is uncommon for transplant teams to encounter actively suicidal candidates. Some transplant candidates who are suicidal, however, have fulminant organ failure following suicide attempts (e.g., acetaminophen-induced hepatic necrosis). These situations warrant consideration of complex ethical and clinical factors. Should transplant be performed, for example, after an effectively lethal acetaminophen overdose in a comatose 18-year-old who has no other chance of awakening?

Transplant programs have no special authority to perform involuntary procedures on protesting patients. Patients who would likely benefit from a transplant but who competently refuse are permitted to make such decisions. Desperately ill patients, whose mental status may preclude participation in decision making, may not protest but also frequently cannot provide meaningful consent. The posttransplant medication regimen and a perpetual patient role, which are epiphenomena of transplantation, impose a very different set of demands on the incompletely assenting patient than a discrete intervention such as cardioversion. These maintenance requirements may tip the scale of ethical considerations away from performing transplants on incompletely assenting patients (Lowy and Martin 1992).

Dementia and Mental Retardation

As mentioned earlier in this chapter, ethical and legal trends, including the Americans With Disabilities Act, increasingly charge gatekeepers of organ transplantation with a responsibility for decision making that does not discriminate against those with mental impairments (Lowy and Martin 1992; Merrikin and Overcast 1987).

A preferable approach recognizes the possible compliance problems associated with dementia and retardation, seeks to characterize current functioning (particularly in the domains critical to successful self-care after organ transplant), and attempts to organize resources necessary for posttransplant care.

Treatment-Refractory Psychiatric Illness

No prospective studies have been done on outcomes in transplant recipients who had pretransplant, treatment-refractory psychiatric illnesses. Surman and Purtillo (1992) published a thoughtful review of a series of patients who were been judged "borderline acceptable" transplant candidates for reasons of age, malignancy, human immunodeficiency virus (HIV) status, mental retardation, or extensive prior treatment for mood, character, and substance abuse problems. The authors emphasized the variable ethical models that consultation-liaison psychiatrists tend to apply to the anticipation of medical-psychiatric risks. They noted the lack of standardized ethical guidelines to determine selection policies among treatment-refractory patients with psychiatric disorders.

In the past, decisions to exclude transplant candidates with nonpsychotic psychiatric illnesses were often based on worries about posttransplant compliance. Reports from the cardiac transplant literature cast doubt on whether patients with prior nonpsychotic psychiatric diagnoses have more medical or psychological morbidity than other transplant patients (Frierson and Lippmann 1987; Maricle et al. 1991; Skotzko et al. 1994; Surman 1989). Personality disorders, however, especially those that coexist with mood disorders or substance abuse, were found to predict postoperative surgical and psychiatric complications (Freeman et al. 1988a; Gastfriend et al. 1989; Kuhn et al. 1988c).

Adherence to Medical Regimen (Compliance)

The complex demands for compliance made on transplant recipients include strict adherence to a medication regimen, active participation in medical surveillance and follow-up regimens, abstinence from substances of abuse, and scrupulous record keeping.

A history of significant medical noncompliance raises concerns about future compliance. Two assumptions support this view: past compliance best predicts future behavior, and noncompliance causes significant morbidity in organ transplant recipients. The latter point is well demonstrated (DeLong et al. 1989; Didlake et al. 1988; Rovelli et al. 1989; Schweizer et al. 1990). Some investigators have shown that past compliance or noncompliance reliably predicts posttransplant behavior. Didlake and colleagues (1988) concluded that reliable predictors of compliance are unavailable for kidney transplant recipients, but other investigators have shown high correlations between pretransplant and posttransplant noncompliance (Rodriguez et al. 1991). Gastfriend and associates (1989) correlated substance abuse history, age younger than 30 years, mood disorder, and socioeconomic duress with noncompliance and graft loss. Other work supports the view that adults have fewer compliance difficulties than do children or adolescents (Hesse et al. 1990; Rovelli et al. 1989; Schweizer et al. 1990).

SELECTION COMMITTEE

The selection process varies from center to center. Most have a chartered working group that meets regularly and follows at least informal rules of operation. Individual candidates are presented, and the medical and surgical indications and contraindications are discussed. Strengths and weaknesses observed in the psychiatric and social work assessments are also presented. Generally, the group arrives at a consensus decision, which may include preconditions for acceptance such as "trials of compliance" or referrals for substance abuse treatment.

TRANSPLANT WAITING PERIOD

Anxiety is a common complaint among individuals awaiting transplantation (Craven 1990b; Mai et al. 1986; Surman et al. 1987a, 1987b; Weems and Patterson 1989). Frustration and demoralization are also commonly seen while an individual awaits transplantation. Pa-

tients' personality traits and ambivalence regarding transplantation may result in pathological behavior (Kuhn et al. 1988a; Phipps 1991). The patient and medical team need encouragement, support, and reassurance to work together effectively. Periodic reevaluation regarding continued commitment to transplantation is important. Some individuals may decide that transplantation, or the quality of life afforded by an inpatient wait for transplantation, is unacceptable (Collins et al. 1990). If these patients do not have any evidence of delirium or treatable psychiatric illness, their wishes should be respected.

Artificial organs function as a bridge to transplantation that increases the number of critically ill patients in the hospital and, ultimately, the number who can survive until transplantation. Cardiac assist devices allow a patient to ambulate and live outside of an intensive care unit (ICU) for months until a suitable donor is found; these devices are likely to become more common (Hravnak and George 1989). The potential for psychological and medical complications for someone maintained with an "artificial organ" is great. These complications include loss of control, adjustment difficulties, delirium, infection, bleeding, and death (Levenson and Glocheski 1991; Levy 1981; Reedy et al. 1990; Ruzevich et al. 1990).

Support groups provide benefit to individuals and families awaiting transplantation (Buchanan 1978; Suszycki 1986). Regional organ procurement associations welcome participation of patients and family members. Active involvement in public organ procurement activities can help patients and their families feel less helpless and hopeless during the waiting period. The Transplant Recipient International Organization (TRIO) provides a forum in which candidates can learn from transplant recipients, hear physicians address topics pertinent to transplantation, and help promote organ donation in the community.

The opportunity to meet with a transplant recipient is a valuable experience for many patients. It provides reassurance and peace of mind that professional intervention may not. Family members can also gain strength from the interaction with the spouse or other family member of a successful transplant patient.

Although not extensively investigated, "beeper" and "telephone" anxiety is often encountered. Beepers may inadvertently go off, signaling a possible summons to the hospital. Telephones ringing in the middle of the night can raise expectations of imminent transplantation. Individuals may develop a sense of dread or foreboding associated with further beeps or calls. Some patients are so concerned that they will miss "the call" that they become homebound and strictly curtail all activity. Treatment interventions aimed at alleviating anxiety are sometimes necessary.

Psychopharmacological Considerations

The major classes of psychopharmacological agents and special considerations in patients with organ dysfunction and failure are reviewed in Table 19–2. Further discussions are available in Stoudemire and Fogel (1987) and Trzepacz et al. (1991, 1993a, 1993b).

When close follow-up is feasible, we advocate efforts to provide relief for psychiatric symptoms whenever safely possible. The side effects of conventional tricyclic antidepressants are often not tolerated in candidates for organ transplant. In addition, new data (Glassman et al. 1993) suggest that tricyclic use in any patient with heart disease is potentially problematic. Newer agents such as the selective serotonin reuptake inhibitors (SSRIs) and bupropion are generally well tolerated by persons with end-organ disease. Special considerations are addressed in Table 19–2.

Profoundly fatigued patients often benefit remarkably from treatment with psychostimulants such as methylphenidate or dextroamphetamine. Time-limited treatment (with the end point often defined by transplant) with 5–10 mg twice daily can vastly improve patients' functioning in and experience of the waiting period.

Clinically significant pretransplant anxiety states can be quite difficult to treat, particularly in patients who have had intermittent delirium. Typically, psychiatrists have invoked the safety of the benzodiazepines oxazepam, temazepam, and lorazepam, which have no active metabolites and are glucuronidated to water-soluble compounds (Greenblatt and Shader 1987). However, benzodiazepines are minimally dialyzable and may worsen confusion in patients with hepatic encephalopathy (Surman 1992, 1994) and low perfusion states associated with cardiac failure. Recent reports implicate endogenous γ-aminobutyric acid (GABA)–ergic compounds in the encephalopathy of liver failure (Basile et al. 1991, 1994; Pomier-Layrargues et al. 1994). Alternatives to careful benzodiazepine dosing include buspirone, which may have special efficacy in the chronic anxiety associated with lung disease (Rapoport 1988), and high-potency neuroleptics such as haloperidol and droperidol. Diphenhydramine should be avoided whenever possible because its anticholinergic effects may exacerbate delirium.

NEUROPSYCHIATRIC PROBLEMS IN THE PERIOPERATIVE PERIOD

Delirium and Disorders of Consciousness

Acute secondary mental disorders are common in the perioperative period. In view of the reported prevalence rate of 20%–30% for clinically evident hepatic encephalopathy before liver transplant (Trzepacz et al. 1989), it is not surprising that up to one-third of all liver transplant recipients have an acute neuropsychiatric syndrome in the perioperative period (Craven 1991; DeGroen and Craven 1992; DeGroen et al. 1987; Surman 1994; Tollemar et al. 1988). As many as 70% of lung transplant recipients may experience postoperative delirium (Craven

Table 19–2. Psychopharmacological considerations in organ failure

Agent	Liver	Heart	Kidney	Lung
Mood stabilizers				
Lithium	1. No effect on clearance or drug levels 2. Ascites associated with lower lithium levels (new fluid compartment) 3. Diuretics will raise lithium levels	1. Rare conduction effects at toxic levels (which can follow lower cardiac output and decreased renal perfusion) 2. Rare sinus node effects limit treatment	May be used as necessary in patients with CRF and in those who are dialysis dependent; monitor levels, oral dosing after dialysis, and lithium in dialysate[a,b]	Unknown
Carbamazepine	1. Delayed metabolism, elevated levels 2. 5% of patients with normal liver function develop benign transaminasemia[c] 3. Risk of acute hepatic necrosis is 1:10,000 4. Known liver disease may increase risk; a relative contraindication to use[a]	Tricyclic antidepressant structure of carbamazepine: conduction effects possible; orthostasis	1. Conjugated OH metabolites accumulate, with tricyclic antidepressants 2. SIADH sometimes occurs in healthy patients; risk in patients with renal disease is unclear[d]	Unknown
Valproate	1. Slight risk of acute hepatic failure 2. Routinely elevated ammonia[e,f] may be intolerable in patients with chronic liver disease			

Anxiolytics				
Benzodiazepines	1. Delayed metabolism, active metabolites, potential oversedation, and exacerbation of encephalopathy 2. Agents requiring only hepatic glucuronidation (oxazepam, temazepam, lorazepam) less affected than those requiring oxidation[g]	Cardiac depressant effects only in overdose	1. At physiological pH, all are lipid-soluble, associated with low dialysance 2. Higher-than-normal levels of glucuronidated metabolites are often found, but these metabolites are inactive 3. In patients with normal liver function, careful dosing is generally safe[h]	Respiratory suppression is a theoretical concern
Buspirone	Delayed clearance in patients with cirrhosis[j]		Clearance also delayed up to 50% in renal disease[j]	May have respiratory stimulant effects[k,l]
Antipsychotics				
Butyrophenones	1. Delayed metabolism 2. Increased free fractions with hypoproteinemia	In high-dose boluses, may be arrhythmogenic[m]	Rare reports of toxicity[h]	Apparently tolerated and effective in patients with agitation
Phenothiazines	1. Delayed metabolism; anticholinergic delirium 2. 1%–2% risk of cholestatic jaundice with chlorpromazine	1. Orthostasis and tachycardia not tolerated 2. Generally benign ECG changes	Rare reports of toxicity[h]	
Clozapine	Delayed metabolism	Orthostasis and tachycardia not tolerated		

(continued)

Table 19–2. Psychopharmacological considerations in organ failure *(continued)*

Agent	Liver	Heart	Kidney	Lung
Antidepressants				
Conventional tricyclic antidepressants	Impaired hepatic oxidative capacity, shunting, and hypoalbuminemia may lead to elevated free blood levels of parent compounds[n]	Quinidine associated with excess arrhythmic morbidity and mortality.[o] Because of quinidine-like action, tricyclic antidepressants are probably contraindicated in all patients with ischemic disease or history of ventricular arrhythmias[p]	Elevated serum levels of conjugated OH metabolites, which may be psychoactive and organotoxic	1. Decreased tissue oxygenation may affect receptor affinity[s] 2. Protriptyline may have unique efficacy in patients with chronic lung disease to increase wake and sleep oxygenation[t,u]
MAOIs	1. Impaired liver function associated with slower clearance 2. Rarely hepatotoxic; hepatotoxicity is more likely with hydrazines (phenelzine and isocarboxazid) than with nonhydrazines (tranylcypromine and pargyline)[v]	1. No known contractility or conduction effects, but orthostasis may not be tolerable 2. Interaction with pressor agents used for surgery or resuscitation may cause severe hypertensive crisis		May be logistically impossible because of need for β-adrenergic bronchodilators
SSRIs	1. Fluoxetine and norfluoxetine half-life tripled in patients with cirrhosis[w] 2. Paroxetine levels elevated in patients with liver disease[x]	No known conduction effects; however, levels elevated and clearance delayed when hemodynamic compromise leads to hepatic congestion	1. Fluoxetine half-life and serum levels reported unchanged in patients with renal disease[y] 2. Elevated paroxetine levels reported in patients with renal disease[x]	

Bupropion	Delayed metabolism	Generally safe with regard to lack of adverse effects on ECG, preexisting arrhythmias, orthostasis, or pulse[z]	Metabolites may accumulate in patients with renal insufficiency and have been associated with delirium, seizure risks, and movement disorders[aa]
Trazodone	Delayed metabolism in elderly patients;[bb] metabolite may cause paradoxical effects[cc]	Metabolite accumulates with left ventricular dysfunction;[cc] ECG effects rare[dd]	mCPP clearance depends on renal function[cc]
Venlafaxine	Significant delays in elimination half-life with cirrhosis[ee]		Elimination half-life prolonged 50% in patients with renal impairment; elimination half-life increased up to 180% in patients on dialysis[ee]
Psychostimulants			
Methylphenidate/ dextroamphetamine	Delayed metabolism	Tachyarrhythmias	

Note. CRF = chronic renal failure; ECG = electrocardiogram; MAOI = monoamine oxidase inhibitor; mCPP = m-Chlorophenylpiperazine; OH = hydroxide; SIADH = syndrome of inappropriate (secretion of) antidiuretic hormone; SSRI = selective serotonin reuptake inhibitor.

Source. [a]Stoudemire and Fogel 1987; [b]Das Gupta and Jefferson 1990; [c]Jeavons 1983; [d]Viewig and Godleski 1988; [e]Eadie et al. 1988; [f]Cotariu and Zaidman 1988; [g]Howden et al. 1989; [h]Sellers and Bendayan 1987; [i]Dalhoff et al. 1987; [j]Gammans et al. 1988; [k]Rapoport 1988; [l]Kiev and Domantay 1988; [m]Metzger and Friedman 1993; [n]Leipzig 1990; [o]Glassman and Preudhomme 1993; [p]Glassman et al. 1993; [q]Lieberman et al. 1985; [r]McCue et al. 1989; [s]Trzepacz 1993a, 1993b; [t]Series et al. 1989; [u]Simonds et al. 1986; [v]Bernstein 1988; [w]Schenker et al. 1988; [x]Tulloch and Johnson 1992; [y]Aronoff et al. 1984; [z]Roose et al. 1991; [aa]Strouse et al. 1993; [bb]Von Moltke et al. 1993; [cc]Caccia et al. 1981; [dd]Spar 1987; [ee]Troy et al. 1994.

1990a). Heart and kidney transplant recipients exhibit acute delirium less frequently. Opportunistic infections of the central nervous system (CNS) are often heralded in transplant recipients by delirium or other mental status changes (Boon et al. 1990; Conti and Tubin 1988; Surman 1994; Surman and Purtillo 1992). Common etiological factors for delirium in transplant recipients include the consequences to the brain of chronic organ failure, the residua of general anesthesia, lengthy transplant surgeries, volume and electrolyte shifts associated with reperfusion of the new organ, cyclosporine loading, postoperative opiate treatment, early graft dysfunction, fever, coagulopathy, infection, and other processes (Dubin et al. 1979; Plevak et al. 1989). Psychoactive substance withdrawal must also be considered.

A growing body of literature implicates cyclosporine and other elements of the transplant pharmacopoeia with postoperative delirium and neurotoxicity (Adams et al. 1987; Berden et al. 1985; Bhatt et al. 1988; Craven 1991; De Bruijn et al. 1989; DeGroen and Craven 1992; DeGroen et al. 1987; Frank et al. 1993; Lopez et al. 1991; Palmer and Toto 1991; C. B. Thompson et al. 1984; Tollemar et al. 1988; Vogt et al. 1988; Wilczek et al. 1984; Winnock et al. 1993). Among patients who have received organ transplants, recipients of liver transplants are most susceptible to these adverse events (Bennett and Norman 1986; Boon et al. 1990; Conti and Tubin 1988; Craven and Rodin 1992; De Bruijn et al. 1989; DeGroen et al. 1987; Lopez et al. 1991; Plevak et al. 1989; Surman and Purtillo 1992; Tollemar et al. 1988; Trzepacz et al. 1993a, 1993b), with large centers reporting some degree of cyclosporine neurotoxicity in 25%–40% of liver recipients in the postoperative phase. There are fewer case series describing these syndromes in recipients of donor hearts (Cooper et al. 1989; Lane et al. 1988; McManus et al. 1992) or kidneys (Palmer and Toto 1991).

The first signs of cyclosporine neurotoxicity are often seen in the ICU. After an early lucid period, patients are lethargic, confused, and require reintubation despite previously adequate respiratory functioning (Craven 1991). Variable symptoms are seen, including seizures, cortical blindness, aphasia, paresthesia, neuropathy, delusions, and agitation (Bennett and Norman 1986; DeGroen et al. 1987). Obtundation, deeper coma, status epilepticus, and neurological death rarely occur (Adams et al. 1987). Diffuse white matter changes are seen on magnetic resonance imaging (MRI), accompanied by symmetric electroencephalographic (EEG) dysrhythmia; cyclosporine holidays have been associated with symptom remission and normalization of white matter changes in some patients (DeGroen et al. 1987).

Although it is generally seen as an acute postoperative complication, cyclosporine neurotoxicity sometimes occurs months after organ transplant (De Bruijn et al. 1989). New-onset cyclosporine-related delirium, complex partial seizures, cortical blindness, frontal-lobe syndromes, and secondary mood syndromes have been observed 3–6 months after liver transplant (T. Strouse, unpublished data, April 1994). A scholarly review of the possible mechanisms of cyclosporine neurotoxicity is found in DeGroen and Craven (1992). Table 19–3 summarizes cyclosporine toxicity symptoms.

Other agents used commonly in organ transplantation that are associated with delirium include corticosteroids (Kershner and Wang-Cheng 1989; Lewis and Smith 1983), OKT3 (Coleman and Norman 1990), and FK 506 (DiMartini et al. 1991; Eidelman et al. 1991). FK 506 is a new immunosuppressant alternative to cyclosporine that in preliminary studies showed less neurotoxicity and fewer neuropathological lesions (Eidelman et al. 1991; Lopez et al. 1991). A recent randomized trial found marginally greater frequency of tremors, sleep disturbance, and seizures in patients taking FK 506 than in those taking cyclosporine (Frank et al. 1993).

Although the general principles of assess-

Table 19–3. Some neuropsychiatric syndromes associated with solid organ transplantation and immune suppression

Delirium
Seizures
Headache/visual symptoms
Cortical blindness
Isolated visual hallucinations
Dementia-like syndromes
Frontal-lobe syndromes
Secondary mood, anxiety, thought disorders
Movement disorders
Central pontine myelinolysis
Impaired taste sensation
Incontinence
Sexual dysfunction

ing and managing delirium (see Wise and Trzepacz, Chapter 7 in this volume) pertain to patients with organ transplants, some special considerations are warranted. For example, benzodiazepines may worsen hepatic encephalopathy or lead to further behavioral disinhibition, presumably via increased GABAergic activity (Basile and Jones 1988; Basile et al. 1991). The benzodiazepine antagonist flumazenil can temporarily reverse the impaired level of consciousness found in advanced hepatic encephalopathy and benzodiazepine intoxication in some patients (Basile et al. 1994; Grimm et al. 1988; Pomier-Layrargues et al. 1994). Heart recipients with delirium may have new CNS vascular insults associated with cardiopulmonary bypass (Shaw et al. 1985).

High-potency neuroleptic agents such as haloperidol and droperidol are effective in treating patients with agitation or post-transplant delirium; however, patients who have received liver transplants may have special vulnerability to extrapyramidal symptoms because of the effects of chronic liver disease on the basal ganglia (Neiman et al. 1990). Heart recipients are possibly sensitive to butyro-phenone-induced hypotension or arrhythmias (Metzger and Friedman 1993).

The practice of combining moderate doses of butyrophenones (haloperidol, 2–4 mg iv every 6–8 hours, or droperidol, 2–4 mg iv every 2–4 hours) with benzodiazepines that do not have active metabolites (lorazepam, 2–4 mg iv every 4–6 hours) often provides sufficient management of the acute symptoms of delirium. The Massachusetts General Hospital group has reported use of 250–2,000 mg/24 hours of intravenous haloperidol in the treatment of patients with postcardiotomy delirium without ill effects (Tesar et al. 1985). Lung recipients also appear to tolerate large cumulative amounts of haloperidol without adverse side effects (Craven 1990a). An extensive review of the differential diagnosis and pharmacological treatment of delirium in transplant recipients is available in reviews by Trzepacz and associates (1991, 1993a, 1993b).

Seizures

At some centers, generalized tonic-clonic seizures and complex partial seizures are the most commonly reported neuropsychiatric complications of transplant; liver recipients may be the most likely to be afflicted (Adams et al. 1987; Estol et al. 1989a, 1989b; C. B. Thompson et al. 1984; Vogt et al. 1988). Seizures were also reported in 10% of patients in a series of lung transplant recipients (Craven 1990a). Cyclosporine is often implicated (Craven 1991; Estol et al. 1989a, 1989b), directly or indirectly: associated CNS lesions, including white matter changes, microinfarcts, central pontine myelinolysis, and edema, are commonly found (Estol et al. 1989a, 1989b). In early studies, both seizure frequency and the severity of the neuropathology appeared to be less with FK 506 than with cyclosporine (Eidelman et al. 1991). Unfortunately, contrary data were published more recently (Frank et al. 1993). OKT3, a drug that is used to prevent rejection, has also been associated with posttransplant seizures (Coleman and Norman 1990), as have acyclovir and ganciclovir (Trzepacz et al. 1993a, 1993b).

Both generalized and partial complex status epilepticus have been described in transplant recipients. These dramatic complications have generally occurred within 2 weeks of transplantation (Surman 1989; C. B. Thompson et al. 1984; Vogt et al. 1988) and may occasionally be refractory to conventional treatment with benzodiazepines and standard antiepileptic agents. Cyclosporine holidays are sometimes necessary to bring seizures under control, in part because correction of magnesium imbalances can be impossible with continued cyclosporine therapy.

Headache and Visual Symptoms

Severe headache is a common complaint among transplant recipients who are taking cyclosporine (Adams et al. 1987). The headache may wax and wane with blood peak levels, and medication compliance can be threatened if this complication is left unattended. Headache occurs less commonly among patients who are taking FK 506.

Severe headache may signal other neurological problems in patients who have received organ transplant. The most dramatic among these is transient cortical blindness, a known complication of cyclosporine therapy (Ghalie et al. 1990; Rubin and Kang 1987; Wilson et al. 1988). After liver transplant, at the peak of headache crisis, we have seen cortical blindness associated with complex partial seizure activity and bilateral occipital abnormalities visible on brain MRI. Seizures, blindness, and edema generally resolve with a cyclosporine holiday. Because cyclosporine is known to induce hypertension, severe headache may also herald a hypertensive crisis.

Isolated visual hallucinations are also attributed to cyclosporine in patients who do not have delirium following transplant (Noll and Kulkarni 1984) and are reported with ganciclovir antiviral therapy (Faulds and Heel 1990; M. N. Thompson and Jeffries 1989) as well as with many of the antibiotics used to treat patients posttransplantation (Trzepacz 1993a, 1993b). Blurred vision is another common complaint; maintenance of lower cyclosporine levels is sometimes helpful.

Secondary Mood, Anxiety, and Thought Disorders

Uncontrolled studies report that the incidence of secondary ("organic") mood syndromes (depressed or manic/hypomanic) and major depression is 68% among recipients of heart transplants (Shapiro and Kornfeld 1989) and 25% among recipients of liver transplants (Surman et al. 1987a, 1987b). Rates among recipients of kidney transplants have not been reported using contemporary criteria.

A variety of case reports and small series describe the full syndrome of mania (Wamboldt et al. 1984), racing thoughts and dense insomnia suggesting hypomania (DeGroen and Craven 1992), and depressive syndromes (Craven 1991; DeGroen and Craven 1992; C. B. Thompson et al. 1984). Many reports temporally link mood symptoms to the initiation of cyclosporine therapy following organ transplantation, with symptom remission after cyclosporine holidays or dose decrements.

Our group has observed transient mania that evolved into fixed frontal-lobe syndromes as part of the clinical presentation of late-onset cyclosporine neurotoxicity in recipients of liver transplants. Mania and depression have been linked to high-dose steroid treatment (Kershner and Wang-Cheng 1989; Lewis and Smith 1983; Ling et al. 1981) and to the prodrome of CNS infection with cytomegalovirus (Surman 1992). FK 506 is associated with "mood changes" (Eidelman et al. 1991), and acyclovir is associated with psychotic major depression (Sirota et al. 1988).

Movement Disorders

Gross tremor is a common problem in organ transplant recipients. High serum cyclosporine levels are often associated with extreme symptoms, although tremor occurs in many patients with normal and low-normal levels. OKT3 also can cause or exacerbate tremor (Coleman and Norman 1990). The chronic brain effects of alcohol may predispose transplant recipients to postsurgical tremor (Neiman et al. 1990). Other potentiating factors may include hypomagnesemia or hypocalcemia (Adams et al. 1987; C. B. Thompson et al. 1984), or the concomitant administration of other drugs that are known to elevate cyclosporine levels, including erythromycin, oral contraceptives, methylprednisolone, ketoconazole, fluconazole, cimetidine, and verapamil (Trzepacz et al. 1993a, 1993b). Some patients experience fasciculations or myoclonic jerking, which may be worse at night and may interrupt sleep. No controlled treatment data exist. When immunosuppressive dosing changes and careful attention to drug interactions are fruitless, clonazepam successfully manages tremor and myoclonic jerking.

Various symptoms of cerebellar dysfunction, such as ataxia, nystagmus, weakness, and dysarthria, are also described in patients following organ transplantation (Adams et al. 1987; Belli et al. 1993; C. B. Thompson et al. 1984; Vogt et al. 1988). As with many of these neuropsychiatric problems, patients who have received donor livers seem most vulnerable. These symptoms, most often described as acute neurotoxic states, can improve or clear entirely despite unclear etiologies but may persist and can become quite disabling. Transient limb paresis, hemiplegia, and spasticity have also been reported (DeGroen and Craven 1992; DeGroen et al. 1987; Martinez et al. 1988).

A syndrome of akinetic mutism, orofacial dyskinesias, pseudobulbar palsy, and MRI-confirmed central pontine myelinolysis in patients following liver transplantation has been described at a number of centers (Bird et al. 1990; Estol et al. 1989a, 1989b; Martinez et al. 1988). A possibly related syndrome of diffuse white matter lesions associated with movement abnormalities and altered consciousness has been described in patients who have undergone heart transplantation (Lane et al. 1988). The dramatic pontine syndrome in patients with donor livers has been convincingly linked to cyclosporine. The syndrome has been reported to clear with cyclosporine holidays or dose reductions, a finding confirmed by the UCLA experience, in which both clinical symptoms and MRI findings have substantially improved or normalized in some of these patients. The risk of recurrence with cyclosporine rechallenge remains unclear. When rechallenge with cyclosporine leads to recurrent neurotoxicity, alternatives include withdrawing cyclosporine entirely and switching to FK 506 or attempting to maximize use of azathioprine and steroids. Unfortunately, akinetic mutism has now also been reported to occur, although rarely, with FK 506 immunosuppression (Eidelman et al. 1991).

POSTOPERATIVE COURSE AND LIFE AFTER TRANSPLANTATION

Compliance

As noted previously in this chapter (see section, "Adherence to Medical Regimen"), some patients' compliance problems may be anticipated. Becker and Maiman (1980) described concrete steps to enhance compliance; these steps are presented in Table 19–4.

Postoperative Adjustment

There is increasing interest in the return of the transplant recipient to a reasonable quality of life. Successful readjustment to life after transplantation generally requires several months or longer. Kuhn et al. (1988b) found that the first anniversary after cardiac transplantation was a major milestone and that full readjustment did not occur until after this point.

Tasks after transplantation and discharge include readjustment to family and vocational roles, changing body image, coping with the persistent fear of rejection and infection, toler-

Table 19–4. Enhancing compliance

1. Improve understanding of medication and follow-up regimen (e.g., provide written instructions).

2. Tailor the regimen to fit the individual's lifestyle (e.g., decrease frequency of dosing, minimize necessary behavioral change).

3. Explore patient's prior experiences with medications and procedures.

4. Maintain a supportive provider-patient relationship.

5. Monitor compliance with medications at every visit.

6. Increase staff awareness of factors that contribute to noncompliance.

7. Use treatment contracts for achieving objectives.

8. Provide continuity of care with transplant team physicians and staff.

9. Establish additional allies (social support network) in supervision of patient's compliance with regimen.

10. Assign roles to team members to better promote adherence to treatment.

Source. Adapted from Becker MH, Maiman LA: "Strategies for Enhancing Patient Compliance." *Journal of Community Health* 6:113–135, 1980. Used with permission.

ating side effects of immunosuppressant medications, meeting the expectations of the medical staff, and coping with continued disability and cost (Craven 1990b). All transplant recipients face these difficulties, which can become the source of major disability. Jones and colleagues (1988) found that individuals were more anxious 4 and 12 months after transplant than they were at the time of discharge posttransplant, underscoring the stress associated with being a convalescing transplant recipient.

Increased autonomy and independence are cited by many transplant recipients as among the reasons for initially seeking transplantation. Actual outcome often falls far short of expectations for immediate recovery and return to health (Stevenson et al. 1990; Walden et al. 1989). This may contribute to distress because the recipient must rely on others for transportation and other tangible needs.

Adverse neurological events, or other complications such as renal failure, can leave individuals with significant unanticipated disability and long-term dependency needs. When these events occur, they inevitably disrupt the social network. For most families, the expectation after the transplant is that the recipient will function independently.

Many barriers exist to the return of patients to gainful employment following organ transplant surgery. Loss of health insurance associated with recovery from disability is among the most pressing issues. Faced with the high cost of health care and the understanding that they will require a lifetime of follow-up visits and expensive immunosuppressant medications, it is not surprising that some patients choose the status quo over aggressively pursuing rehabilitation.

Employers are often unwilling to hire an individual with such an unusual medical condition. In addition, employers fear the recipient as a potential liability to the company health insurance policy. If an employer wishes to hire a transplant recipient, the presence of a preexisting condition may disqualify that individual from participating in the company health insurance plan.

Paris et al. (1993) documented six predictors for return to employment: 1) feeling physically able to work, 2) no risk of losing health insurance, 3) longer length of time since transplant, 4) education beyond high school, 5) maintenance of disability income, and 6) shorter period of disability pretransplant.

CONCLUSION

Although OTP has made impressive early progress, and although the scope and sophistication of the OTP research literature have grown rapidly in the early 1990s, many challenges remain to the continued growth and vitality of OTP.

In addition to fostering specialized clinical competence in its practitioners (which ultimately may require the development of a small number of formal fellowship training programs in OTP) and to developing sophisticated strategies to ensure its long-term economic survival, OTP as a field faces significant research challenges. Table 19–5 summarizes a number of areas in which further knowledge is needed.

OTP is a dynamically developing field of clinical and research activity. Psychiatrists, along with psychologists, social workers, and other mental health care professionals who may be team members, need to work closely and effectively with the wide variety of health care professionals who compose the organ transplant team. This collaborative spirit, and the specific skills that psychiatrists and other mental health care professionals bring to organ transplant programs, often make critically important contributions to successful transplant recipient outcomes.

Table 19–5. Areas of organ transplant psychiatry in which further research is needed

Neuropsychiatric sequelae and neuropsychiatric management of patients who develop end-stage organ failure and who undergo organ transplantation

Indications for, safety of, and efficacy of psychopharmacological treatments of psychiatric disorders in patients in this population

Pretransplantation predictors of important psychiatric, behavioral, and psychosocial outcomes among patients who receive organ transplants

Assessment and management of patients with substance-related disorders who are candidates for and recipients of transplants

Pretransplantation psychosocial variables that may predict critical medical (as opposed to psychiatric) outcomes in patients who receive transplants (e.g., survival status or duration)

Predictors of critical transplant recipient rehabilitation, adaptation, and quality of life outcomes

Efficacy of specific psychiatric interventions, including psychotherapy, in targeted or high-risk transplant recipients

Effects of organ donation on living donors

REFERENCES

Adams DH, Ponsford S, Gunson B, et al: Neurological complications following liver transplantation. Lancet 1:949–951, 1987

Alter M, Favero MS, Miller JK: National surveillance of dialysis-associated diseases in the United States. Transactions of the American Society of Artificial Internal Organs 35:820–831, 1989

Aronoff GR, Bergstrom RF, Pottratz ST, et al: Fluoxetine kinetics and protein binding in normal and impaired renal function. Clin Pharmacol Ther 36:138–144, 1984

Basile AS, Jones E: Hepatic encephalopathy and the GABA\benzodiazepine receptor chloride ionophore complex: an update. J Gastroenterol Hepatol 3:387–398, 1988

Basile AS, Hughes RD, Harrison PM, et al: Elevated concentration of 1,4 benzodiazepines in fulminant liver failure. N Engl J Med 327:473–478, 1991

Basile AS, Harrison PM, Hughes RD, et al: Relationship between plasma benzodiazepine receptor ligand concentrations and severity of hepatic encephalopathy. Hepatology 19:112–121, 1994

Becker MH, Maiman LA: Strategies for enhancing patient compliance. J Community Health 6:113–135, 1980

Belli LS, De Carlis L, Romani F, et al: Dysarthria and cerebellar ataxia: late occurrence of severe neurotoxicity in a liver transplant recipient. Transpl Int 6:176–178, 1993

Bennett WM, Norman DJ: Action and toxicity of cyclosporine. Annu Rev Med 37:215–224, 1986

Berden JHM, Hoitsma AJ, Merx JL, et al: Severe central nervous system toxicity associated with cyclosporine. Lancet 1:219–220, 1985

Bernstein JG: Monoamine oxidase inhibitors, in Handbook of Drug Therapy in Psychiatry. Edited by Bernstein JG. Littleton, MA, PSG Publishing, 1988, pp 161–188

Bhatt BD, Meriano FV, Buchwald D: Cyclosporine associated central nervous system toxicity (letter). N Engl J Med 318:788, 1988

Bird FLA, Meadows J, Goka J, et al: Cyclosporin-associated akinetic mutism and extrapyramidal syndrome after liver transplantation. J Neurol Neurosurg Psychiatry 53:1068–1071, 1990

Boon AP, Adams DH, Buckels J, et al: Cerebral aspergillosis in liver transplantation. J Clin Pathol 43:114–118, 1990

Broelsch CE, Whitington PF, Edmond JC: Evolution and future perspectives for reduced-size hepatic transplantation. Surg Gynecol Obstet 171:353–360, 1990

Buchanan DC: Group therapy for chronic physically ill patients. Psychosomatics 19:425–431, 1978

Burdine J, Fischel RJ, Bolman RM: Cardiac transplantation. Crit Care Clin 6:927–945, 1990

Caccia S, Ballabio M, Samanin R, et al: m-Chlorophenyl-piperazine, a central 5-hydroxytryptamine agonist, is a metabolite of trazodone. J Pharm Pharmacol 33:477–478, 1981

Coleman AE, Norman DJ: OKT3 encephalopathy. Ann Neurol 28:837–838, 1990

Collins JA, Skidmore MA, Melvin DB, et al: Home intravenous dobutamine therapy in patients awaiting heart transplantation. J Heart Lung Transplant 9:205–208, 1990

Conti DJ, Tubin RH: Infection of the central nervous system in organ transplant recipients. Neurosurg Clin N Am 6:241–260, 1988

Cooper DK, Novitzky D, Davis L, et al: Does central nervous system toxicity occur in transplant patients with hypocholesterolemia receiving cyclosporine? J Heart Lung Transplant 8:221–224, 1989

Cotariu D, Zaidman JL: Valproic acid and the liver. Clin Chem 34:890–897, 1988

Craven JL: Postoperative organic mental syndromes in lung transplant recipients: the Toronto Lung Transplant Group. J Heart Lung Transplant 9:129–132, 1990a

Craven J: Psychiatric aspects of lung transplant: the Toronto Lung Transplant Group. Can J Psychiatry 35:759–764, 1990b

Craven JL: Cyclosporine-associated organic mental disorders in liver transplant recipients. Psychosomatics 32:94–102, 1991

Craven J, Rodin G: Introduction, in Psychiatric Aspects of Organ Transplantation. Edited by Craven J, Rodin GJ. Oxford, UK, Oxford University Press, 1992, pp 1–5

Dalhoff K, Poulsen HE, Garrard P, et al: Buspirone pharmacokinetics in patients with cirrhosis. Br J Pharmacol 24:547–550, 1987

Das Gupta K, Jefferson JW: The use of lithium in the medically ill. Gen Hosp Psychiatry 12:83–97, 1990

De Bruijn KM, Klompmaker IJ, Slooff MJH, et al: Cyclosporine neurotoxicity late after liver transplantation. Transplantation 47:575–576, 1989

DeGroen P, Craven J: Organic brain syndromes in transplant patients, in Psychiatric Aspects of Organ Transplantation. Edited by Craven J, Rodin G. Oxford, UK, Oxford University Press, 1992, pp 67–88

DeGroen PC, Aksamit AJ, Rakela J, et al: Central nervous system toxicity after liver transplantation: the role of cyclosporine and cholesterol. N Engl J Med 317:861–866, 1987

DeLong P, Trollinger JH, Fox N, et al: Noncompliance in renal transplant recipients: methods for recognition and intervention. Transplant Proc 21:3982–3984, 1989

Didlake RH, Dreyfus K, Kerman RH, et al: Patient noncompliance: a major cause of late graft failure in cyclosporine treated renal transplant. Transplant Proc 20:63–69, 1988

DiMartini A, Twillman R: Organ transplantation and paranoid schizophrenia. Psychosomatics 35:159–160, 1994

DiMartini A, Pajer K, Trzepacz P, et al: Psychiatric morbidity in liver transplant patients. Transplant Proc 23:3179–3180, 1991

Dubin WR, Field HL, Gastfriend DR: Postcardiotomy delirium: a critical review. J Thorac Cardiovasc Surg 77:586–594, 1979

Eadie MJ, Hooper WD, Dickinson RG: Valproate-associated hepatotoxicity and its biochemical mechanisms. Medical Toxicology Adverse Drug Experiences 3:85–106, 1988

Eidelman B, Abu-Elmagd K, Wilson J, et al: Neurologic complication of FK-506. Transplant Proc 23:3175–3178, 1991

Eisendrath RM, Guttmann RD, Murray JE: Psychologic considerations in the selection of kidney transplant donors. Surg Gynecol Obstet 129:243–248, 1969

Estol CJ, Faris AA, Martinez AJ, et al: Central pontine myelinolysis after liver transplantation. Neurology 39:493–498, 1989a

Estol CJ, Lopez O, Brenner RP, et al: Seizures after liver transplantation: a clinicopathologic study. Neurology 39:1297–1301, 1989b

Faulds D, Heel RC: Ganciclovir: a review of its antiviral activity, pharmacokinetic properties, and therapeutic efficacy in cytomegalovirus infections. Drugs 39:597–638, 1990

Fellner CH: Selection of living kidney donors and the problem of informed consent. Seminars in Psychiatry 3:79–85, 1971

Fox RC, Swazey JP: Leaving the field. Hastings Cent Rep 22:9–15, 1992

Frank B, Perdrizet GA, White HM, et al: Neurotoxicity of FK-506 in liver transplant recipients. Transplant Proc 25:1887–1888, 1993

Freeman AM, Folks DG, Sokol RS, et al: Cardiac transplantation: clinical correlates of psychiatric outcome. Psychosomatics 29:47–54, 1988a

Freeman AM, Sokol RS, Folks DG, et al: Psychiatric characteristics of patients undergoing cardiac transplantation. Psychiatr Med 6:8–23, 1988b

Freeman A, Davies L, Libb JW, et al: Assessment of transplant candidates and prediction of outcome, in Psychiatric Aspects of Organ Transplantation. Edited by Craven J, Rodin G. Oxford, UK, Oxford University Press, 1992, pp 9–19

Freeman AM, Westphal JR, Davis LL, et al: The future of organ transplant psychiatry. Psychosomatics 36:429–437, 1995

Frierson RL, Lippmann SB: Heart transplantation patients rejected on psychiatric indication. Psychosomatics 28:347–355, 1987

Gammans PE, Mayoe RF, La Budde SA: Metabolism and disposition of buspirone. Am J Med 80(suppl):S41–S51, 1988

Gastfriend DR, Surman OS, Gaffey G, et al: Substance abuse and compliance in organ transplantation. Substance Abuse 10:149–153, 1989

Gellman RN: Divided loyalties: a physician's responsibility in an information age. Soc Sci Med 23:817–826, 1989

Ghalie R, Fitzsimmons WE, Bennette D, et al: Cortical blindness: a rare complication of cyclosporine therapy. Bone Marrow Transplant 6:147–149, 1990

Glassman AH, Preudhomme XA: Review of the cardiovascular effects of heterocyclic antidepressants. J Clin Psychiatry 54(suppl):16–22, 1993

Glassman AH, Rose SP, Bigger JT: The safety of tricyclic antidepressants in cardiac patients: risk benefit reconsidered. JAMA 269:2673–2675, 1993

Goldman LS: Liver transplantation using living donors: preliminary donor psychiatric outcomes. Psychosomatics 34:235–240, 1993

Greenblatt DJ, Shader R: Pharmacokinetics of antianxiety agents, in Psychopharmacology: The Third Generation of Progress. Edited by Meltzer HY. New York, Raven, 1987, pp 387–401

Grimm G, Ferenci P, Katzenschlager R, et al: Improvement of hepatic encephalopathy treated with flumazenil. Lancet 2:1392–1394, 1988

Hesse UJ, Roth B, Knuppertz G, et al: Control of patient compliance in outpatient steroid treatment of nephrologic disease and renal transplant recipients. Transplant Proc 22:1405–1406, 1990

House R, Thompson RL: Psychiatric aspects of organ transplantation. JAMA 260:535–539, 1988

Howden CW, Birnie GG, Brodie MJ: Drug metabolism in liver disease. Pharmacol Ther 40:439–474, 1989

Hravnak M, George E: Nursing considerations for the patient with a total artificial heart. Critical Care Nursing Clinics of North America 1:495–513, 1989

Jeavons PM: Hepatotoxicity in antiepileptic drugs, in Chronic Toxicity of Antiepileptic Drugs. Edited by Oxley J, Janz D, Meinardi H. New York, Raven, 1983, pp 1–46

Jones BM, Chang VP, Esmore D, et al: Psychological adjustment after cardiac transplantation. Med J Aust 149:118–122, 1988

Jonsen AR: Ethical issues in organ transplantation, in Medical Ethics. Edited by Veatch RM. Boston, MA, Jones & Bartless, 1989, pp 181–204

Kahn JP, Drusin RE, Klein DF: Idiopathic cardiomyopathy and panic disorder: clinical association in cardiac transplant candidates. Am J Psychiatry 144:1327–1330, 1987

Kellner R, Samet J, Pathak D: Dyspnea, anxiety, and depression in chronic respiratory impairment. Gen Hosp Psychiatry 14:20–28, 1992

Kershner P, Wang-Cheng R: Psychiatric side effects of steroid therapy. Psychosomatics 30:135–139, 1989

Kiev A, Domantay AG: A study of buspirone coprescribed with bronchodilators in 82 anxious ambulatory patients. J Asthma 25:281–284, 1988

Kuhn WF, Myers B, Davis MH: Ambivalence in cardiac transplantation candidates. Int J Psychiatry Med 18:305–314, 1988a

Kuhn WF, Davis MH, Lippmann SB: Emotional adjustment to cardiac transplantation. Gen Hosp Psychiatry 10:108–113, 1988b

Kuhn WF, Myers B, Brennan AF, et al: Psychopathology in heart transplant candidates. J Heart Transplant 7:223–226, 1988c

Kuhn WF, Brennan AF, Lacefield PK, et al: Psychiatric distress during stages of the heart transplant protocol. J Heart Lung Transplant 9:25–29, 1990

Lane RJ, Roche SW, Leung AA, et al: Cyclosporin neurotoxicity in cardiac transplant recipients. J Neurol Neurosurg Psychiatry 51:1434–1437, 1988

Leipzig RM: Psychopharmacology in patients with hepatic and gastrointestinal disease. Int J Psychiatry Med 202:109–139, 1990

Levenson JL, Glocheski S: Psychological factors affecting end-stage renal disease: a review. Psychosomatics 32:382–389, 1991

Levenson JL, Olbrisch ME: Shortage of donor organ and long waits. Psychosomatics 28:399–403, 1987

Levenson JL, Olbrisch ME: Psychiatric aspects of heart transplantation. Psychosomatics 34:114–123, 1993a

Levenson JL, Olbrisch ME: Psychosocial evaluation of organ transplant candidates: a comparative survey of process, criteria, and outcomes in heart, liver, and kidney transplantation. Psychosomatics 34:314–323, 1993b

Levy NB: Psychological reactions to machine dependency: hemodialysis. Psychiatr Clin North Am 4:351–363, 1981

Lewis DA, Smith RE: Steroid-induced psychiatric syndromes. J Affect Disord 5:319–332, 1983

Lieberman JA, Cooper TB, Suckow RF, et al: Tricyclic antidepressant and metabolite levels in chronic renal failure. Clin Pharmacol Ther 37:301–307, 1985

Ling MHM, Perry PJ, Tsuang MT: Side effects of corticosteroid therapy: psychiatric aspects. Arch Gen Psychiatry 38:471–477, 1981

Loewy EH: Drunks, livers, and values: should social value judgments enter into liver transplant decisions? J Clin Gastroenterol 9:436–441, 1987

Lopez OL, Martinez AJ, Torre-Cisneros J: Neuropathologic cyclosporine and FK-506. Transplant Proc 23:3181–3182, 1991

Lowry MR: Frequency of depressive disorder in patients entering home hemodialysis. J Nerv Ment Dis 167:199–204, 1979

Lowy F, Martin D: Ethical consideration in transplantation, in Psychiatric Aspects of Organ Transplantation. Edited by Craven J, Rodin G. Oxford, UK, Oxford University Press, 1992, pp 212–230

Lucey MR, Beresford TP: Alcoholic liver disease: to transplant or not to transplant. Alcohol Alcohol 27:103–108, 1992

Lucey MR, Kolars JC, Merio RM, et al: Cyclosporin toxicity, therapeutic blood levels and cytochrome P-450 IIIA. Lancet 335:11–15, 1990

Mai FM: Liaison psychiatry in the heart transplant unit. Psychosomatics 28:44–46, 1987

Mai FM, McKenzie FN, Kostuk WJ: Psychiatric aspects of heart transplantation: preoperative. BMJ 292:311–313, 1986

Maricle RA, Hosenpud JD, Norman DJ, et al: The lack of predictive value of preoperative psychologic distress for postoperative medical outcome in heart transplant recipients. J Heart Lung Transplant 10:942–947, 1991

Martinez AJ, Estol C, Faris A: Neurologic complication of liver transplantation. Neurol Clin 6:327–348, 1988

McCue RE, Georgotas A, Suckow RF, et al: 10-hydroxy nortriptyline and treatment effects in elderly depressed patients. J Neuropsychiatry Clin Neurosci 1:176–180, 1989

McManus RP, O'Hair DP, Schweiger J, et al: Cyclosporine-associated central neurotoxicity after heart transplantation. Ann Thorac Surg 53:326–327, 1992

Merrikin KJ, Overcast TD: Patient selection for heart transplantation: when is a discriminating choice discrimination? Journal of Politics, Policy, and the Law 10:7–32, 1987

Metzger E, Friedman R: Prolongation of the corrected QT and torsades de pointes cardiac arrhythmia associated with intravenous haloperidol in the medically ill. J Clin Psychopharmacol 13:128–132, 1993

Murray TH: Divided loyalties for physicians: social context and moral problems. Soc Sci Med 23:827–832, 1989

Neiman J, Lang AE, Fornazzari L, et al: Movement disorders in alcoholism: a review. Neurology 40:741–746, 1990

Nissenson AR, Levin ML, Klawans HL, et al: Neurological sequelae of end stage renal disease. Journal of Chronic Disease 30:705–733, 1987

Noll RB, Kulkarni R: Complex visual hallucination and cyclosporine. Arch Neurol 41:329–330, 1984

Olbrisch ME, Levenson JL: Psychosocial evaluation of heart transplant candidates: an international survey of process, criteria, and outcomes. J Heart Lung Transplant 10:948–955, 1991

Olbrisch ME, Levenson J, Hamer R: The PACT: a rating scale for the study of clinical decision-making in psychosocial screening criteria for organ transplant candidates. Clin Transpl 3:164–169, 1989

Palmer BF, Toto RD: Severe neurologic toxicity induced by cyclosporine A in three renal transplant patients. Am J Kidney Dis 1:116–121, 1991

Paris W, Woodbury A, Thompson S, et al: Returning to work after heart transplantation. J Heart Lung Transplant 12:46–53, 1993

Phipps L: Psychiatric aspects of heart transplantation. Can J Psychiatry 36:563–568, 1991

Plevak DJ, Southorn PA, Narr BJ, et al: Intensive care unit experience in the Mayo liver transplantation program: the first 100 cases. Mayo Clin Proc 64:433–445, 1989

Pomier-Layrargues G, Giguere JF, Lavoie J, et al: Flumazenil in cirrhotic patients in hepatic coma: a randomized double-blind placebo-controlled crossover trial. Hepatology 19:32–37, 1994

Rapoport DM: Buspirone: anxiolytic treatment with respiratory implications. Fam Pract Res J 11:32–37, 1988

Reedy JE, Swartz MT, Termuhlen DF, et al: Bridge to heart transplantation: importance of patient selection. J Heart Transplant 9:473–480, 1990

Regier DA, Narrow WE, Rae DS, et al: The de facto US mental and addictive disorders services system. Arch Gen Psychiatry 50:85–94, 1993

Robins LN, Helzer JE, Croughan J, et al: National Institute of Mental Health Diagnostic Interview Schedule: its history, characteristics, and validity. Arch Gen Psychiatry 38:381–389, 1981

Rodin G, Voshart K: Depressive symptoms and functional impairment in the medically ill. Gen Hosp Psychiatry 9:251–258, 1987

Rodriguez A, Diaz M, Colon A, et al: Psychosocial profile of noncompliant transplant patients. Transplant Proc 23:1807–1809, 1991

Roose SP, Dalack GW, Glassman AH, et al: Cardiovascular effects of bupropion in depressed patients with liver disease. Am J Psychiatry 148:512–516, 1991

Rovelli M, Palmeri D, Vossler E, et al: Noncompliance in organ transplant recipients. Transplant Proc 21:833–834, 1989

Rubin AN, Kang H: Cerebral blindness and encephalopathy with cyclosporin A toxicity. Neurology 37:1072–1076, 1987

Ruzevich SA, Swartz MT, Reedy JE, et al: Retrospective analysis of the psychologic effects of mechanical circulatory support. J Heart Lung Transplant 9:209–212, 1990

Schall RR, Petrucci RJ, Brozena SC, et al: Cognitive function in patients with symptomatic dilated cardiomyopathy before and after cardiac transplantation. J Am Coll Cardiol 14:1666–1672, 1989

Schenker S, Bergstrom RF, Wolen RL, et al: Fluoxetine disposition and elimination in cirrhosis. Clin Pharmacol Ther 44:353–359, 1988

Schweizer RT, Rovelli M, Palmeri D, et al: Noncompliance in organ transplant recipients. Transplantation 49:374–377, 1990

Sellers EM, Bendayan R: Pharmacokinetics of psychotropic drugs in selected patient populations, in Psychopharmacology: The Third Generation of Progress. Edited by Meltzer HY. New York, Raven, 1987, pp 1397–1406

Series F, Cormier Y, Laforge J: Changes in day and night time oxygenation with protriptyline in patients with chronic obstructive pulmonary disease. Thorax 44:275–279, 1989

Shapiro PA, Kornfeld DS: Psychiatric outcome of heart transplantation. Gen Hosp Psychiatry 11:352–357, 1989

Shaw PJ, Bates D, Cartlide NEF: Early neurological complication of coronary artery bypass surgery. BMJ 291:1384–1386, 1985

Sills LM, Popkin MK: Elective removal of a transplanted organ. Psychosomatics 33:461–465, 1992

Simonds AK, Parker RA, Branthwaite MA: Effects of protriptyline on sleep-related disturbances of breathing in restrictive chest wall disease. Thorax 41:586–590, 1986

Sirota P, Stoler M, Meshulam B: Major depression with psychotic features associated with acyclovir therapy. Drug Intelligence and Clinical Pharmacy 22:306–308, 1988

Skotzko CE, Brownfield E, Kobashigawa J, et al: Non-psychotic DSM-III-R Axis I psychiatric disorders and the outcome after cardiac transplantation (abstract). Psychosomatics 35:200, 1994

Smith MD, Hong BA, Robson AM: Diagnosis of depression in patients with end-stage renal disease: comparative analysis. Am J Med 79: 160–166, 1985

Spar JE: Plasma trazodone concentration in elderly depressed inpatients: cardiac effects and short-term efficacy. J Clin Psychopharmacol 7:406–409, 1987

Stevenson LW, Sietsema K, Tillisch JH, et al: Exercise capacity for survivors of cardiac transplantation or sustained medical therapy for stable heart failure. Circulation 81:78–85, 1990

Stoudemire A, Fogel BS: Psychopharmacology in the medically ill, in Principles of Medical Psychiatry. Edited by Stoudemire A, Fogel BS. Orlando, FL, Grune & Stratton, 1987, pp 79–112

Strouse TB, Salehmoghaddam S, Spar JE: Acute delirium and parkinsonism in a bupropion-treated liver transplant recipient (letter). J Clin Psychiatry 54:489–490, 1993

Surman OS: Psychiatric aspects of organ transplantation. Am J Psychiatry 146:972–982, 1989 (published erratum appears in Am J Psychiatry 146:1523, 1989)

Surman OS: Liver transplantation, in Psychiatric Aspects of Organ Transplantation. Edited by Craven J, Rodin G. Oxford, UK, Oxford University Press, 1992, pp 177–188

Surman OS: Psychiatric aspects of liver transplantation. Psychosomatics 35:297–307, 1994

Surman OS, Purtilo R: Reevaluation of organ transplantation criteria: allocation of scarce resources to borderline candidates. Psychosomatics 33:202–212, 1992

Surman OS, Dienstag JL, Cosimi AB, et al: Liver transplantation: psychiatric considerations. Psychosomatics 28:615–618, 621, 1987a

Surman OS, Dienstag JL, Cosimi AB, et al: Psychosomatic aspects of liver transplantation. Psychother Psychosom 48:26–31, 1987b

Suszycki LH: Social work groups on a heart transplant program. J Heart Lung Transplant 5:166–170, 1986

Tarter RE, Switala J, Plail J, et al: Severity of hepatic encephalopathy before liver transplantation is associated with quality of life after transplantation. Arch Intern Med 152:2097–2101, 1992

Tesar GE, Murray GB, Cassem NH: Use of high-dose intravenous haloperidol in the treatment of agitated cardiac patients. J Clin Psychopharmacol 5:344–347, 1985

Thompson CB, June CH, Sullivan KM, et al: Association between cyclosporin neurotoxicity and hypomagnesemia. Lancet 2:1116–1120, 1984

Thompson MN, Jeffries DJ: Ganciclovir therapy in iatrogenically immunosuppressed patients with cytomegalovirus disease. J Antimicrob Chemother 23:61–70, 1989

Tollemar J, Ringden O, Ericzon BG, et al: Cyclosporin associated central nervous system toxicity. N Engl J Med 318:788–789, 1988

Troy SM, Schultz RW, Parker VD, et al: The effect of renal disease on the disposition of venlafaxine. Clin Pharmacol Ther 56:14–21, 1994

Trzepacz PT, Brenner RP, Coffman G, et al: Delirium in liver transplantation candidates: discriminant analysis of multiple test variables. Biol Psychiatry 24:3–14, 1988

Trzepacz PT, Brenner R, Van Thiel DH: A psychiatric study of 247 liver transplantation candidates. Psychosomatics 30:147–153, 1989

Trzepacz PT, Levenson JL, Tringali RA: Psychopharmacology and neuropsychiatric syndromes in organ transplantation. Gen Hosp Psychiatry 13:233–245, 1991

Trzepacz PT, DiMartini A, Tringali R: Psychopharmacologic issues in organ transplantation, part I: pharmacokinetics in organ failure and psychiatric aspects of immunosuppressants and anti-infectious agents. Psychosomatics 34:199–207, 1993a

Trzepacz PT, DiMartini A, Tringali RD: Psychopharmacologic issues in organ transplantation, part II: psychopharmacologic medications. Psychosomatics 34: 290–298, 1993b

Tulloch IF, Johnson AM: The pharmacologic profile of paroxetine, a new serotonin-specific reuptake inhibitor. J Clin Psychiatry 53 (no 2, suppl):7–12, 1992

Twillman RK, Manetto C, Wolcott DL: The transplant evaluation scale: a revision of the psychosocial levels system for evaluating organ transplant candidates. Psychosomatics 34: 144–153, 1993

Vaillant GE: The Natural History of Alcoholism. Cambridge, MA, Harvard University Press, 1983

Vidt DG: Selection and preparation of patients for renal transplantation. Surg Clin North Am 51:1105–1121, 1971

Viewig WVR, Godleski LS: Carbamazepine and hyponatremia. Am J Psychiatry 145: 1323–1324, 1988

Vogt DP, Lederman RJ, Carey WD, et al: Neurologic complication after liver transplantation. Transplantation 45:1057–1061, 1988

von Moltke LL, Greenblatt DJ, Shader RI: Clinical pharmacokinetics of antidepressants in the elderly: therapeutic implications. Clin Pharmacokinet 24:141–160, 1993

Walden JA, Stevenson LW, Dracup K, et al: Heart transplantation may not improve quality of life for patients with stable heart failure. Heart Lung 18:497–506, 1989

Wamboldt FW, Weiler SV, Kalin NH: Cyclosporin-associated mania (letter). Biol Psychiatry 19: 1161–1162, 1984

Weems J, Patterson ET: Coping with uncertainty and ambivalence while awaiting a cadaveric renal transplant. ANNA J 16:27–31, 1989

Wells KB, Golding JM, Burnam MA: Affective, substance use, and anxiety disorders in persons with arthritis, diabetes, heart disease, high blood pressure, or chronic lung conditions. Gen Hosp Psychiatry 11:320–327, 1989

Wilczek H, Rigden O, Tyden G: Cyclosporine associated central nervous system toxicity after renal transplantation (letter). Transplantation 39:110, 1984

Wilson SE, DeGroen PC, Aksamit AJ, et al: Cyclosporine A induced reversible cortical blindness. Clinical Neuro-Ophthalmology 8: 215–220, 1988

Winnock S, Janvier G, Parmentier F, et al: Pontine myelinolysis following liver transplantation: a report of two cases. Transpl Int 6:26–28, 1993

Wolcott DL: Organ transplant psychiatry: psychiatry's role in the second gift of life. Psychosomatics 1:388–394, 1990

Wolcott DL: Psychiatric aspects of renal dialysis and organ transplantation. Psychiatr Med 9: 623–640, 1991

Chapter 20

Oncology

Fawzy I. Fawzy, M.D.
Donna B. Greenberg, M.D.

Today, many patients with cancer are completely cured; others live far longer than they did before. In the past, meeting the psychosocial needs of most patients with cancer involved only the care of the terminally ill. Now the tasks of clinicians in psychooncology include facilitating life after a cancer diagnosis, combating increasing tolerance to treatment, and managing psychiatric complications in patients and families. A life-threatening disease such as cancer prematurely interrupts a forward life trajectory, disrupting an individual's assumptive world (Fawzy and Fawzy 1982; Fawzy and Natterson 1994; Holland and Rowland 1989). Patients who are in great distress may seek out a psychiatrist as they adjust their assumptions, find adaptive and maladaptive coping strategies, and move forward. The psychiatrist's task is to diagnose and treat patients who have syndromes that impair psychological function, to facilitate the patient's strengths and adaptive capacity, and to bolster the patient's outside resources (Breitbart 1995).

The experience of cancer includes distinct chronological phases: prediagnosis, diagnosis, initial treatment, posttreatment, recurrence, progressive disease, and terminal/palliation. These phases are accompanied by adaptive and maladaptive responses. In the prediagnostic phase, when the question of cancer is first pursued medically, patients face fears of pain, disfigurement, isolation, and death. Ideally, in the diagnostic phase, the physician delivers the news of cancer in an unhurried and honest manner, with realistic hope and the commitment to stand by the patient. In this early phase, the patient faces the existential plight (Weisman and Worden 1976–1977), and most often he or she adjusts to the tasks at hand with hope for the future. Frequently, however, repetition of clinical information is necessary as anxiety blocks complete comprehension and assimilation of information. Sleep may be disrupted; shock and disbelief come with the normal defense of denial.

Treatment brings fears of surgical pain, death, or loss of control and vulnerability. Patients may grieve the loss of a breast, uterus, arm, or leg. They may lose the activities of the healthy world of work, social contact, and the ability to move easily. Physical changes such as weight gain and hair loss come with chemotherapy. Sexual function and fertility are at risk. Neuropsychiatric complications of treatment must be identified, treated, and, if possible, prevented.

When initial treatment has been completed, patients face the threat of recurrence of the cancer. Just when it seems as if a patient could be rejoicing at the completion of treatment, the anxiety of the posttreatment phase becomes prominent. Many patients fear that cancer will recur while doctors are not watching as closely and while the treatment is not actively killing the tumor. With that fear, the patient may feel that he or she must become the guardian over every ache and pain. For many patients who proceed through a schedule of the checkups that structure life in remission, each visit and follow-up scan provokes significant anticipatory anxiety.

Recurrent cancer produces great distress and disappointment, especially when recurrence signals that the tumor will not be curable. Patients may search desperately for new information, new doctors, and alternative therapies. The terminal/palliation phase signals the patient's awareness of the irreversible nature of the illness. He or she fears abandonment, loss of bodily dignity, and pain. Concerns include unfinished business, children left without care, and grief over losses.

ANXIETY

Anticipatory Nausea and Vomiting

Nausea and vomiting constitute a profound stimulus, a "one-time-is-enough" (Ellis et al. 1979), vivid visceral memory that is tightly bound to associated stimuli. Patients who vomit with chemotherapy frequently develop an aversion to the hospital, nurse, or the sight and smell of medical implements. Nausea or vomiting may be the most obvious manifestation, but the entire array of anticipatory symptoms is mediated by the severity of anxiety before treatment, and the conditioned anxiety is linked to these memories (Andrykowski 1990). Paradoxically, the patient is trapped by visceral dread of the very treatment that may preserve his or her life (Greenberg 1991).

There are several ways to manage this clinical phenomenon. The first strategy is to prevent this condition by optimal antiemetic treatment (Stefanek et al. 1988). The second strategy is to minimize anxiety just before treatment by use of benzodiazepines such as alprazolam or lorazepam (Greenberg 1991; Holland et al. 1991; Razavi et al. 1993; Triozzi et al. 1988), systematic desensitization (Morrow and Morrell 1982), hypnosis, or distraction. Benzodiazepines should continue through the period of nausea after chemotherapy, but with an end point for their use agreed on in advance by physician and patient.

Claustrophobia

Patients with clinical anxiety in closed spaces have great difficulty with the magnetic resonance imaging (MRI) equipment (Meléndez and McCrank 1993) and occasionally with other diagnostic tests. Antianxiety premedication helps, as does having the patient come to the laboratory with a significant other. Special attention by the technicians helps. If the phobia is recognized as a problem in advance, the physician may be able to tailor and shorten the test by, for example, focusing the MRI study on the section of the patient's body that poses the most immediate diagnostic question.

Akathisia

The restlessness and need to walk around that is associated with neuroleptics—akathisia—can be mistaken for anxiety in the oncology setting. Restlessness, insomnia, and inner discomfort may be mistaken for agitated depression. Because phenothiazines such as perphenazine and prochlorperazine are used so commonly to prevent nausea, patients may not even report their usage when asked about drug intake. Usually one of the phenothiazines or metoclopramide is the hidden culprit. Drug elimination resolves the problem.

Pulmonary Embolus or Pulmonary Edema

Pulmonary edema and, in particular, pulmonary embolus are medical causes of anxiety due to hypoxia; these conditions should cross a consultant's mind in the first moments of anxiety symptom evaluation. Emboli are commonly seen with many types of cancer.

■ DEPRESSION

The American tradition to believe in the power of positive thinking has a strong appeal to patients with cancer. Positive thinking offers hope and implies a means to control directly the course of the cancer. Depression and cancer were linked by Galen, and patients who learn of the growing field of psychoimmunology sometimes have the impression that negative thoughts or admission of demoralization has the power to make tumor cells grow (Greenberg 1989). In psychotherapy, the task may be to put a patient's negative thoughts, anger, and sadness in perspective and to clarify that these thoughts do not correlate simply with tumor growth.

The prevalence of current major depression in patients in cancer centers is 5%–8% (Derogatis et al. 1983; Lansky et al. 1985; Valente et al. 1994), about the same as rates reported among patients with other medical illnesses. The prevalence of adjustment disorder is higher, perhaps 25% (Derogatis et al. 1983). Those with a history of depression, panic disorder, or bipolar disorder are at greater risk. Those in chronic pain are also more likely to

have associated depressive features. One cancer in particular, pancreatic cancer, has been associated with a disproportionate incidence of dysphoria as a presenting and associated feature (Holland et al. 1986). Steroids and biological treatments such as interferon are the most common anticancer medications associated with affective instability.

Suicide is rare among patients with cancer. Epidemiological studies in Finland (Louhivuori and Hakama 1979) and Connecticut (Fox et al. 1982), as well as studies of death certificates, have demonstrated only a slightly higher suicide rate among patients with cancer compared with persons in the general population. Some patients will hold out the option of suicide as an escape from the specter of unremitting pain and suffering, which preserves the sense that they can be in control. Most patients wish to receive continuing care and symptomatic relief even if the disease is progressing (Massie et al. 1994).

The diagnosis of depression in the medically ill is always confounded by similar physical symptoms in both depression and somatic illness (McDaniel et al. 1995). The unrelenting awareness of the diagnosis, inability to concentrate, guilt of being a burden, suicidal thoughts, insomnia not due to pain, and awakening in the morning with dread all argue differentially in favor of primary depression.

In general, antidepressant choice depends on target symptoms and the need to avoid undesirable side effects in a given patient. In patients without cardiac conduction defects, tricyclic antidepressants may be beneficial, especially if effects on sleep and pain are sought. However, because many patients with cancer—including those with breast cancer, for example, who are taking adjuvant chemotherapy—will gain weight (Demark-Wahnefried et al. 1993), the tendency for patients on tricyclic medication to crave sweets may be an undesirable side effect. A trial of a psychostimulant, such as dextroamphetamine (Fernandez et al. 1987), methylphenidate, or pemoline (Breitbart and Mermelstein 1992), is appropriate for a rapid effect in those patients who are systemically ill and who are depressed, apathetic, and not eating. A course of treatment lasting 1–2 months has been shown to provide lasting benefit in patients with cancer.

Trazodone is widely used among medically ill patients, including patients with cancer. This drug has the distinct advantage of addressing the troublesome target symptoms of insomnia and appetite disturbance.

Selective serotonin reuptake inhibitors (SSRIs) are commonly used in medical-surgical populations because of their favorable adverse-effect profile. Fluoxetine does not have the disadvantage of anticholinergic and sedative side effects. However, it can add to anorexia, jitteriness, and agitation, and, as with the tricyclic medications, the antidepressant response is delayed by several weeks (Massie et al. 1991; Shuster et al. 1992). Fluoxetine inhibits metabolism by the P-450 enzyme system. It is fortunate, however, that this is unlikely to affect other chemotherapy regimens. The initial appetite-suppressant effect of fluoxetine, along with nausea, diarrhea, and agitation, makes this drug a poor choice for some debilitated patients but an advantage for those who have gained too much weight. Sertraline and paroxetine, each of which has a shorter half-life than fluoxetine, do not typically cause an increase or decrease in weight but can have similar initial gastrointestinal (GI) side effects.

Neither tricyclic medications nor SSRIs typically interact with chemotherapeutic agents. However, procarbazine, used primarily for Hodgkin's disease, is a mild monoamine oxidase inhibitor (MAOI) and disulfiram-like drug that delays metabolism of other psychotropic medications. Most oncologists proscribe alcohol but not tyramine-containing foods when prescribing procarbazine. Fortunately, it is unlikely for a hypertensive crisis to occur even if the patient is concurrently given a tricyclic antidepressant (DeVita et al. 1965); hypertensive crisis has never been reported.

However, procarbazine's use with fluoxetine or other SSRI should probably be avoided.

MANIA

Mania is rarely related to cancer itself. Although in rare cases diencephalic tumors and cerebral metastases have led to secondary mania, corticosteroids are the most frequent cause of syndromes resembling mania among patients with cancer (Greenberg and Brown 1985).

As cancer treatment progresses, lithium treatment remains appropriate for patients with primary bipolar disorder (Greenberg et al. 1993b). Lithium will favorably increase the patient's white blood cell count by stimulating granulocyte-stimulating factor and interleukin-6.

Lithium should be withheld on days that the patient receives chemotherapy. Lithium may expose more than the desired number of bone marrow cells to cell death at the time of chemotherapy; therefore, chemotherapy protocols that have included lithium have withheld lithium for 2 days before chemotherapy. The nausea, vomiting, and relative dehydration that may occur on days of chemotherapy make lithium toxicity both more likely to occur and more difficult to recognize.

Lithium may be continued during radiation treatment. White blood cell death is not more likely for the patient taking lithium during radiation treatment because radiation-induced cell death is not cell-cycle specific. During cranial radiation, it is best to stop lithium because of the risk of neurotoxicity and seizures from the tumor or edema.

The consultation-liaison psychiatrist should remain alert for renal compromise or brain injury that would increase the risk of lithium toxicity in a patient who is otherwise stable on the medication. The first alternative to lithium is a neuroleptic medication. Carbamazepine may also be useful for its affect-stabilizing and anticonvulsant effect. The mild leukopenia that can occur in the early treatment with carbamazepine must be evaluated in light of bone marrow reserves.

PSYCHOTHERAPEUTIC TREATMENTS

In systematic studies, individual psychotherapy (Massie et al. 1989; Watson 1983; Weisman 1976), behavioral treatment, and group therapy have been shown to reduce distress in patients with cancer. Behavioral programs and hypnosis have resulted in decreased anxiety, pain, nausea, and vomiting (Trijsburg et al. 1992). Researchers have evaluated not only the role of psychotherapy in reducing distress but also whether psychotherapy in patients with cancer can prolong life (Fawzy et al. 1995). Women with metastatic breast cancer were randomized to receive 1 year of weekly support group sessions (Spiegel et al. 1981, 1989). The investigators found that the intervention group had less mood disturbance, fewer phobic responses, and half the pain of the control group. The treated group also lived an average of 36.6 months, compared with 18.9 months for the control group.

In another series, newly diagnosed patients with stage I or II malignant melanoma who were randomized to a 6-week psychoeducational intervention experienced less turmoil than did the control group following diagnosis (Fawzy et al. 1990a, 1990b, 1993). At 6 years, significantly fewer patients in the group who received psychiatric intervention had died. The depth of the original lesions in the two groups did not account for the difference in prognosis.

COMMON NEUROLOGICAL COMPLICATIONS OF CANCER

Metastatic Brain Tumors

When a psychiatric consultant evaluates a patient with cancer for change in mental status, he or she considers the possibility that a tumor would metastasize to the brain (Cascino 1993; Hochberg and Pruitt 1987). Lung cancer, both small cell and non-small cell, metastasizes to the brain most frequently and accounts for a majority of metastatic brain tumors. Ten percent of lung cancer patients have brain metastases at diagnosis, and as many as 30% develop them later. Breast cancer metastasizes to the brain in 6%–20% of patients. In patients with metastatic melanoma, metastases to the central nervous system (CNS) are also common. Kidney cancer, typically a tumor with a very variable course, metastasizes to the brain in 11%–13% of patients. Other tumors—thyroid, pancreas, ovary, uterus, prostate, testes, bladder, and sarcoma—metastasize to the brain more rarely. The most acute management issues are treatment of brain edema with dexamethasone and seizures with anticonvulsants. Metastatic brain lesions are identified best by computed tomography (CT) scan with high doses of iodinated contrast material and delayed scanning. When a metastatic tumor appears to be isolated, surgical resection is considered. Otherwise, the treatment is whole brain radiation.

Leptomeningeal Disease

Consider leptomeningeal disease when mental status changes are associated with a normal CT scan (Wasserstrom 1982). Cytological examination of cerebrospinal fluid (CSF) may reveal malignant cells. This finding is most likely with non-Hodgkin's lymphoma, leukemia, melanoma, and adenocarcinoma of the lung, breast, or GI system. In addition to mental status changes, patients usually have cranial nerve deficits or radicular signs. The nonspecific signs that may prompt psychiatric referral include headache, balance difficulty, and seizures.

Complex Partial Seizures

Patients with cancer are prone to seizures not only because of brain tumors but also because of leptomeningeal carcinomatoses, treatment-related brain injury, hyponatremia, hypomagnesemia, hyperviscosity syndrome (Gilbert and Armstrong 1995; Stern et al. 1985), and infections seen in immunocompromised hosts. Patients without motor symptoms but with primary psychiatric manifestations may be referred to the psychiatrist. Delirium, catatonia, transient focal symptoms, minor tremors, vocalization and speech arrest, simple hallucinations, tingling, light flashes, buzzing, episodic autonomic changes, epigastric sensations, distortions of time, strong emotions, dreamy states, panic attacks, illusions, and the pathognomonic symptom of bad smells should suggest partial seizures. Of note, phenytoin levels decrease in patients receiving chemotherapy (Grossman et al. 1989).

Paraneoplastic Syndromes

Delirium in patients with cancer may be related to distant, nonmetastatic effects of tumors. Subacute cerebellar degeneration, encephalomyopathy, and Eaton-Lambert myasthenic syndrome form a spectrum of neurological insults that are frequently associated with delirium and dementia. Limbic encephalopathy results in a prominent memory defect, anxiety, depression, and seizures. The mechanism is thought to be autoimmune and to be associated with antineuronal antibodies (Cornelius et al. 1986; Moll et al. 1990; Newman et al. 1990; Posner 1989).

Ectopic production of hormone by tumors can alter mental status by 1) increasing antidiuretic hormone production and causing low sodium levels, 2) increasing parathyroid hormone production and causing high calcium levels, or 3) increasing adrenocorticotropic hormone production and causing Cushing's syndrome, characterized by excess cortisol production that is often associated with affective change. Paraneoplastic phenomena are most common with small cell carcinoma of the lung; however, breast, stomach, uterine, renal,

testicular, thyroid, and colon cancers may also be associated with paraneoplastic syndromes (Minotti et al. 1994; Peterson et al. 1994; Schiller and Jones 1993).

Other Causes of Delirium

Delirium secondary to hypercalcemia is an oncological emergency and is often secondary to bone metastases. The treatment is rehydration, administration of diphosphonates (specific anticalcium agents), and possibly a change in antitumor regimen. Subtle signs of hypercalcemia, such as fatigue, nausea, or cognitive impairment, may be mistaken for depression. Calcium is bound to albumin, and total serum calcium values that are within normal limits may be significant if the albumin is low.

Hypomagnesemia in patients with cancer is most commonly secondary to the tubular defect caused by cisplatin or secondary to impaired nutrition (Schilsky and Anderson 1979). Hypomagnesemia has been associated with lethargy and depression, hypocalcemia, hypokalemia, and increased risk for seizures.

Hyperviscosity syndrome, with a sudden onset of confusion or seizures, occurs in patients with lymphoma, Waldenström's macroglobulinemia, and myeloma (Crawford et al. 1985). Paraproteins increase blood viscosity and impair circulation in the brain. A level above 4.0 centipoise (cp) (normal is between 1.56 and 1.68 cp) has been associated with symptoms. Classic symptoms of hyperviscosity syndrome are bleeding, visual signs and symptoms, and delirium. Plasmapheresis, along with primary anticancer treatment, may be indicated.

COMPLICATIONS OF TREATMENT

Complications of Radiation Treatment

In addition to medical side effects of skin inflammation and bone marrow suppression, patients may develop fatigue or nausea. Side effects are related to the volume radiated, and nausea is related to radiation over viscera (Greenberg 1991; Greenberg et al. 1992, 1993a). After the course of treatment is complete, fatigue diminishes over several weeks. Patients who receive radiation to the CNS take dexamethasone to reduce swelling. The required dosage of dexamethasone is commonly associated with insomnia and agitation. Brain radiation causes much more profound fatigue than does radiation to other sites. Radiation treatment near the neck presents the risk of hypothyroidism. Radiation to the brain may also affect pituitary function.

Neuropsychiatric Side Effects of Anticancer Agents

Neuropsychiatric side effects are among the most important potential clinical complications of anticancer agents. Table 20–1 describes some of the important side effects that consultation-liaison psychiatrists may encounter.

Treatment-Related Dementia

Cancer treatment sometimes causes a late dementia. The most common lesion is disseminated necrotizing leukoencephalopathy. These white matter lesions, seen better on MRI than on CT scans, may be transient or progressive. Their onset may be marked by ataxia, confusion, somnolence, spasticity, and dementia. Gray matter and basal ganglia are spared. Cerebral atrophy is common after brain radiation but correlates poorly with neurological function and may be reversible (Frytak et al. 1985; Lee et al. 1986; Rottenberg 1991).

Anorexia

When patients with cancer lose their appetite, their refusal to eat often becomes a focus for family conflict (Holland et al. 1977). Some appetite loss may be due to chemotherapy, radiation, or progression of a systemic tumor. Major depressive disorder, conditioned taste aversion (Bernstein 1978), and/or anxiety about pain or

diarrhea that will follow food intake may also contribute. In the setting of medical illness, appetite may be stimulated by increasing the patient's energy with agents such as dextroamphetamine. Megestrol acetate (Loprinzi 1995; Loprinzi et al. 1990, 1994a), cyproheptadine, prednisone, and cannabinoids have all been used to foster weight gain (Nelson et al. 1994).

Sexual Dysfunction and Infertility

Cancer can cut life short. Initially, mortality eclipses all other issues, but as the hope for survival increases, younger patients consider their sexual attractiveness, sexual function, and ability to have children. In women who have ovarian cancer or endometrial cancer, which requires surgical resection of the organs of parturition, the loss of fertility is immediate (Flay and Matthews 1995). After breast cancer, the hormones of pregnancy may promote micrometastases, so a woman must feel confident of cure as she faces pregnancy.

Procarbazine and alkylating agents are the chemotherapeutic agents most apt to cause infertility (Thachil et al. 1981), but many regimens do not affect fertility. Men with Hodgkin's disease or testicular cancer may have low sperm counts at diagnosis. With procarbazine and alkylating agents, men become sterile as treatment progresses but may become fertile again years later. Some men may choose to preserve sperm before chemotherapy treatment.

■ FAMILIES OF PATIENTS WITH CANCER

Longer survival times for patients with cancer bring greater demands for families. The course of cancer involves many emotional ups and downs that still, in some cases, end in loss. The manner in which a particular family deals with this turmoil depends on the ages and number of family members, their coping resources, their stability before the patient's diagnosis, their ethnic and cultural background, and the

Table 20–1.   Neuropsychiatric side effects of chemotherapeutic agents

Hormones

Tamoxifen[a]
1. Syndrome mimics menopausal symptoms: hot flashes, sleep disorder, irritability
2. Occasionally associated with hypercalcemia early in treatment
3. One report of confusion that began after 2 days and remitted in 7–10 days

Aminoglutethimide
1. Initial syndrome of rash, malaise, fatigue
2. Congener of glutethimide
3. May minimize symptoms by increasing dose gradually

Megestrol acetate[b]
1. Progestogen
2. Increases appetite; useful in patients with cachexia; weight gain and side effects are dose related
3. Low doses (20 mg qid) are useful for hot flashes[c]

Fluoxymesterone
1. Androgen
2. Irritability, increased libido, hirsutism

Corticosteroids[d]
1. Graded by Rome and Braceland (1952): grade I, mild to more severe; grade II, hyperactivity and insomnia; grade III, lability, anxiety, agitation; grade IV, psychosis with prominent affective features
2. Dose related; more common with the equivalent of 60 mg/day or more of prednisone
3. Manic and depressive features prominent
4. History of psychosis apparently does not increase risk
5. In repeated cycles of chemotherapy, the affective response may vary
6. Cessation of steroid may be associated with muscle aching and letdown
7. If a major organic affective syndrome has occurred, then remission does not occur immediately with stopping steroids and patient should be treated with psychotropic medication
8. Treatment for hyperactivity and insomnia is with major tranquilizers, such as perphenazine and haloperidol; clonazepam may also be helpful
9. Lithium has been used prophylactically in the setting of steroid treatment of patients with multiple sclerosis

Chemotherapy

Procarbazine[e]
1. Mechanism unclear; likely inhibits DNA, RNA, and protein synthesis
2. Causes somnolence, psychosis, and delirium with immediate onset, rapid resolution
3. Weak MAO effect: no clinical reports of drug interaction leading to hypertensive crisis; most oncologists do not recommend a tyramine-restricted diet; no reports of hypertensive crisis
4. One case of mania has been reported
5. Delays metabolism of barbiturates and phenothiazines
6. Disulfiram-like effect; do not mix with alcohol

L-Asparaginase[f]
1. Mechanism: deprives acute lymphocytic leukemia cells of aspartate, a required amino acid that these cells cannot synthesize
2. Somnolence, lethargy, delirium, of immediate onset and rapid resolution; not dose related, common
3. Rare late-onset (day 8) delirium; may be related to lack of asparagine

Pyrimidine analogues (inhibit DNA synthesis)

Cytosine arabinoside[g]
1. High dose causes delirium; dose related, age related
2. Onset on days 2–4, lasting a week
3. May be due to toxic metabolite, uracil arabinoside
4. Leukoencephalopathy may result from high dose: syndrome of personality change, drowsiness, dementia, psychomotor retardation, ataxia
5. Periventricular white matter signal densities on MRI: discrete, multifocal, coagulative necrosis in periventricular white matter and centrum semiovale bilaterally; demyelination occurs
6. Cerebellar syndrome

5-Fluorouracil[h]
1. Fatigue
2. Rare delirium or seizure (especially with break in blood-brain barrier or aberrant metabolic pathway)
3. Cerebellar syndrome

(continued)

Table 20–1. Neuropsychiatric side effects of chemotherapeutic agents (*continued*)

Folate antagonist

Methotrexate[i,j]

1. Inhibits reduction of dihydrofolate and thereby inhibits DNA, RNA, and protein synthesis
2. More neurological toxicity with high-dose or intrathecal regimens
3. More toxicity with concomitant radiation treatment
4. Transient delirium—days 10–13
5. Leucovorin rescue—5-hydrofolinic acid
6. High-dose or intrathecal administration may cause leukoencephalopathy

Metaphase inhibitors[k]

Vincristine, vinblastine

1. Dysphoria, lethargy
2. Dose related
3. Consider risk of seizures, inappropriate ADH (low sodium)
4. Vincristine inhibits dopamine hydroxylase; more dysphoria in small cell lung cancer protocol when added to complex regimen
5. Myelotoxic effects of vinblastine are more limited so neurotoxicity is less common than with vincristine

Alkylating agents[l]

Ifosfamide

1. Related to cyclophosphamide, which is not associated with neurotoxicity
2. Urinary toxicity related to metabolite acrolein-related hemorrhagic cystitis; now toxicity is blocked by concomitant use of mesna, which binds acrolein, so ifosfamide can be used at higher doses
3. CNS toxicity ranges from lethargy to seizures, coma, and death; includes delirium, cerebellar signs, weakness, and cranial nerve deficit
4. EEG shows delta rhythmic slowing consistent with metabolic or toxic syndrome
5. Usually patients return to normal in 3 days
6. Attributed to chloracetaldehyde (metabolite of ifosfamide) but not to cyclophosphamide
7. Degraded by alcohol dehydrogenase
8. Renal impairment (e.g., from nephrectomy, previous DDP toxicity) is a risk factor for CNS toxicity
9. Mimics alcohol intoxication
10. Ifosfamide associated with inappropriate ADH, so check sodium

Biologicals

Interferon[m]

1. Most get flulike syndrome, with fever, myalgias, malaise, which dissipates
2. Diffuse encephalopathy noted at high doses
3. Syndrome of fatigue, difficulty in concentration, psychomotor retardation, and general disinterest at 3 million units/day im; affective changes not prominent
4. Two reports of patients with psychotic reactions, two reports of patients with manic symptoms; four other cases of psychosis reported in patients on more than 20 million units/m^2
5. Among 58 patients treated with interferon for chronic viral hepatitis: 4 had marked irritability and short temper (organic personality syndrome); 3 had tearfulness, depression, and hopelessness (organic affective syndrome); 3 had delirium (delirium occurred in those with a history of brain injury or more severe liver disease)

Interleukin-2 (IL-2) and lymphokine-activated killer cells (LAK)[n]

1. Delirium is dose related
2. Mostly at end of course of IL-2 or several days after onset of combined treatment
3. Delirium in IL-2 phases did not predict delirium in next phase
4. Recovery in 2–3 days
5. Other factors such as hypoxia or sepsis can contribute to delirium
6. Most patients have flulike syndrome, with malaise, chills, anorexia, fatigue with treatment (fever and chills are effectively treated with 50 mg meperidine iv)
7. Affective changes other than delirium not prominent
8. Hypothyroidism posttreatment (mostly in women with preexisting antibodies suggesting autoimmune thyroiditis)

Note. ADH = antidiuretic hormone; CNS = central nervous system; DDP = diamminedichloroplatinum (cisplatin); DNA = deoxyribonucleic acid; EEG = electroencephalogram; MAO = monoamine oxidase; MRI = magnetic resonance imaging; qid = four times a day; RNA = ribonucleic acid.
Source. [a]Pluss and DiBella 1984; [b]Loprinzi et al. 1990; [c]Loprinzi et al. 1994b; [d]Ling et al. 1981; [e]DeVita et al. 1965; [f]Holland et al. 1974; [g]Lazarus et al. 1981; [h]Lynch et al. 1981; [i]Mulhern et al. 1987; [j]Walker et al. 1986; [k]Silberfarb et al. 1983; [l]Zalupski and Baker 1988; [m]Adams et al. 1984; [n]Denicoff et al. 1987.

roles and responsibilities of each family member (Lewis 1993).

In the best scenarios, the cohesiveness and emotional closeness of the family will actually increase, creating a sense of joy and appreciation for their home life and living in general. Such families communicate openly with both the patient and the physician throughout the patient's illness. The patient's ability to discuss feelings openly with the physician and family, and to participate in future family plans, gives meaning and continuity to all concerned (Fawzy et al. 1983).

However, emotional and financial drains may disrupt families. Family caretakers must deal with their own emotional distress while also meeting the needs of the patient and other family members, whose needs usually increase as well. Caretakers may benefit from permission to meet their own needs for food, rest, and relaxation without guilt for leaving the patient at times. Caretakers need to know that they can and should ask for help from staff members, from other family members, and from friends. Rather than viewing requests as an imposition, many family members and friends are relieved and grateful to be able to do something to help (Rait and Lederberg 1989). The patient with cancer and his or her partner often hide their feelings of helplessness and fear in an effort to appear optimistic and reassuring. Studies suggest that a conspiracy of silence is not helpful, but expression of feelings and shared involvement in decision making improve adjustment. Support groups are an excellent resource for partners and are emerging at many medical centers.

Cancer in a child invariably results in a high level of stress on the parents. Because family disintegration, substance abuse, and serious psychopathology are common among parents of seriously ill or dying children, early psychiatric referral may be offered even without overt symptoms. When a parent is the patient, preschool and school-age children often act out their emotional distress at school. The child should know what is happening to his or her parent; the explanation should match the child's level of understanding. Older children and adolescents often experience role reversal as they become caregivers (Fawzy and Natterson 1994).

Many families will appreciate the physician letting them know or confirming their impression that the patient's death is near. The death of a loved one may often be met with relief, both personal and projected, and with the rationalization that at least the suffering is over. The physician can offer a close family member the opportunity to visit the office a few weeks after the patient's death to ask questions about the course of the illness or autopsy results. This meeting often gives the family member a chance to discuss guilt or anxiety over something he or she feels was done that may have contributed to the patient's discomfort or early death. Talking with a physician who knew and respected the patient, who assisted the patient and family during the final days of the illness, can help to resolve familial grief (Fawzy et al. 1983).

ONCOLOGY STAFF

Often, the psychiatric consultant to the oncology center will be asked to help medical and other center staff cope with the stresses of caring for patients with cancer. For instance, the strain of being a target of a patient's rage can weigh heavily on the oncology nurse. When family members are absent, patients tend to direct their rage primarily toward nurses, who not only are seen as maternal figures but are unconsciously viewed perhaps as more expendable than physicians and hence as more appropriate objects of anger. The consultation psychiatrist may help staff members to see that the patients' rage is at the illness, not the result of criticism of staff inadequacy.

One method to help the oncology staff to deal with the stressors of working with patients with cancer is to have clearly identified goals for each patient and then to strive to meet those goals. Patients fall into one of three categories: 1) those for whom treatment will result in a cure or long-term, disease-free survival, 2) those for whom the goal is long-term control and good quality of life (those patients who need good supportive symptom therapy, including pain control), and 3) those for whom death is fairly imminent. Patients in the third group need to know that they will not be abandoned. They need increased human contact. Recognition that the needs of each group of patients are of equal importance can go a long way toward helping staff members to feel a sense of helpfulness and satisfaction with their work.

■ REFERENCES

Adams R, Quesada JR, Gutterman JU: Neuropsychiatric manifestations of human leukocyte interferon therapy in patients with cancer. JAMA 252:938–941, 1984

Andrykowski MA: The role of anxiety in the development of anticipatory nausea in cancer chemotherapy: a review and synthesis. Psychosom Med 52:458–475, 1990

Bernstein IL: Learned taste aversions in children receiving chemotherapy. Science 200: 1302–1303, 1978

Breitbart W: Identifying patients at risk for, and treatment of, major psychiatric complications of cancer. Support Care Cancer 3:45–60, 1995

Breitbart W, Mermelstein H: Pemoline: an alternative psychostimulant in the management of depressive disorders in cancer patients. Psychosomatics 33:352–356, 1992

Cascino TL: Neurologic complications of systemic cancer. Med Clin North Am 77:265–278, 1993

Cornelius JR, Soloff PH, Miewald BK: Behavioral manifestations of paraneoplastic encephalopathy. Biol Psychiatry 21:686–690, 1986

Crawford J, Cox EB, Cohen HJ: Evaluation of hyperviscosity in monoclonal gammopathies. Am J Med 79:13–22, 1985

Demark-Wahnefried W, Winer EP, Rimer BK: Why women gain weight with adjuvant chemotherapy for breast cancer. J Clin Oncol 11: 1418–1429, 1993

Denicoff KD, Rubinow DR, Papa MZ, et al: The neuropsychiatric effects of treatment with interleukin-2 and lymphokine-activated killer cells. Ann Intern Med 107:293–300, 1987

Derogatis LR, Morrow RG, Fetting J, et al: The prevalence of psychiatric disorders among cancer patients (abstract). JAMA 249:751, 1983

DeVita VT, Hahn MA, Oliverio VT: Monoamine oxidase inhibition by a new carcinostatic agent, N-isopropyl a-(2-methylhydrazino)-p-toluamide. Proc Soc Exp Biol Med 118: 561–565, 1965

Ellis HC, Bennett TC, Daniel TC, et al: Psychology of Learning and Memory. Monterey, CA, Brooks Cole Publishing, 1979, pp 33–34

Fawzy FI, Fawzy NW: Psychosocial aspects of cancer, in Diagnosis and Management of Cancer. Edited by Nixon D. Menlo Park, NJ, Addison-Wesley, 1982, pp 111–123

Fawzy FI, Natterson B: Psychological care of the cancer patient, in Clinical Oncology: A Lange Clinical Manual. Edited by Cameron R. San Mateo, CA, Simon and Schuster Higher Education Group, 1994, pp 40–44

Fawzy FI, Pasnau RO, Wolcott DL, et al: Psychosocial management of cancer. Psychiatric Medicine 1:165–180, 1983

Fawzy FI, Cousins N, Fawzy NW, et al: A structured psychiatric intervention for cancer patients, I: changes over time in methods of coping and affective disturbance. Arch Gen Psychiatry 47:720–725, 1990a

Fawzy FI, Kemeny ME, Fawzy NW, et al: A structured psychiatric intervention for cancer patients, II: changes over time in immunological measures. Arch Gen Psychiatry 47:729–735, 1990b

Fawzy FI, Fawzy NW, Hyun CS, et al: Malignant melanoma, effects of an early structured psychiatric intervention, coping, and affective state on recurrence and survival 6 years later. Arch Gen Psychiatry 50:681–689, 1993

Fawzy FI, Fawzy NW, Arndt LA, et al: Critical review of psychosocial interventions in cancer care. Arch Gen Psychiatry 52:100–113, 1995

Fernandez F, Adams F, Holmes VF, et al: Methyl-phenidate for depressive disorders in cancer patients. Psychosomatics 28:455–461, 1987

Flay LD, Matthews JH: The effects of radiotherapy and surgery on the sexual function of women treated for cervical cancer. Int J Radiat Oncol Biol Phys 31:399–404, 1995

Fox BH, Stanek EJ, Boyd SC, et al: Suicide rates among cancer patients in Connecticut. Journal of Chronic Disease 35:85–100, 1982

Frytak S, Earnest F IV, O'Neill BP, et al: Magnetic resonance imaging for neurotoxicity in long-term survivors of carcinoma. Mayo Clin Proc 60:803–812, 1985

Gilbert MR, Armstrong TS: Management of seizures in the adult patient with cancer. Cancer Practice 3:143–149, 1995

Greenberg DB: Depression and cancer, in Depression and Coexisting Disease. Edited by Robinson RG, Rabins PV. New York, Igaku-Shoin Medical Publishers, 1989, pp 103–115

Greenberg DB: Strategic use of benzodiazepines in cancer patients. Oncology 5:83–88, 1991

Greenberg DB, Brown GL: Single case study: mania resulting from brain stem tumor. J Nerv Ment Dis 173:434–436, 1985

Greenberg DB, Sawicka J, Eisenthal S, et al: Fatigue syndrome due to localized radiation. J Pain Symptom Manage 7:38–45, 1992

Greenberg DB, Gray JL, Mannic CM, et al.: Treatment related fatigue and serum interleukin 1 levels in patients during external beam irradiation for prostate cancer. J Pain Symptom Manage 8:196–199, 1993a

Greenberg DB, Younger J, Kaufman SD: Management of lithium in patients with cancer. Psychosomatics 34:388–394, 1993b

Grossman SA, Sheidler VR, Gilbert MR: Decreased phenytoin levels in patients receiving chemotherapy. Am J Med 87:505–510, 1989

Hochberg F, Pruitt A: Neoplastic diseases of the central nervous system, in Harrison's Principles of Internal Medicine, 11th Edition. Edited by Braunwald E, Isselbacher KJ, Petersdorf RG, et al. New York, McGraw-Hill, 1987, pp 1968–1980

Holland JC, Rowland JH (eds): Handbook of Psychooncology: Psychological Care of the Patient With Cancer. New York, Oxford University Press, 1989

Holland J, Fasanello S, Ohnuma T: Psychiatric symptoms associated with L-asparaginase administration. J Psychiatr Res 10:105–113, 1974

Holland JCB, Rowland J, Plumb M: Psychological aspects of anorexia in cancer patients. Cancer Res 37:2425–2428, 1977

Holland JC, Korzun AH, Tross S, et al: Comparative psychological disturbance in patients with pancreatic and gastric cancer. Am J Psychiatry 143:982–986, 1986

Holland JC, Morrow G, Schmale A, et al: A randomized clinical trial of alprazolam versus progressive muscle relaxation in cancer patients with anxiety and depressive symptoms. J Clin Oncol 9:1004–1011, 1991

Lansky SB, List MA, Herrman CA, et al: Absence of major depressive disorder in female cancer patients. J Clin Oncol 3:1553–1560, 1985

Lazarus HM, Herzig RH, Herzig GP, et al: Central nervous system toxicity of high-dose systemic cytosine arabinoside. Cancer 48:2577–2582, 1981

Lee Y, Nauert C, Glass JP: Treatment related white matter changes in cancer patients. Cancer 57:1473–1482, 1986

Lewis FM: Psychosocial transitions and the family's work in adjusting to cancer. Semin Oncol Nurs 9:127–129, 1993

Ling MHM, Perry PJ, Tsuang MT: Side effect of corticosteroid therapy. Psychiatric aspects. Arch Gen Psychiatry 38:471–477, 1981

Loprinzi CL: Management of cancer anorexia/cachexia. Support Care Cancer 3:120–122, 1995

Loprinzi CL, Ellison NM, Schaid DJ, et al: Controlled trial of megestrol acetate for the treatment of cancer anorexia and cachexia. J Natl Cancer Inst 82:1127–1132, 1990

Loprinzi CL, Bernath AM, Schaid DJ, et al: Phase III evaluation of 4 doses of megestrol acetate as therapy for patients with cancer anorexia and/or cachexia. Oncology 51 (suppl 1):2–7, 1994a

Loprinzi CL, Michalak JC, Quella SK, et al: Megestrol acetate for the prevention of hot flashes. N Engl J Med 331:347–352, 1994b

Louhivuori KA, Hakama J: Risk of suicide among cancer patients. Am J Epidemiol 109:59–65, 1979

Lynch HT, Droszcz CP, Albano WA, et al: Organic brain syndrome secondary to 5-fluorouracil toxicity. Dis Colon Rectum 24:130–131, 1981

Massie MJ, Holland JC, Straker N: Psychotherapeutic interventions, in Handbook of Psychooncology: Psychological Care of the Patient With Cancer. Edited by Holland JC, Rowland JH. New York, Oxford University Press, 1989, pp 455–469

Massie MJ, Heiligenstein E, Lederberg MS: Psychiatric complications in cancer patients, in American Cancer Society Textbook of Clinical Oncology. Edited by Holleb AI, Fink DJ, Murphy GP. Atlanta, GA, American Cancer Society, 1991, pp 576–586

Massie MJ, Gagnon P, Holland JC: Depression and suicide in patients with cancer. J Pain Symptom Manage 9:325–340, 1994

McDaniel JS, Musselman DL, Porter MR, et al: Depression in patients with cancer: diagnosis, biology, and treatment. Arch Gen Psychiatry 52:89–99, 1995

Meléndez JC, McCrank E: Anxiety-related reactions associated with magnetic resonance imaging examinations. JAMA 270:745–747, 1993

Minotti AM, Kountakis SE, Stiernberg CM: Paraneoplastic syndromes in patients with head and neck cancer. Am J Otolaryngol 15: 336–343, 1994

Moll JWB, Henzen-Logmans SC, Splinter TAW, et al: Diagnostic value of anti-neuronal antibodies for paraneoplastic disorders of the nervous system. J Neurol Neurosurg Psychiatry 53: 940–943, 1990

Morrow GR, Morrell C: Behavioral treatment for the anticipatory nausea and vomiting induced by cancer chemotherapy. N Engl J Med 307: 1476–1480, 1982

Mulhern RK, Ochs J, Fairclough D, et al: Intellectual and academic achievement status after CNS relapse: a retrospective analysis of 40 children treated for acute lymphoblastic leukemia. J Clin Oncol 5:933–940, 1987

Nelson K, Walsh D, Deeter P, et al: A phase II study of delta-9-tetrahydrocannabinol for appetite stimulation in cancer-associated anorexia. J Palliat Care 10:14–18, 1994

Newman NJ, Bell IR, McKee AC: Paraneoplastic limbic encephalitis: neuropsychiatric presentation. Biol Psychiatry 27:529–540, 1990

Peterson K, Forsyth PA, Posner JB: Paraneoplastic sensorimotor neuropathy associated with breast cancer. J Neurooncol 21:159–170, 1994

Pluss JL, DiBella NJ: Reversible central nervous system dysfunction with tamoxifen in a patient with breast cancer (letter). Ann Intern Med 101:652, 1984

Posner JB: Central nervous system synthesis of autoantibodies in paraneoplastic syndromes. Neurology 39 (suppl 1):244–245, 1989

Rait D, Lederberg M: The family of the cancer patient, in Handbook of Psychooncology: Psychological Care of the Patient With Cancer. Edited by Holland JC, Rowland JH. New York, Oxford University Press, 1989, pp 585–597

Razavi D, Delvaux N, Fravacques C, et al: Prevention of adjustment disorders and anticipatory nausea secondary to adjuvant chemotherapy: a double-blind, placebo-controlled study assessing the usefulness of alprazolam. J Clin Oncol 11:1384–1390, 1993

Rottenberg DA: Acute and chronic effect of radiation therapy on the nervous system, in Neurological Complications of Cancer Treatment. Edited by Rottenberg DA. Boston, MA, Butterworth-Heinemann, 1991, pp 3–19

Schiller JH, Jones JC: Paraneoplastic syndromes associated with lung cancer. Curr Opin Oncol 5:335–342, 1993

Schilsky RI, Anderson T: Hypomagnesemia and renal magnesium wasting in patients receiving cisplatin. Ann Intern Med 90:929–931, 1979

Shuster JL, Stern TA, Greenberg DB: Pros and cons of fluoxetine for the depressed cancer patient. Oncology 6:45–56, 1992

Silberfarb PM, Holland JCB, Anbar D, et al: Psychological response of patients receiving two drug regimens for lung carcinoma. Am J Psychiatry 140:110–111, 1983

Spiegel D, Bloom JR, Yalom I: Group support for patients with metastatic cancer. Arch Gen Psychiatry 38:527–533, 1981

Spiegel D, Bloom JR, Kraemaer HC, et al: Effect of psychosocial treatment on survival of patients with metastatic breast cancer. Lancet 2:888–891, 1989

Stefanek ME, Sheidler VR, Fetting JH: Anticipatory nausea and vomiting: does it remain a significant clinical problem? Cancer 62:2654–2657, 1988

Stern TA, Purcell JJ, Murray GB: Complex partial seizures associated with Waldenstrom's macroglobulinemia. Psychosomatics 26: 890–892, 1985

Thachil JV, Jewitt MAS, Rider WD: The effects of cancer and cancer therapy on male fertility. J Urol 126:141–145, 1981

Trijsburg RW, van Knippenberg FCE, Rijpma SE: Effects of psychological treatment on cancer patients: a critical review. Psychosom Med 54: 489–517, 1992

Triozzi PL, Goldstein D, Laszlo J: Contributions of benzodiazepines to cancer therapy. Cancer Invest 6:103–111, 1988

Valente SM, Saunders JM, Cohen MZ: Evaluating depression among patients with cancer. Cancer Practice 2:65–71, 1994

Walker RW, Allen JC, Rosen G, et al: Transient cerebral dysfunction secondary to high dose methotrexate. J Clin Oncol 4:1845–1850, 1986

Wasserstrom WR: Diagnosis and treatment of leptomeningeal metastases from solid tumors: experience with 90 patients. Cancer 49: 759–763, 1982

Watson M: Psychosocial intervention with cancer patients: a review. Psychol Med 13:839–846, 1983

Weisman AD: Early diagnosis of vulnerability in cancer patients. Am J Med Sci 271:187–196, 1976

Weisman A, Worden W: The existential plight in cancer: significance of the first 100 days. Int J Psychiatry Med 7:1–15, 1976–1977

Zalupski M, Baker LH: Ifosfamide. J Natl Cancer Inst 80:556–566, 1988

Chapter 21

Neurology and Neurosurgery

Gregory Fricchione, M.D.
Jeffrey B. Weilburg, M.D.
George B. Murray, M.D.

In this chapter, we focus on the consultative evaluation, diagnosis, and management of neurological and neurosurgical disorders in patients who also have psychiatric or neurobehavioral signs and symptoms. These patients may have primary or secondary psychiatric disorders that account for their problems.

EPIDEMIOLOGY AND CLINICAL FEATURES

A knowledge of disease frequency is essential to the psychiatric consultant to the neurology and neurosurgery service. Tables 21–1 and 21–2 summarize the prevalence and incidence of certain neuropsychiatric disorders (Black et al. 1988; Kurtzke 1984; Malaspina et al. 1992; Regier et al. 1988).

Structural Lesions

Cerebrovascular Disease

Cerebrovascular disease is the most common neurological disorder in the world and the third leading cause of morbidity and mortality in the United States after cardiac disease and cancer (Hachinski and Norris 1985; Starkstein and Robinson 1992). Ischemia accounts for 85% of cerebrovascular disease. Hemorrhagic phenomena account for the remaining 15%.

Poststroke depression (PSD). The major psychiatric sequela of cerebrovascular disease is depression. Robinson and colleagues (1983; Sinyor et al. 1986), as part of a 2-year longitudinal study, confirmed that depression (DSM-III [American Psychiatric Association 1980] major depression and dysthymia) occurs in 30%–50% of patients immediately following a stroke. These investigators reported that 26% of patients demonstrated a clinical picture that was consistent with major depression, whereas another 20% had dysthymia or minor depression. Other studies corroborate these prevalences of PSD in various treatment settings (Eastwood et al. 1989; Ebrahim et al. 1987).

Follow-up longitudinal natural history

Table 21–1. Prevalence of neuropsychiatric disorders in the general population

Disease	Population prevalence per 100,000
Dyslexia	5,000–10,000
Dementia (Alzheimer's disease)	7,700
Major depression	2,200
Seizure disorder	650–1,700
Schizophrenia	600–900
Brain injury	800
Cerebrovascular accident	600
Panic disorder	500
Bipolar illness	500
Parkinson's disease	133–200
Narcolepsy	10–100
CNS tumors (primary and secondary)	80
Persistent postconcussive syndrome	80
Multiple sclerosis	60
Subarachnoid hemorrhage	50
Transient postconcussive syndrome	50
Tourette's syndrome	28.7
Dementia (Pick's disease)	24
Huntington's disease	19
Lesch-Nyhan disease	10
Wilson's disease	10
Myotonic dystrophy	5.5
Metachromatic leukodystrophy	2.5
Acute intermittent porphyria	2
Acquired immunodeficiency syndrome (AIDS)	
Prevalence of CNS dysfunction in AIDS population	30%–75%[a]
Prevalence of AIDS dementia complex in AIDS population	16%–33%[b]

Note.   CNS = central nervous system.
Data obtained from [a]Levy and Bredesen 1988; [b]Portegies et al. 1993.
Source.   Adapted from Black DW, Yates WR, Andreasen NC, et al: "Schizophrenia, Schizophreniform Disorder and Delusional (Paranoid) Disorders," in *The American Psychiatric Press Textbook of Psychiatry.* Edited by Talbott JA, Hales RE, Yudofsky SC. Washington, DC, American Psychiatric Press, 1988, pp. 357–402; Kurtzke JF: "Neuroepidemiology." *Annals of Neurology* 16:265–277, 1984. Copyright 1984, Little, Brown; Malaspina D, Quitkin HM, Kaufmann CA: "Epidemiology and Genetics of Neuropsychiatric Disorders," in *The American Psychiatric Press Textbook of Neuropsychiatry,* 2nd Edition. Edited by Yudofsky SC, Hales RE. Washington, DC, American Psychiatric Press, 1992, pp. 187–226; Regier DA, Boyd JH, Burke JD Jr, et al: "One-Month Prevalence of Mental Disorders in the United States." *Archives of General Psychiatry* 45:977–986, 1988. Copyright 1988, American Medical Association. Used with permission.

studies suggest that average duration of major PSD is approximately 1 year. Dysthymia may last longer, often more than 2 years (Robinson et al. 1983, 1987).

Starkstein and colleagues (1988a) argued that there are two possible influences on the natural course of PSD. One is lesion location, with those recovered from depression having a higher proportion of subcortical and cerebellar brain stem lesions relative to cortical ones. An-

Table 21–2. Incidence of neuropsychiatric disorders in the general population

Disease	Annual incidence per 100,000
Brain injury	200
Cerebrovascular accident	150
Transient postconcussive syndrome	150
Schizophrenia	11–70
Seizure disorder	50
Dementia	50
Brain tumors (benign, metastatic, malignant)	30
Parkinson's disease	30
Persistent postconcussive syndrome	20
Subarachnoid hemorrhage	15
Multiple sclerosis	3

Source. Adapted from Black DW, Yates WR, Andreasen NC, et al: "Schizophrenia, Schizophreniform Disorder and Delusional (Paranoid) Disorders," in *The American Psychiatric Press Textbook of Psychiatry.* Edited by Talbott JA, Hales RE, Yudofsky SC. Washington, DC, American Psychiatric Press, 1988, pp. 357–402; Kurtzke JF: "Neuroepidemiology." *Annals of Neurology* 16:265–277, 1984. Copyright 1984, Little, Brown and Company; Malaspina D, Quitkin HM, Kaufmann CA: "Epidemiology and Genetics of Neuropsychiatric Disorders," in *The American Psychiatric Press Textbook of Neuropsychiatry,* 2nd Edition. Edited by Yudofsky SC, Hales RE. Washington, DC, American Psychiatric Press, 1992, pp. 187–226; Regier DA, Boyd JH, Burke JD Jr, et al: "One-Month Prevalence of Mental Disorders in the United States." *Archives of General Psychiatry* 45:977–986, 1988. Copyright 1988, American Medical Association. Used with permission.

other is the degree of impairment in activities of daily living (ADLs), with patients who have good depression outcome also having less severe impairments. Antidepressant medication shortens the duration of PSD.

Studies support the contention that the risk of depression is higher the closer the lesion is to the left frontal (and right posterior) pole, with left anterior frontal lesions being most highly associated with depression (Robinson and Starkstein 1990; Robinson et al. 1984). It should be noted, however, that some researchers have not found a relation between left- versus right-hemispheric stroke lesion location and risk of depression (Ebrahim et al. 1987; Sinyor et al. 1986).

Psychiatric consultants are sometimes called to see patients who are thought to be depressed but who actually have aprosodia. Aprosodia is a disorder of the affective components of language, and it can be classified in the same manner as aphasia. In aprosodia, a group of assessments analogous to those used to assess dysphasia are used to observe spontaneous prosody, prosodic repetition, prosodic comprehension, and comprehension of emotional gesturing (Ross 1981).

Some patients, who at first appear to have PSD, may simply be aprosodic and unable to mount appropriate affective responses to the treatment team. A helpful marker for depression in the poststroke patient population is lack of motivation in physical therapy (Ross and Rush 1981).

A major risk factor for developing PSD other than lesion location is an increased ventricular area-to-brain ratio caused by subcortical atrophy. In addition, a family or premorbid history of affective illness appears to confer a predisposition to PSD (Starkstein et al. 1988b, 1989).

A wide range of mood changes may occur following lacunar strokes, including emotional incontinence and depression. Lacunar infarcts are small lesions, often the result of hypertension, that occur in the deeper subcortical parts of the cerebrum and in the brain stem (Fisher 1982).

Poststroke mania. Starkstein and Robinson (1992) saw only 3 cases of poststroke mania in a series of 300 consecutive patients who had had a stroke. Nevertheless, poststroke mania can be seen with orbitofrontal, basotemporal, basal ganglia, and thalamic lesions, especially in the right hemisphere (Robinson and Starkstein 1990). Genetic vulnerability, suggested by family history of mood disorder, and subcortical atrophy may also increase the risk of poststroke mania.

Poststroke anxiety. In a series of 98 patients with acute first stroke, only 6 met adapted criteria for generalized anxiety disorder. On the other hand, almost half (23/47) of one series of patients with PSD had comorbid anxiety symptoms (Starkstein et al. 1990).

Brain Tumors

Brain neoplasms account for almost 10% of nontraumatic neurological disease (Silver et al. 1990). Between 1% and 2% of patients with a psychiatric disorder may actually have unrecognized brain neoplasms (Price et al. 1992).

Frontal-lobe neoplasms are especially likely to be associated with neuropsychiatric symptoms, up to 90% of the time in one survey of 85 subjects (Strauss and Keschner 1935). Three types of frontal-lobe dysfunction have been suggested (Cummings 1985a, 1985b, 1985c):

1. The *orbitofrontal syndrome* is characterized by disinhibition, impulsivity, emotional lability with inappropriate jocularity and euphoria, and inattention with poor insight and judgment.
2. The hypothesized *frontal convexity syndrome* is characterized by apathy, indifference and psychomotor retardation, angry outbursts, motor perseveration, impersistence, lack of congruity between motor and verbal behavior, deficits in motor programming, concreteness, and poor categorization.
3. The *medial frontal syndrome* is associated frequently with akinetic presentations. There is loss of spontaneous gesturing, decreased speech production, leg weakness, sensation loss, and incontinence in the medial frontal syndrome (Cummings 1985a, 1985b, 1985c). The akinetic mutism seen with anterior

cingulate lesions is sometimes considered a medial frontal syndrome.

Emotional alterations noted in patients with temporal-lobe tumors include depression, irritability, apathy, or elation. Episodic dyscontrol and affective lability may also be present.

Parietal- and occipital-lobe neoplasms are less likely to cause psychiatric symptoms than are tumors in other locations. However, visual hallucinations occur in patients with occipital tumors (Lohr and Cadet 1987). Agitation, paranoid trends, and affective disturbances can occur in patients with parietal tumors.

Midline diencephalic tumors involve subcortical, limbically related structures, such as thalamus, hypothalamus, and periventricular regions. Schizophreniform psychoses have been reported in patients with such tumors (Malamud 1967). Mood and personality changes and akinetic mutism have also been reported (Burkle and Lipowski 1978; Cairns and Mosberg 1951). Hypothalamic neoplasms may produce eating disorders and hypersomnia, including excessive daytime sleepiness (Climo 1982; Coffey 1989); problems with thirst and temperature regulation can also be seen. Up to 90% of corpus callosum tumors produce neurobehavioral abnormalities (Selecki 1964).

Pituitary tumors are responsible for endocrinopathies associated with psychiatric sequelae. Basophilic pituitary adenomas can lead to Cushing's syndrome, which can cause depression and other secondary psychiatric syndromes. Acidophilic pituitary adenomas can present with acromegaly, which is associated with depression and anxiety (Price et al. 1992). A visual field loss such as bitemporal hemianopsia should immediately implicate a pituitary or hypothalamic lesion as the etiology of mental status change.

Paraneoplastic processes affect the central nervous system (CNS) as a consequence of the remote effects of a tumor and not because of direct invasion. CNS paraneoplastic syndromes often result from an immune reaction directed against antigens shared by the underlying neoplasm and certain neurons. The most common tumor associated with CNS paraneoplastic disease is small cell lung cancer. Other associated tumors include breast, stomach, uterine, renal, testicular, thyroid, and colon cancers (Skuster et al. 1992). Sometimes cancer patients can be admitted to psychiatry units for the onset of a syndrome that includes depression, anxiety, personality disturbances, hallucinations, catatonia, and memory impairment with or without delirium. Psychiatrists should have a high index of suspicion for CNS paraneoplastic syndromes when psychiatric signs and symptoms occur in patients with cancer.

Seizure Disorder

The original definition of epilepsy by Hughlings Jackson remains current: Epilepsy is an "occasional, excessive and disorderly electrical discharge of nerve tissue" (qtd. in Browne et al. 1983, p. 414). The electroencephalogram (EEG) may corroborate the seizure activity via spikes, spike and wave complexes, or other findings (Mendez et al. 1984). Focal sharp and slow waves suggest seizure activity in patients with a clinical picture of epilepsy. It should be noted, however, that of the estimated 2 million or more Americans who have epilepsy, 60% have nonconvulsive seizures free of any body motor symptoms and signs that otherwise herald the end of a seizure (Goldensohn 1983). As Murray (1985) pointed out, the majority of patients with nonconvulsive epilepsy have partial seizures, and 40% of these patients do not show focal spiking on their EEGs (Klass 1975; Murray 1985).

Generalized seizures are characterized by simultaneous involvement of both cerebral hemispheres. In partial seizures, focal signs and symptoms emerge from excitation in a limited site in one hemisphere. Simple partial seizures occur without impaired consciousness and usually stem from primary motor, sensory, or visual cortical regions. Complex partial seizures are associated with impairment of consciousness and most often originate from limbic system foci in the medial temporal lobe. This may explain why psychiatric signs and symptoms—including cognitive auras (depersonalization, forced thinking, déjà vu), affective auras (fear, depression, pleasure), perceptual changes (illusions, hallucinations), and memory dysfunction (amnesia)—are so common (Mendez et al. 1984). Complex partial status epilepticus appears to have two separate behavioral phases. A continuous twilight state with partial and amnestic responsiveness, partial speech, and reactive complex automatisms cycles with the other phase of total unresponsiveness, speech arrest, staring, and stereotyped automatisms (Treiman and Delgado-Escueta 1983).

Psychiatric consultants may be called by neurologists to evaluate patients with possible pseudoseizures. A significant number of patients will have both true seizures and pseudoseizures (or nonepileptic seizures).

Depression is common in patients with epilepsy. Mendez et al. (1986) suggested that depression in some epileptic patients may be due to a specific epileptic psychosyndrome secondary to limbic dysfunction. Compared with 7% of control subjects, 30% of patients with epilepsy had histories of suicide attempts. The suicide rate in one series of patients with epilepsy was five times that of the general population (Barraclough 1981). In patients with temporal-lobe epilepsy, the incidence of suicide is 25 times that of the general population (Robertson and Trimble 1983).

A schizophreniform psychosis is also described in patients with epilepsy, usually in those with temporal-lobe epilepsy (McKenna et al. 1985; Mendez et al. 1984). Symptoms may include thought disorder, paranoid ideations, hallucinations, and mood changes in the context of preserved affect. Persistent psychoses are well-known concomitants of epilepsy, again often attributed to subictal temporal-lobe dysrhythmias. Incidence studies suggest that the psychosis risk in patients with epilepsy is 6–12 times greater than in the population without epilepsy (McKenna et al. 1985).

Bear and Fedio (1977) have written about the so-called interictal behavioral syndrome (humorless sobriety, dependence, obsessionalism) seen in patients with temporal-lobe epilepsy. Hyperreligiosity, hypergraphia, and hyposexuality are associated with the temporal-lobe epileptic interictal personality (Waxman and Geschwind 1975), although these associations are controversial (Rodin and Schmaltz 1984). There does seem to be, however, a clear and distinctive verbosity in patients with complex partial seizures that gives them a viscous interpersonal quality (Hoeppner et al. 1987).

Head Trauma

Head trauma is an important public health problem, with 750,000 to 3 million cases occurring each year in the United States (Jennett and Teasdale 1981; Kwentus et al. 1985). Head trauma can produce significant changes in personality. Whether there is damage to frontal lobes or whether these structures remain unharmed, psychiatric consultants can encounter the frontal-lobe syndrome, which is characterized by lability, irritability, shallowness, and inappropriateness. Patients may have diminished ability to utilize language, calculation skills, and logical analysis, as well as reduced ability to concentrate and abstract (Silver et al. 1990).

Premorbid mood disorders are often worsened by brain injuries, but depression or mania can emerge after head injury without any prior personal or family history (Robinson et al. 1988). Significant head injury before a first psychotic episode has been found in up to 15% of patients with schizophrenia (Lishman 1987).

Symptoms of *postconcussion syndrome* include headache, dizziness, tiredness, and insomnia. Patients may exhibit memory dysfunction, lack of concentration, perceptual changes, dysthymia, anxiety, irritability, and

personality changes (Lishman 1988; Silver et al. 1990). Postconcussion syndrome is not correlated with head injury severity or degree of loss of consciousness.

Degenerative Diseases

A wide variety of degenerative diseases cause neuropsychiatric signs and symptoms. *Parkinson's disease* is a degenerative disorder with high psychiatric comorbidity (Fogel 1993)—65% of patients with Parkinson's disease develop an associated dementia by age 85 (Mayeux et al. 1990). About 40% of patients with Parkinson's disease can expect to eventually have at least one major depressive syndrome (Cummings 1992). This degree of comorbidity and the added risk of psychiatric dysfunction as a result of antiparkinsonian medications suggest the need for psychiatric as well as neurological management for optimal patient care.

Patients with Parkinson's disease have tremor, bradykinesia, rigidity, gait dysfunction, and/or postural unsteadiness. Drugs are a frequent cause of parkinsonism; neuroleptics are the most common offenders. Metoclopramide (Albibi and McCallum 1983) and fluoxetine (Bouchard et al. 1989), as well as amoxapine and lithium, may also cause extrapyramidal syndromes.

The psychiatric side effects of antiparkinsonian medications, such as psychosis and confusion, often lead to treatment alterations. If slow withdrawal of one antiparkinsonian medication at a time does not resolve psychotic symptoms, then clozapine can be tried (Fogel 1993).

Depression seems to be more common in patients with Parkinson's disease who have more severe bradykinesia and gait disturbance than in those who have a more dominant tremor presentation. Depression in patients with Parkinson's disease is not merely a reaction to degree of disability; Parkinson's disease is complicated by the presence of physical signs (apathy, bradykinesia, rigidity) that mimic the psychomotor and vegetative symptoms of depression. Focusing on the psychological symptoms of depression can help with diagnosis of a depressive syndrome.

Huntington's disease is an autosomal-dominant, degenerative, basal ganglia disease in which psychiatric issues are often dominant until the late stages of illness (Maricle 1993). Patients with Huntington's disease have involuntary choreic movements, abnormal voluntary movements, cognitive deficits, and psychiatric dysfunction. Common psychiatric syndromes in patients with Huntington's disease include conduct disorder, antisocial personality disorder, other personality syndromes, mood disorder (in more than 50%), schizophrenia-like conditions (with more negative than positive symptoms), and alcoholism (Maricle 1993). Suicidal behavior occurs in 30% of patients, with completed suicide in 2%–7% (Maricle 1993). A subcortical dementia eventually strikes all those with Huntington's disease and progresses at a variable rate.

The most important example of a demyelinating degenerative disease is *multiple sclerosis*. The etiology of multiple sclerosis remains unknown, but recent discoveries seem to point to an autoimmune component. Multiple sclerosis is diagnosed most often in young women, with onset between ages 20 and 40. At least early on, neuropsychiatric symptoms tend to remit and recur. Lesions most commonly affect the optic nerve, cerebellum, brain stem, and long tracts of the spinal cord, causing ataxic gait, intention tremor, dysarthria, dissociation of lateral conjugate gaze, paraparesis, sensory loss in limbs, and urinary incontinence.

Some studies suggest a physiological basis for depression in patients with multiple sclerosis. In one study comparing 30 patients with multiple sclerosis with equally disabled, neurologically ill control subjects, patients with multiple sclerosis were more likely to be depressed before they showed signs of their disease as well as during the illness phase (Whitlock and Suskind 1980).

Amyotrophic lateral sclerosis (ALS) is a degenerative motor neuron disease characterized by loss of strength and muscle atrophy. It is sometimes associated with dementia (Wikstrom et al. 1982). Personality changes may occur before the onset of motor neuron disease, sometimes in association with frontotemporal atrophy.

CNS Infections

CNS infections are part of the potential differential diagnosis any consultation-liaison psychiatrist will consider. *Neurosyphilis* is becoming more common because of immunodeficiency related to the human immunodeficiency virus (HIV). Neurosyphilis symptoms may start with headache, lethargy, poor concentration, forgetfulness, and poor judgment. Early neuropsychiatric evidence of neurosyphilis may include ophthalmoplegia, pupillary abnormalities, and, rarely, the fully developed Argyll Robertson pupil (small irregular pupils reacting normally to convergence but not at all to light and only partly to a mydriatic agent). The cerebrospinal fluid (CSF) shows a moderate leukocytosis (200 cells/mL) of mostly mononuclear cells. The clinical picture may, over time, deteriorate to a dementia.

Acute bacterial, fungal, and *viral meningitis* may sometimes be seen in hospitalized medical-surgical patients. Immunocompromised populations on hospital units serving patients who have acquired immunodeficiency syndrome (AIDS) or on oncology units, as well as patients who have indwelling ventriculoperitoneal shunts, sometimes develop acute meningitis. Headache, meningismus, and CSF abnormalities are associated with a wide variety of mental status changes in patients with meningitis.

Encephalitis is a generalized CNS infection that usually has an acute onset with fever, meningeal signs, focal neurological findings, and delirium sometimes progressing to stupor (Skuster et al. 1992). The most frequently encountered focal encephalitis is caused by herpes simplex virus, which has a predilection for temporal lobes and the inferomedial portions of the frontal lobes. Associated findings may include anosmia, olfactory or gustatory perceptual changes, simple or complex partial seizures, personality changes, and psychosis. Unless encephalitis is treated early with antiviral agents such as acyclovir, there is significant morbidity and mortality. Long-standing sequelae of encephalitis include personality alteration, affective lability, cognitive dysfunction, and hallucinations (Baker 1988).

DIFFERENTIAL DIAGNOSIS

Examination for Conversion Disorder

Conversion disorder is often diagnosed prematurely (Boffeli and Guze 1992). In one 10-year follow-up study, 10 of 40 men who originally received a diagnosis of conversion disorder were later found to have recognizable neurological disease, most commonly a CNS degenerative disease (Watson and Buranen 1979). In a more recent study, 11 of 56 conversion patients were found to have neurological disorders 10 years later (Mace and Trimble 1996). The prognosis for chronic symptomatology often of the somatization type remains poor. In another provocative study, Gould and colleagues (1986) found at least one feature of a nonphysiological sensory examination, such as nonanatomical anesthesia or a midline split of pain or vibration, in 29 of 30 neurology inpatients with documented CNS injury, 25 of whom had acute strokes.

Delirium versus conversion disorder.   In conversion disorder, orientation is usually preserved, or when "disorientation" occurs, it often includes person as well as place and time. Cognition is also usually intact, but if poor, it commonly is out of proportion to alertness and responsiveness. Hallucinations are rare in patients who have conversion delirium.

Stupor versus conversion stupor.   In conversion stupor, variable awareness is possible. For example, the patient is often motionless but can respond to command or pain. He or she is completely mute (usually a sign of conversion stupor) or may utter monosyllabic or short phrases.

"Focal" findings versus conversion disorder.   Psychogenic ptosis usually fails to have accompanying frontalis muscle overcompensation. The patient with psychogenic hemiplegia will not adduct the weak arm or leg when asked; however, if these limbs are placed in the adducted position bilaterally and tested against resistance, adductor contraction on both sides is present. In psychogenic paraplegia, sphincter dysfunction is not found. Hoover's sign is often present in cases of conversion weakness. Normally, when a supine individual flexes his or her thigh to lift the leg, there is downward leg movement contralaterally, which is easily appreciated by the examiner who has placed his or her hand beneath that heel or leg. A patient with psychogenic hemiparesis has no downward movement in the contralateral normal leg when attempts are made to raise the "paretic" leg (Wells and Duncan 1980).

Complaints of sensory deficits are seen in patients with somatoform disorders. Suspicion of somatization is aroused when there is a well-defined, abrupt border between an area of sensory loss and another of normal sensation. Unilateral sensory loss with a midline border is highly unusual especially if it is persistent along the nose and genitalia. Similarly, a midline loss of vibration sense over the skull or sternum has no physiological etiology. Conversion disorders often coincide with neurological illnesses, so they are by no means mutually exclusive (Wells and Duncan 1980).

Movement disorders versus conversion movement disorder.   Conversion myoclonus, consisting of atypical movements responsive to distraction or suggestion, is the most frequent somatoform symptom in a movement disorder clinic population (Monday and Jankovic 1993).

Seizures versus conversion seizures (pseudoseizures). Several useful diagnostic approaches are available to differentiate actual seizures from conversion seizures (pseudoseizures). Conversion seizures should be suspected when seizures are unusual or variable in presentation, when there is absence of epileptiform activity on ictal and of slowing activity on postictal EEG monitoring, and when seizure frequency does not change despite decreased plasma concentration of anticonvulsants (Desai et al. 1982). Provocative tests using suggestion can sometimes initiate or terminate a conversion "spell." Weeping has recently been suggested as a common element of pseudoseizures, but it is an extremely rare ictal phenomenon, except in dacrystic epilepsy (Bergen and Ristanovic 1993). Of patients with seizures, 20%–25% have both seizures and pseudoseizures (Ramani et al. 1980).

It is sometimes diagnostically helpful to study serum prolactin levels in patients after a seizure. A twofold or greater increase in serum prolactin is usually seen in generalized and complex partial seizure patients 15–20 minutes postictus, but no such increase is seen in patients with pseudoseizures (Dana-Haeri and Trimble 1984; Pritchard et al. 1985; Trimble 1978).

Syncope versus conversion syncope. Conversion syncope usually occurs in the presence of witnesses, is dramatic in presentation, may carry some sexual association, and is rarely associated with personal injury or with autonomic changes.

Suggestions for the management of conversion disorders can be found in Table 21–3.

Laboratory Evaluation

The CSF does not normally contain more than five lymphocytes or monocytes per cubic milli-

meter. An elevation in white blood cells reflects an inflammation brought on by bacteria, viruses, other infectious agents, blood, chemicals, or neoplastic disease. Bacterial and fungal CNS infection may precipitate CSF polymorphonuclear cell response, whereas tuberculosis sparks lymphocytic pleocytosis. A white blood cell count less than $50/mm^3$ suggests a noninfectious etiology, such as sarcoidosis, vasculitis, or carcinomatous meningitis.

The protein content of CSF is normally 45 mg/dL or less. CSF protein levels are typically elevated in bacterial meningitis and to a lesser extent in viral meningitis, brain and spinal cord tumors, diabetes mellitus, syphilis, multiple sclerosis, Guillain-Barré syndrome, lupus cerebritis, myxedema, and Cushing's syndrome. CSF protein can be low (less than 15 mg/dL) in meningismus and in hyperthyroidism. The normal range of CSF glucose is 45–80 mg/dL. Abnormal CSF glucose levels, usually lower than 40 mg/dL, occur in the presence of pleocytosis and usually signify a pyogenic, tubercular, or fungal meningitis.

Cytology can be diagnostic in carcinomatosis meningitis, with 45%–75% of patients diagnosed on the first lumbar puncture (LP) and 80%–90% after three LPs (Coyle 1991).

Imaging and Electrophysiology

Computed Tomography of the Head

The head computed tomography (CT) scan is useful in the diagnosis of arteriovenous malformations, hydrocephalus, herpes encephalitis, parasitic infestations, and progressive neurodegenerative diseases. It is also sometimes of benefit in the search for causes of partial or focal seizure disorders (Goodstein 1985). If contrast media is used, CT scans can demonstrate a small primary brain neoplasm. Metastatic tumors of the brain can also be visualized. Up to 95% of brain tumors can be seen on CT. The CT can also distinguish between ischemic and hemorrhagic cerebrovascular lesions, along with a reasonable percentage of subarachnoid

Table 21–3.   Management of conversion disorder in neurology and neurosurgery settings

Abreaction and positive suggestion

Engage in one-to-one discussion; alone without family, friends; discuss experience and events surrounding onset of symptoms. Use sympathetic, patient, supportive encouragement of emotion.

Allow for saving face in explaining diagnosis; avoid statements such as "it's all in your head" and "there's nothing wrong."

Avoid confrontation; use direct, nonthreatening explanation of role of emotional difficulties in physical symptoms.

Make use of patient's characteristic suggestibility by suggesting a reasonable timetable for improvement of patient's particular condition.

Conduct an interview with patient under the influence of amobarbital, pentobarbital, a benzodiazepine, or hypnosis, which may be useful in uncovering conflict and leading to abreaction.

Behavioral approaches

Teach simple behavioral coping techniques that are more appropriate as a response in dealing with emotional problems than having physical symptom (e.g., seizure). Can be done in individual or group sessions.

Use behavioral approach aimed at rewarding "well behavior" in some patients with chronic problem.

Family involvement

Demonstrate appropriate "well behavior" to family and friends.

Minimize, through education, convenient sources of secondary gain in the family.

Begin family therapy, which may be helpful, especially in patients with chronic problem.

Chronically ill patient care

Employ systematic, reeducative type of psychotherapy based on personality profile and psychosocial variables.

Use behavioral therapy.

Use family therapy.

Require (infrequently) inpatient hospitalization to prevent consequences of conversion disorder (e.g., muscle atrophy).

hemorrhages. Decreased density is seen on CT scan when there is an infarct. A CT scan with contrast can increase the amount of cerebrovascular lesions found.

Magnetic Resonance Imaging

Magnetic resonance imaging (MRI) provides greater contrast between gray and white matter than CT scans are able to provide (Gilman 1992). In addition, there is increased sensitivity to white matter lesions that occur in demyelinating diseases such as multiple sclerosis. Particularly when contrast (gadolinium) is used, the visualization of certain tumors such as meningiomas and acoustic neuromas is improved. AVMs, gliomas, and cerebral anomalies, on the other hand, are well delineated with noncontrast MRI. MRI is particularly effective in showing posterior fossa pathology that may occur in brain stem and cerebellar lesions. MRI requires that patients be placed in a tightly confined receptacle; claustrophobia is a significant problem in approximately 5% of patients who undergo MRI.

MRI is superior to CT in evaluating most cerebral parenchymal lesions. Nevertheless, CT is preferable in certain situations, such as when patients have equipment needs, are unable to remain immobile, have head or spine injuries that require rapid evaluation, are uncooperative, or have pacemakers, mechanical valves, or intracranial clips.

Electroencephalogram

Although the EEG generally lacks diagnostic specificity, it is still a helpful test in certain clinical states. The EEG with generalized slowing can help establish the diagnosis of delirium. A patient with paroxysmal spells of behavioral symptoms in whom the diagnosis of epilepsy is being considered should undergo EEG testing. It should be emphasized that the EEG may be read as normal in a high percentage of patients with complex partial seizure disorder; that diagnosis ultimately rests on clinical grounds.

Neuropsychological Testing

Neuropsychological testing can help delineate suspected neurological illnesses that escape detection with other neurodiagnostic procedures; help differentiate "organic" from "functional" illness; monitor mental status after medical or surgical treatment; assess cognitive capacities of the brain-injured patient to determine needs for rehabilitation, placement, or competence; and help identify learning disorders and guide remediation efforts.

■ TREATMENT AND MANAGEMENT

Psychopharmacology

The practical use of psychopharmacological agents for some neuropsychiatric syndromes and their target symptoms requires specific knowledge (Silver et al. 1990).

Neuroleptics

When psychotic thought and behavior occur in the neurology or neurosurgery patient and offending causes such as antiparkinsonian drugs cannot be removed or diminished, patients can be treated with neuroleptic medications (Silver et al. 1990). However, neuroleptics have sedative, anticholinergic, and hypotensive side effects that must be carefully monitored (Dubovsky 1992).

Neurological side effects must also be considered, including extrapyramidal symptoms such as akathisia, dystonia, parkinsonism, neuroleptic malignant syndrome (NMS), perioral tremor, tardive dystonia, and tardive dyskinesia. In general, higher potency neuroleptics carry a higher risk for these side effects. Thus, patients with Parkinson's disease are not likely to tolerate haloperidol or fluphenazine, whereas they may do well on clozapine or thioridazine in low doses. There is a great deal of recent success with the atypical neuroleptic clozapine controlling psychotic symptoms without worsening parkinsonism signs (Fogel

1993). Clozapine is usually started at a low dose, such as 25 mg/day, with the patient being monitored closely for sedation, anticholinergic side effects, and blood dyscrasia, especially agranulocytosis. Patients often respond to doses as low as 25 mg/day (Kahn et al. 1991).

Psychotic symptoms can occur interictally in epilepsy patients. Anticonvulsants may not control these symptoms, so neuroleptics must be used. Molindone and fluphenazine may be best because they have the lowest potential for lowering seizure threshold (Silver and Yudofsky 1988). Clinicians should keep seizure potential in mind in patients with agitated delirium secondary to brain dysfunction. Anticonvulsant medications are sometimes necessary when psychotropics that lower seizure threshold must be used (Ojemann 1987).

Psychostimulants and Dopaminergics

Methylphenidate and dextroamphetamine have been used successfully in medically ill depressed patients without causing anorexia or worsening confusion, even in patients with dementia or other primary brain disorders (Woods et al. 1986). Patients with PSD frequently respond to psychostimulants (Masand et al. 1991). Average daily doses required are about 10–15 mg for methylphenidate and about 10 mg for dextroamphetamine. Psychostimulants also strengthen attention, concentration, and performance on neuropsychological testing in some patients with AIDS, as well as decrease depression (Fernandez et al. 1988).

Antidepressants

Silver et al. (1990) suggested that patients with "clinically significant depressed mood," amotivation, apathy, poor compliance, and impaired progress in physical rehabilitation therapy should be strongly considered for an antidepressant trial. A cyclic antidepressant with the most favorable risk-benefit ratio can be chosen. Among the tricyclics, secondary amines are generally preferred. Therapeutic levels of nortriptyline are effective in relieving PSD (Lipsey et al. 1984). Nortriptyline has relatively little anticholinergicity and is the least likely to cause orthostatic hypotension. Oversedation, hypotension, confusion and worsening cognition, other anticholinergic effects, cardiotoxicity, and a lowered seizure threshold sometimes require discontinuation of cyclic antidepressants.

Trazodone has also been reported to benefit patients with PSD (Reding et al. 1986). Bupropion in doses greater than 450 mg/day appears to be particularly prone to lowering seizure threshold in predisposed patients. Patients with brain tumors, bulimia, and EEG abnormalities are at greatest risk for problems related to bupropion's potential to lower seizure threshold. Fluoxetine, sertraline, paroxetine, fluvoxamine, trazodone, and monoamine oxidase inhibitors (MAOIs) appear to lower seizure threshold less than tricyclic antidepressants (TCAs), bupropion, maprotiline, and amoxapine (McNamara 1993). In one unblinded study, fluoxetine actually showed anticonvulsant properties, lowering seizure frequency by 30% (Favale et al. 1995). Careful use of selective serotonin reuptake inhibitors (SSRIs), trazodone, MAOIs, or secondary amine TCAs can be justified in this population (McNamara 1993).

For patients with Parkinson's disease and depression, clinicians favor the use of the TCAs (e.g., nortriptyline and imipramine), especially if anxiety or panic symptoms are present. However, anticholinergic effects can be problematic because most of these patients are elderly (Dubovsky 1992; Fogel 1993). Bupropion is theoretically a good choice because of its dopaminergic action, especially if apathy and anhedonia are prominent (Fogel 1993). However, experience with bupropion in this clinical setting is limited, especially in combination with L-dopa (an increased risk of psychosis) or selegiline. Amoxapine should be avoided because it may worsen extrapyramidal side effects (Dubovsky 1992). Trazodone and SSRIs (e.g., fluoxetine, sertraline, and paroxetine) may be useful, especially when the patient has a prominent negative affect. However, a worsening of parkinsonian symptoms may occur, especially with fluoxetine (Fogel 1993). Selegiline itself has proven for some patients to be an effective antidepressant, at least at higher doses. It selectively inhibits MAO (monoamine oxidase)-B at a dose of 10 mg, but at doses greater than 30–40 mg, it also inhibits MAO-A, and therefore, diet and drug restrictions must be observed.

Antidepressants have a number of specific uses in certain neurological patient groups. Serotonin reuptake inhibitors (SRIs) have been shown to relieve the pathological crying that can occur after a cerebrovascular accident (Andersen et al, 1993). TCAs have been used with some success in reducing the depression associated with Huntington's disease, and SSRIs are also now being tested (Maricle 1993). The same can be said about the use of antidepressants in patients with multiple sclerosis. Patients with chronic pain may benefit from treatment with antidepressants such as amitriptyline, desipramine, and doxepin. SSRIs are also used for pain management, sometimes in combination with TCAs. Tinnitus may be improved with nortriptyline. Amitriptyline and nortriptyline have been anecdotally reported to be effective in reducing pathological laughing and crying. Amitriptyline and doxepin have been used widely in headache management, especially for migraine prophylaxis. Trazodone has been used to control agitation in patients with a brain injury or disease. Neurogenic bladder with urinary retention, common in several neurological illnesses, is a challenge when treatment of depression is required. Drugs that are low in anticholinergic potency, such as sertraline, paroxetine, fluoxetine, trazodone, bupropion, and methylphenidate, are reasonable choices for patients who have urinary retention (Dubovsky 1992).

Anticonvulsants (Including Benzodiazepines)

Carbamazepine has proven antimanic efficacy, especially in patients who are more severely manic at onset, more dysphoric, more rapidly cycling, and with less family loading for the disease. There is also an emerging consensus that carbamazepine offers effective long-term prophylaxis for both mania and depression. Secondary manias may be carbamazepine responsive, especially if they are secondary to a seizure disorder. (For further information about the treatment of manic disorders, see McDaniel et al., Chapter 10, in this volume.)

Carbamazepine is also effective for aggression and violence related to neuropsychiatric illnesses such as complex partial seizure disorder and head trauma. It can be given in divided doses of 600–1,200 mg/day to maintain serum levels at 4–12 μg/nL (Silver et al. 1990). Carbamazepine is also beneficial for paroxysmal neuropathic pain syndromes such as trigeminal neuralgia.

Sodium valproate is as effective as carbamazepine in treating generalized seizures but less effective for complex partial seizure disorder (Mattson et al. 1992). Nevertheless, valproate has clinically important acute and prophylactic effects in manic and depressive illness (Post 1989). Valproate may block mania more than depression. Newer anticonvulsants such as lamotrigine and Neurontin are also being used in affective disorder treatment.

Clonazepam is a benzodiazepine anticonvulsant that has antimanic and limited antidepressant properties. Clonazepam is helpful in the management of manic breakthroughs and for sleep hygiene in the patient with mania (Post 1989). Lorazepam has been found to be a useful agent in the treatment of patients who are in catatonic states (Fricchione 1989).

Lithium Carbonate

There is some evidence that lithium can reduce aggressive, impulsive, and destructive behaviors in patients with mood lability secondary to brain syndromes (Silver and Yudofsky 1988).

When a patient with an underlying CNS disorder who is taking lithium becomes delirious, lithium is often the etiology, sometimes even at therapeutic levels. Thus, lithium must be withheld and the clinician must search for other potential contributors. Lithium can also worsen secondary psychiatric disorders. Lithium-induced hypothyroidism may cause mental status changes and may also exacerbate lithium toxicity. Lithium may occasionally even lower seizure threshold and initiate seizure activity, even in nonepileptic patients (Massey and Folger 1984). Patients with epilepsy may require increased anticonvulsant doses when taking lithium. Extrapyramidal side effects sometimes occur on lithium.

Neurotoxicity syndromes have been reported with combinations of lithium and neuroleptics, carbamazepine, calcium channel blockers, and clonazepam. The use of lithium should be limited to patients with mania and recurrent depressions that preceded brain disease (Silver et al. 1990) and to patients with aggression related to mania. If lithium is used in patients with CNS disease, a strategy that is used with elderly patients seems reasonable: doses should be started low and increased slowly, and treatment should be aimed at lower therapeutic levels. Neurological status should be monitored closely.

β-Blockers

Anecdotal evidence indicates that β-blockers, including propranolol, nadolol, pindolol, and metoprolol, are effective in the treatment of aggression related to neurological illnesses such as epilepsy, head trauma, Huntington's disease, Wilson's disease, and dementia (Silver et al. 1990). Silver et al. (1990) recommended a test dose of propranolol of 20 mg/day, especially if there are concerns about hypotension or bradycardia. The dosage can be increased by 20 mg/day every 3 days. Dosage increases should be stopped when the pulse rate falls below 50 beats/minute or when systolic blood pressure is less than 90 mm Hg. β-Blockers may take 4–6 weeks at maximum dosage to work, which is a major drawback when acute agitation requires control.

Electroconvulsive Therapy

In addition to its well-known efficacy in mania and primary major depression, electroconvulsive therapy (ECT) is an effective treatment for PSD (Murray et al. 1986) and for major depression associated with epilepsy, Parkinson's disease, and multiple sclerosis (Dubovsky 1986). In addition, it is the most powerful treatment for catatonic states (Fink and Taylor 1991). Confusional states and short-term memory dysfunction are the main neurological side effects of ECT (Weiner 1990).

Psychotherapy

Most neurologically ill patients do not initiate their own psychiatric referrals (Minden 1992). Depression, lack of motivation, overelaborated symptomatology, or family discord may prompt the neurologist or neurosurgeon to seek psychiatric consultation. These patients will vary in their willingness to go to a psychiatrist. For this reason, Minden wrote that one of the chief goals of the evaluation is to establish a therapeutic alliance. A related goal is to pay attention to the patient's skepticism about psychiatry, typically coupled with a lack of "psychological-mindedness."

The psychiatrist should use a medical consultation model, gathering detailed medical data involving neurological function and pain, while in an easygoing and natural way inquiring about the psychological concomitants of illness. "How has this illness affected your life?" is often a successful question and a way of improving compliance and participation in the process. Psychological jargon should be avoided, and the patient's emotional experience should be validated, emphasizing normality.

The psychotherapy evaluation should end with a simple, clear summary of the patient's problems and the factors that may be contributing (Minden 1992). A discussion of available effective treatments can then follow. If the neurologically ill patient does not want to enter psychotherapy, it is best to react neutrally and to offer help in the future.

Couples, family, group, and behavioral psychotherapies are helpful for many patients with neurological disorders (Forrest 1992; Minden 1992). Patients with a degenerative disease such as multiple sclerosis often benefit from the shared experience of others with the disease in a support or educational group setting. Family approaches can establish healthy communication among the designated patient and family members involved in the patient's care. Caregiver groups help reduce caregiver "burnout" syndromes.

Ward Management

Environmental management is important for many neuropsychiatric patients. Patients with delirium require close observation. Restraints are sometimes required for patient protection. The need should be reevaluated every few hours. Patients who have lost independence because of their neurological illness can gain some sense of control if they are permitted to schedule activities and request medications and are taught autohypnosis or deep relaxation techniques to control anxiety. Firm structure consistently applied by all staff members is frequently required for patients plagued by impulsive behaviors and low frustration tolerance (e.g., frontal-lobe syndrome patients).

Staff members who work on neurological and neurosurgical units, particularly if there are a substantial number of chronic care patients, sometimes have a tendency to become demoralized and discouraged by the lack of patient progress or the degree of functional loss. Group support enables the staff to ventilate these feelings and to make constructive suggestions. An excellent model is the consultation-liaison nurse as group leader for these meetings supervised by the consultation-liaison psychiatrist.

■ REFERENCES

Albibi R, McCallum RW: Metoclopramide: pharmacology and clinical application. Ann Intern Med 98:86–95, 1983

American Psychiatric Association: Diagnostic and Statistical Manual of Mental Disorders, 3rd Edition. Washington, DC, American Psychiatric Association, 1980

Andersen G, Vestergaard K, Rus JO: Citalopram for post-stroke pathological crying. Lancet 342:837–839, 1993

Baker AB: Viral encephalitis, in Clinical Neurology. Edited by Baker AB. Philadelphia, PA, JB Lippincott, 1988, pp 1–147

Barraclough B: Suicide and epilepsy, in Epilepsy and Psychiatry. Edited by Reynolds EH, Trimble MR. New York, Churchill Livingstone, 1981, pp 72–76

Bear DM, Fedio P: Quantitative analysis of interictal behavior in temporal lobe epilepsy. Arch Neurol 34:454–467, 1977

Bergen D, Ristanovic R: Weeping as a common element of pseudoseizures. Arch Neurol 50:1059–1060, 1993

Black DW, Yates WR, Andreasen NC: Schizophrenia, schizophreniform disorder, and delusional (paranoid) disorders, in The American Psychiatric Press Textbook of Psychiatry. Edited by Talbott JA, Hales RE, Yudofsky SC. Washington, DC, American Psychiatric Press, 1988, pp 357–402

Boffeli TJ, Guze SB: The simulation of neurologic disease. Psychiatr Clin North Am 15:301–309, 1992

Bouchard RH, Pourcher E, Vincent P: Fluoxetine and extrapyramidal side effects. Am J Psychiatry 146:1352–1353, 1989

Browne TR, Feldman RG, Buchanan RA, et al: Methsuximide for complex partial seizures: efficacy, toxicity, clinical pharmacology, and drug interactions. Neurology 33:414–418, 1983

Burkle FM, Lipowski ZJ: Colloid cyst of the third ventricle presenting as psychiatric disorder. Am J Psychiatry 135:373–374, 1978

Cairns H, Mosberg WH: Colloid cysts of the third ventricle. Surg Gynecol Obstet 92:545–570, 1951

Climo LH: Anorexia nervosa associated with hypothalamic tumor: the search for clinical-pathological correlations. Psychiatric Journal of the University of Ottawa 7:20–25, 1982

Coffey RJ: Hypothalamic and basal forebrain germinoma presenting with amnesia and hyperphagia. Surg Neurol 31:228–233, 1989

Coyle P: Chronic meningitis, in Infections of the Nervous System. Boston, MA, American Academy of Neurology Annual Courses, 1991

Cummings JL: Clinical Neuropsychiatry. Orlando, FL, Grune & Stratton, 1985a

Cummings JL: Psychosomatic aspects of movement disorders. Adv Psychosom Med 13:111–132, 1985b

Cummings JL: Organic delusions: phenomenology, anatomical correlations and review. Br J Psychiatry 146:184–197, 1985c

Cummings JL: Depression and Parkinson's disease. Am J Psychiatry 149:443–454, 1992

Dana-Haeri J, Trimble MR: Prolactin and gonadotrophin changes following partial seizures in epileptic patients with and without psychopathology. Biol Psychiatry 19:329–336, 1984

Desai BT, Porter RJ, Kiffin-Penry J: Psychogenic seizures. Arch Neurol 39:202–209, 1982

Dubovsky SL: Using electroconvulsive therapy for patients with neurological disease. Hosp Community Psychiatry 37:819–825, 1986

Dubovsky SL: Psychopharmacological treatment in neuropsychiatry, in The American Psychiatric Press Textbook of Neuropsychiatry, 2nd Edition. Edited by Yudofsky SC, Hales RE. Washington, DC, American Psychiatric Press, 1992, pp 663–701

Eastwood MR, Rifat SL, Nobbs H, et al: Mood disorder following cerebrovascular accident. Br J Psychiatry 154:195–200, 1989

Ebrahim S, Barer D, Nouri F: Affective illness after stroke. Br J Psychiatry 151:52–56, 1987

Favale E, Rubino V, Mainardi P, et al: Anticonvulsant effect of fluoxetine in humans. Neurology 45:1926–1927, 1995

Fernandez F, Adams F, Levy JK, et al: Cognitive impairment due to AIDS-related complex and its response to psychostimulants. Psychosomatics 29:38–46, 1988

Fink M, Taylor MA: Catatonia: a separate category in the DSM-IV? Integrative Psychiatry 7:2–7, 1991

Fisher CM: Lacunar strokes and infarcts: a review. Neurology 32:871–876, 1982

Fogel BS: Parkinson's disease: recent developments of psychiatric interest, in Medical-Psychiatric Practice, Vol 2. Edited by Stoudemire A, Fogel BS. Washington, DC, American Psychiatric Press, 1993, pp 447–469

Forrest DV: Psychotherapy of patients with neuropsychiatric disorders, in The American Psychiatric Press Textbook of Neuropsychiatry, 2nd Edition. Edited by Yudofsky SC, Hales RE. Washington, DC, American Psychiatric Press, 1992, pp 703–739

Fricchione GL: Catatonia: a new indication for benzodiazepines? Biol Psychiatry 26:761–765, 1989

Gilman S: Advances in neurology I. N Engl J Med 326:1608–1616, 1992

Goldensohn ES: Symptomatology of non-convulsive seizures; ictal and post-ictal. Epilepsia 24(suppl):505–521, 1983

Goodstein RK: Guide to CAT scanning in hospital psychiatry. Gen Hosp Psychiatry 7:367–376, 1985

Gould R, Miller BL, Goldberg MA, et al: The validity of hysterical signs and symptoms. J Nerv Ment Dis 174:593–597, 1986

Hachinski V, Norris JW: The Acute Stroke. Philadelphia, PA, FA Davis, 1985

Hoeppner JB, Garron DC, Wilson RS, et al: Epilepsy and verbosity. Epilepsia 28:35–40, 1987

Jennett B, Teasdale J: Management of Head Injuries. Philadelphia, PA, FA Davis, 1981

Kahn N, Freeman A, Juncos JL, et al: Clozapine is beneficial for psychosis in Parkinson's disease. Neurology 41:1699–1700, 1991

Klass DW: Electroencephalographic manifestations of complex partial seizures, in Complex Partial Seizures and Their Treatment. Advances in Neurology, Vol 2. Edited by Penry JK, Daly DD. New York, Raven, 1975, pp 113–140

Kurtzke JF: Neuroepidemiology. Ann Neurol 16:265–277, 1984

Kwentus JA, Hart RP, Peck ET, et al: Psychiatric complications of closed-head trauma. Psychosomatics 26:8–15, 1985

Levy R, Bredesen DE: Central nervous system dysfunction in acquired immunodeficiency syndrome. J Acquir Immune Defic Syndr 1:46–64, 1988

Lipsey JR, Robinson RG, Pearlson GD, et al: Nortriptyline treatment of post-stroke depression: a double blind study. Lancet 1:297–300, 1984

Lishman WA: Organic Psychiatry: The Psychological Consequences of Cerebral Disorder, 2nd Edition. Oxford, UK, Blackwell Scientific, 1987

Lishman WA: Physiogenesis in the "post-concussional syndrome." Br J Psychiatry 153:460–469, 1988

Lohr JB, Cadet JL: Neuropsychiatric aspects of brain tumors, in The American Psychiatric Press Textbook of Neuropsychiatry. Edited by Hales RE, Yudofsky SC. Washington, DC, American Psychiatric Press, 1987, pp 351–364

Mace CJ, Trimble MR: Ten year prognosis of conversion disorder. Br J Psychiatry 169:282–288, 1996

Malamud N: Psychiatric disorder with intracranial tumors of the limbic system. Arch Neurol 17:113–123, 1967

Malaspina D, Quitkin HM, Kaufmann CA: Epidemiology and genetics of neuropsychiatric disorders, in The American Psychiatric Press Textbook of Neuropsychiatry, 2nd Edition. Edited by Yudofsky SC, Hales RE. Washington, DC, American Psychiatric Press, 1992, pp 187–226

Maricle RA: Psychiatric disorders in Huntington's disease, in Medical-Psychiatric Practice, Vol 2. Edited by Stoudemire A, Fogel BS. Washington, DC, American Psychiatric Press, 1993, pp 471–512

Masand P, Murray GB, Pickett P: Psychostimulants in post-stroke depression. J Neuropsychiatry Clin Neurosci 3:23–27, 1991

Massey EW, Folger WN: Seizures activated by therapeutic levels of lithium carbonate. South Med J 77:1173–1175, 1984

Mattson RH, Cramer JA, Collins JF, et al: A comparison of valproate with carbamazepine for the treatment of complex partial seizures and secondarily generalized tonic-clonic seizures in adults. N Engl J Med 327:765–771, 1992

Mayeux R, Chen J, Mirabello E, et al: An estimate of the incidence of dementia in idiopathic Parkinson's disease. Neurology 40:1513–1517, 1990

McKenna PJ, Kane JM, Parrish K: Psychotic syndromes in epilepsy. Am J Psychiatry 142:895–904, 1985

McNamara ME: Clinical neurology, in Psychiatric Care of the Medical Patient. Edited by Stoudemire A, Fogel BS. New York, Oxford University Press, 1993, pp 455–483

Mendez MF, Cummings JL, Benson DF: Epilepsy: psychiatric aspects and use of psychotropics. Psychosomatics 25:883–894, 1984

Mendez MF, Cummings JL, Benson DF: Depression in epilepsy: significance and phenomenology. Arch Neurol 43:766–770, 1986

Minden SL: Psychotherapy for people with multiple sclerosis. J Neuropsychiatry Clin Neurosci 4:198–213, 1992

Monday K, Jankovic J: Psychogenic myoclonus. Neurology 43:349–352, 1993

Murray GB: Psychiatric disorders secondary to complex partial seizures. Drug Therapy 4:21–26, 1985

Murray GB, Shea V, Conn DK: Electroconvulsive therapy for post-stroke depression. J Clin Psychiatry 47:258–260, 1986

Ojemann R: Effect of psychotropic medication on seizure control in patients with epilepsy. Neurology 37:1525–1527, 1987

Portegies P, Enting RH, de Gans J, et al: Presentation and cause of AIDS dementia complex: 10 years of follow up in Amsterdam, The Netherlands. AIDS 7:669–675, 1993

Post RM: Use of anticonvulsants in the treatment of manic-depressive illness, in Clinical Use of Anticonvulsants in Psychiatric Disorders. Edited by Post RM, Trimble MR, Pippenger CE. New York, Demos, 1989, pp 113–152

Price TRP, Goetz KL, Lovell MR: Neuropsychiatric aspects of brain tumors, in The American Psychiatric Press Textbook of Neuropsychiatry, 2nd Edition. Edited by Yudofsky SC, Hales RE. Washington, DC, American Psychiatric Press, 1992, pp 473–497

Pritchard PB III, Wannamaker BB, Sagel J, et al: Serum prolactin and cortisol levels in evaluation of pseudoepileptic seizures. Ann Neurol 18:87–89, 1985

Ramani SV, Quesney LF, Olson D, et al: Diagnosis of hysterical seizures in epileptic patients. Am J Psychiatry 137:705–709, 1980

Reding MJ, Orto LA, Wanter SW, et al: Antidepressant therapy after stroke: a double blind trial. Arch Neurol 43:763–765, 1986

Regier DA, Boyd JH, Burke JD Jr, et al: One-month prevalence of mental disorders in the United States. Arch Gen Psychiatry 45:977–986, 1988

Robertson MM, Trimble MR: Depressive illness in patients with epilepsy: a review. Epilepsia 24 (suppl 2):S109–S116, 1983

Robinson RG, Starkstein SE: Current research in affective disorders following strokes. J Neuropsychiatry Clin Neurosci 2:1–14, 1990

Robinson RG, Starr LB, Kubos KL, et al: A two-year longitudinal study of post-stroke mood disorders: findings during the initial evaluation. Stroke 14:736–741, 1983

Robinson RG, Kubos KL, Starr LB, et al: Mood disorders in stroke patients: importance of lesion location. Brain 107:81–93, 1984

Robinson RG, Bolduc PL, Price TR: Two-year longitudinal study of post-stroke mood disorders: diagnosis and outcome at one and two years. Stroke 18:837–843, 1987

Robinson RG, Boston JD, Starkstein SE: Comparison of mania and depression after brain injury: causal factors. Am J Psychiatry 145:172–178, 1988

Rodin E, Schmaltz S: The Bear-Fedio personality inventory and temporal lobe epilepsy. Neurology 34:591–596, 1984

Ross ED: The aprosodias: functional-anatomic organization of the affective components of language in the right hemisphere. Arch Neurol 38:561–569, 1981

Ross ED, Rush AJ: Diagnosis and neuroanatomical correlates of depression in brain damaged patients. Arch Gen Psychiatry 38:1344–1354, 1981

Ross ED, Stewart RM: Akinetic mutism from hypothalamic damage: successful treatment with a dopamine agonist. Neurology 31:1435–1439, 1981

Selecki BR: Cerebral mid-line tumors involving the corpus callosum among mental hospital patients. Med J Aust 2:954–960, 1964

Silver JM, Yudofsky SC: Psychopharmacology and electroconvulsive therapy, in The American Psychiatric Press Textbook of Psychiatry. Edited by Talbott JA, Hales RE, Yudofsky SC. Washington, DC, American Psychiatric Press, 1988, pp 767–853

Silver JM, Hales RE, Yudofsky SC: Psychiatric consultation to neurology, in the American Psychiatric Press Review of Psychiatry, Vol 9. Edited by Tasman A, Goldfinger SM, Kaufmann CA. Washington, DC, American Psychiatric Press, 1990, pp 433–465

Sinyor D, Jacques P, Kaloupek DA, et al: Post-stroke depression and lesion location: an attempted replication. Brain 109:537–546, 1986

Skuster DZ, Digre KB, Corbett JJ: Neurologic conditions presenting as psychiatric disorders. Psychiatr Clin North Am 15:311–333, 1992

Starkstein SE, Robinson RG: Neuropsychiatric aspects of cerebral vascular disorders, in The American Psychiatric Press Textbook of Neuropsychiatry, 2nd Edition. Edited by Yudofsky SC, Hales RE. Washington, DC, American Psychiatric Press, 1992, pp 449–472

Starkstein SE, Robinson RG, Price TR, et al: Comparison of patients with and without post-stroke major depression matched for size and location of lesion. Arch Gen Psychiatry 45:247–252, 1988a

Starkstein SE, Robinson RG, Price TR: Comparison of spontaneously recovered versus non-recovered patients with post-stroke depression. Stroke 19:1491–1496, 1988b

Starkstein SE, Robinson RG, Honig MA, et al: Mood changes after right hemisphere lesions. Br J Psychiatry 155:79–85, 1989

Starkstein SE, Cohen BS, Federoff P, et al: Relationship between anxiety disorders and depressive disorders in patients with cerebrovascular injury. Arch Gen Psychiatry 47:246–251, 1990

Strauss I, Keschner M: Mental symptoms in cases of tumor of the frontal lobe. Archives of Neurology and Psychiatry 33:986–1005, 1935

Treiman DM, Delgado-Escueta AV: Complex partial status epilepticus, in Advances in Neurology, Vol 34: Status Epilepticus. Edited by Delgado-Escueta AV, Wasterlain CG, Treiman DM, et al. New York, Raven, 1983, pp 69–81

Trimble M: Serum prolactin in epilepsy and hysteria (letter). BMJ 2:1682, 1978

Watson CG, Buranen C: The frequency and identification of false positive conversion reactions. J Nerv Ment Dis 167:243–247, 1979

Waxman SG, Geschwind N: The interictal behavior syndrome of temporal lobe epilepsy. Arch Gen Psychiatry 32:1580–1586, 1975

Weiner RD: Does ECT cause brain damage? Behav Brain Res 7:1–53, 1990

Wells CE, Duncan GW: Neurology for Psychiatrists. Philadelphia, PA, FA Davis, 1980

Whitlock FA, Suskind MM: Depression as a major symptom of multiple sclerosis. J Neurol Neurosurg Psychiatry 43:861–865, 1980

Wikstrom J, Paetau A, Palo J, et al: Classic amyotrophic lateral sclerosis with dementia. Arch Neurol 39:681–683, 1982

Woods S, Tesar G, Murray GB, et al: Psychostimulant treatment of depressive disorders secondary to medical illness. J Clin Psychiatry 47:12–15, 1986

Chapter 22

Obstetrics and Gynecology

Nada L. Stotland, M.D.

Obstetrician/gynecologists work with the most affect-laden processes, situations, and interventions in medicine. They must comprehend highly complex physiological processes and master surgical and other technical skills. They tend to have a large patient load, with little time in the outpatient or inpatient setting to spend with each patient.

Obstetrician/gynecologists also find themselves involved in social changes and discontent surrounding women's roles and women's health care (Stotland 1988). These changes differ from subculture to subculture and patient to patient. One patient, mindful of the questions about the high rate of cesarean deliveries or hysterectomies in the United States, regards a well-founded recommendation for a procedure with suspicion. Another woman with similar symptoms and clinical indications may demand a procedure that is not medically advisable.

Medical school and residency training in obstetrics and gynecology offer far too little information about psychological, cultural, social, and psychiatric issues (Weissberg 1990). The risk is that the physician who is poorly trained to handle anxiety evoked by affect-laden situations will react by blaming or stigmatizing patients by overgeneralizing from his or her own experiences and imposing his or her own values, and/or by ignoring clinically significant findings.

Psychiatrists and other mental health professionals are often unfamiliar with obstetrics and gynecology. Psychiatrists may neglect to inquire or counsel about Papanicolaou tests, use of contraception, sexual function, sexual side effects of medications, sexual concerns, protection against sexually transmitted diseases, anniversary reactions, unresolved guilt and grief, and the relation between psychiatric symptoms and recent reproductive events in patients' lives (Lesko et al. 1982).

■ REPRODUCTIVE PHYSIOLOGY AND PSYCHOLOGY THROUGH THE LIFE CYCLE

So much is now known about the physiology of reproduction that vital aspects of it can be manipulated in vivo and effectively duplicated in vitro. Hormonal concomitants of the menstrual cycle are mapped not only in daily but in hourly detail. However, vexing physiological mysteries remain and result in unsolved clinical problems. Even more relevant to consultation-liaison psychiatrists is the current lack of knowledge sufficient to bridge the gap between physiological and psychosocial factors in symptoms related to the reproductive system. This chapter addresses important aspects of reproductive psychology, as well as psychiatric diagnoses, situations, and treatments specific to obstetrics and gynecology.

Gender identity, now believed to be established during the second year of life, is closely linked to the capacity for sexual relationships and reproduction (Notman 1991). The assignment of gender at—or even before, with the use of prenatal testing—birth has a significant effect on virtually every aspect of the child's social experience. Most people experience considerable discomfort when they cannot identify someone's gender. Because gender is determined for most people by genitalia, conditions, illnesses, and treatments affecting the genitalia impinge on an individual's core identity and roles in society.

The powerful feelings evoked by reproductive organs underlie social conventions and, at least partially, determine emotional experiences, including modesty and shame, sexual desirability, envy, status, and self-esteem. A cholecystectomy does not carry the same emotional valence or interpersonal implications as does a hysterectomy—the emotional meaning of the latter surgery varies extensively from woman to woman and from context to context.

Women's reproductive lives are marked by distinct milestones: menarche, first intercourse, conception, first and subsequent deliveries, and menopause. Most cultures mark many of these milestones with rituals and/or changes in status, roles, and responsibilities, which shape the meaning of these events. For example, menarche is identified in most cultures as the formal borderline between girl-

hood and womanhood; young girls await it as proof of their normality. In some societies, first menstruation makes a girl marriageable. At the same time, the sense of shame and the taboos associated with menstruation in most cultures are dreaded by many girls. Because bleeding is otherwise associated with injury and pain, girls who are not prepared for menarche as a normal function often experience considerable fear.

Like menstruation, first intercourse tends to evoke mixed feelings (Lewis and Volkmar 1990). Because girls' genitalia are internal, casual visual inspection cannot evoke either competition or reassurance of normality as it does in boys. Anticipation of first intercourse evokes fear of physical pain and the revelation of defectiveness. First intercourse causes a permanent anatomical change; conflicts about having engaged in intercourse may therefore complicate the prospect of gynecological examination. On the other hand, the ability to engage in coitus confirms anatomical normality and is another significant symbol of maturity.

The next developmental stage is conception, pregnancy, and childbirth. The desire to actually conceive, gestate, bear, and raise children is not precisely the same as the desire to know that one is capable of doing so. Some women report becoming pregnant deliberately, to prove their fertility, with no intention of carrying the pregnancy to term. The gynecologist may assume that a woman who has a certain number of children, has reached a certain age, and/or has expressed a desire to curtail further childbearing will have little emotional reaction to a medical or surgical intervention resulting in sterility. These faulty assumptions can result in serious miscommunication, psychological turmoil, and malpractice suits. The tendency of gynecologists to assume that all women are heterosexual has resulted in an unwillingness of lesbians to obtain gynecological care.

The cessation of monthly bleeding signifies entry of a woman into an "older" category. Powerful social influences shape the woman's experience of menopause and confound research into the relation between menopause and psychiatric symptoms. Generations of psychiatrists were taught that menopause frequently precipitated a developmental crisis or psychiatric illness. More recent studies indicate that there is no association between clinical depression and menopause as a physiological event (Matthews et al. 1990; McKinlay et al. 1987).

The hormonal changes that occur during the climacteric (see Table 22–1) are associated with vasomotor episodes commonly referred to as "hot flashes" and changes in vaginal lubrication and other functions. For some women, hot flashes may interfere with sleep, secondarily leading to psychological symptoms. It has been extremely tempting to simply "replace" the "missing" hormones with exogenous ones (Ravnikar 1992). Many gynecologists now believe that the prescription of hormones is the single most beneficial intervention they have to offer their patients. The use of unopposed estrogen necessitates periodic uterine biopsies; the addition of progesterone causes periodic bleeding that can be inconvenient and embarrassing. Sixty percent of women for whom hormone "replacement therapy" is prescribed do not continue taking hormones after the first year (Ravnikar 1992). There are no data on the long-term effects of any currently prescribed hormonal regimen. Advertisements aimed at physicians and at consumers, however, continue to convey the message that "replacement" therapy will prolong youth and sexual attractiveness (Apfel and Palmund 1992).

Women whose chief gratification and status were derived from their youthful attractiveness and their ability to bear children, as well as women who desired but were not able to achieve gratifying childbearing and mothering, are both vulnerable to depression at menopause (Apfel and Handel 1993). When women's resources and environment allow them to make a gratifying and acknowledged contribution to society after parenting tasks have ended, menopause is usually experienced as a relief from monthly bleeding, childbearing, and child rearing, as well as an opportunity for the expression of other interests and talents. Nevertheless, negative images of menopause persist not only among psychiatrists but also among gynecologists, who often view menopause as a deficiency state.

WOMEN'S HEALTH AND HEALTH CARE: TRADITION AND CHANGE

Women's health care has recently become a legislative, marketing, and research focus (Cotton 1992a, 1992b). The government and other major social institutions, including foundations and health care managers, have highlighted the need for increased numbers and availability of primary care—rather than specialty and subspecialty—providers. Obstetrician/gynecologists, whose training focuses on the aggressive management of disease, are now considered primary care physicians.

Only a minority of women in the United States obtain regular gynecological care. Almost a quarter of all pregnant women receive no first trimester prenatal care (Muller 1990). Many women lack the language to explain and locate their symptoms. Contraceptive care is not obtained; diaphragms are incorrectly placed. Sexually transmitted diseases are pandemic. Breast masses and cervical lesions often are not diagnosed when still treatable (Ciotti

Table 22–1. Hormonal changes during the climacteric

Estrogen production is decreased.

Progesterone levels are unchanged.

Follicle-stimulating hormone production is increased.

Luteinizing hormone levels are unchanged.

Prolactin levels are decreased.

Androgen production is unchanged.

Source.   Adapted from Droegemueller et al. 1987.

1992; Rimer and King 1992). Consultation-liaison psychiatrists can reinforce the need for patient education, improve obstetrician/gynecologists' empathy, and thus enhance patients' knowledge and comfort.

SYNDROME DEFINITIONS AND EPIDEMIOLOGY

The belief is widespread in both lay and medical communities that a relation exists between female reproductive events and psychopathology. This belief is associated with the designation of specific nosological entities, including postpartum depression, postpartum psychosis, and premenstrual tension. In addition, some disorders, such as pseudocyesis and hyperemesis gravidarum, are unique to the obstetrics/gynecology setting.

Research in these areas has unfortunately had methodological problems. Discontinuities in care make it difficult to track responses to reproductive events and interventions. Patients may receive only perfunctory care after a brief hospitalization for surgery or delivery. A subsequent treating psychiatrist may be unaware of a patient's obstetric/gynecological status. Perhaps most serious is the failure to take critical psychosocial variables into account. Nevertheless, there have been attempts to delineate incidence, prevalence, associated hormonal changes, risk factors, and characteristic signs and symptoms.

Mood Disorders

It has been estimated that up to 80% of women who have recently delivered a baby develop a relatively mild, self-limited mood disturbance often called "baby blues" (Bagedahl-Strindlund 1992; Rosenthal and O'Grady 1992). Tearfulness, emotional lability, and anxiety begin approximately 3 days postpartum and usually abate by the seventh day. Theoretical links exist to the hormonal changes of the postpartum period, but no hormonal risk marker or effective treatment has been identified.

Approximately 10% of parturients experience a major depressive episode during the postpartum period (Apfel and Handel 1993). Opinions differ as to whether postpartum psychiatric illness is a distinct entity or the same disorders that occur at other stages of life (Hamilton 1992).

Obstetrics-Specific Psychiatric Issues

Requests for psychiatric consultation by obstetrician/gynecologists are precipitated by the patient's behavior, the patient's failure to accept or comply with medical recommendations, the presence of symptoms that are unresponsive to standard diagnosis and treatment, medical-legal questions, or conflicts between patient and staff. Some outpatient clinic staffs include a mental health practitioner who provides screening, support, and treatment and who may conduct research.

Consultation requests in obstetrics/gynecology settings often involve profound decisions about fertility and parenthood. Psychiatric treatment in the peripartum period can have a long-lasting impact on mother-child attachment and outcome. The interests of the fetus may come into conflict with the interests of the mother. Professional specialty organizations, including the American College of Obstetricians and Gynecologists and the American Psychiatric Association, have developed positions addressing conflicts between fetal and maternal rights. Both organizations advise that a woman's autonomy must not be violated because she is pregnant (Brown et al. 1991). Clinical realities, however, strain physicians' abilities to adhere to these ethical guidelines (e.g., a woman abusing substances).

Voluntary sterilization. Female sterilization is an extremely common form of birth control. Psychiatric consultation in such cases usually involves issues of competency to consent.

Anxieties about "irreversible" sterilization are somewhat relieved by the availability of increasingly reversible procedures, such as the placement of elastic bands around the fallopian tubes. However, reversibility is never guaranteed.

Barriers to voluntary sterilization often derive from the assumption that other forms of contraception exist that are effective and reversible. Lack of knowledge and/or the presence of significant psychological, interpersonal, and medical complications actually render them ineffective for some women. Sterilization offers women assurance against pregnancy, frees them from concern about contraception, and removes the fear that an unplanned pregnancy will force them into a choice between abortion and undesired motherhood. The consultant psychiatrist should be alert to the possibility that a male partner has pressured the patient into requesting tubal ligation. In some situations, the possibility of conception is the only motivation for the use of condoms, which protects both partners against infection with sexually transmitted diseases.

Gynecologists often request psychiatric consultation when a patient with a major psychiatric illness requests sterilization. Clinicians without psychiatric training may assume that a psychotic illness, per se, renders a patient incompetent to consent. (See Simon, Chapter 6, in this volume for further discussion of legal and ethical issues.) The psychiatrist can also alert the gynecology staff that patients who are in the throes of depression or labor may request or agree to sterilization and regret it afterward.

Issues in infertility treatment. Infertility is believed to affect approximately 10% of couples in the United States (Kraft et al. 1980). Infertility is no longer thought to have an unconscious psychodynamic basis. In most cases, anatomical and physiological etiologies are identified. Psychiatric consultation might be requested in cases of 1) infertility in patients with amenorrhea related to eating disorders and 2) infertility in patients whose sexual practices are responsible for the failure to conceive. Generally, psychiatric consultants now focus on helping patients with the results, not the causes, of infertility. The inability to conceive or to carry a pregnancy to term is a narcissistic injury and a profound psychological loss.

Men are more likely to want to keep infertility secret, and women are more likely to talk about it with friends and relatives (Myers 1990). Both women and men report that infertility is stressful; however, women are more likely to describe it as the worst life crisis they have experienced. Simple office counseling can be helpful in opening lines of communication and support.

Media coverage of new reproductive technologies has not only informed the public about new possibilities but may have raised expectations beyond what technologies can provide. Patients are uncertain about when to seek treatment, what provider to see, and when to proceed from a primary practitioner to a specialist or subspecialist. Treatments such as in vitro fertilization are unsuccessful more often than not. Diagnosis and treatment are extremely expensive, intense, and intrusive. Sexual intercourse must be performed according to a prescribed regimen, the menstrual cycle and ovulation are manipulated with exogenous hormones, ova are retrieved from women, and semen must be produced from men by masturbation.

Infertile women and their mates often feel deprived of sexual intimacy and reduced to procreative objects. Each menstrual cycle or cycle of treatment is a crescendo of hope and excitement, often ending in disappointment.

The consultation-liaison psychiatrist may assist the infertility team in dealing with patients—or staff members—who are unwilling to discontinue treatments despite repeated failures. Increasing numbers of infertility centers are also devising guidelines for entry to and exit from treatment programs. Counseling can enhance patients' abilities to communicate with and utilize their own sources of psychosocial support; support groups are particularly helpful (Stewart 1992).

The quest for parenthood may entail the establishment of new family constellations. For example, mothers may gestate embryos for their daughters, women may gestate pregnancies and donate ova for unrelated couples, and divorcing couples may even fight for "custody" of frozen embryos. Mental health professionals are sometimes consulted and asked to serve as gatekeepers in the context of these and other emotionally demanding, physically risky, and/or unorthodox avenues to parenthood. Unfortunately, very little scientific literature is available to guide consultations. Common sense would indicate that the consultant should determine whether the patient has any condition interfering with her ability to make an informed decision, facilitate access to all relevant information, and help the patient to review her options, values, and circumstances.

Adolescent pregnancy.   Approximately 10% of women in the United States conceive during their high school years (Children's Defense Fund 1988; Hayes 1987). This is the highest frequency of adolescent pregnancy in the developed world. Although in some other societies pregnancy in adolescents is normative and supported, in the United States, it demands psychological and material resources that the environment seldom provides. The most effective preventive interventions are school health clinics. At present, few adolescents use contraceptives regularly before the first conception.

In all states, pregnant minors may obtain obstetric care and make decisions about that care without parental notification or consent. The psychiatrist who sees a young pregnant woman should work with her to decide whether it is in her best interest to involve her parents or guardian. Often, the parents will respond more constructively than the patient had anticipated, but sometimes she appropriately

fears abuse or exile from the family home. Approximately half of all adolescent pregnancies end in spontaneous or therapeutic abortion, 45% result in the birth of a child that the mother will raise, and only 5% result in the birth of child who is put up for adoption (Hayes 1987).

Abortion.   There is no evidence that most women who undergo induced abortion—including those under the age of majority—need psychiatric services or experience adverse psychiatric sequelae (Russo and Zierk 1992; Stotland 1992). Nevertheless, both counseling and psychiatric referral should be available. A woman may experience a sense of loss despite the fact that an abortion is her choice. Women who experience paralyzing ambivalence, are subjected to outside pressure, have a history of and/or experience ongoing psychiatric disorders, or have abortions because of genetic or other medical indications are at increased risk for postabortion psychiatric illness (Blumenthal 1991). Consultation must include an assessment of the circumstances that surrounded the abortion. A woman may have been abandoned or abused, or abortion may have been available only under illegal, unsafe, and financially and psychologically punishing conditions.

Psychiatric Complications of Pregnancy

Pseudocyesis.   Pseudocyesis, which was described by Hippocrates, is a condition characterized by a woman's belief that she is pregnant and the manifestation of the related signs and symptoms of pregnancy, including nausea and vomiting, increasing abdominal girth, amenorrhea, and objective changes in the appearance of the breasts and cervix. There are no other associated delusions or hallucinations and no single characteristic psychiatric diagnosis or patient population. Findings are consistent, in some cases, with the persistence of a corpus luteum (i.e., gonadotropins, luteinizing hormone, and prolactin may be elevated). Psychodynamic factors may play a role as well.

The staff must empathically share with the patient the negative results of pregnancy tests and ultrasound examinations; abrupt confrontations may lead her to seek care elsewhere.

Hyperemesis gravidarum. In the absence of methodologically adequate, prospective studies, it is difficult to know whether negative feelings about pregnancy cause nausea and vomiting or vice versa. Vomiting associated with electrolyte changes and inability to maintain adequate hydration and nutrition is characterized as hyperemesis and may require hospitalization and parenteral administration of fluids and electrolytes. It is now believed that neurohormonal and emotional factors are involved and interrelated in this condition. Supportive psychotherapy, relaxation techniques, and symptomatic treatment are usually helpful.

Noncompliance with obstetric advice. Complicated pregnancies can pose substantial maternal risks, which patients misunderstand or deny. Their decisions or behavior may seem bizarre or self-destructive to care providers. It is also difficult to provide care for a woman whose behavior may threaten the well-being of her fetus.

The clinician is sometimes tempted to coerce a patient into interventions during pregnancy. In more than one state, women have been incarcerated and criminally charged for their use of illicit substances during pregnancy. Obstetrics services may try to pressure the psychiatric consultant to hospitalize patients involuntarily on fetal, rather than maternal, grounds. Such action may not be found legal; the right of an individual to refuse a procedure necessary to the health or even life of another has been upheld. The American Psychiatric Association has adopted a stance urging therapeutic, rather than punitive, approaches to substance abuse during pregnancy.

Morbid anxieties associated with pregnancy. Given the tendency of contemporary Western society to overvalue thinness in women, it is not surprising that some women fear the bodily expansion of pregnancy. This fear can interfere with a woman's ingestion of a nourishing diet. Patients with a history of or with current eating disorders are at higher risk. In mild cases, patients are reassured. Patients with more severe anxiety may require psychotherapy or hospitalization, if normal weight gain cannot be achieved.

Noncompliance or paralyzing anxiety during pregnancy can result from a morbid fear of the process of childbirth. Although childbirth preparation courses are useful in reducing the fear of helplessness through active mastery (Walcher 1992), the realities of labor and delivery may precipitate acute anxiety in the vulnerable patient. A complete history, including cultural and familial attitudes and myths, and the patient's previous experience of obstetric/gynecological care will generally reveal the source of the problem. Relaxation techniques and hypnosis are often helpful.

Acute psychiatric decompensation in the gravid patient. Despite the prevalence of psychiatric disorders, routine histories taken on obstetrics/gynecology care services typically omit any questions about psychiatric symptoms. Therefore, psychiatric syndromes often "erupt" as emergencies—pregnant patients stab themselves in the abdomen, patients in labor become psychotic and combative, or newly delivered mothers are unable to assume the care of their newborns. Problems are sometimes exacerbated by the tendency of obstetricians to discontinue psychotropic medications—without psychiatric consultation or the use of alternative means of management—for fear of teratogenicity. A consultation-liaison psychiatrist can avert many such disasters by convincing obstetrics/gynecology staff to include in the initial workup a brief series of psychiatric screening questions.

Decisions about the use of psychoactive medications during pregnancy (see Table

22–2) are made in consultation with the patient. The risks of medication and the untreated psychiatric illness are weighed against the benefits of treatment. Psychotic, mood, and anxiety disorders have significant effects on fetal development and obstetric outcome (Chang and Renshaw 1986); they influence maternal nutrition, sleep, circulation, substance abuse, adherence to medical advice, exercise, and other physiological and behavioral parameters (Apfel and Handel 1993). Whereas some patients or their physicians may insist on continuing or discontinuing medication, most will prefer a plan that combines a minimum of medication with an enhancement of other treatment modalities, including careful attention by family members, frequent outpatient visits, and hospitalization if necessary.

Table 22–3 contains guidelines for psychiatric consultation during labor. Even under the stress of an active labor, it is usually possible to "reach" and calm a patient.

Postpartum grief.   Aside from postpartum depression and psychosis, women may have grief reactions after complicated and/or operative deliveries, the birth of a child with a congenital defect, or the death of an embryo, fetus, or newborn. Postpartum grief is sometimes complicated by a sense that the woman's body did not function normally, putting her child at risk, or by the experience of unacceptable rage at the child for causing her so much emotional and physical suffering. The delivery of a defective, dead, or dying child, at any gestational age, also precipitates feelings of disgust, failure, guilt, and shame.

The support offered by health care providers at the time of a perinatal death is a key factor in helping the mother and father adjust to the loss (Benfield et al. 1978; Knapp and Peppers 1979; Murray and Callan 1988). A physician may complicate the emotional situation by asking questions about family history and prenatal behaviors that compound the sense of responsibility and increase familial tensions. The parents should be allowed and even encouraged to see and hold a dead or dying baby. The infant can be draped in such a way as to emphasize its most normal features, and the parents may unwrap the infant if they wish. A knowledgeable professional should be present at all times to explain the physical findings and to point out areas of normalcy but not to intrude on the family's own assimilation of the event.

The obstetrician and the consulting psychiatrist can review the events of the delivery with the family to absorb the family's emotional responses without defensiveness and to elicit from the patient/mother her preferences: Does she wish to be left alone, to have visitors and family excluded, to have someone always with her, or some combination? Would she like to see a member of the clergy and to make funeral arrangements?

Parents find that holding and speaking to their baby, even one who is dead, fulfills some of their sense of parental obligation. Counseling the couple at the time of the loss and at intervals, such as 6 weeks, 6 months, and 1 year later, will enhance communication and recovery and permit the identification and treatment of psychological complications.

Parents of a "defective" child cannot grieve and get on with life, as painful as that might be. They must live with and constantly be reminded of their "reproductive failure." The degree of distress this imposes depends on their religion, their financial and social resources, their personal coping skills, their relationships, and the nature of the child's defect and treatment.

Postpartum custody issues.   Postpartum psychiatric consultations are frequently sought when a patient's history or behavior raises questions about her ability to care for the newborn. Quality foster care is in short supply in most areas of the United States and is likely to disrupt the child's attachment to parental figures (American Academy of Pediatrics, Committee on Early Childhood, Adoption, and

Table 22–2. Psychotropic drug use in pregnancy: risks of selected agents

Agent	FDA risk factor	Comments
Antidepressants		
Lithium	D	Suspected teratogen in first trimester, especially cardiovascular abnormalities, including Ebstein's anomaly
		Self-limited toxicity in newborn
		Avoid during first trimester, near term
		Contraindicated during lactation
Fluoxetine	ND	?Increased risk of miscarriage
		No reported risk of major malformations
Amitriptyline	D	No reported teratogenicity
		?Withdrawal in neonate
		Avoid in first trimester
Imipramine	D	Few rare malformations reported
		Neonate withdrawal
		Avoid in first trimester
Clomipramine	D	Neonatal toxic morbidity
Phenelzine (MAOI)	C	Increased risk of malformations
		Avoid in pregnancy because of possibility of hypertensive crises
Neuroleptics		
Chlorpromazine (phenothiazine)	C	No conclusive evidence of teratogenicity
		Avoid during labor; possible hypotension
		Avoid near term; neonatal withdrawal
		Safe if used occasionally in small doses
		Not recommended in first trimester
Haloperidol (butyrophenone)	C	Reported use without negative effects
Sedative-hypnotics		
Diazepam (benzodiazepine)	D	May be teratogenic; two major syndromes
		• Floppy baby syndrome (hypotonia, lethargy, sucking difficulties)
		• Withdrawal syndrome (tremors, irritability, vigorous sucking, hypertonicity)
		Not recommended during lactation

Note. MAOI = monoamine oxidase inhibitor; ND = not designated.
FDA risk factors (A, B, C, D, X) are assigned by the U.S. Food and Drug Administration (FDA) to all drugs based on the risks posed to a fetus.
Category C indicates that animal studies show an adverse affect on the fetus or that no studies in animals or women are available. Drug should only be used if potential benefit justifies the potential risk to the fetus.
Category D indicates that there is evidence of human risk, but the benefits may be worth the risk in some situations.
Source. Briggs et al. 1990; Mortola 1989; Pastuszak et al. 1993.

Table 22–3. Keys to psychiatric consultation during labor

1. Determine the patient's premorbid level of intelligence, psychological health, and psychosocial functioning.

2. Observe the interaction between the patient and staff.

   Is the patient being left alone, physically or psychologically?

   Are others focused only on monitoring devices?

   Has the patient's behavior provoked irritation in staff?

   Have the patient's coping mechanisms been overwhelmed?

3. Evaluate for signs and symptoms of acute intoxication or withdrawal from psychoactive substances.

4. Help the patient to focus on one calm, consistent care provider.

   Stand or sit in the direct line of vision of the patient.

   Hold the patient's hand, if indicated.

   Speak in a soft, soothing cadence.

   Ask her to state what is bothering her and what help she needs.

   Perform a simple, formal mental status examination if the patient does not seem to understand.

5. Ascertain from the obstetrical staff the stage of labor, complications, treatment plan, and prognosis.

   Make sure the patient understands this information.

Dependent Care 1993). The existence of a psychiatric disorder, even a severe one, does not preclude adequate mothering. In some cases, the consulting service and psychiatrist may conclude that a mother with a psychiatric disorder is unable to parent her child. Even so, children's service agencies are usually reluctant to take custody unless or until some damage has befallen the child.

In addition to the standard psychiatric history and mental status examination, the consultation must focus on an assessment of the patient's ability to recognize her newborn's needs and provide for them. Unless there is evidence of immediate danger to the child, mother-child interaction in the hospital should be maximized, closely observed, and carefully documented by the obstetrics and pediatric nursing staff as well as by the psychiatrist. Every effort should be made to mobilize social, psychiatric, and medical support for the mother-infant dyad after discharge. Hospitals have legal authority to assume protective custody in cases of suspected child abuse.

Patients with a history of psychiatric illness. In some cases, the history of psychiatric illness is the precipitant for a psychiatric consultation. Psychiatric illness carries a stigma that distances many practitioners from patients.

Acute care/emergencies. Psychiatrists are probably not called often enough to the acute care setting by obstetrician/gynecologists; unless a patient manifests grossly disturbed behavior, the demands of the emergency situation distract clinicians' attention from the psychiatric issues. A patient's allusion to suicide is sometimes the only cue for an emergency psychiatric referral.

Many cases of victimization, rape, abuse, and violence appear in the outpatient or emergency room setting. Until very recently, the care that rape victims received exacerbated their psychological injuries; many were disbelieved, interrogated, and overexamined. Data indicate that relatively few unfounded accusations of rape are made (Hursch 1977). The risk of false accusation, although real, is far less than the risk of retraumatizing the victims by insinuating that the accusation is unfounded.

Many health care settings now have improved systems for dealing with rape. These approaches may include a trained patient advocate who accompanies the patient (if she wishes) throughout the procedures, regardless of the time of day or night. The advocate is available to her afterward, and referral for professional counseling is made if necessary. The advocate helps the patient to understand the examination process; medical care must include the systematic gathering of forensic information such as samples of fluids present in the genitalia, pubic hairs of victim and assailant, and documentation of injuries. The process, even if sensitively carried out, is unpleasant to the traumatized patient but is vital to the subsequent identification and prosecution of the perpetrator. Screening for infection with human immunodeficiency virus (HIV) and other sexually transmitted diseases is also a painful reminder of the possible infectious sequelae of the assault.

Care providers' misconceptions and insensitivities are related to the widespread lack of knowledge about the typical behavior of assault victims. Emotional shock and desperate attempts at self-control, such as the patient's reluctance to undergo examination, are sometimes misinterpreted as evidence that no trauma took place. Medical and law enforcement professionals may be visibly annoyed by the loss of evidence when victims bathe, douche, or destroy objects bearing stigmata of the assault. Victims' tendency to blame themselves—for past sexual behavior, for being "in the wrong place at the wrong time," for failing to take safety precautions, for allowing themselves to be alone with the perpetrator—is synergistic with some care providers' denial and tendency to believe that the victim "asked for it."

Rape victims are at significant risk of leading constricted, isolated lives. Psychotherapy can forestall severe complications (Rose 1993).

Victims of sexual, psychological, and/or physical abuse may present in the acute care setting with symptoms of pelvic inflammatory disease, other gynecological infections, and nonspecific or seemingly unrelated injuries. Emergency care providers frequently fail to ask about domestic violence (Kurz and Stark 1988; Warshaw 1989). Some may accept explanations for injuries, no matter how unlikely. The patient is sent back to the abusive environment, which puts her at significant risk of further injury and even death. The incidence of domestic violence increases during pregnancy.

Patients who present with injuries of dubious origin are interviewed in private—away from the partner suspected of abuse, who may hover over her—by an empathic care provider who asks specifically about violence and offers information about shelters and other resources for battered women. Many such women frustrate care providers by denying the violence and refusing the help at first, although they are able to free themselves from the abusive situation at a later date. The interest and information provided can be lifesaving.

Human immunodeficiency virus and other sexually transmitted diseases. Besides their implications in the emergency setting, HIV and other sexually transmitted diseases may occasion psychiatric consultation because of the anxiety they engender. Although women constitute the fastest growing group with HIV infection, relatively little is known about the differential manifestations and natural courses between the sexes. Women, in general, die sooner after diagnosis than do men (American College of Obstetricians and Gynecologists 1992). Women tend to be diagnosed later in the course of illness, have decreased access to or use of antiviral therapy, are older at the time of infection, or have other concurrent risk factors (Lemp et al. 1992). Gynecological presentations are frequently unrecognized. AIDS and HIV infection may also present with neuropsychiatric symptoms (see Worth and Halman, Chapter 26, in this volume).

Because women with HIV infection are at risk for transmitting the virus to their unborn children, they are sometimes regarded as vectors rather than as patients. Society's efforts to discourage HIV-infected women from childbearing may conflict with their psychological need to enjoy the normal pleasures of parenthood and to produce offspring who will survive after they are gone. Women infected with

HIV are often impoverished and abused and may find it difficult to obtain birth control or abortion services when they desire them. Patients and care providers, including the consultation-liaison psychiatrist, may experience feelings of rage, resentment, longing, and despair precipitated by the ravages of HIV disease.

Transmission of HIV infection to women generally occurs through the sharing of intravenous needles and through heterosexual contact with bisexual and/or intravenous substance-abusing men. Although clean needles and condoms can help to prevent transmission, their use presupposes not only knowledge but also access and psychological assertiveness. The woman who is addicted to crack cocaine frequently resorts to prostitution and is in no position to demand the use of condoms by her drug-supplying sexual partners. Many women who are well-educated, well-informed, and well-off find themselves unable to insist that their sexual partners use condoms. It is incumbent on the psychiatrist to ask patients about contraception and protection from sexually transmitted diseases and to work with them to master any reluctance to protect themselves.

Psychological aspects of gynecological neoplasia.   Gynecological neoplasms range in lethality and incidence from the common, benign myomata of the uterus to rare teratomas and ovarian carcinomas. Patients react with the usual responses to cancer: fear, denial, anger, shame, and coping skills. Neoplasms of the reproductive organs provoke guilt and shame about past sexual behavior as well as current sexual and reproductive dysfunction. Medical inattention to the psychological significance of individual organs is reflected in terms like total hysterectomy; the fact that the ovaries and fallopian tubes are also removed is not always clear to patients, who may subsequently feel betrayed and castrated.

Gynecological cancer treatment may be complicated in some women by a sense of mu-

tilation and loss of gender identity. Involvement of the sexual partner in counseling is advised. They must be reassured that cancer is not contagious and taught alternative sexual skills for the recovery period.

Menopause.   As mentioned earlier in this chapter, menopause is not associated with an increased incidence of psychiatric disorders (Holte 1992; Sherwin 1993). However, patients may be referred for psychiatric consultation under the assumption that their symptoms are related to this reproductive phase. A full gynecological, medical, and psychiatric evaluation is indicated.

Eating disorders.   Patients with a history of eating disorders may present in the obstetrics/gynecology setting, either because the obstetrician/gynecologist is their primary physician or because the eating disorder affects the reproductive system. A classic presentation is the amenorrheic patient in the gynecological endocrinology/infertility clinic. Most patients in the acute phases of anorexia and bulimia deny that they are ill. Given the societal pressures on women to become and remain slim, even physicians may fail to notice that patients are wasting away until the situation becomes emergent.

CONCLUSION

Psychiatric consultation and liaison with obstetrics and gynecology encompasses a fascinating array of ethical, scientific, educational, and clinical challenges. Issues literally range from birth to death. The central psychological significance of sexuality and reproduction heightens the emotional response of every aspect of gynecological and obstetrical care. A number of allied organizations and publications can serve as resources to the consultant, consultee, and patient. Obstetrician/gynecologists learn and practice under extreme pressures of time, legal liability, and impending medical emergency, in addition to the psychological needs of their patients. Consultation-liaison psychiatrists, who are knowledgeable about the medical and psychological aspects of obstetrics/gynecology and empathic to the situations of both the obstetrician/gynecologist and the patient, can forestall crises, relieve suffering and disability, and enhance the health of future generations.

■ REFERENCES

American Academy of Pediatrics, Committee on Early Childhood, Adoption, and Dependent Care: Developmental issues in foster care for children. Pediatrics 91:1007–1009, 1993

American College of Obstetricians and Gynecologists: Issues in women's health: media kit. Washington, DC, American College of Obstetricians and Gynecologists, 1992

Apfel RJ, Handel MH: Madness and Loss of Motherhood: Sexuality, Reproduction, and Long-Term Mental Illness. Washington, DC, American Psychiatric Press, 1993

Apfel RJ, Palmund I: Medical advertising images of menopausal women. Paper presented at the 10th International Congress of Psychosomatic Obstetrics and Gynecology, Stockholm, Sweden, June 1992

Bagedahl-Strindlund M: Postpartum mental illness: cross-cultural and social anthropological aspects—a review, in Reproductive Life: Advances in Research in Psychosomatic Obstetrics and Gynecology. Edited by Wijma K, von Schoultz B. Park Ridge, NJ, Parthenon Publishers, 1992, pp 121–140

Benfield DG, Leib SA, Vollman JH: Grief response of parents and parental participation in deciding care. Pediatrics 62:171–177, 1978

Blumenthal SJ: Psychiatric consequences of abortion: overview of research findings, in Psychiatric Aspects of Abortion. Edited by Stotland NL. Washington, DC, American Psychiatric Press, 1991, pp 17–37

Briggs GG, Freeman RK, Yaffe SJ: Drugs in Pregnancy and Lactation: A Reference Guide to Fetal and Neonatal Risk, 3rd Edition. Baltimore, MD, Williams & Wilkins, 1990

Brown D, Andersen HF, Elkins TF: An analysis of the ACOG and AAP ethics statements on conflicts in maternal-fetal care. J Clin Ethics 2: 19–24, 1991

Chang S, Renshaw D: Psychosis and pregnancy. Compr Ther 12:36–41, 1986

Children's Defense Fund: Teenage Pregnancy: Advocate's Guide to the Numbers. Washington, DC, Children's Defense Fund, 1988

Ciotti MC: Screening for gynecologic and colorectal cancer: is it adequate? Women's Health Issues 2(2):83–93, 1992

Cotton P: Women's health initiative leads way as research begins to fill gender gaps. JAMA Medical News and Perspectives 267:469–473, 1992a

Cotton P: Women scientists explore more ways to smash through the "glass ceiling." JAMA Medical News and Perspectives 268:173, 1992b

Droegemueller W, Herbst AL, Mishell DR Jr, et al: Comprehensive Gynecology. St Louis, MO, CV Mosby, 1987

Hamilton JA: The issue of unique qualities, in Postpartum Psychiatric Illness: A Picture Puzzle. Edited by Hamilton JA, Harberger PN. Philadelphia, PA, University of Pennsylvania Press, 1992, pp 135–162

Hayes C: Risking the Future: Adolescent Sexuality, Pregnancy and Childbearing, Vol 1. Washington, DC, National Academy Press, 1987

Holte A: The search for a climacteric mood disorder: methodological problems and recent results, in Reproductive Life: Advances in Research in Psychosomatic Obstetrics and Gynecology. Edited by Wijma K, von Schoultz B. Park Ridge, NJ, Parthenon Publishers, 1992, pp 214–233

Hursch CJ: The Trouble With Rape. Chicago, IL, Nelson-Hall, 1977

Knapp RJ, Peppers LG: Doctor-patient relationships in fetal/infant death encounters. Journal of Medical Education 54:775–780, 1979

Kraft AD, Palombo J, Mitchell D, et al: The psychological dimensions of infertility. Am J Orthopsychiatry 50:618–628, 1980

Kurz D, Stark E: Not-so-benign neglect: the medical response to battering, in Feminist Perspectives on Wife Abuse. Edited by Yllo K, Bograd M. Newbury Park, NJ, Sage, 1988, pp 54–72

Lemp GF, Hirozawa AM, Cohen JB, et al: Survival for women and men with AIDS. J Infect Dis 166:74–79, 1992

Lesko LM, Stotland NL, Seagraves RT: Three cases of female anorgasmia associated with MAOIs. Am J Psychiatry 139:1353–1354, 1982

Lewis M, Volkmar FR: Clinical Aspects of Child and Adolescent Development: An Introductory Synthesis of Developmental Concepts and Clinical Experience, 3rd Edition. Philadelphia, PA, Lea & Febiger, 1990

Matthews KA, Wing RR, Kuller LH, et al: Influences of natural menopause on psychological characteristics and symptoms of middle-aged healthy women. J Consult Clin Psychol 58: 345–351, 1990

McKinlay JB, McKinlay SM, Brambilla DJ: Health status and utilization behavior associated with menopause. Am J Epidemiol 125:110–121, 1987

Mortola J: The use of psychotropic agents in pregnancy and lactation. Psychiatr Clin North Am 12:69–87, 1989

Muller C: Health Care and Gender. New York, Russell Sage Foundation, 1990

Murray J, Callan V: Predicting adjustment to perinatal death. Br J Med Psychol 61:237–244, 1988

Myers MF: Male gender-related issues in reproduction and technology, in Psychiatric Aspects of Reproductive Technology. Edited by Stotland NL. Washington, DC, American Psychiatric Press, 1990, pp 25–35

Notman MT: Gender development, in Women and Men: New Perspectives on Gender Differences. Edited by Notman MT, Nadelson CC. Washington, DC, American Psychiatric Press, 1991, pp 117–127

Pastuszak A, Schick-Boschetto B, Zuber C, et al: Pregnancy outcome following first trimester exposure to fluoxetine (Prozac). JAMA 269:2246–2248, 1993

Ravnikar VA: Compliance with hormone replacement therapy: are women receiving the full impact of hormone replacement therapy preventive health benefits? Women's Health Issues 2:75–82, 1992

Rimer BK, King E: Why aren't older women getting mammograms and clinical breast exams? Women's Health Issues 2:94–101, 1992

Rose DS: Sexual assault, domestic violence, and incest, in Psychological Aspects of Women's Health Care: The Interface Between Psychiatry and Obstetrics and Gynecology. Edited by Stewart DE, Stotland NL. Washington, DC, American Psychiatric Press, 1993, pp 447–483

Rosenthal M, O'Grady JP: Affective and anxiety disorders, in Obstetrics: Psychological and Psychiatric Syndromes. Edited by O'Grady JP, Rosenthal M. New York, Elsevier, 1992, pp 109–138

Russo NF, Zierk KL: Abortion, childbearing and women's well-being. Professional Psychology, Research and Practice 23:269–280, 1992

Sherwin BB: Menopause: myths and realities, in Psychological Aspects of Women's Health Care: The Interface Between Psychiatry and Obstetrics and Gynecology. Edited by Stewart DE, Stotland NL. Washington, DC, American Psychiatric Press, 1993, pp 227–248

Stewart DE: A prospective study of the effectiveness of brief professionally led infertility support groups, in Reproductive Life: Advances in Research in Psychosomatic Obstetrics and Gynecology. Edited by Wijma K, von Schoultz B. Park Ridge, NJ, Parthenon Publishers, 1992, pp 151–165

Stotland NL: Social change and women's reproductive health care, in Psychiatric Aspects of Reproductive Technology. Edited by Stotland NL. New York, Praeger, 1988, pp 89–104

Stotland NL: The myth of the abortion trauma syndrome (commentary). JAMA 268:2078–2079, 1992

Walcher W: Results of holistic childbirth preparation, in Reproductive Life: Advances in Research in Psychosomatic Obstetrics and Gynecology. Edited by Wijma K, von Schoultz B. Park Ridge, NJ, Parthenon Publishers, 1992, pp 101–119

Warshaw C: Limitations of the medical model in the care of battered women. Gender and Society 3(4):506–517, 1989

Weissberg M: The meagerness of physicians' training in emergency psychiatric intervention. Acad Med 65:747–750, 1990

Chapter 23

Physical Medicine and Rehabilitation

Duane S. Bishop, M.D.
L. Russell Pet, M.D.

Rehabilitation medicine is a rapidly expanding area of medicine that requires effective and efficient attention by consultation-liaison psychiatrists. Forty million Americans have some physical impairment, disability, or handicap (Hahn 1983). The rate of disability increases with age and is higher among ethnic minorities (Group for the Advancement of Psychiatry, Committee on Handicaps, 1993). Contrary to common belief, disability benefits generally are going to the right people (i.e., people with genuine disabilities) (International Center for the Disabled 1986). In this chapter, we focus on consultation-liaison psychiatry issues that are salient to inpatient and outpatient rehabilitation treatment settings.

Rehabilitation medicine is not acute medicine, and consultation-liaison psychiatry in rehabilitation settings demands a different conceptualization. Rehabilitation staff are intensely invested, remain motivated, and may receive little immediate return for their efforts. When they ask for psychiatric assistance, they want more than a diagnosis and medication recommendations. Members of the staff have detailed observations and knowledge they wish to share and a need to understand behavior in the context of their interventions. They want feedback and demand an integrated, consistent team plan for patient problems. Psychiatric credibility is gained only by addressing these expectations.

DEFINITIONS

The terms *impairment, disability,* and *handicap* (World Health Organization 1980) are not always used appropriately. *Impairment* is loss of psychological, physiological, or anatomical structure or function. *Disability* is a loss in ability to perform activities of daily living. *Handicap* is the sum of social and environmental disadvantage arising out of disease, impairment, or disability. A direct relation among the three does not always exist, and interventions are different for each. Rehabilitation focuses on minimizing disability and handicap.

■ CONTEXT OF REHABILITATION

Effective psychiatric consultation on rehabilitation units requires considering many contextual issues.

Rehabilitation Versus Acute Medicine and Surgery

In acute medical settings, patients are acutely ill and are passive recipients of care. During rehabilitation, patients and their families assume more responsibility for the patient's progress.

Time and Patient Stability

Rehabilitation generally involves a longer stay in a facility than is required for acute inpatient medical-surgical care. Patients referred for rehabilitation are also usually medically stable and physically active. This facilitates both initial psychiatric consultation and follow-up care.

Three-Hour Rule

Patients must be able to tolerate and receive 3 hours a day of any combination of physical therapy, occupational therapy, and speech therapy. Therapists are usually assigned for the entire period, and this consistent contact provides reliable information about behavior, mood, and cognition.

Psychiatric comorbidity can make meeting the 3-hour rule difficult, and psychiatric intervention in such situations may prevent premature discharge. Programs have formal scheduling systems that can assist the psychiatric consultant in choosing the most efficient time for consultation.

Rehabilitation Teams

The rehabilitation staff members function in interdisciplinary teams that are usually larger than an inpatient psychiatry treatment team.

Consultation-liaison psychiatrists should schedule visits in order to meet briefly with the team. If this is not possible, the team should be asked to designate an individual who will serve as liaison with the psychiatrist for a given patient.

Comprehensive Evaluation

Good assessment is good management. Careful review of the record is a must. The psychiatric examination must be thorough. Psychiatrically significant vegetative signs and symptoms must be differentiated from signs and symptoms of concurrent medical conditions. During the evaluation, patients may indicate medical symptoms to the psychiatrist that have not been previously noted; this information must be passed on to the consulting physiatrist and/or primary care physician.

Management Protocols

Psychiatric interventions may be most effectively delivered in rehabilitation settings if presented in protocol form similar to what rehabilitation staff use for bowel and bladder control.

Cultural Sensitivity

Cultural values play a significant role in rehabilitation (Group for the Advancement of Psychiatry, Committee on Handicaps, 1993). Cultures vary in their values and views regarding issues such as dependence/independence, pain, acceptance of body deformities, sexuality, caregiving expectations, and other issues that influence course and outcome.

Functional Assessment

Psychiatric consultants should become familiar with functional capacity assessment methods used in rehabilitation. Maximal functioning is a central goal, and all programs document detailed assessments. These functional measures provide crucial information, point to areas of discrepancy between expected and observed functioning, and suggest when psychosocial factors may be affecting a patient's progress. If the patient is not achieving expected improvement goals, the suspicion should be raised that undetected medical and/or significant psychosocial factors may be involved.

◼ REASONS FOR PSYCHIATRIC CONSULTATION

The most frequent problems that consultation-liaison psychiatrists are asked to address in patients in rehabilitation units include depression, cognitive changes, adjustment problems, and behavioral difficulties.

Depression

Depression is one of the most frequent reasons for psychiatric consultation in rehabilitation medicine. Yet the diagnosis of depression is overlooked in 70%–80% of depressed inpatients in acute medical settings and in up to 68% of depressed patients in rehabilitation settings (Schubert et al. 1992a). Major depression is associated with longer duration of inpatient rehabilitation, deficient self-care (Malec and Neimeyer 1983; Schubert et al. 1992b; Tiller 1992), and delay in resumption of premorbid social activities (Tiller 1992). On the other hand, at least one research team (Starkstein and Robinson 1989) found that depression does not appear to be related to severity of neurological impairment in patients who have had a stroke. The reported incidences of depression and dysthymia in rehabilitation-related disorders in different medical disorder groups are outlined in Table 23–1.

Depression syndromes have many etiologies that include but are not limited to 1) primary major depression, 2) dysthymia, 3) exacerbation of dysthymic features under stress, 4) adjustment disorder with depressed mood, 5) the general malaise of being ill, 6) a secondary disorder resulting from medical conditions such as hypothyroidism and Addison's disease, 7) a side effect of medications, and 8) central nervous system (CNS) deficits (Bishop 1980).

Table 23–1. Rates of depression in rehabilitation diagnostic groups

Diagnostic group	Rate of depression (%)
Amputation	35–58[a,b,c]
Chronic pain	28 dysthymia[d]
	8–87 major depression[d,e]
Multiple sclerosis	6–27[f]
Oncology	6–25[g,h]
Rheumatoid arthritis	19–50[i]
Spinal cord injury	2–30[j,k]
Stroke	25–30[l]
Traumatic brain injury	25[m]

Source. [a]Gerhardt et al. 1984; [b]Rybarczyk et al. 1992; [c]Shukla et al. 1982; [d]Large 1986; [e]Lindsay and Wyckoff 1981; [f]Lishman 1987; [g]Holland 1987; [h]Massie and Holland 1990; [i]Beckham et al. 1992; [j]MacDonald et al. 1987; [k]Fullerton et al. 1981; [l]Tiller 1992; [m]Federoff et al. 1992.

Depression is often the result of a mixture of at least two or three of these etiologies in rehabilitation settings.

The principles of depression assessment in the patient undergoing rehabilitation do not vary significantly from those that apply to other medical settings. Reports of depressed mood by the patient may be misleading because of cognitive deficits, lack of awareness, or aphasia. Depressed mood must also be differentiated from organic labile affect (Caplan and Shechter 1987).

The suicide rate is higher among patients in rehabilitation settings than in the general population and among patients with other types of medical illness (Table 23–2). Missel (1978) reported that concerns about suicide risk led to 15% of requests for psychiatric consultation in one series. Suicidal rehabilitation patients may not always have traditional suicide risk factors. Suicidal thinking and behaviors can sometimes be a reaction to life circumstances in patients who have no concurrent active psychiatric disorder (Sakinofsky 1980; Whitlock 1986). Some patients choose to die when quality of life or burden on others reaches a point of critical personal crisis.

Table 23–2. Suicide prevalence among patients with illnesses compared with general population

Diagnosis	Suicide prevalence
Cancer	15–20 times greater
Cerebrovascular accident	2–6 times greater
Multiple sclerosis	14 times greater
Musculoskeletal diseases (excluding rheumatoid arthritis)	No greater prevalence
Rheumatoid arthritis	2–3 times greater
Spinal cord injury	15 times greater

Source. Adapted from Whitlock 1986.

Mania

Patients previously diagnosed with bipolar disorder are at greatest risk for developing mania or hypomania after a CNS event or injury. Mania is relatively rare in patients with head injury (Reiss et al. 1987; Starkstein et al. 1987) and other CNS disorders. In contrast, early classic reports of euphoria or manic syndromes in multiple sclerosis (e.g., Cottrell and Wilson 1926) have been substantiated by more recent studies suggesting a prevalence of 6%–26% (Lishman 1987). Steroids often precipitate or exacerbate mania in patients with multiple sclerosis (S. Minden, personal communication, July 1990).

Cognitive and Neurobehavioral Problems

Cognitive and neurobehavioral deficits occur in 25%–64% of patients undergoing rehabilitation (Caplan 1987; Luxenberg and Feigenbaum 1986) and many rehabilitation programs have special programs for patients with traumatic brain injury. Delirium is less common among patients in rehabilitation settings than in acute care because delirium is usually an exclusion criterion for admission except for patients with head injury. Frequently encountered cognitive problems in rehabilitation medicine include problems with memory, vision, intellect, neglect, apraxia, aprosodia, aphasia, agnosia, distractibility, impulsivity, poor judgment and safety awareness, and orientation difficulties. Unrecognized cognitive and neurobehavioral problems may be mislabeled as poor motivation (Goodstein 1984).

Careful assessment of cognitive factors is essential in psychiatric consultation to patients undergoing rehabilitation (Caplan 1987; Gordon et al. 1985). The need is obvious following head injury and stroke. Occult head injury occurs in up to 50% of patients with spinal cord injury (Wilmot et al. 1985). Fortunately, in rehabilitation medicine, diagnosis-related group (DRG)-exempt, CARF (Certified Acute Rehabilitation Facility), and CORF (Certified Outpatient Rehabilitation Facility) accreditations all require adequate neuropsychology services for both assessment and cognitive rehabilitation efforts.

Adjustment and Coping Problems

Most patients in rehabilitation settings cope well, even when they have major and disfiguring injuries (Bowden et al. 1980). Nevertheless, it is common for consultation-liaison psychiatrists to be asked to see patients whom staff members designate as having adjustment problems. These difficulties may represent a true DSM-IV (American Psychiatric Association 1994) adjustment disorder; a major depression, an anxiety disorder, or other major psychiatric disorders that have been misidentified by staff as adjustment problems; cognitive problems (e.g., receptive dysphasia or aprosodia); reactions by staff to the problem the patient is facing; and adjustment problems because the disability prevents the use of personally preferred coping strategies. Personality, temperament, and coping also affect rehabilitation outcome.

Etiology—that is, congenital problem, trauma, medical disorder, or cancer—as well as course, prognosis, and age at onset of the disability can affect physical, emotional, social, and occupational adjustment in unique ways.

Conditions seen in rehabilitation have varying clinical courses. The patient's and family's understanding, experience, and perceptions of expected course and prognosis all must be assessed during a psychiatric consultation.

Patients can have difficulty maintaining the commitment and drive required of them. The pace of the rehabilitation program may be much faster than expected for any given individual. The financial stress of health care costs, loss of work, and changes in contribution to household management can be stressful.

Occupational retraining may be necessary for patients who previously worked. Vocational rehabilitation counselors are usually available and will assist in the mechanics of job retraining, funding, new job searches, and so forth.

Body Image Changes

We all have a body image, a highly individualized, subjective, and integrated sense of what we look like and what we feel (Group for the Advancement of Psychiatry, Committee on Handicaps, 1993). Rehabilitation staff and psychiatric consultants may be confronted by malformed bodies, which can trigger strong and painful reactions.

Changes in body image and other emotional aspects of catastrophic events can trigger significant boundary and vulnerability issues and lead to primitive, unrealistic patient fantasies about how caregivers should relate. For example, patients can split staff into "good" and "bad." Families can be divided and compete with staff to be the "good" caregiver. These regressive, splitting, boundary, responsibility, powerlessness, and "whose life is it anyway?" issues are well described in the Group for the Advancement of Psychiatry (GAP) report (1993).

Three body image changes that are frequently seen in rehabilitation settings deserve additional consideration. First, 30%–70% of pa-

tients with amputations will experience a phantom limb syndrome (Gerhardt et al. 1984; Katz 1992), which persists in some patients for up to 25 years (Katz 1992). Etiological mechanisms are not well understood, and treatments have a low success rate (Katz 1992). Second, in our experience, patients with hand and finger amputations present special problems. These patients present with anxiety, apprehension, and obsessive ruminations that are seemingly out of proportion to the circumstance. They have difficulty when others look at their hands and often have sexual difficulties related to loss of or changes in touch. Third, "hemineglect" is a neurologically based body image problem seen particularly in patients after a nondominant parietal stroke. In severe cases, these patients do not recognize the left side of their body, have major problems with safety (e.g., they will allow their arm to dangle in wheelchair spokes), do not recognize their deficits, are impulsive, and have anosognosia that can be misinterpreted as a psychiatric symptom.

Nonadherence to Treatment

One manifestation of poor adjustment to loss of body function is nonadherence to treatment. Bradley (1985) reported nonadherence rates of 22%–67% for medications and 38%–66% for physical therapy instructions in patients with rheumatoid arthritis. Factors predicting lack of adherence in this study included type of medication, duration of illness, disease severity, and patient beliefs about efficacy. Similar patterns are seen in patients with other disorders.

Loss and Mourning

Loss, mourning, and stages of recovery historically are important concepts in rehabilitation medicine (Group for the Advancement of Psychiatry, Committee on Handicaps, 1993; Krueger 1984; Wortman and Silver 1989). However, disability is not death! Disabling conditions provide a different set of challenges, and every step of recovery poses new challenges. Research indicates that specific stages do not occur in adjustment to spinal cord injury (Craig et al. 1994; S. Harasymin, personal communication, August 1981). Although "staff may be motivated to seek staged mourning models by their desire to have specific interventions to handle difficult situations, the application of stages of mourning in the context of disability can lead to premature closure and a failure to fully appreciate the course of any given individual with a disability" (Bishop 1980, p. 7).

Consultation-liaison psychiatrists are sometimes asked to see patients "in denial." Yet, especially during early stages of rehabilitation, a balance between denial and reality is required (Caplan and Shechter 1987; Group for the Advancement of Psychiatry, Committee on Handicaps, 1993).

Behavior Problems

Behavior problems seen in patients in rehabilitation settings include aggression, yelling out, and inappropriate sexual behavior. These behaviors can be expressions of depression, cognitive dysfunction, adjustment problems, anxiety, or personality problems. In general, fewer problems occur on units that have an experienced staff and a well-integrated psychosocial program that includes consultation-liaison psychiatry.

Active aggression may lead staff to 1) punish the patient, 2) capitulate to the patient's demands, or 3) withdraw from important aspects of care. Unfortunately, these reactions escalate the aggressive behavior. Passive forms of aggression include inaction, interfering actions, dependency, displacement, and projections.

Some patients undergoing rehabilitation may be identified by staff as splitting, noncompliant, unmotivated, dependent, needy, or otherwise "difficult." Vanderpool (1984) described six concepts that are useful in addressing behavioral problems among "difficult" patients (Table 23–3).

There are many conceptual approaches to

rehabilitation unit behavior problems, including team processes, special interviewing techniques, and psychological assessment methods (Group for the Advancement of Psychiatry, Committee on Handicaps, 1993; Guenther et al. 1993; Vanderpool 1984). Psychiatric consultants can most effectively address character and behavior problems by assisting rehabilitation staff 1) to operationally define the "difficult behavior," 2) to know when, where, and in whose presence it is most likely to occur, and 3) to clarify expected responses to specific staff and family interventions.

A range of troublesome externalized (seductiveness, obscene language, and aggression) and internalized (denial and repression) sexual behavior problems may occur among patients undergoing rehabilitation (Crewe 1980b). These difficulties should be addressed in an open manner, and firm limits should be set with patients. Sexual issues should be addressed with all patients. Treatment should be offered to patients and partners who desire it.

Table 23–3. Concepts for managing rehabilitation in "difficult patients"[a]

Recognize neuropsychiatric syndromes early[a]

Make a careful, complete, and inclusive diagnosis[a]

Know what may or may not work[a]

Ask "Can the patient be helped?" (Is status quo all that may be expected?)[a]

Know the patient mix on the unit and the effect on staff working with them[a]

Avoid inappropriate "over-helping" that may do more harm than good for the patient or treatment team[a]

Work toward prevention—primary, secondary, and tertiary[b]

Staff members should strive for an understanding of

- Themselves
- Their specific treatment center
- The effect of program on different types of patients[b]

Source. [a]Vanderpool 1984; [b]Crewe 1980a.

Anxiety

The paucity of information about anxiety disorders in patients in rehabilitation settings is surprising because, in our experience, aspects of anxiety, fears, apprehension, and worry are very common, underrecognized, and the underlying cause of many behavior difficulties.

Anxiety may present as a symptom or a disorder. DSM-IV anxiety disorders are all seen. Careful assessment by the consultation-liaison psychiatrist is needed to separate posttraumatic stress disorder (PTSD) and acute stress disorder from other anxiety and adjustment disorders. Whenever possible, the treatment of patients with PTSD and acute stress disorder in rehabilitation settings should not include psychopharmacological therapy—medications that may interfere with the patient's ability to participate in exercise and other unit treatment activities. Psychotherapy may be started while the patient is on the inpatient service and must usually be continued into the outpatient setting.

Anxiety may lead to anticipatory avoidance and phobias. The apprehension of falling is common and normal and frequently interferes with rehabilitation therapies. Patients may also have claustrophobic responses to closed bedside curtains, halos, traction devices, and wheelchairs. Despite their significant personal distress, it is surprising that patients often do not easily volunteer information about anxiety and phobias. Patients seem to talk about these issues only if they are brought up by others and if it is suggested that these are "normal" reactions. In general, these problems respond well to appropriate and brief supportive psychotherapy and relaxation training.

Patients with Guillain-Barré syndrome can also develop generalized anxiety, especially when progression leads to respirator use. They often develop a "terror" associated with the progressive loss of function and the slow recovery and become hypervigilant for any symptoms of returning paralysis. Generally, they resist use of medications because they fear any upset in their recovery. They respond well to reframing their experience as "normal," to imagery, and to relaxation and pain control techniques that improve their sense of autonomy.

Pervasive anxiety may also be seen in patients who have coronary artery bypass grafts and sustain an intraoperative or postoperative stroke. Patients with cognitive deficits can experience catastrophic anxiety when their deficits are confronted, and this anxiety may initiate avoidance behavior.

Physical, occupational, and speech therapists see patients daily and can help to identify increasing anxiety and the specific situations in which it occurs. Anxiety occurring in only one therapy setting is likely to be related to a particular staff member or specific aspects of that situation. Anxiety that occurs across all therapies suggests an anxiety syndrome.

Substance-Related Problems

The epidemiology of alcohol and drug abuse among patients in rehabilitation settings has not been well studied. This is surprising because alcohol and drug abuse can cause disabling conditions and may represent a maladaptive adjustment to such disabilities (Greenwood 1984). It has been reported that 78% of patients undergoing rehabilitation who have a history of premorbid drug or alcohol use resume use late in rehabilitation or a few months after discharge (Donahue et al. 1986; Gorelick and Kelly 1992; O'Donnell et al. 1981/1982). Patients may arrive in the rehabilitation setting receiving large quantities of narcotics after major surgical procedures and may require a tapering of their medication.

Accurate identification of a premorbid substance use history is crucial, especially in patients with trauma, head injury, spinal cord injury, or hemorrhagic stroke. Traditional alcohol and drug abuse programs have difficulty handling patients with a major disability and, to an even greater extent, patients with cognitive deficits. Fortunately, some rehabilitation programs are beginning to develop specialized substance disorders treatment programs.

Sleep Problems

Sleep problems are common among patients undergoing rehabilitation (Kryger et al. 1989). Hypersomnia is usually the result of problems of arousal or neuropsychiatric effects of medications. Insomnia is often caused by a primary or secondary psychiatric disorder, neurological disorder, or exacerbation of long-standing primary insomnia. A number of other problems may also interfere with sleep, including pain, opioid dependence, nighttime opioid withdrawal symptoms, sedative-hypnotic tolerance, the activating quality of some antidepressants, urinary tract problems, and incontinence. As a group, patients with spinal cord injury have proportionately less stage 4 sleep. This lack of sleep may contribute to spasticity problems, possibly triggered by pathophysiological mechanisms similar to those seen in patients with fibromyalgia (Bishop 1980). Sleep charts, detailed sleep histories, and sleep monitoring systems are all helpful.

Pain

Pain of various types is common among patients in rehabilitation settings (Fey and Williamson-Kirkland 1987; Steger and Brockway 1980; Steger et al. 1980; Tunks and Merskey 1980). Pain during rehabilitation occurs for many reasons.

Patients who are dependent on narcotic analgesics pose special problems. It is useful to have the patient formally rate his or her pain and to keep 24-hour diaries of major pain episodes and circumstances. Charting for 2–3 days usually is sufficient to establish the pain pattern. The patient's medication use should not be challenged immediately, but he or she should ask the patient to indicate his or her un-

derstanding of the symptoms of dependence. Most are surprised to learn that pain itself is a significant medication withdrawal symptom. This process has allowed us, in almost all cases, to obtain active collaboration for a tapering and detoxification program (for more details see Bouckoms, Chapter 31, in this volume).

Sexual Dysfunction

Although sexual activity is a vital part of normal life, society tends to ignore the sexuality of both elderly and disabled individuals. From 25% to 55% of men with spinal cord injury cannot achieve an erection (Ducharme 1987; Trieschman 1980). Ejaculation and conception are possible for most men with spinal cord injuries with the assistance of special techniques. In women, spinal cord injury may result in an inability to experience orgasm; this teaches them to see themselves as less attractive and desirable (Vrey and Henggeler 1987). Women with spinal cord injuries respond to audiovisual stimulation in a manner similar to that of able-bodied women but require manual stimulation for reflex genital vasocongestion (Sipski et al. 1995).

Sexual dysfunction also may occur in patients with other diagnoses. For example, sexual activity decreased in 46% of patients with rheumatoid arthritis (Deyo et al. 1982). Sexual dysfunction is reported in 50% of women and 75% of men with multiple sclerosis (Valleroy and Kraft 1984). Studies have also documented a decline in sexual activity after stroke (Bray et al. 1981; Fugl-Meyer and Jaasko 1980). Touch impairment is more of a factor than motor dysfunction (Fugl-Meyer and Jaasko 1980).

Despite these findings, patients undergoing rehabilitation and their partners generally do not receive sexual counseling (Sjogren et al. 1983). Information about these and related issues can be obtained from several sexuality and disability centers listed by Ducharme (1987, p. 436).

FAMILIES AND CAREGIVERS

Most patients have one primary person who provides the majority of assistance for them (i.e., their primary caregiver). Caregivers can provide a great deal of information to the psychiatrist and assist by following through when care reverts to the outpatient setting. Caregivers appear to experience similar degrees of burden and similar levels of psychological morbidity whether dealing with disabilities or dementias (Gwyther and George 1986; Lichtenberg and Gibbons 1993). Attention must be paid, therefore, to caregiver mood, function, family life, and health. Consultation for a patient undergoing rehabilitation often involves psychiatric assessment and treatment of a spouse, partner, or other caregiver.

The majority of home care for disabled patients is in fact provided by partners or adult children (Lichtenberg and Gibbons 1993). Partners who serve as caregivers generally receive less assistance (e.g., homemakers) than do adult children (Pruchno 1990); they also have poorer health (Cantor 1983). Fifty percent of caregivers can expect to develop major depression (Schulz et al. 1990). A large number of employed caregivers must quit their jobs to provide care (Brocklehurst et al. 1981).

Families provide information that is crucial for accurate diagnosis, notice changes in behavior, and often have a intuitive sense of why the patient has a response to a particular situation. Table 23–4 summarizes research findings on how families function following the onset of disability in one of its members.

STAFF PROBLEMS

In general, staff problems arise out of situations that confront and threaten a staff member's sense of professional and personal self (Crewe 1980a; Gans 1987; Group for the Advancement

Table 23–4. Summary of family functioning and disability research findings

In the general population, 25% of families function at a level that places them at risk for significant family problems if a family member becomes disabled.[a]

Many families function well despite a member's disability.[a]

Family functioning during the acute crisis does not predict later functioning, which is similar to what is found in nonclinical community samples.[b]

The relations between family functioning and other variables in one diagnostic group do not necessarily apply in another diagnostic group (i.e., findings and observations cannot be generalized).[a]

Families have more difficulty dealing with cognitive dysfunction than with the loss of other functions.[a]

The presence of a family, the patient's perception of a significant family role to return to, and the family's support of the rehabilitation process positively affect outcomes.[b]

Families require education and follow-up.[c] Families who receive education have reduced anxiety and cooperate better with the health team.[b]

Families with a disabled member face changes in roles, leisure, activities, and health statuses of other members.[b]

Depression is common among patients undergoing rehabilitation. Depression has a negative effect on rehabilitation patients' families, which is worsened if patients also have a medical disorder.[d,e]

Source. [a]Bishop and Miller 1988; [b]Bishop et al. 1984; [c]Evans et al. 1988; [d]Keitner et al. 1989; [e]Keitner et al. 1991.

of Psychiatry, Committee on Handicaps, 1993; Gunther 1987; Romano 1984). Staff problems often arise when events, circumstances, colleagues, and especially patients lead staff members to feel inefficient or ineffective. The greatest staff problems arise within the intimacy of the staff-patient relationship and the need for the staff to be successful.

◼ TREATMENT AND MANAGEMENT

Medical Interventions

Medical interventions include the usual attention to diagnosis and management of correctable medical causes for primary and secondary psychiatric symptoms and syndromes. Rehabilitation-related guidelines from the Agency for Health Care Policy and Research cover urinary incontinence, pain, pressure sores, stroke rehabilitation (pending), depression in primary care, and other topics.[1]

Clinical Psychopharmacology

Psychopharmacological medications can effectively treat primary and secondary psychiatric disorders in patients undergoing rehabilitation, and new approaches are advancing rapidly (Cook 1984; McLean et al. 1993; Murray 1987; Silver and Yudofsky 1993). However, psychopharmacology can be a double-edged sword. Some side effects can worsen specific functions in patients who are already compromised. A recent report suggested that impaired motor recovery is seen in stroke patients who receive commonly used medications (e.g., haloperidol, α_1- and α_2-receptor antagonists, and benzodiazepines) that have been shown to impair recovery in animal stroke models (Goldstein et al. 1995). Table 23–5 shows various medications and their beneficial uses and potential adverse effects in rehabilitation settings.

Most psychopharmacological medications should be used in lower-than-usual dosages in patients with brain injuries (Finklestein et al. 1987; Goodstein 1984).

Patients undergoing rehabilitation may have been taking narcotic analgesics for weeks or months. Consultation-liaison psychiatrists may be asked to help taper patients off their pain medications. A calculated and gradual narcotic withdrawal protocol is essential. (For further information on psychopharmacology, see Jachna et al., Chapter 30, in this volume.)

Psychotherapy

Supportive and brief psychotherapy.
Brief psychotherapy is best suited for patients in acute medical and surgical situations (Blacher 1991). It is also helpful for patients in rehabilitation with physical trauma and illness (Murdaugh 1984). Brief psychiatric treatment can often be completed within a single rehabilitation inpatient program and not require additional sessions in the outpatient setting. Frieden and Cole (1984) have provided an approach to creative problem solving that is also useful in brief psychotherapy in rehabilitation.

Behavioral and cognitive therapies. A number of behavioral and cognitive therapy approaches are useful in rehabilitation settings (Ince 1980). Social skills training (Dunn 1987) is useful when patients need assistance in asserting themselves in new contexts such as wheelchairs, access problems, stairs, and other barriers to maximal functioning. Biofeedback (Brucker 1980; Gianutsos and Eberstein 1987; Harris 1980; Sachs 1980) is widely used by both physical and occupational therapists. Interviewing patients who are already wearing biofeedback apparatus provides a visual display of muscle tension changes as various issues are covered during the psychiatric evaluation. This technique can be used to identify conflicts that are closely tied to disability-related physiological responses.

---

[1]Each guideline is provided as a book, a physician's guide, and a consumer pamphlet. These books provide a succinct update in each area and are available from the Department of Health and Human Services, Public Health Service, Agency for Health Care Policy and Research, Executive Office Center, 2101 East Jefferson Street, Suite 501, Rockville, MD 20852.

Table 23–5. Psychopharmacological medications: unique indications, benefits, and risks in patients undergoing rehabilitation

Medication	Unique indications	Specific benefits	Risks in patients undergoing rehabilitation
Analgesics			
Methadone	Pain; opiate tapering	Long half-life	Anticholinergic effects; tolerance; withdrawal; sedation
Morphine sulfate concentrate	Pain; opiate tapering	Can be given via nasogastric tube; can be mixed with juices to disguise dosage	Anticholinergic effects; tolerance; withdrawal; sedation
NSAIDs	Inflammation and bone pain	No tolerance, withdrawal, sedation, or anticholinergic effects	Gastrointestinal distress
Anticonvulsants			
Carbamazepine	Seizure disorder; trigeminal neuralgia;[a] peripheral neuropathic pain;[b] rapid cycling mood syndrome; secondary mania[b]	Partial seizures; seizure treatment and prophylaxis	Bone marrow suppression; sedation for some patients; hepatic enzyme induction
Phenytoin	Seizure disorder	Seizure treatment and prophylaxis	Ataxia with drug toxicity; hepatic enzyme induction
Valproic acid	Same as carbamazepine except for peripheral neuropathic pain[b]	Partial seizures; seizure treatment and prophylaxis	Hepatotoxicity[b]
Antidepressants	Aggression;[b] primary or secondary depression (e.g., poststroke depression);[c] pain; sleep disturbances		
Amitriptyline	Insomnia; peripheral neuropathic pain;[b] mood lability;[d] cancer pain;[a] fibrositis pain;[a] poor appetite	Helps with sleep; stimulates appetite; effective with some patients who are incontinent	Anticholinergic effects;[b] oversedation; lowered seizure threshold; paradoxical agitation in patients with CNS disorders; hypotension; heart block; tachycardia
Desipramine	Pain,[a] including neuropathic pain[d]	Secondary amine tricyclic	Lowered seizure threshold; heart block
Doxepin	Pain; insomnia; poor appetite	Helps with sleep; stimulates appetite; effective analgesic;[a] H$_2$-receptor blockade in patients with gastrointestinal distress	Anticholinergic effects; oversedation; lowered seizure threshold; hypotension; heart block; tachycardia
Imipramine	Spasticity	Secondary amine tricyclic	Lowered seizure threshold; heart block

(continued)

Table 23–5. Psychopharmacological medications: unique indications, benefits, and risks in patients undergoing rehabilitation (*continued*)

Medication	Unique indications	Specific benefits	Risks in patients undergoing rehabilitation
MAOIs	Pain[a]	No anticholinergic activity	Hypotension; hypertensive crisis
Nortriptyline	Labile affect; pathological laughing and crying;[e] poststroke depression;[f] pain[a]	As a secondary amine tricyclic, is not overly sedating and has minimal anticholinergic effects	Lowered seizure threshold; heart block
SSRIs	Mood lability;[b] pain;[a] body dysmorphia	Lack of anticholinergic activity; not sedating; sertraline metabolized by conjugation	Potential for extrapyramidal side effects, dystonia, and sexual dysfunction; may be associated with a discontinuation syndrome
Trazodone	Insomnia; agitation; pain[a]	No anticholinergic activity	Sedation; priapism; hypotension
Antiparkinsonian medications			
Amantadine	Parkinson's disease; fatigue in patients with multiple sclerosis[b,g]	No anticholinergic effects	Anxiety; agitation; psychosis
Benztropine	Parkinson's disease	Not as likely as amantadine to cause agitation or psychosis	Memory and mood changes, especially in elderly patients[g]
Benzodiazepines			
Clonazepam	Myoclonus; partial seizure disorder	Can be used for tapering patients off alprazolam	Tolerance; withdrawal; impaired short-term memory; sedation
Diazepam	Aggression;[b] muscle tension; spasticity	Muscle relaxant; antispasticity effect	Tolerance; withdrawal; impaired short-term memory; sedation; paradoxical rage[b]
Lorazepam	Aggression;[b] acute agitation in delirium	Short-acting; metabolized by hepatic conjugation (can be used for alcohol withdrawal in patients with hepatic impairment)	Tolerance; withdrawal; impaired short-term memory; sedation; accumulation in patients with renal impairment
β-Blockers	Chronic or recurrent agitation[b,h,i]	May help patients with chronic anxiety	4–6 weeks latency of response for agitation;[b] hypotension; depression[a]
Buspirone	Anxiety;[b] agitation in patients with closed-head injury;[j,k] agitation in patients with major depression[b]	No tolerance or withdrawal; lacks benzodiazepines' memory effects; nonsedating	3–4 weeks latency of response[b]

Lithium	Mania;[b] aggression[b]	Does not induce hepatic enzymes	Tremor; gastrointestinal symptoms; ataxia
Neuroleptics			
Haloperidol	Psychosis and psychosis-related aggression[b]		Extrapyramidal signs; dystonia; akathisia; tardive dyskinesia
	Agitation following head injury;[l] experience with intravenous use	Little anticholinergic activity; effective analgesic adjuvant	Possible impaired recovery following stroke[b,m]
Thioridazine	Agitation; delirium; insomnia	Helps agitated patients sleep	Oversedation; anticholinergic effects; hypotension; short-term memory impairment; must be used in very small doses
Stimulants	Disorders of attention, concentration, arousal, and memory[n,o,p]	May diminish anger[n,p]	Agitation; anxiety; psychosis[b]
Other			
Bromocriptine	Antimotivational states resulting from nondominant parietal stroke;[q] nonfluent aphasia[r]	May improve "hemineglect" in patients with nondominant-hemisphere stroke[q]	Psychotic symptoms
Clonidine	Mania;[b] spasticity[s]	Can be used in patients with substance withdrawal syndromes	Hypotension
Physostigmine	Arousal disorder following traumatic head injury[g]	Improves memory following head injury in conjunction with other medications and memory training	Nausea; vomiting; salivation; can precipitate cholinergic crisis in overdose
Experimental			
CDP-choline	Closed-head trauma[g]	Reduced neuropsychiatric signs and symptoms	
Gangliosides	Spinal cord injury; stroke[g]	Improved recovery potential	
Pramiracetam	Head injury	Enhanced memory recovery with and without memory training	

Note. CNS = central nervous system; MAOIs = monoamine oxidase inhibitors; NSAIDs = nonsteroidal antiinflammatory drugs; SSRIs = selective serotonin reuptake inhibitors.

Source. [a]Block 1993; [b]Silver and Yudofsky 1993; [c]Finklestein et al. 1987; [d]Max et al. 1992; [e]Robinson et al. 1993; [f]Lipsey et al. 1984; [g]McEvoy 1987; [h]Greendyke et al. 1986; [i]Petrie et al. 1982; [j]McLean et al. 1993; [k]Gualtieri 1991; [l]Rao et al. 1985; [m]Feeney et al. 1982; [n]Evans et al. 1987; [o]Brooke et al. 1992; [p]Mooney and Haas 1993; [q]Fleet et al. 1987; [r]Gupta Sudha and Milcoch 1992; [s]Nance et al. 1985.

Operant conditioning (Friedlander 1980; Guenther et al. 1993; Levenkron 1987; Rapoff et al. 1984) has been widely used. However, these interventions require a high degree of integration and consistency by all staff members if they are to be effective.

Relaxation and imagery techniques are used for stress management and are also helpful with speech therapy (Marshall and Watts 1976), anxiety, spasticity, increased muscle tone, and pain management. Deficits require attention, and techniques are most effective when they maximize the patient's control. Many generic relaxation tapes and standard group approaches do not work well.

Cognitive therapy (Larcombe and Wilson 1984), cognitive restructuring, and attribution-altering techniques are effective for treating patients with depression or anxiety, for those who are adjusting to major life changes, and for some inpatients with personality disorders.

Cognitive rehabilitation and retraining.
Patients with traumatic brain injury, stroke, brain tumor, or other CNS insult require neuropsychological assessment. The focus of cognitive rehabilitation varies depending on the presentation of neuropsychiatric disorders in specific individuals (Gualtieri 1988, 1993; Kikmen et al. 1986; Levin et al. 1982; Lovell and Starratt 1992).

Family treatment.
The consultation-liaison psychiatrist should involve the family and work with the family. Families respond well to structure and to formalized assessments. Open, loosely defined meetings lead families to feel "under the microscope" and defensive about interpretations. Problems must be clarified and agreed on and action plans developed that are consistent with the given family's structure, usual approach, and culture. Family education is crucial (Evans and Held 1984). Evans and co-workers (1988) have demonstrated that follow-up counseling sessions focusing on key elements of the education lead to more sustained benefits than does education alone. Families usually also require assistance and advocacy to negotiate the system and to obtain appropriate care and resources.

Group psychotherapy.
Group psychotherapy approaches used in rehabilitation settings include 1) ward groups, to deal with the issues on the unit; 2) predischarge groups; 3) education groups (Evans and Held 1984); 4) sexuality groups; 5) family groups (Gonzalez et al. 1989; Rohrer et al. 1980); 6) peer counseling and self-help groups; 7) support groups in the community; and 8) specific intervention groups (Salhoot 1984). Occupational therapists increasingly use groups for their therapy.

The psychiatrist who provides consultation on a rehabilitation unit should be aware of the type, focus, and frequency of groups.

Ward management.
Ward management issues include milieu staff problems, transfers to a psychiatric ward, and restraints for safety.

At times, the psychiatric condition of the patient will require transfer to a psychiatric unit, but this is rare. It usually happens at the end of the physical rehabilitation phase when a psychiatric condition contraindicates discharge, yet inpatient rehabilitation interventions can no longer be justified. This is frequently the result of major depression occurring late in rehabilitation and not remitting rapidly. In general, it is possible to manage the treatment of most suicidal patients on a rehabilitation unit. If the suicidality continues for longer than a few days and interferes with rehabilitation, then transfer to a psychiatric ward or medical-psychiatric unit should be considered.

Medication restraint is rarely needed and usually is not helpful in rehabilitation settings because it may sedate the patient to the point that he or she is no longer able to be actively involved in rehabilitation.

OUTPATIENT CONSULTATION-LIAISON PSYCHIATRY AND REHABILITATION

As with virtually all other medical specialties, more and more rehabilitation is being provided on an outpatient basis. Patients and families describe two nodal time periods that are most likely to be associated with psychosocial problems. The first is the initial period after the patient returns home. Patients and families are often, despite education, shocked by the impact of the disability. The burden of care shifts and falls almost totally on the patient, family, or other intimate caregivers. The second risk period usually occurs some time later and is in response to those situations in which patients and caregivers are faced with the realization that "this is it, and it may not get a whole lot better."

Outpatient follow-up appointments, therefore, must extend through the expected recovery curves for any given disorder (e.g., 6–12 months for functional improvement in stroke and longer for aphasia).

REFERENCES

American Psychiatric Association: Diagnostic and Statistical Manual of Mental Disorders, 4th Edition. Washington, DC, American Psychiatric Association, 1994

Beckham JC, D'Amico CJ, Rice JR, et al: Depression and level of functioning in patients with rheumatoid arthritis. Can J Psychiatry 37:538–543, 1992

Bishop D: Behavior and disability: challenges for assessment and management, in Behavior Problems and the Disabled: Assessment and Management. Edited by Bishop D. Baltimore, MD, Williams & Wilkins, 1980, pp 1–16

Bishop DS, Miller IW: Traumatic brain injury: empirical family assessment techniques. Journal of Head Trauma Rehabilitation 3:16–30, 1988

Bishop DS, Baldwin LM, Epstein NB, et al: Assessment of family functioning, in Functional Assessment in Rehabilitation Medicine. Edited by Granger C, Gresham G. Baltimore, MD, Williams & Wilkins, 1984, pp 305–323

Blacher R: Brief psychotherapy for medical and surgical patients, in Handbook of Studies on General Hospital Psychiatry. Edited by Judd F, Burroughs G, Lipsitt D. Amsterdam, The Netherlands, Elsevier, 1991, pp 149–162

Block B: Antidepressants in the treatment of pain. Resident and Staff Physician, February 1993, pp 17–26

Bowden ML, Feller I, Tholen D, et al: Self-esteem of severely burned patients. Arch Phys Med Rehabil 61:449–452, 1980

Bradley LA: Psychological aspects of arthritis. Bull Rheum Dis 35:1–12, 1985

Bray GP, DeFrank RS, Wolfe TL: Sexual functioning in stroke survivors. Arch Phys Med Rehabil 62:286–288, 1981

Brocklehurst JC, Morris P, Andrews K, et al: Social effects of stroke. Soc Sci Med 15:35–39, 1981

Brooke M, Patterson D, Questad K, et al: The treatment of agitation during initial hospitalization after traumatic brain injury. Arch Phys Med Rehabil 73:917–921, 1992

Brucker B: Biofeedback and rehabilitation, in Rehabilitation Medicine. Edited by Ince L. Baltimore, MD, Williams & Wilkins, 1980, pp 188–217

Cantor M: Strain among caregivers: a study of experience in the United States. Gerontologist 23:597–604, 1983

Caplan B: Neuropsychological assessment in rehabilitation, in Rehabilitation Psychology Desk Reference. Edited by Caplan B. Rockville, MD, Aspen, 1987, pp 247–280

Caplan B, Shechter J: Denial and depression in disabling illness, in Rehabilitation Psychology Desk Reference. Edited by Caplan B. Rockville, MD, Aspen, 1987, pp 133–170

Cook L: Psychopharmacology in rehabilitation medicine, in Rehabilitation Psychology: A Comprehensive Textbook. Edited by Krueger D. Rockville, MD, Aspen, 1984, pp 139–147

Cottrell S, Wilson S: The affective symptomatology of disseminated sclerosis: a study of 100 cases. Journal of Neurology and Psychopathology 7:1–30, 1926

Craig AR, Hancock KM, Dickson HG: A longitudinal investigation into anxiety and depression in the first 2 years following a spinal cord injury. Paraplegia 32:675–679, 1994

Crewe N: The difficult patient, in Behavior Problems and the Disabled: Assessment and Management. Edited by Bishop D. Baltimore, MD, Williams & Wilkins, 1980a, pp 98–119

Crewe N: Sexually inappropriate behavior, in Behavior Problems and the Disabled: Assessment and Management. Edited by Bishop D. Baltimore, MD, Williams & Wilkins, 1980b, pp 120–141

Deyo RA, Inui TS, Leininger J, et al: Physical and psychosocial function in rheumatoid arthritis: clinical use of a self-administered health status instrument. Arch Intern Med 142:879–882, 1982

Donahue RP, Abbott RD, Reed DM, et al: Alcohol and hemorrhagic stroke: the Honolulu heart program. JAMA 255:2311–2314, 1986

Ducharme S: Sexuality in physical disability, in Rehabilitation Psychology Desk Reference. Edited by Caplan B. Rockville, MD, Aspen, 1987, pp 419–436

Dunn M: Social skills in rehabilitation, in Rehabilitation Psychology Desk Reference. Edited by Caplan B. Rockville, MD, Aspen, 1987, pp 345–359

Evans RL, Held S: Evaluation of family stroke education. Int J Rehabil Res 7:47–51, 1984

Evans RW, Gualtieri CT, Patterson D: Single case study: treatment of chronic closed head injury with psychostimulant drugs: a controlled case study and an appropriate evaluation procedure. J Nerv Ment Dis 175:106–110, 1987

Evans RL, Matlock A, Bishop D, et al: Family intervention after stroke: does counseling or education help? Stroke 19:1243–1249, 1988

Federoff JP, Starkstein SE, Forrester AW, et al: Depression in patients with acute traumatic brain injury. Am J Psychiatry 149:918–923, 1992

Feeney D, Gonzalez A, Law W: Amphetamine, haloperidol, and experience interact to affect rate of recovery after motor cortex injury. Science 217:855–857, 1982

Fey S, Williamson-Kirkland: Chronic pain: psychology and rehabilitation, in Rehabilitation Psychology Desk Reference. Edited by Caplan B. Rockville, MD, Aspen, 1987, pp 247–280

Finklestein SP, Weintraub RJ, Karmouz N, et al: Antidepressant drug treatment for poststroke depression: retrospective study. Arch Phys Med Rehabil 68:772–776, 1987

Fleet WS, Valenstein E, Watson RT, et al: Dopamine agonist therapy for neglect in humans. Neurology 37:1765–1770, 1987

Frieden L, Cole J: Creative problem solving, in Rehabilitation Psychology: A Comprehensive Textbook. Edited by Krueger D. Rockville, MD, Aspen, 1984, pp 69–80

Friedlander B: Automated operant methods for assessment and treatment in physical rehabilitation, in Rehabilitation Medicine. Edited by Ince L. Baltimore, MD, Williams & Wilkins, 1980, pp 25–63

Fugl-Meyer A, Jaasko L: Post stroke hemiplegia and sexual intercourse. Scand J Rehabil Med Suppl 7:158–166, 1980

Fullerton DT, Harvey RF, Klein MH, et al: Psychiatric disorders in patients with spinal cord injuries. Arch Gen Psychiatry 38:1369–1371, 1981

Gans J: Facilitating staff/patient interaction in rehabilitation, in Rehabilitation Psychology Desk Reference. Edited by Caplan B. Rockville, MD, Aspen, 1987, pp 185–218

Gerhardt F, Florin I, Knapp T: The impact of medical, reeducational, and psychological variables on rehabilitation outcome in amputees. Int J Rehabil Res 7:379–388, 1984

Gianutsos J, Eberstein A: Computer-augmented feedback displays: treatment of hemiplegic motor deficits as a paradigm, in Rehabilitation Psychology Desk Reference. Edited by Caplan B. Rockville, MD, Aspen, 1987, pp 241–264

Goldstein LB: Common drugs may influence motor recovery after stroke: the Sygen in Acute Stroke Study investigators. Neurology 45:865–871, 1995

Gonzalez S, Steinglass P, Reiss D: Putting the illness in its place: discussion groups for families with chronic medical illnesses. Fam Process 28: 69–87, 1989

Goodstein R: Cerebrovascular accident: a multidimensional clinical problem, in Emotional Rehabilitation of Physical Trauma and Disability. Edited by Krueger D. New York, Spectrum Publications, 1984, pp 111–140

Gordon WA, Hibbard MR, Egelko S, et al: Perceptual remediation in patients with right brain damage: a comprehensive program. Arch Phys Med Rehabil 66:353–359, 1985

Gorelick PB, Kelly MA: Alcohol as a risk factor for stroke. Heart Disease and Stroke 1:255–258, 1992

Greendyke RM, Kanter DR, Schuster DB, et al: Propranolol treatment of assaultive patients with organic brain disease: a double-blind crossover, placebo-controlled study. J Nerv Ment Dis 174:290–294, 1986

Greenwood W: Alcoholism: a complicating factor in the rehabilitation of disabled individuals. Journal of Rehabilitation 7:51–52, 72, 1984

Group for the Advancement of Psychiatry, Committee on Handicaps: Report #135: Caring for People With Physical Impairment: The Journey Back. Washington, DC, American Psychiatric Press, 1993

Gualtieri CT: Pharmacotherapy and the neurobehavioral sequelae of traumatic brain injury. Brain Inj 2:101–109, 1988

Gualtieri CT: Buspirone for the behavior problems of patients with organic brain disorders. J Clin Psychopharmacol 11:280–281, 1991

Gualtieri CT: Traumatic brain injury, in Psychiatric Care of the Medical Patient. Edited by Stoudemire A, Fogel BS. New York, Oxford University Press, 1993, pp 517–535

Guenther R, Frank R, McAdams C: Management of behavior on a spinal cord injury unit. NeuroRehabilitation 3:50–59, 1993

Gunther M: Catastrophic illness and the caregiver: real burdens and solutions with respect to the role of behavioral sciences, in Rehabilitation Psychology Desk Reference. Edited by Caplan B. Rockville, MD, Aspen, 1987, pp 219–240

Gupta Sudha R, Milcoch AG: Bromocriptine treatment of nonfluent aphasia. Arch Phys Med Rehabil 73:373–376, 1992

Gwyther LP, George LK: Caregivers of dementia patients: complex determinants of well-being and burden. Gerontologist 26:245–247, 1986

Hahn H: Paternalism and public policy. Society 20:36–46, 1983

Harris F: Exteroceptive feedback of position and movement in remediation for disorders of coordination, in Rehabilitation Medicine. Edited by Ince L. Baltimore, MD, Williams & Wilkins, 1980, pp 87–156

Holland JC: Managing depression in the patient with cancer. CA Cancer J Clin 37:366–371, 1987

Ince L (ed): Behavioral Psychology in Rehabilitation Medicine. Baltimore, MD, Williams & Wilkins, 1980

International Center for the Disabled: ICD Survey of Disabled Americans: Bringing Disabled Americans Into the Mainstream. New York, ICD—International Center for the Disabled (in cooperation with the National Council on the Handicapped), 1986

Katz J: Psychophysiological contributions to phantom limbs. Can J Psychiatry 37:282–298, 1992

Keitner GI, Miller IW, Ryan CE, et al: Compounded depression and family functioning during the acute episode and 6-month follow-up. Compr Psychiatry 30:512–521, 1989

Keitner GI, Ryan CE, Miller IW, et al: 12-month outcome of patients with major depression and comorbid psychiatric or medical illness (compound depression). Am J Psychiatry 148: 345–350, 1991

Kikmen S, McLean A, Temkin N: Neuropsychological and psychosocial consequences of minor head injury. J Neurol Neurosurg Psychiatry 49:1227–1232, 1986

Krueger D: Psychological rehabilitation of physical trauma and disability, in Rehabilitation Psychology: A Comprehensive Textbook. Edited by Krueger D. Rockville, MD, Aspen, 1984, pp 3–14

Kryger M, Roth T, Dement W (eds): Principles of Sleep Medicine. Philadelphia, PA, WB Saunders, 1989

Larcombe NA, Wilson PH: An evaluation of cognitive-behaviour therapy for depression in patients with multiple sclerosis. Br J Psychiatry 145:366–371, 1984

Large RG: DSM-III diagnoses in chronic pain: confusion or clarity? J Nerv Ment Dis 174:295–303, 1986

Levenkron J: Behavior modification in rehabilitation: principles and clinical strategy, in Rehabilitation Psychology Desk Reference. Edited by Caplan B. Rockville, MD, Aspen, 1987, pp 383–416

Levin HS, Benton AL, Grossman RG: Neurobehavioral Consequences of Closed Head Injury. New York, Oxford University Press, 1982

Lichtenberg PA, Gibbons TA: Geriatric rehabilitation and the older adult family caregiver: stages of caregiving. NeuroRehabilitation 3:62–71, 1993

Lindsay PG, Wyckoff M: The depression-pain syndrome and its response to antidepressants. Psychosomatics 22:571–577, 1981

Lipsey J, Robinson R, Pearlson G, et al: Nortriptyline treatment of post-stroke depression: a double-blind study. Lancet 11:297–300, 1984

Lishman WA: Other disorders affecting the nervous system, in Organic Psychiatry: The Psychological Consequences of Cerebral Disorder, 2nd Edition. Boston, MA, Blackwell Scientific, 1987, pp 588–650

Lovell MR, Starratt C: Cognitive rehabilitation and behavior therapy of neuropsychiatric disorders, in The American Psychiatric Press Textbook of Neuropsychiatry, 2nd Edition. Edited by Yudofsky SC, Hales RE. Washington, DC, American Psychiatric Press, 1992, pp 741–754

Luxenberg J, Feigenbaum L: Cognitive impairment on a rehabilitation service. Arch Phys Med Rehabil 67:796–798, 1986

MacDonald MR, Nielson WR, Cameron MGP: Depression and activity patterns of spinal cord injured persons living in the community. Arch Phys Med Rehabil 68:339–343, 1987

Malec J, Neimeyer R: Psychologic prediction of duration of inpatient spinal cord injury rehabilitation and performance of self-care. Arch Phys Med Rehabil 64:359–363, 1983

Marshall RC, Watts MT: Relaxation training: effects on the communicative ability of aphasic adults. Arch Phys Med Rehabil 57:464–467, 1976

Massie M, Holland J: Depression and the cancer patient. J Clin Psychiatry 51 (suppl 7):12–17, 1990

Max M, Lynch S, Muir J, et al: Effects of desipramine, amitriptyline, and fluoxetine on pain in diabetic neuropathy. N Engl J Med 326: 1250–1256, 1992

McEvoy JP: A double-blind crossover comparison of antiparkinson drug therapy: amantidine versus anticholinergics in 90 normal volunteers, with an emphasis on differential effects on memory function. J Clin Psychiatry 48 (suppl 9):20–23, 1987

McLean A, Cardenas D, Haselkorn J, et al: Cognitive psychopharmacology. NeuroRehabilitation 3(2):1–14, 1993

Missel JL: Suicide risk in the medical rehabilitation setting. Arch Phys Med Rehabil 59:371–376, 1978

Mooney GF, Haas L: Effect of methylphenidate on brain injury-related anger. Arch Phys Med Rehabil 74:153–160, 1993

Murdaugh J: Psychotherapeutic intervention in physical trauma and illness, in Rehabilitation Psychology: A Comprehensive Textbook. Edited by Krueger D. Rockville, MD, Aspen, 1984, pp 37–42

Murray P: Clinical pharmacology in rehabilitation, in Rehabilitation Psychology Desk Reference. Edited by Caplan B. Rockville, MD, Aspen, 1987, pp 501–526

Nance P, Shears A, Nance D: Clonidine in spinal cord injury. Can Med Assoc J 133:41–43, 1985

O'Donnell J, Cooper J, Gessner J, et al: Alcohol, drugs, and spinal cord injury. Alcohol Health and Research World 3:27–29, 1981/1982

Petrie WM, Maffucci RJ, Woosley RL: Propranolol and depression (letter). Am J Psychiatry 139:92–94, 1982

Pruchno R: The effects of help patterns on the mental health of spouse caregivers. Research on Aging 12:57–71, 1990

Rao N, Jellinek H, Woolston D: Agitation in closed head injury: haloperidol effects on rehabilitation outcome. Arch Phys Med Rehabil 66:30–33, 1985

Rapoff MA, Lindsley CB, Christophersen ER: Improving compliance with medical regimens: case study with juvenile rheumatoid arthritis. Arch Phys Med Rehabil 65:267–269, 1984

Reiss H, Schwartz CE, Klerman GL: Manic syndrome following head injury: another form of secondary mania. J Clin Psychiatry 48:29–30, 1987

Robinson RG, Parikh RM, Lipsey JR, et al: Pathological laughing and crying following stroke: validation of a measurement scale and a double-blind treatment study. Am J Psychiatry 150:286–293, 1993

Rohrer K, Adelman B, Puckett J, et al: Rehabilitation in spinal cord injury: use of a patient-family group. Arch Phys Med Rehabil 61:225–229, 1980

Romano M: The therapeutic milieu in the rehabilitation process, in Rehabilitation Psychology: A Comprehensive Textbook. Edited by Krueger D. Rockville, MD, Aspen, 1984, pp 43–50

Rybarczyk BD, Nyenhuis DL, Nicholas JJ, et al: Social discomfort and depression in a sample of adults with leg amputations. Arch Phys Med Rehabil 73:1169–1173, 1992

Sachs D: Behavioral feedback techniques for rehabilitation of motor problems, in Rehabilitation Medicine. Edited by Ince L. Baltimore, MD, Williams & Wilkins, 1980, pp 157–187

Sakinofsky I: Depression and suicide in the disabled, in Behavior Problems and the Disabled: Assessment and Management. Edited by Bishop D. Baltimore, MD, Williams & Wilkins, 1980, pp 17–51

Salhoot J: Group therapy in rehabilitation, in Rehabilitation Psychology: A Comprehensive Textbook. Edited by Krueger D. Rockville, MD, Aspen, 1984, pp 61–68

Schubert DSP, Taylor C, Lee S, et al: Detection of depression in the stroke patient. Psychosomatics 33:290–294, 1992a

Schubert DSP, Burns R, Paras W, et al: Increase of medical hospital length of stay by depression in stroke and amputation patients: a pilot study. Psychother Psychosom 57:61–66, 1992b

Schulz R, Visintainer P, Williamson G: Psychiatric and physical morbidity effects of caregiving. J Gerontol 45:181–191, 1990

Shukla GD, Sahu SC, Tripathi RP, et al: A psychiatric study of amputees. Br J Psychiatry 141:50–53, 1982

Silver J, Yudofsky S: Pharmacologic treatment of neuropsychiatric disorders. NeuroRehabilitation 3:15–25, 1993

Sipski ML, Alexander CJ, Rosen RC: Physiological parameters associated with psychogenic sexual arousal in women with complete spinal cord injuries. Arch Phys Med Rehabil 76:811–818, 1995

Sjogren K, Damber J, Liliequist B: Sexuality after stroke with hemiplegia: I. Scand J Rehabil Med 4:80–87, 1983

Starkstein SE, Robinson RG: Affective disorders and cerebral vascular disease. Br J Psychiatry 154:170–182, 1989

Starkstein SE, Pearlson GD, Boston J, et al: Mania after brain injury: a controlled study of causative factors. Arch Neurol 44:1069–1073, 1987

Steger H, Brockway J: Management of chronic pain in the disabled, in Behavior Problems and the Disabled: Assessment and Management. Edited by Bishop D. Baltimore, MD, Williams & Wilkins, 1980, pp 272–301

Steger H, Fox C, Fienberg S: Behavioral evaluation and management of chronic pain, in Behavior Problems and the Disabled: Assessment and Management. Edited by Bishop D. Baltimore, MD, Williams & Wilkins, 1980, pp 302–336

Tiller J: Post-stroke depression. Psychopharmacology 106(suppl):S130–S133, 1992

Trieschman R: Spinal Cord Injuries: The Psychological, Social, and Vocational Adjustment. Elmsford, NY, Pergamon, 1980

Tunks E, Merskey H: Psychiatric treatment in chronic pain, in Behavior Problems and the Disabled: Assessment and Management. Edited by Bishop D. Baltimore, MD, Williams & Wilkins, 1980, pp 195–217

Valleroy ML, Kraft GH: Sexual dysfunction in multiple sclerosis. Arch Phys Med Rehabil 65:125–128, 1984

Vanderpool J: Stressful patient relationships and the difficult patient, in Rehabilitation Psychology: A Comprehensive Textbook. Edited by Krueger D. Rockville, MD, Aspen, 1984, pp 167–174

Vrey JR, Henggeler SW: Marital adjustment following spinal cord injury. Arch Phys Med Rehabil 68:69–74, 1987

Whitlock FA: Suicide and physical illness, in Suicide. Edited by Roy A. Baltimore, MD, Williams & Wilkins, 1986, pp 151–170

Wilmot CB, Cope DN, Hall KM, et al: Occult head injury: its incidence in spinal cord injury. Arch Phys Med Rehabil 66:227–231, 1985

World Health Organization: International Classification of Impairments, Disabilities, and Handicaps: A Manual of Classification Relating to the Consequences of Disease. Geneva, Switzerland, World Health Organization, 1980

Wortman CB, Silver RC: The myths of coping with loss. J Consult Clin Psychol 57:349–357, 1989

Chapter 24

Intensive Care Units

John L. Shuster, Jr., M.D.
Theodore A. Stern, M.D.

Consultation-liaison psychiatry in the critical care setting is a challenging and rewarding activity that forces the psychiatrist to manage a wide variety of clinical problems under the pressure of time and to make decisions about and implement biological, psychological, and behavioral interventions at a rapid pace.

PSYCHIATRIC EVALUATION OF THE CRITICALLY ILL PATIENT

General Approach

When called on to see a patient in the intensive care unit (ICU), the psychiatric consultant often assumes the role of medical detective. Performing a consultation in the ICU usually requires piecing together scattered clues. Patients in the ICU are often too ill to provide detailed history or to participate in a complete mental status examination. Psychiatric evaluation in the ICU is complicated by lack of privacy and by noises, distractions, and interruptions created by the provision of intensive medical care. Physical barriers (e.g., placement of an endotracheal tube) or pharmacological barriers (e.g., use of paralytic agents or sedatives) to psychiatric evaluation are frequently present. Family members, when available, are sometimes too emotionally overwhelmed to contribute much to the history. ICU staff members are typically so focused on treatment of the patient's critical illness that they have a limited awareness of the patient's affect, behavior, or cognition. Medical records of ICU patients often contain massive amounts of data, only a portion of which is pertinent to the psychiatric evaluation. One important task of the psychiatric consultant is to determine which information is relevant. Consultation-liaison psychiatrists who are comfortable playing the role of medical detective are effective in the ICU.

Gathering Historical Information

As with any medical evaluation, the patient's history is the most helpful guide to diagnosis. Unfortunately, the patient in the ICU is often unable to provide an extensive history. Thus, collateral history, obtained from family, ICU staff, and consulting physicians, is of greater importance in the ICU than it is in other settings. At the time of initial assessment and recommendations, little reliable history may be known. Persistence often pays off; additional history is often obtained from the patient as he or she becomes more alert, family members can provide additional data after the consultation is initiated, and staff members can refine the physical diagnoses and provide ongoing history.

The ICU chart is unrivaled in the hospital as a source of information. The consultant should review the physicians' and nurses' progress notes, especially admission, consultation, and summary notes. The ICU flowsheet, with graphic representations of many physiological parameters (including vital signs), pertinent laboratory values, medications administered, and notes about patient behavior, will often help establish temporal relations between interventions and symptoms. Laboratory sheets should be reviewed to identify electrolyte, metabolic, hematological, or infectious disturbances that may contribute to or cause neuropsychiatric symptoms. Medication orders for the patient should be reviewed—with special attention given to medications recently discontinued or prescribed, as well as all medications currently administered. In patients who have undergone surgery, the operative records should also be reviewed for adverse intraoperative events such as reactions to intraoperatively administered medications, prolonged intraoperative hypoxia, or hypotension; these events can lead to behavioral symptoms in the postoperative phase. The anesthesia record provides thorough moment-to-moment documentation of important events that can alter central nervous system (CNS) function.

Patient Examination

The evaluation of patients who are intubated poses a problem for many clinicians. Although verbal responses to open-ended questions are obviously impossible, a full examination is possible. The first step is an assessment of the patient's level of alertness and concentration. Inquiry into a patient's subjective sense of confusion and an assessment of his or her ability to follow commands gives the interviewer a chance to assess alertness. If intubation is the only obstacle to the interview, the patient is usually able to write answers out on paper and to convey information with facial expressions. If the patient cannot write, information is obtained by asking a series of binary (yes or no) questions aimed at symptom identification or by using nonverbal techniques to facilitate communication—for example, having patients point to letters on a letter board or reading the patients' lips.

Assessing Cognitive Function

A formal assessment of cognitive function is necessary for every patient evaluated in the ICU. The Mini-Mental State Exam (MMSE; Folstein et al. 1975) is commonly used for this purpose and allows rapid assessment of orientation, registration of information, attention, calculation ability, recall, language functions, reading, writing, and design construction. The chief advantages of the MMSE are its ease of use, brevity, and usefulness for serial examinations. Its chief drawbacks are its low sensitivity (patients with mild to moderate impairment may score well on the test) and its unfortunate name (many nonpsychiatrists confuse the test with the full mental status examination).

Making a Diagnosis

Given the sketchy information about psychiatric history and current psychiatric symptoms that is often available to the ICU psychiatrist, a definitive psychiatric diagnosis is sometimes difficult to establish. It is best to label diagnoses as provisional when incomplete information is available. As soon as a diagnosis is possible, the psychiatrist should communicate it clearly and without jargon in the chart. The dynamic state of the patient in the ICU necessitates frequent diagnostic reassessments and revisions.

PSYCHIATRIC TREATMENT OF THE CRITICALLY ILL PATIENT: GENERAL CONCEPTS

Changes in Medical-Surgical Management

All patients in ICUs have serious physical illnesses. A large proportion of the psychiatric symptoms and disorders seen in the ICU setting are secondary to these medical disorders and/or their treatments. Consequently, the first step in the management of psychiatric disorders in the ICU setting is the consideration of whether changes in the medical management of a disorder would alleviate or treat the psychiatric symptoms. For example, it is not logical (and will not be effective) to treat delirium that is caused by hypoxia or hypoglycemia with neuroleptics alone. Whenever possible, delirium should be treated specifically (e.g., reversal of hypoxia with oxygen or hypoglycemia with glucose). A physical cause for mental symptoms in the patient in the ICU must always be considered first. A useful framework for remembering the life-threatening causes of delirium in patients in ICUs is the WWHHHIMP mnemonic (Tesar and Stern 1986), found in Chapter 7 in this volume.

Temporal correlations between the onset of mental symptoms and changes in the medical-surgical management of the patient are important to detect. The ICU flowchart or laboratory summary sheet may reveal a metabolic or infectious problem that accounts for an altered mental status. The medication list should be reviewed for medications added just before symptom onset or discontinued long enough before symptom onset to induce a withdrawal reaction. These and other temporal correlations are often the primary (or only) clues available to help identify the cause of psychiatric symptoms in ICU patients.

When a physical problem (e.g., hypoxia, intracranial hemorrhage, medication side effect) is suspected as a cause of psychiatric symptoms, recommendations for changes in the medical-surgical management of the patient are included in the consultation report. Missing a physical problem is potentially embarrassing for the referring physician, so the consultant's note is best written in a direct, helpful manner, without gloating or being critical. In such cases, a telephone call to the referring physician is often more appreciated (and better tolerated) than an extensive note with a remedial tone. Clinical one-upmanship or hurt feelings should not supersede or jeopardize the provision of excellent patient care.

Psychopharmacological Treatments

As Townsend and Reynolds (1991) pointed out, the dynamic physiological state of the critically ill patient can lead to rapid changes in pharmacokinetic parameters. Decrements in hepatic or renal function brought on by the patient's illness (or its treatment) may adversely affect drug clearance. Serious physical illness may also render the patient more sensitive to drug side effects (Stoudemire et al. 1990).

The guidelines proposed by Jenike (1989) for prescription of psychotropic drugs to the elderly are useful for critically ill patients (Table 24–1). These guidelines also remind us to make every effort to achieve an accurate diagnosis before the initiation of treatment. Symptomatic treatment alone may not solve the targeted problem; it may even create new problems.

A thorough knowledge of the pharmacological properties of psychotropic agents is crucial to successful use of these drugs in the intensive care setting. Most psychotropics are metabolized in the liver; most are cleared through the liver or kidneys. Therefore, alteration in hepatic or renal function clearly influences the choice and dosing of psychotropic drugs. Before administering a psychotropic drug, the clinician must consider known or po-

Table 24–1. Guidelines for prescription of psychotropic drugs to critically ill patients

1. Take a careful psychiatric history (do not base treatment on assumptions).
2. Diagnose before initiation of treatment.
3. Optimize the patient's environment.
4. Know the pharmacology of the drugs prescribed (consider effects of the alterations in hepatic or renal function, interactions with other drugs, side effects in light of patient's current illness).
5. Use a low dosage initially, advance dosage slowly (if the clinical situation warrants it).
6. Avoid polypharmacy whenever possible.
7. Monitor drugs and response to target symptoms on a regular basis (remember that physiological parameters in the critically ill patient may change rapidly).
8. Observe for drug side effects.
9. Evaluate potential for noncompliance in both the patient and the referring physician.
10. Do not avoid the use of psychotropic agents simply because the patient is critically ill.

Source. Adapted from Jenike MA: *Geriatric Psychiatry and Psychopharmacology.* Chicago, IL, Year Book Medical, 1989. Used with permission.

tential drug interactions (Dec and Stern 1990; Lipson and Stern 1991; Shuster et al. 1992; Stoudemire et al. 1990, 1991). In addition, the side-effect profile of the psychotropic drug must be considered in light of the patient's physical problems. For example, patients in a cardiac care unit who have cardiac conduction system abnormalities may have difficulty with the quinidine-like effects of tricyclic antidepressants and low-potency neuroleptics. Because the kinetic and dynamic behavior of psychotropic drugs in critically ill patients is somewhat unpredictable, low doses are, in general, initially appropriate. Unless the clinical situation requires prompt treatment, doses should be advanced slowly to maximize patient tolerance. Clinical experience shows that doses below the standard therapeutic range are often effective in patients with medical ill-

nesses. This is particularly true when drug interactions or renal or hepatic impairment slows drug clearance.

The consultation-liaison psychiatrist must monitor medications given to the patient in the ICU because nonpsychiatric physicians may have ordered psychotropics before consultation, and additional medications are sometimes ordered by cross-covering physicians.

Drug side effects are sometimes troublesome to critically ill patients and can complicate the diagnostic picture. For example, neuroleptic-induced akathisia can cause restlessness and agitation that is in some cases extreme. In patients for whom the neuroleptic was initially prescribed to treat agitation, this creates a vexing clinical problem. It is best not to neglect the common side effects of psychotropics in the setting of critical illness, even when low doses are used.

It is unwise to avoid the use of psychotropic drugs simply because the patient is critically ill. At times, it might seem that using psychiatric medications in critically ill patients is not worth the trouble. However, when used appropriately, psychotropic drugs are generally well tolerated and effective. The presence of psychiatric symptoms adds to the suffering of critically ill patients; it is inconsistent with excellent clinical care to neglect these symptoms and/or disorders when effective treatments are available.

Nonpharmacological Measures

Nonpharmacological measures may also help reduce the patient's suffering. For example, patients with confusion, delirium, or dementia can benefit from efforts to provide a calming environment, with frequent reassurance and reorientation. Anxious or fearful patients are often reassured by frequent visits from trusted relatives or friends. Although confusional states in the ICU are sometimes attributed to exposure to a stressful and noisy environment (so-called ICU psychosis), severe psychiatric symptoms are much more commonly caused by brain dysfunction related to the patient's physical disorder(s) and/or treatment. Environmental manipulations are helpful in such patients, but they do not address the cause of the symptoms.

Psychotherapeutic Treatments

Psychotherapeutic interventions are woven into the treatment of most psychiatric problems in the ICU (Stein et al. 1969). Occasionally, a patient's stay in the ICU is long enough for brief psychotherapy. Treatment of a patient's family, when indicated and possible, almost always involves psychodynamic issues that are activated by the critical illness.

Ward Management

Treatment recommendations sometimes include changes in the way patients are managed in the ICU. Such interventions are often effective in reducing psychiatric symptoms. For example, provision of as much calm, quiet, and protection from interruptions in sleep as possible, in combination with reassurance and reorientation, may help to calm a patient with delirium. Patients who are depressed or fearful are usually reassured by more frequent contact with ICU staff. Patients who are anxious or confused can benefit from having a supportive friend or relative nearby.

Use of Restraints

Mechanical restraint is required when explosive outbursts of agitation or a serious threat to self or others is present. Some staff members, who are fearful of litigation, may object to the use of physical restraint. Mechanical restraints are associated with injuries in some reports (Francis 1989). However, when indicated for the prevention of injury and used with appropriate safety measures and close supervision, use of mechanical restraint is consistent with the goal of excellent medical care. It is much

easier to defend an ICU staff member against charges of battery resulting from restraint when restraint is indicated for safety than to defend him or her against charges of negligence resulting from failure to protect a patient or bystander from harm (Hackett and Stern 1991).

Keys to the proper use of restraints in the ICU are thorough documentation of the current need for such safety measures and close clinical supervision of the patient while he or she is in restraints. Implementation of these principles is facilitated by development of a restraint protocol, which outlines the intensity of clinical supervision by ward staff, the frequency of examination used to prevent injury resulting from restraint, and the frequency of reassessment for continued restraint.

Frequent Follow-Up Visits

For the reasons already described, frequent follow-up is a key to effective psychiatric consultation in the ICU. Ongoing medical evaluation may reveal new clues to the etiology and proper treatment of the patient with a mental disorder that were not initially available to the consultant. Improvements in the patient's condition may allow a more thorough examination. As previously discussed, the condition of a patient in the ICU may change dramatically; factors affecting the safety, effectiveness, and tolerability of recommended treatments often vary. Even without rapid changes in a patient's overall condition, treatment response is less predictable in a patient with severe medical illness, thereby necessitating close monitoring. Finally, referring physicians appreciate the consultant's diligence and availability to assist in the ongoing care of critically ill patients.

◼ PSYCHIATRIC DISTURBANCES IN THE CRITICALLY ILL PATIENT

Anxiety

Anxiety may interrupt sleep or interfere with the patient's ability to comply with treatment in the ICU. Anxiety can also have adverse physiological consequences for the critically ill patient because anxiety and stress are associated with sympathetic arousal, elevated catecholamine levels, and electrical and ischemic cardiac events (Charney and Redmond 1983; Hickam et al. 1948; Jewitt et al. 1969; Reich et al. 1981).

The differential diagnosis of anxiety in the patient in the ICU leans heavily toward medical and substance-induced causes (MacKenzie and Popkin 1983; Strain et al. 1981), especially in patients with no personal or family history of anxiety disorders. Common causes include hypoxia (often associated with confusion and agitation), metabolic abnormalities, sepsis, and medication side effects. Intoxication and drug withdrawal states should always be considered, including iatrogenically induced intoxication and withdrawal. Because a complete history is often unavailable in ICU patients, a history of substance use is often not discovered until symptoms of drug withdrawal appear. Neurological disorders, such as complex partial seizures, can also present with anxiety symptoms. Patients with preexisting anxiety disorders or a predisposition to anxiety disorders may have an exacerbation of such symptoms under the stress of critical illness.

Fear is differentiated from anxiety primarily in that it is a reaction to an identifiable—and, in the ICU, an often understandable—stressor. Fear can present in a manner identical to anxiety and may range in severity from mild worry (not evident unless the patient is directly questioned) to extreme emotional upset, agitation, or irrational behavior (e.g., refusing needed medical treatment).

Fear also implies a different diagnosis and prognosis. When fear is the primary symptom, it is much more likely that the patient is manifesting a time-limited, reasonable response to a severe stressor, an adjustment disorder, or a maladaptive reaction to the stress of serious illness resulting from limited or inflexible coping skills rather than a true anxiety disorder. Anecdotal evidence based on clinical experience

suggests that a trial of low-dose neuroleptic medication may be especially helpful in treating patients who have severe fearfulness.

Treatment of patients with anxiety in the ICU setting begins with correction of any underlying physical disorder or imbalance that is producing the symptom, if possible. Anxiety is reduced as these symptomatic treatments progress, but this is not a substitute for addressing the primary problem. This approach is not always feasible; if the physical problem does not respond to treatment or if the putative offending agent (e.g., corticosteroids in patients who have undergone transplantation, parenteral antibiotics in patients being treated for sepsis) cannot safely be discontinued, symptomatic treatment should be initiated to reduce the patient's suffering.

Benzodiazepines and neuroleptics are the mainstays of anxiolytic therapy for patients in the ICU. These agents are typically underprescribed and are given in inadequate doses when they are ordered for anxiety relief in the medical setting. In the ICU, providing anxiolytics on an as-needed basis, rather than scheduled dosing, is usually inadequate for treatment of anxiety because as-needed anxiolytics are not reliably administered by ICU staff (Stern et al. 1987).

Although all benzodiazepines are effective anxiolytics, lorazepam is often favored because it is available in oral and injectable forms, is reliably absorbed by the intramuscular route, and is more rapidly and simply metabolized. Lorazepam is not oxidatively metabolized, but it is conjugated and then excreted without the formation of active metabolites.

If anxiety or fearfulness is severe or is complicated by psychotic symptoms or confusion, time-limited use of a neuroleptic is usually effective. Additionally, some patients exhibit paradoxical disinhibitory reactions to benzodiazepines (common in elderly individuals or in those who are brain injured). These patients also tend to respond preferentially to neuroleptics. In the ICU, high-potency agents such as haloperidol are preferred over low-potency agents because the higher-potency agents cause less sedation, have fewer anticholinergic and adverse cardiac effects, and have a long history of use in the ICU setting (Settle and Ayd 1983).

Depression

Depression (see also Rouchell et al., Chapter 9, in this volume) can present in patients in the ICU as apathy, withdrawal, helplessness, tearfulness, decreased cooperation with treatment, or suicidal ideation or behavior (Cassem 1990; Cohen-Cole and Stoudemire 1987; Geringer and Stern 1991; Kathol et al. 1990; Rodin and Voshart 1986). Discouragement and worry about medical problems are very frequently seen in patients in the ICU, and these are often mistaken as symptoms of a formal depressive disorder. Anger, fear, apathetic states, and nonagitated delirium are at times misdiagnosed as depression. Depression is usually the result of major depressive disorder, dysthymia, or a medically or substance-induced mood disorder. ICU admission frequently results when depressed mood leads to a suicide attempt or extreme inattention to self-care.

Another cause of depressed mood among patients in the ICU is grief. Many patients have visited an ICU before, usually during the critical (often terminal) illness of a friend or relative—possibly during a past personal episode of illness. If the ICU setting reminds the patient of past experience, feelings of dread or grief are sometimes aroused. This is especially true if the grief was not dealt with appropriately at the time.

Critical illness may be perceived as a narcissistic injury. Particularly when the illness necessitating admission to the ICU is sudden in onset (e.g., myocardial infarction), the resultant change in self-perception is sometimes devastating. Stern (1985) described a modification of the Draw-a-Person Test, in which the patient is asked to draw a picture of a person and a picture of what the patient thinks is wrong, as a useful technique to access and monitor such changes in self-perception.

Treatment of patients with major depression usually includes pharmacological agents. In the ICU, the selective serotonin reuptake inhibitors (SSRIs) and psychostimulants are used more often than tricyclic antidepressants and monoamine oxidase inhibitors (MAOIs). SSRIs, including fluoxetine, sertraline, and paroxetine, are generally well tolerated, even by critically ill patients. Awareness of drug interactions is important (Shuster et al. 1992), particularly the inhibitory effect that SSRIs have on the cytochrome P-450 system. Levels of drugs metabolized via these pathways are commonly raised by the concomitant administration of an SSRI.

Psychostimulants are generally safe and useful in the treatment of depression in medically ill patients (Kaufman et al. 1982; Woods et al. 1986). The ICU setting allows close monitoring of the response to psychostimulant administration. The chief advantages of stimulants for depression in the ICU are rapid therapeutic response, rapid clearance of the drug if side effects emerge, and safety and tolerability at the low doses usually required. Initially, dosing begins with 2.5–5.0 mg of dextroamphetamine in the morning or 5.0 mg of methylphenidate in the morning and early afternoon, with an increase of 2.5 mg/dose/day until the desired therapeutic benefit is achieved, intolerable side effects emerge, or a dose of 15–20 mg/day of dextroamphetamine or 15–20 mg/dose with twice-daily dosing of methylphenidate is reached. Side effects that may limit psychostimulant treatment include hypertension, tachycardia, arrhythmia, agitation, confusion, insomnia, and appetite suppression. Low doses of stimulants often increase appetite in medically ill patients with depression. The clinician should screen for each of these side effects before each dose increase.

Confusion

Confusion is so common in the ICU that psychiatric consultation is often not requested unless the patient is also agitated. The quietly confused patient is often mistakenly referred by his or her physicians for depression, anxiety, or an unpleasant personality. At the other extreme, when patients become agitated, combative, or otherwise uncooperative, psychiatric assistance is urgently required.

All instances of confusion in the ICU merit attention and evaluation because a confusional state is usually a sign of an underlying medical complication. Moreover, because alert and cognitively intact patients are better able to cooperate with treatment and comply with specific instructions (e.g., use of incentive spirometers, ambulation), aggressive screening and treatment of delirium are cost-effective in that they reduce the length of ICU stay and utilization of resources (Levenson et al. 1990).

Treatment of delirium in the ICU, as outlined in Table 24–2 (Lipowski 1990), begins with a thorough search for causative medical or substance-induced problems (e.g., infections, head trauma, metabolic abnormalities). Medications, as listed in Table 24–3, or interactions between drugs should also be considered, and any offending agents should be discontinued whenever possible. Withdrawal states, particularly those related to alcohol and sedative-hypnotic medications, are always possible, even when the admitting history indicates no problem with substance use—patients typically underreport substance-use patterns (Hackett et al. 1991; Khantzian and McKenna 1979). Sensory overstimulation should be minimized to help patients sleep, although adequate interpersonal contact and stimulation should be maintained—admittedly a difficult task in the ICU. General supportive care with frequent reassurance and reorientation is very helpful to the patient who is recovering from delirium.

Medications used to treat patients with agi-

Table 24–2. Guidelines for treatment of patients with delirium in the intensive care unit

1. Monitor the patient's mental state and behavior closely.
2. Search for causative physical problems and correct them when possible.
    Consider adverse effects of medications.
    Consider interactions between medications.
    Consider withdrawal states.
3. Use medications (e.g., neuroleptics, benzodiazepines) to treat agitation and psychotic symptoms.
4. Structure the patient's environment to provide adequate contact with others, without overstimulation.
5. Maintain nutrition, fluid and electrolyte balance, and vitamin intake.
6. Provide general nursing care aimed at reorienting the patient, observing and reporting his or her behavior, and providing emotional support.
7. Provide supportive psychotherapy at the bedside, which may help calm the patient and aid adaptation after resolution of delirium.

Source. Adapted from Lipowski ZJ: *Delirium: Acute Confusional States.* New York, Oxford University Press, 1990. Copyright 1990, Oxford University Press. Used with permission.

tation in the ICU include neuroleptics, benzodiazepines, narcotics, and paralytic agents (Sos and Cassem 1980; Tesar and Stern 1988; Thompson and Thompson 1983). The pharmacological properties of medications commonly used to treat confusion and agitation in patients in the ICU are outlined in Table 24–4.

Neuroleptics are usually the drugs of first choice in the ICU setting, although benzodiazepines are commonly used alone or in combination with neuroleptics (Salzman et al. 1986). Haloperidol, a high-potency butyrophenone, is the most commonly used neuroleptic agent in the ICU setting because of its long record of safety and utility (Cameron 1978; Donlon et al. 1979; Settle and Ayd 1983). Another feature of

Table 24–3. Common delirium-inducing drugs used in the intensive care unit

Group	Agent
Antiarrhythmics	Lidocaine
	Mexiletine
	Procainamide
	Quinidine
Antibiotics	Penicillin
	Rifampin
Anticholinergics	Atropine
Antihistamines	Nonselective
	Diphenhydramine
	Promethazine
	H_2-blockers
	Cimetidine
	Ranitidine
β-Blockers	Propranolol
Narcotic analgesics	Meperidine
	Morphine
	Pentazocine

Source. Adapted from Tesar GE, Stern TA: "Evaluation and Treatment of Agitation in the Intensive Care Unit." *Journal of Intensive Care Medicine* 1:137–148, 1986. Copyright 1986, Little, Brown, and Company. Used with permission.

haloperidol that makes it appealing for use in the ICU is its safety and efficacy when it is administered intravenously (Cassem and Hackett 1991; Fernandez et al. 1988). Pharmacological treatments for delirium can usually be safely discontinued once the patient is symptom-free for 24–48 hours, unless habituating agents such as benzodiazepines were used long enough to induce tolerance and withdrawal, in which case drug tapering is appropriate.

Psychosis

The ICU is potentially a frightening and distressing place for patients with psychosis. Patients with schizophrenia or other psychotic disorders, delusional disorder, bipolar disorder, or psychotic depression can have problems adapting to the stress of critical illness and ICU treatment (Goff et al. 1991). This is particularly true if the patient has paranoia or active psychotic symptoms.

The patient with psychosis is treated in the ICU much as he or she would be treated in other settings. Neuroleptic agents are the mainstays of treatment. If the patient takes a neuroleptic that has proven effective as outpatient therapy, this medication is generally continued if the patient can tolerate it while critically ill. In some cases, low-potency neuroleptics are discontinued and high-potency agents (e.g., haloperidol) are substituted at equivalent doses. Depot preparations are almost always avoided in the ICU. Benzodiazepines (e.g., lorazepam, clonazepam) are helpful adjuncts to neuroleptics for psychosis. The patient in the ICU with psychotic agitation may be treated with a range of agents, as listed in Table 24–4.

Personality

Most patients in the ICU who are alert enough to interact with staff members tolerate their stay without major interpersonal conflicts. Unfortunately, patients with maladaptive personality traits or full-blown personality disorders rely on familiar maladaptive patterns of behavior when challenged by stressors such as severe illness (Groves 1975; Wool et al. 1991). In fact, personality styles are usually amplified in the ICU because these traits are the patient's best or only defense against such stress (e.g., the paranoid person becomes more hostile, withdrawn, and suspicious when admitted to the cardiac care unit after a myocardial infarction). Obviously, such patterns of behavior impede the delivery of care by rendering the patient less able to cooperate with ICU staff in a mature and appropriate manner and by rendering the staff less able (and sometimes less willing) to deliver needed care.

Before behavior is attributed to personality, a careful evaluation of substance-induced and medical causes (e.g., confusion, delirium)

Table 24–4. Pharmacology of drugs used to treat patients with confusion and agitation

Drug	Route	Onset (minutes)	Peak effect (minutes)	Starting dosage	Comments
Neuroleptics					
Haloperidol	iv,[a] im	5–20	15–45	Mild agitation: 0.5–2 mg	Generally considered the first line of treatment, especially when confusion is prominent
	po	30–60	120–240	Moderate agitation: 5–10 mg	
				Severe agitation: ≥10 mg	
Droperidol	iv, im	3–10	15–45	2.5–10 mg	
Chlorpromazine	im, iv[b]	5–40	10–30	25 mg	
Benzodiazepines					
Diazepam	iv	2–5	5–30	2–5 mg	Useful alone or in combination with neuroleptics; especially useful when symptoms of anxiety predominate
	po	10–60	30–180		
Lorazepam	iv, im	2–20	60–120	1–2 mg	
	sl	2–20	20–60	0.5–1 mg	
	po	20–60	20–120	0.5–1 mg	
Midazolam	im, iv	1–2	30–40	0.05–0.15 mg/kg	
Narcotic					
Morphine	im, iv	1–2	20	4–10 mg	ICU staff familiar with use; reversible with naloxone if necessary; very useful if pain is prominent
Paralytic agents					
Metocurine	iv	1–4	2–10	0.2–0.4 mg/kg	Generally considered treatment of last resort to prevent patient self-injury; requires intubation
Pancurium	iv	0.5–1	5	0.04–0.10 mg/kg	

Note. ICU = intensive care unit; im = intramuscular; iv = intravenous; po = per os (orally); sl = sublingual.
[a]Intravenous haloperidol is not approved for routine use by the U.S. Food and Drug Administration; permission for its use should be requested from the hospital's formulary.
[b]Intravenous administration of chlorpromazine is more likely to cause cardiovascular disturbance (e.g., hypotension) than intramuscular administration.
Source. Adapted from Tesar GE, Stern TA: "Rapid Tranquilization of the Agitated Intensive Care Unit Patient." *Journal of Intensive Care Medicine* 3:195–201, 1988. Copyright 1988, Little, Brown, and Company. Used with permission.

should be performed. Confusional states may render the patient irritable, paranoid, combative, or unable to cooperate with treatment, although this behavior is not intentional, and the patient may have little awareness of or control over the behavior. The consulting psychiatrist should next screen for other Axis I disorders (e.g., severe anxiety, psychosis), as well as physical problems (e.g., pain) and interpersonal difficulties (e.g., anger at staff or family members). If this search for other explanations of maladaptive behavior is unrevealing, characterological problems should be considered. A life-threatening illness often causes regressive behaviors in many patients; this behavior does not necessarily reflect baseline (premorbid) functioning.

CLINICAL SITUATIONS UNIQUE TO THE INTENSIVE CARE UNIT

Clinical situations or procedures unique to the ICU setting and worth special mention include mechanical ventilation, placement of an intra-aortic balloon pump (IABP), and cardiac surgery.

Respirators

Anxiety is very commonly associated with mechanical ventilation. In addition, the underlying respiratory problems often produce sufficient hypoxia to produce or exacerbate anxiety symptoms. Although ventilatory support usually resolves such anxiety by correcting hypoxia, patients are at times made more anxious by intubation and ventilation. The endotracheal tube is often uncomfortable, and ventilation is sometimes suboptimal even with aggressive respiratory therapy. In addition, the constant rhythmic noise of the respirator can serve as a nerve-racking reminder to the patient of his or her critical state. Alert patients may worry about their prognosis or may feel helpless and out of control.

Anxiety is particularly common when the patient is weaned from the ventilator. Several factors can play a role in the anxiety: patients may experience at least brief periods of relative hypoxia during weaning trials; prolonged ventilation usually leads to deconditioning of muscles of respiration, so patients become frightened by the unfamiliar difficulty they experience with breathing until these muscles are reconditioned; and patients often become psychologically dependent on the ventilator and fearful when the device is disconnected.

Intra-Aortic Balloon Pumps and Cardiac Surgery

Delirium commonly complicates cardiac procedures in the critically ill patient. An association between placement of the IABP and delirium occurred in 34% of 198 patients undergoing this procedure at Massachusetts General Hospital (Sanders et al. 1992). Delirium usually developed acutely—on the first or second day after IABP insertion—and resolved rapidly after the IABP was removed. Although in-hospital mortality was nearly identical between patients with delirium and those without delirium, the patients who became delirious had significantly longer hospital stays and a greater likelihood of developing residual neuropsychiatric deficits.

Cardiac surgery is also associated with a high rate of delirium during the postoperative phase, estimated at 32% in a literature review and meta-analysis by Smith and Dimsdale (1989). Factors that contribute to delirium following cardiac surgery are outlined in Table 24–5. Preexisting brain dysfunction and the duration and complexity of the operative procedure are the most important factors.

STAFF STRESS

The task of providing intensive care for patients with critical illness is very stressful (Gonzales and Stern 1991). Patients in ICUs are very ill. Treatment of acute and often rapidly changing illnesses puts pressure on the ICU staff to produce good clinical results in very difficult situations under great time pressure. Family members, themselves burdened by concern about their critically ill loved one, may express fears and frustrations to or at ICU staff members. Some members of the treatment team, who are also under pressure, can withdraw, be less supportive, or inappropriately direct feelings of frustration, anger, or helplessness toward one another or toward the patient or his or her family. Clearly, intensive care is aptly named from the perspective of the caregiver. The intensity, the fast pace, and the action inherent in ICU medicine are part of the appeal of this field for those who choose it. These same factors, however, place clinicians who work in the ICU at great risk for burnout.

Prevention or intervention measures require recognition of the potential sources of stress related to provision of intensive care. Table 24–6 lists some stressors for ICU staff.

Group interventions for ICU physicians, nurses, and other staff members are very effective in reducing work stress in the ICU (Cassem and Hackett 1975; Siegal and Donnelly 1978; Simon and Whitely 1977; Weiner et al. 1983). Stern et al. (1993) reported on autognosis rounds, a group stress reduction and self-knowledge intervention that has been an ongoing part of the medical house staff's experience in the medical ICU at Massachusetts General Hospital for more than 15 years. The goals for the house staff participants are

to 1) identify their subjective reactions to clinical situations, 2) learn to use their emotions in clinical practice, 3) learn how to minimize possible disruptive effects of their reactions to patients (e.g., manage their angry feelings toward patients so they can be expressed during the rounds and not interfere with patient care), and 4) share their reactions with each other and thereby learn that they are not alone with their feelings. (Stern et al. 1993, p. 2)

Stern has also maintained The Red Book, a sort of community journal, as an adjunct to autognosis rounds. Participants are invited to contribute as they see fit. The Red Book, now in its fifteenth year, contains an impressive and often enlightening collection of jokes, reflections, slogans, and even impromptu essays. These interventions are valued and well attended by the medical house staff.

Table 24–5. Factors contributing to the development of delirium following cardiac surgery

Time course	Factor
Preoperative	History of MI
	Preexisting CNS dysfunction
	Psychiatric disorders and factors
	Panic-level anxiety
	Major depression
	Alcohol or drug abuse
	Poor understanding of or reluctance to undergo planned procedure
	Severe physical illness
Intraoperative	Body temperature $\leq 28°C$
	Complexity of surgical procedure
	Systolic blood pressure ≤ 50–60 mm Hg
	Total anesthesia time
	Type of oxygenator used in the bypass device (?)
Postoperative	Complications during recovery
	Environment (e.g., sensory overload or deprivation)
	Intraaortic balloon pump (?)
	Medications administered (e.g., excess anticholinergic agents, narcotics, sedative-hypnotics)

Note. CNS = central nervous system; MI = myocardial infarction.
Source. Adapted from Tesar GE, Stern TA: "Evaluation and Treatment of Agitation in the Intensive Care Unit." *Journal of Intensive Care Medicine* 1:137–148, 1986. Copyright 1986, Little, Brown, and Company. Used with permission.

Table 24–6. Common stressors for intensive care unit staff

Physician stressors	Nurse stressors
Being sleep-deprived	Having an excessive workload (high patient-to-nurse ratio)
Having long on-duty assignments	
Providing high-technology care	Having too little time to deal with patients' or their families' emotional needs
Dealing with chronically and/or severely ill patients	
	Dealing with death
Feeling a responsibility to patients' families	Dealing with the unnecessary prolongation of life
Having limited training in ethics	Providing high-technology care
Being exposed to contagious and/or deadly diseases (e.g., AIDS)	Having unpredictable schedules
	Being subjected to environmental disturbances (e.g., noise)
Performing complex or invasive procedural tasks	
Being overloaded with information	Having administrative conflicts
Having a large financial debt	Feeling powerless or insecure
Anxiety about malpractice	

Note. AIDS = acquired immunodeficiency syndrome.
Source. Reprinted from Gonzales JJ, Stern TA: "Recognition and Management of Staff Stress in the ICU," in *Intensive Care Medicine,* 2nd Edition. Edited by Rippe JM, Irwin RS, Alpert JS, et al. Boston, MA, Little, Brown, 1991, pp. 1916–1922. Copyright 1991, Little, Brown, and Company. Used with permission.

CONCLUSION

Although consultation-liaison psychiatry in the ICU is challenging and intense, it is not qualitatively different from other areas of consultation psychiatry. Compared with other settings, the patients to be treated are sicker, the pace is faster, and the stress level is higher. The same mental disorders that are seen in other settings are seen in the ICU, especially the secondary mental disorders, but these are complicated by the severity and dynamic state of the patients' physical problems. The consultation-liaison psychiatrist can offer help by focusing efforts on clinical care of ICU patients and by focusing liaison efforts on helping members of the ICU staff care for the critically ill while preventing burnout.

REFERENCES

Cameron OG: Safe use of haloperidol in a patient with cardiac dysrhythmia (letter). Am J Psychiatry 135:1244, 1978

Cassem NH: Depression and anxiety secondary to medical illness. Psychiatr Clin North Am 13:597–612, 1990

Cassem NH, Hackett TP: Stress on the nurse and therapist in the intensive care unit and the coronary care unit. Heart Lung 4:252–259, 1975

Cassem NH, Hackett TP: The setting of intensive care, in Massachusetts General Hospital Handbook of General Hospital Psychiatry, 3rd Edition. Edited by Cassem NH. St Louis, MO, CV Mosby, 1991, pp 373–399

Charney DS, Redmond DE Jr: Neurobiological mechanisms in human anxiety: evidence supporting noradrenergic hyperactivity. Neuropharmacology 22:1531–1536, 1983

Cohen-Cole S, Stoudemire A: Major depression and physical illness. Psychiatr Clin North Am 10:1–17, 1987

Dec GW, Stern TA: Tricyclic antidepressants in the intensive care unit. Journal of Intensive Care Medicine 5:69–81, 1990

Donlon PT, Hopkin J, Schaffer CB, et al: Cardiovascular safety of rapid treatment with intramuscular haloperidol. Am J Psychiatry 136:233–234, 1979

Fernandez F, Holmes VF, Adams F, et al: Treatment of severe, refractory agitation with a haloperidol drip. J Clin Psychiatry 49:239–241, 1988

Folstein MF, Folstein SE, McHugh PR: Mini-Mental State: a practical method for grading the cognitive state of patients for the clinician. J Psychiatr Res 12:189–198, 1975

Francis J: Using restraints in the elderly because of fear of litigation (letter). N Engl J Med 320:870, 1989

Geringer ES, Stern TA: Recognition and treatment of depression in the ICU, in Intensive Care Medicine, 2nd Edition. Edited by Rippe JM, Irwin RS, Alpert JS, et al. Boston, MA, Little, Brown, 1991, pp 1887–1902

Goff DC, Manschreck TC, Groves JE: Psychotic patients, in Massachusetts General Hospital Handbook of General Hospital Psychiatry, 3rd Edition. Edited by Cassem NH. St Louis, MO, CV Mosby, 1991, pp 217–236

Gonzales JJ, Stern TA: Recognition and management of staff stress in the ICU, in Intensive Care Medicine, 2nd Edition. Edited by Rippe JM, Irwin RS, Alpert JS, et al. Boston, MA, Little, Brown, 1991, pp 1916–1922

Groves JE: Management of the borderline patient on a medical surgical ward: the psychiatric consultant's role. Int J Psychiatry Med 6: 337–348, 1975

Hackett TP, Stern TA: Suicide and other disruptive states, in Massachusetts General Hospital Handbook of General Hospital Psychiatry, 3rd Edition. Edited by Cassem NH. St Louis, MO, CV Mosby, 1991, pp 281–307

Hackett TP, Gastfriend DR, Renner JA: Alcoholism: acute and chronic states, in Massachusetts General Hospital Handbook of General Hospital Psychiatry, 3rd Edition. Edited by Cassem NH. St Louis, MO, CV Mosby, 1991, pp 9–22

Hickam JB, Cargill WH, Golden A: Cardiovascular reactions to emotional stimuli: effect on the cardiac output, arteriovenous oxygen difference, arterial pressure, and peripheral resistance. J Clin Invest 27:290–298, 1948

Jenike MA: Geriatric Psychiatry and Psychopharmacology. Chicago, IL, Year Book Medical, 1989

Jewitt DE, Mercer CJ, Reid D, et al: Free noradrenaline and adrenaline excretion in relation to the development of cardiac arrhythmias and heart failure in patients with acute myocardial infarction. Lancet 1:635–641, 1969

Kathol RG, Noyes R, Williams J, et al: Diagnosing depression in patients with medical illness. Psychosomatics 31:434–440, 1990

Kaufman MW, Murray GB, Cassem NH: Use of psychostimulants in medically ill depressed patients. Psychosomatics 23:817–819, 1982

Khantzian EJ, McKenna GJ: Acute toxic and withdrawal reactions associated with drug use and abuse. Ann Intern Med 90:361–372, 1979

Levenson JL, Hamer RM, Rossiter LF: Relation of psychopathology in general medical inpatients to use and cost of services. Am J Psychiatry 147:1498–1503, 1990

Lipowski ZJ: Delirium: Acute Confusional States. New York, Oxford University Press, 1990

Lipson RE, Stern TA: Management of monoamine oxidase inhibitor-treated patients in the emergency and critical care setting. Journal of Intensive Care Medicine 6:117–125, 1991

MacKenzie TB, Popkin MK: Organic anxiety syndrome. Am J Psychiatry 140:342–344, 1983

Reich P, deSilva RA, Lown B, et al: Acute psychological disturbances preceding life-threatening ventricular arrhythmias. JAMA 246:233–235, 1981

Rodin G, Voshart K: Depression in the medically ill: an overview. Am J Psychiatry 143:696–705, 1986

Salzman C, Green AI, Rodriguez-Villa F, et al: Benzodiazepines combined with neuroleptics for management of severe disruptive behavior. Psychosomatics 27(suppl):17–22, 1986

Sanders KM, Stern TA, O'Gara PT, et al: Delirium during intra-aortic balloon pump therapy: incidence and management. Psychosomatics 33:35–44, 1992

Settle EC, Ayd FJ: Haloperidol: a quarter century of experience. J Clin Psychiatry 44:440–448, 1983

Shuster JL, Stern TA, Greenberg DB: Pros and cons of fluoxetine for the depressed cancer patient. Oncology 6:45–50, 1992

Siegal B, Donnelly JC: Enriching personal and professional development: the experience of a support group for interns. Journal of Medical Education 53:908–914, 1978

Simon NM, Whitely S: Psychiatric consultation with MICU nurses: the consultation conference as a working group. Heart Lung 6:497–504, 1977

Smith LW, Dimsdale JE: Postcardiotomy delirium: conclusions after 25 years? Am J Psychiatry 146:452–458, 1989

Sos J, Cassem NH: Managing postoperative agitation. Drug Therapeutics 10:103–106, 1980

Stein EH, Murdaugh J, MacCleod JA: Brief psychotherapy of psychiatric reactions to physical illness. Am J Psychiatry 125:1040–1047, 1969

Stern TA: The management of depression and anxiety following myocardial infarction. Mt Sinai J Med 52:623–633, 1985

Stern TA, Caplan RA, Cassem NH: Use of benzodiazepines in a coronary care unit. Psychosomatics 28:19–23, 1987

Stern TA, Prager LM, Cremens MC: Autognosis rounds for medical house staff. Psychosomatics 34:1–7, 1993

Stoudemire A, Moran MG, Fogel BS: Psychotropic drug use in the medically ill: part I. Psychosomatics 31:377–391, 1990

Stoudemire A, Moran MG, Fogel BS: Psychotropic drug use in the medically ill: part II. Psychosomatics 32:34–44, 1991

Strain JJ, Leisowitz MR, Klein DF: Anxiety and panic attacks in the medically ill. Psychiatr Clin North Am 4:333–350, 1981

Tesar GE, Stern TA: Evaluation and treatment of agitation in the intensive care unit. Journal of Intensive Care Medicine 1:137–148, 1986

Tesar GE, Stern TA: Rapid tranquilization of the agitated intensive care unit patient. Journal of Intensive Care Medicine 3:195–201, 1988

Thompson TL, Thompson WL: Treating postoperative delirium. Drug Therapeutics 13:30–43, 1983

Townsend PL, Reynolds JR: Applied pharmacokinetics: an overview, in Intensive Care Medicine, 2nd Edition. Edited by Rippe JM, Irwin RS, Alpert JS, et al. Boston, MA, Little, Brown, 1991, pp 1695–1707

Weiner MF, Caldwell T, Tyson J: Stresses and coping in ICU nursing: why support groups fail. Gen Hosp Psychiatry 5:179–183, 1983

Woods SW, Tesar GE, Murray GB, et al: Psychostimulant treatment of depressive disorders secondary to medical illness. J Clin Psychiatry 47:12–15, 1986

Wool C, Geringer ES, Stern TA: The management of behavioral problems in the ICU, in Intensive Care Medicine, 2nd Edition. Edited by Rippe JM, Irwin RS, Alpert JS, et al. Boston, MA, Little, Brown, 1991, pp 1906–1916

Chapter 25

Psychiatric Issues in the Care of Dying Patients

Ilona Wiener, M.D.
William Breitbart, M.D.
Jimmie Holland, M.D.

The consultation-liaison psychiatrist faces one of the greatest challenges of the field when treating terminally ill patients. The task is to assist each person to achieve the personal death that is "appropriate" for that individual (Weisman 1972). To help patients achieve an appropriate death requires that the consultation-liaison psychiatrist be knowledgeable about the psychological aspects of care, be familiar with the principles of symptom control, and be personally comfortable in dealing with issues around mortality.

▮ THE CONCEPT OF AN APPROPRIATE DEATH

Weisman (1972) and his colleagues, through his work with Project Omega in the 1970s, developed the first extensive treatises concerning the psychological care of the dying patient. He described four goals for what he called an "appropriate" death:

1. Internal conflicts, such as fears about loss of control, should be reduced as much as possible.
2. The individual's personal sense of identity should be sustained.
3. Critical relationships should be enhanced or at least maintained; conflicts should be resolved, if possible.
4. The person should be encouraged to establish and attempt to reach meaningful goals—even though limited—such as attending a graduation, marriage, or birth of a child as a way to provide a sense of continuity into the future.

These four goals can serve as general guidelines for the consultation-liaison psychiatrist.

PSYCHOLOGICAL ISSUES AND MANAGEMENT

Patients who face death, especially when it entails a slow downhill course, experience anticipatory grief that is manifested differently among individual patients. The primary psychological issues in anticipatory grieving are those of facing losses brought on by illness and anticipated losses related to death (Barton 1977). A sense of loss of control is felt with worsening of illness and increasing symptoms that do not remit. Hope that control of the illness will be reestablished diminishes. The impending loss of life and continuity with the future and with those who will live on becomes painfully real. The sense of being isolated and alone, despite closeness of others, adds to distress. Continuing evidence of affection from others mitigates some of the pain of loss (Lieber et al. 1976).

Psychotherapy with terminally ill patients differs in significant ways from therapy provided in traditional settings (Sourkes 1982). The psychiatrist must be willing to visit the patient in the hospital, clinic, or home. The visits must be shortened to accommodate the patient's medical condition. The visits may need to be more frequent, providing an opportunity for the patient to explore the feelings of loss.

The primary psychological issues for the family are similar in that they are responding to the changes in the patient's physical condition and, at the same time, beginning the anticipatory grieving for the impending loss. Questions in their minds are "When and how will the loved one die?" "What will the moment of death be like?" "How will I be able to manage it?" As more patients, especially those with cancer and acquired immunodeficiency syndrome (AIDS), choose to die at home, the family caregiver must be prepared to handle an increasingly heavy burden of care and the terminal event itself. Support for the family as well as the patient is important (Schachter 1992).

PSYCHIATRIC DISORDERS

The most common psychiatric disorders encountered in patients who are dying include anxiety disorders, depression, and delirium. Often, these psychiatric complications of the dying process are a consequence of progression of the disease, physical debilitation, and distressing, uncontrolled symptoms, particularly pain.

Anxiety Disorders

As outlined in Table 25–1, anxiety occurs in patients who are terminally ill as 1) an adjustment disorder with anxious mood alone or in combination with depressed mood; 2) a disease- related or treatment-related condition; and 3) an exacerbation of a preexisting anxiety disorder (Massie 1989). Adjustment disorder with anxiety is related to adjusting to the existential crisis and the uncertainty of the prognosis and the future (Holland 1989). Anxiety related to medical causes is frequently a consequence of poorly controlled pain. The patient who is in pain appears restless, appears tense, and may be agitated. Once the pain is controlled, the secondary anxiety subsides. Metabolic abnormalities such as hypoxia, sepsis with fever, and delirium can produce anxiety and restlessness. A sudden onset of anxiety with respiratory distress or chest pain may signal pulmonary embolism or an acute cardiac event. Among the drugs used in terminal states, corticosteroids occasionally cause anxiety. Antiemetic neuroleptics, such as metoclopramide and prochlorperazine, often cause profound akathisia and anxiety. Bronchodilators used for dyspnea can produce tremulousness and anxiety. Withdrawal states from opioid analgesics, benzodiazepines, alcohol, and barbiturates produce anxiety and agitation. Use of short-acting benzodiazepines, such as lorazepam and alprazolam, may be associated with rebound anxiety.

When faced with a terminal illness, patients with preexisting anxiety disorders are at risk for reactivation of symptoms. A generalized anxiety disorder or panic disorder is apt to recur, especially in the presence of shortness of breath or pain. Persons with a history of phobias, especially a phobia of death, will have anxiety symptoms that will require medication and reassurance. Posttraumatic stress disorder may be activated in dying patients as they relate their situation to some prior near-death experience and the terror associated with it, such as memories of the Holocaust or a combat experience.

The management of significant anxiety in dying patients is likely to require pharmacological intervention, along with psychological support or behavioral interventions. Short-acting benzodiazepines, such as lorazepam and alprazolam, are used most often. Lorazepam is metabolized by conjugation in the liver and, therefore, is safer to use in patients with hepatic disease. Alprazolam is me-

Table 25–1. Common causes of anxiety in dying patients

Types of anxiety	Causes
Reactive anxiety/adjustment disorder	Awareness of terminal condition
	Fears and uncertainty about death
	Conflicts with family or staff
	DNR discussion
Disease- and treatment-related anxiety	Poor pain control
	Related metabolic disturbances
	Hypoxia
	Hypoglycemia
	Delirium
	Sepsis
	Bleeding
	Pulmonary embolus
Substance-induced anxiety	Anxiety-producing drugs
	Corticosteroids
	Dexamethasone
	Prednisone
	Antiemetic neuroleptics
	Metoclopramide
	Prochlorperazine
	Bronchodilators
	Withdrawal states
	Opioids
	Benzodiazepines
	Alcohol

Preexisting anxiety disorders
  General anxiety disorder
  Panic
  Phobias
  Posttraumatic stress disorder
	Exacerbation of symptoms related to fears and distressing medical symptoms

Note. DNR = do not resuscitate.

tabolized through oxidative mechanisms in the liver and can exacerbate liver damage. Midazolam, a very-short-acting benzodiazepine, administered intravenously, is used to achieve rapid sedation in patients who are agitated or anxious. In an intensive care setting, midazolam is most often administered intravenously; it is also useful and safe when administered subcutaneously (Bottomley and Hanks 1990). Starting doses should be low (i.e., 10–60 mg over 24 hours), and the patient should be carefully monitored (DeSousa and Jepson 1988). Clonazepam, a longer acting benzodiazepine, is used in patients who experience breakthrough anxiety on short-acting drugs. It is also useful in tapering patients from alprazolam. Diazepam can be administered rectally to control anxiety and restlessness when oral administration is not possible (Twycross and Lack 1984).

Neuroleptics such as haloperidol or thioridazine, given in low doses, are used when benzodiazepines are contraindicated or do not control anxiety. Haloperidol, 0.5–5 mg given every 2–12 hours orally, intravenously, or subcutaneously, controls anxiety without causing sedation. The combination of haloperidol and a benzodiazepine is often used to control the anxiety and agitation associated with delirium. Thioridazine or chlorpromazine, both low-potency neuroleptics, are effective anxiolytics that also promote sedation. Doses for thioridazine are 10–25 mg orally three times a day; 12.5–50 mg of chlorpromazine should be given orally every 4–12 hours. Because of the side effects of hypotension and anticholinergic symptoms, these drugs must be used with caution. When using neuroleptics, one must keep in mind that these drugs are associated with extrapyramidal side effects and the possibility of neuroleptic malignant syndrome.

Buspirone, a nonbenzodiazepine anxiolytic, has limited usefulness in terminally ill patients because of its delayed onset of action.

For providing psychological support, supportive, crisis-oriented psychotherapy is the best model. The consultation-liaison psychiatrist must be able to discuss the meaning of information about the medical condition and treatment plan, listen to the patient's fears and concerns, and support adaptive ways of coping. Cognitive-behavioral techniques seek to reduce anxiety by providing information and by teaching self-monitoring techniques, distraction, and relaxation. Cognitive approaches focus on thought processes and perceptions; behavioral approaches focus on modifying behavior. The behavioral techniques most often use elements of muscular relaxation and cognitive distraction, passive breathing followed by passive or active muscle relaxation, and pleasant imagery (Mastrovito 1989).

Depression

Prevalence rates for major depressive syndromes in patients with cancer range from 4.5% to 58%, according to psychiatric consultation database studies (Hinton 1972; Levine et al. 1978; Massie and Holland 1987; Massie et al. 1979) and research-based prevalence studies (Bukberg and Holland 1980; Bukberg et al. 1984; Chochinov et al. 1994; Dean 1987; Derogatis et al. 1983; Evans et al. 1986; Kathol et al. 1990; Lansky et al. 1985; Morton et al. 1984; Plumb and Holland 1977; Weddington et al. 1986). Only a limited number of these studies examined the prevalence of depression in patients with greatly advanced disease (Bukberg and Holland 1980; Bukberg et al. 1984; Chochinov et al. 1994; Derogatis et al. 1983; Hinton 1972; Kathol et al. 1990), and the data from these studies suggested that depression is more common in later stages of the disease, ranging in prevalence from 23% to 58%. Family history of depression and history of previous depressive episodes further suggest the reliability of a diagnosis. Evaluation of cancer-related organic factors that can present as depression must precede initiation of treatment. These factors include administration of corticosteroids (Stiefel et al. 1989); use of chemotherapeutic agents, including vincristine, vinblastine, asparaginase, intrathecal methotrexate, interferon, and interleukin-2 (Adams et al. 1984; Denicoff et al. 1987; Holland et al. 1974; Young 1982); use of amphotericin B (Weddington 1982); whole brain radiation (DeAngelis et al. 1989); central nervous system (CNS) metabolic-endocrine complications (Breitbart 1989); and paraneoplastic syndromes (Patchell and Posner 1989; Posner 1988).

Depressed mood and sadness can be appropriate responses as the terminally ill patient faces death. These emotions can be manifestations of anticipatory grief over the impending loss of one's life, health, loved ones, and autonomy. Terminal illness itself can produce many of the physical symptoms that are characteristic of major depression in the physically healthy population.

Management of Depression in Patients Who Are Terminally Ill

Depression in patients with advanced disease is optimally managed with a combination of supportive psychotherapy, cognitive-behavioral techniques, and antidepressant medications (Massie and Holland 1990). Psychotherapy and cognitive-behavioral techniques are useful in the management of psychological distress in patients with cancer and have been applied to the treatment of depressive and anxious symptoms related to cancer and cancer pain. Psychotherapeutic interventions, in the form of either individual or group counseling, have been shown to effectively reduce psychological distress and depressive symptoms in patients with cancer (Massie et al. 1989; Spiegel and Bloom 1983; Spiegel et al. 1981). Cognitive-behavioral interventions, such as relaxation and distraction with pleasant imagery, have also been shown to decrease depressive symptoms in patients with mild to moderate levels of depression (Holland et al. 1987). However, psychopharmacological interven-

tions such as antidepressant medications are the mainstay of treatment of terminally ill patients with severe depressive symptoms who meet criteria for a major depressive episode (Massie and Holland 1990). The efficacy of antidepressants in the treatment of depression in patients with cancer has been established (Costa et al. 1985; Massie and Holland 1990; Popkin et al. 1985; Purohit et al. 1978; Rifkin et al. 1985). However, few controlled studies of antidepressant drug therapy focus specifically on the treatment of patients who are terminally ill (Mermelstein and Lesko 1992).

Pharmacological Treatment of Depression in Patients Who Are Terminally Ill

Factors such as prognosis and the time frame for treatment may play important roles in determining the type of pharmacotherapy that is chosen for depression. A patient with depression whose life expectancy is several months can afford to wait the 10–14 days it may take to respond to a tricyclic antidepressant. The dying patient with depression who has less than 3 weeks to live may do best with a rapid-acting psychostimulant (Breitbart 1988). Patients who are within hours to days of death and in distress are likely to benefit most from the use of sedatives or narcotic analgesic infusions.

Tricyclic antidepressants. Treatment should be initiated at low doses (10–25 mg at bedtime), especially in patients who are debilitated and have advanced disease; the doses should be increased slowly, in increments of 10–25 mg every 1–2 days until a beneficial effect is achieved. Patients with cancer who have depression often have a therapeutic response at much lower doses (25–125 mg/day orally) than are usually required in patients who do not have medical illness (150–300 mg/day) (Massie and Holland 1990). It is often useful to monitor plasma drug levels of tricyclics (desipramine, nortriptyline, amitriptyline, imipramine) because patients who are medically ill in general, and those with advanced cancer in particular, are often found to have therapeutic plasma levels at modest dosages (Stoudemire and Fogel 1987). Moreover, typical regimens of the tricyclics (100–250 mg/day) can cause toxic effects in these patients, and plasma levels obtained on a serial basis can guide the physician in effective and safe administration.

The selection of tricyclic depends on the side-effect profile, the existing medical problems, the nature of depressive symptoms, and past response to specific antidepressants. Sedating tricyclics such as amitriptyline or doxepin are prescribed for the patient with agitation and depression accompanied by insomnia. Desipramine or nortriptyline have relatively low anticholinergic potential and so are useful when one must avoid exacerbating urinary retention, decreased intestinal motility, or stomatitis. Patients who are receiving multiple drugs with anticholinergic properties (e.g., meperidine, atropine, diphenhydramine, phenothiazines) are at risk for developing an anticholinergic delirium, and so tricyclics with potent anticholinergic properties should be avoided in these patients.

Second-generation antidepressants. The second-generation antidepressants are generally considered to be less cardiotoxic than the tricyclic antidepressants (Glassman 1984). Trazodone is strongly sedating and, in low doses (50–100 mg at bedtime), is helpful in the treatment of depression in patients with insomnia. Trazodone is highly serotonergic, and its use should be considered when the patient requires analgesia in addition to antidepressant effects. Trazodone has been associated with priapism and, therefore, should be used with caution in male patients (Sher et al. 1983).

At present, bupropion is not the drug of first choice for patients with depression in a medical setting; however, we would consider prescribing bupropion for patients who have a poor response to a reasonable trial of other an-

tidepressants. Bupropion may have a role in the treatment of the terminally ill patient with psychomotor retardation because this drug has energizing effects similar to those of psychostimulant drugs (Peck et al. 1983; Shopsin 1983). However, because of the increased incidence of seizures in patients with CNS disorders, bupropion has a limited role in the oncology population.

Selective serotonin reuptake inhibitors. Fluoxetine, a selective inhibitor of neuronal serotonin uptake, has fewer sedative cardiac and autonomic effects than the tricyclic antidepressants (Cooper 1988). These aspects of its side-effect profile have made fluoxetine an attractive antidepressant for use in patients who are medically ill. However, certain other common side effects seen with fluoxetine may limit its usefulness in patients with cancer who are terminally ill or dying. Fluoxetine can cause mild nausea and a brief period of increased anxiety, as well as appetite suppression that usually lasts for several weeks. Some of our patients have experienced transient weight loss, but weight usually returns to baseline level. Furthermore, fluoxetine and its active metabolite, norfluoxetine, have long half-lives. The half-life of the parent compound averages 1–4 days, and the metabolite, 7–14 days. Until it has been further studied in patients who are medically ill, we suggest cautious use of fluoxetine, particularly in patients who are debilitated and dying.

Two newer selective serotonin reuptake inhibitors (SSRIs)—sertraline and paroxetine—have shorter half-lives, and their metabolites are not significantly active (Boyer and Feighner 1991). They have been useful additions to the list of choices of antidepressants for patients who are terminally ill. Paroxetine may have the additional benefit of being a potent analgesic agent for the management of neuropathic pain (Sindrup et al. 1990). Fluvoxamine is a newly released SSRI, but little clinical experience with its use has been accumulated in patients who are medically ill. Similarly, venlafaxine, a serotonin and norepinephrine reuptake inhibitor, is newly available, and experience with its use in patients who are medically ill is being established (Feighner 1994; Khan et al. 1991). Because of its mild side-effect profile (nausea, somnolence, insomnia, elevation of blood pressure), venlafaxine might prove to be useful in medical settings.

Psychostimulants. The psychostimulants (dextroamphetamine, methylphenidate, and pemoline) offer an alternative and effective pharmacological approach to the treatment of depression in patients with terminal illnesses (Chiarillo and Cole 1987; Fernandez et al. 1987; Fisch 1985–1986; Katon and Raskind 1980; Kaufmann et al. 1982; Satel and Nelson 1989; Woods et al. 1986). These drugs have a more rapid onset of action than do the tricyclics, and they are often energizing. They are most helpful in the treatment of depression in patients with advanced disease and in those in whom dysphoric mood is associated with severe psychomotor slowing and even mild cognitive impairment. Psychostimulants have been shown to improve attention, concentration, and overall performance on neuropsychological testing in patients who are medically ill (Fernandez et al. 1988). In relatively low doses, psychostimulants improve appetite, promote a sense of well-being, and counteract feelings of weakness and fatigue. Treatment with dextroamphetamine or methylphenidate usually begins with a dose of 2.5 mg at 8:00 A.M. and at noon. The dosage is slowly increased over several days until a desired effect is achieved or side effects (overstimulation, anxiety, insomnia, paranoia, confusion) intervene. Typically, a dose greater than 30 mg/day is not necessary, although patients occasionally require up to 60 mg/day. Patients usually are maintained on methylphenidate for 1–2 months, and approximately two-thirds will be able to be withdrawn from methylphenidate without a recurrence of depressive symptoms. Those whose symptoms

do recur can be maintained on a psychostimulant for up to 1 year without significant abuse problems. Tolerance will develop, and adjustment of dose may be necessary. Additional benefits of stimulants such as methylphenidate and dextroamphetamine are that they have been shown to reduce sedation secondary to opioid analgesics, and they provide adjuvant analgesia in patients with cancer (Bruera et al. 1987). Common side effects of stimulants include nervousness, overstimulation, mild increase in blood pressure and pulse rate, and tremor. Less common side effects include dyskinesia or motor tics as well as paranoid psychosis or exacerbation of an underlying and unrecognized confusional state.

Pemoline is a unique psychostimulant that is chemically unrelated to amphetamine. It is a less potent stimulant that has little abuse potential (Chiarillo and Cole 1987). The advantages of pemoline as a psychostimulant in patients with advanced illness include the lack of abuse potential, the lack of federal regulations requiring special triplicate prescriptions, the mild sympathomimetic effects, and the fact that the drug comes in a chewable tablet form that can be absorbed through the buccal mucosa and be used by patients who have difficulty swallowing or who have intestinal obstruction. In our clinical experience, pemoline is as effective as methylphenidate or dextroamphetamine in the treatment of depressive symptoms in patients who are terminally ill (Breitbart and Mermelstein 1992). Pemoline can be started at a dose of 18.75 mg in the morning and at noon and increased gradually over days. Typically, patients require 75 mg/day or less for adequate symptom relief. Pemoline should be used with caution in patients with liver impairment, and liver function tests should be monitored periodically with longer-term treatment regimens (Stein et al. 1980).

Monoamine oxidase inhibitors. Monoamine oxidase inhibitors (MAOIs), if considered, must be used with great caution. Avoidance of tyramine-containing foods during MAOI treatment is poorly received by severely ill patients who already have dietary and nutritional restrictions. One must be extremely cautious when using narcotic analgesics in patients taking MAOIs because myoclonus and delirium have been reported with such combinations (Breitbart 1988). The concomitant use of meperidine and an MAOI is absolutely contraindicated and can lead to hyperpyrexia and cardiovascular collapse. Sympathomimetic drugs and other less obvious MAOIs, such as the chemotherapeutic agent procarbazine, can cause a hypertensive crisis in patients taking an MAOI. If a patient has responded well to an MAOI for depression in the past, its continued use is warranted but again with caution.

Lithium carbonate. Patients who were taking lithium before their illness should continue lithium therapy, if necessary, with close monitoring in the preoperative and postoperative periods when fluids and salt may be restricted. Maintenance doses of lithium may need to be reduced in patients who are seriously ill. Lithium should be prescribed with caution for patients receiving cisplatin because of the potential nephrotoxicity of both drugs. Several authors have reported that lithium can transiently stimulate leukocyte production in leukopenic cancer patients. It is unclear, however, whether such lithium-stimulated leukocytes function normally. No mood changes have been noted in such patients (Stein et al. 1980).

Electroconvulsive therapy. Occasionally, it is necessary to consider electroconvulsive therapy (ECT) for patients who have depression with psychotic features or in whom treatment with antidepressants poses unacceptable side effects. The safe, effective use of ECT in patients who are medically ill has been reviewed by others (Massie and Holland 1990).

Nonpharmacological Treatment of Depression in Patients Who Are Terminally Ill

Supportive psychotherapy is a useful treatment approach to depression in the patient who is terminally ill. Psychotherapy with the dying patient consists of active listening with supportive verbal interventions and occasional interpretation (Cassem 1987). Despite the seriousness of the patient's plight, it is not necessary for the psychiatrist or psychologist to appear overly solemn or emotionally restrained. Often, it is only the psychotherapist, of all the patient's caregivers, who is comfortable enough to converse lightheartedly and allow the patient to talk about his or her life and experiences rather than to focus solely on impending death. The dying patient who wishes to talk or ask questions about death should be allowed to do so freely, with the therapist maintaining an interested, interactive stance. It is not uncommon for the dying patient to benefit from pastoral counseling. If a chaplaincy service is available, it should be offered to the patient and family.

SUICIDE AND PATIENTS WHO ARE TERMINALLY ILL

Patients in terminal stages of illness with multiple complications such as pain, depression, delirium, and deficit symptoms are at increased risk for suicide compared with the general population. Factors associated with increased risk of suicide in patients with advanced disease (Breitbart 1987, 1990) are listed in Table 25–2.

Patients with cancer commit suicide most frequently in the advanced stages of disease (Bolund 1985; Farberow et al. 1963; Fox et al. 1982; Louhivuori and Hakama 1979). A reported 86% of suicides studied by Farberow et al. (1963) occurred in the preterminal or terminal stages of illness, despite the patient's greatly reduced physical capacity. Several studies showed that the vast majority of patients with cancer who committed suicide had

Table 25–2. Risk factors for suicide among patients with terminal illnesses

Depression and hopelessness
Debilitating illness
Uncontrolled pain
Delirium and disinhibition
Previous depression or suicide attempts
Family history of depression
Lack of social supports
History of substance abuse
Feeling of being a burden on others
Recent loss or bereavement

severe pain that was often inadequately controlled and poorly tolerated (Bolund 1985; Farberow et al. 1971).

Management of Problems in Terminally Ill Suicidal Patients

Analgesic, neuroleptic, or antidepressant medications should be utilized when appropriate to treat pain, agitation, psychosis, or major depression. Underlying causes of delirium or pain should be addressed specifically when possible. Initiation of a crisis intervention-oriented psychotherapeutic approach, mobilizing as much of the patient's support system as possible, is important.

Psychiatric hospitalization can sometimes be helpful; however, it is usually not desirable in the patient who is terminally ill. Thus, the medical hospital or home is the setting in which management most often takes place. Although it is appropriate to intervene when medical or psychiatric factors are clearly the driving force for suicidal ideation, in some circumstances, usurping control from the patient and his or her family with overly aggressive intervention may be less helpful. This is most evident in patients with advanced illness, for whom comfort and control of symptoms are the primary concerns.

The goal of the intervention should not be to prevent suicide at all cost, but to prevent suicide that is driven by desperation. Prolonged suffering because of poorly controlled symptoms leads to such desperation, and it is the consultant's role to provide effective management of such problems as an alternative to suicide in the patient who is terminally ill.

COGNITIVE IMPAIRMENT DISORDERS

Delirium is common in patients who are dying. Massie et al. (1983) found that more than 75% of terminally ill cancer patients they studied had delirium. Delirium can result from either the direct effects of cancer on the CNS or indirect CNS effects of the disease or treatments (medications, electrolyte imbalance, failure of a vital organ or system, infection, vascular complications and preexisting cognitive impairment, or dementia). Because of the large number of drugs that patients with cancer require and the fragile state of their physiological functioning, even routinely ordered hypnotics are enough to cause a delirium. Narcotic analgesics such as levorphanol, morphine sulfate, and meperidine are common causes of confusional states, particularly in elderly and terminally ill patients (Bruera et al. 1989). Chemotherapeutic agents known to cause delirium include methotrexate, fluorouracil, vincristine, vinblastine, bleomycin, carmustine, cisplatin, asparaginase, procarbazine, and the glucocorticosteroids (Adams et al. 1984; Denicoff et al. 1987; Holland et al. 1974; Stiefel et al. 1990; Weddington 1982). Except for steroids, most patients receiving these agents will not develop prominent CNS effects. The spectrum of mental disturbances related to steroids includes minor mood lability, affective disorders (mania or depression), cognitive impairment (reversible dementia), and delirium (steroid psychosis). The incidence of these disorders ranges from 3% to 57% in populations of patients without cancer, and they occur most commonly with higher doses. Symptoms usually develop within the first 2 weeks that the patient is taking steroids but can occur at any time, on any dose, even during the tapering phase. Prior psychiatric illness or prior disturbance on steroids is not a good predictor of susceptibility to or the nature of mental disturbance with steroids. These disorders are often rapidly reversible on dose reduction or discontinuation of the medication (Stiefel et al. 1989).

The treatment of delirium in the dying patient is unique because 1) most often, the etiology of terminal delirium is multifactorial or may not be found; 2) when a distinct cause is found, it is often irreversible (such as hepatic failure or brain metastases); 3) the workup may be limited by the setting (home, hospice); and 4) the consultant's focus is usually on the patient's comfort, and ordinarily helpful diagnostic procedures that are unpleasant or painful (e.g., computed tomography scan, lumbar puncture) may be avoided. When confronted with delirium in the patient with cancer who is terminally ill or dying, a differential diagnosis should always be formulated; however, studies should be pursued only when a suspected factor can be identified easily and treated effectively.

In addition to seeking out and correcting the underlying cause for delirium, symptomatic and supportive therapies are important (Lipowski 1987). In fact, in the dying patient, they may be the only steps taken. Fluid and electrolyte balance, nutritional support, and vitamins may be helpful. Measures to help reduce anxiety and disorientation (e.g., structure and familiarity) may include a quiet, well-lit room with familiar objects, a visible clock or calendar, and the presence of family. Judicious use of physical restraints, along with one-to-one nursing observation, may also be necessary and useful. Often, these supportive techniques alone are not effective, and symptomatic treatment with neuroleptic or sedative medications is necessary.

The use of neuroleptics in the management of delirium in the dying patient remains controversial in some circles. Some have argued that pharmacological interventions with

neuroleptics or benzodiazepines are inappropriate in the dying patient. Delirium is viewed as a natural part of the dying process that should not be altered. Another rationale that is often presented is that these patients are so close to death that aggressive treatment is unnecessary. Parenteral neuroleptics or sedatives may be mistakenly avoided because of exaggerated fears that these drugs might hasten death through hypotension or respiratory depression. Many clinicians are unnecessarily pessimistic about the possible results of neuroleptic treatment for delirium. They argue that because the underlying pathophysiological process (such as hepatic or renal failure) often continues unabated, no improvement can be expected in the patient's mental status. Physicians may be concerned that neuroleptics or sedatives may worsen a delirium by making the patient more confused or sedated. Our clinical experience in managing delirium in patients with cancer who are dying suggests that the use of neuroleptics in the management of agitation, paranoia, hallucinations, and altered sensorium is safe, effective, and quite appropriate. Management of delirium on a case-by-case basis seems most wise. The agitated patient with delirium who is dying should probably be given neuroleptics to help restore calm. A "wait and see" approach before using neuroleptics may be most appropriate with patients who have a lethargic or somnolent presentation of delirium. The consultant must educate staff, patients, and families and weigh each of these issues in making the decision whether to use pharmacological interventions for the dying patient who presents with delirium.

PAIN

From 60% to 90% of patients with advanced cancer experience pain (Foley 1985). Pain is also frequent in patients with advanced AIDS. Pain usually symbolizes advancing disease and is therefore experienced with more dread and suffering because of this meaning. Depression and anxiety also increase the experience of pain. In the evaluation of pain, the first step is to assess quality of pain, time course, fluctuations, and factors that exacerbate or relieve it. Mental status examination and medical and neurological evaluations are performed. Pain is also assessed repeatedly because the analgesic dosage is titrated against the level of pain and alertness (Elliott and Foley 1990).

Management of Pain in Patients Who Are Terminally Ill

Pharmacological therapy is central to the management of physiologically based pain. The nonnarcotic analgesics, opioids, and adjuvant analgesic drugs have specific indications. The nonopioid analgesics—that is, the nonsteroidal anti-inflammatory drugs (NSAIDs)—are prescribed for mild to moderate pain. Opioid analgesics are prescribed for moderate to severe pain. Opioids are a diverse group of compounds that bind to specific opioid receptors. They are subdivided into agonists, antagonists, and agonist-antagonists (this last group having both analgesic and antagonist properties). The narcotic agonists morphine, hydromorphone, and levorphanol are the preferred analgesics.

To treat pain adequately, clinicians should observe the following principles (Portenoy and Foley 1989):

1. Choose a specific drug for the specific level of pain—for example, codeine or oxycodone for moderate pain, morphine or a morphinelike agonist for moderate to severe pain.
2. Know the duration of effect and the pharmacokinetics of the drug chosen—for example, morphine and hydromorphone have short half-lives, and methadone and levorphanol have long half-lives.
3. Prescribe analgesics around the clock. As-needed dosing, which requires the pa-

tient's request, results in considerable time loss, anxiety, and increased pain.
4. Remember that combinations of drugs, such as opioids and nonnarcotic analgesics, have additive effects.
5. Treat patients who have analgesic-induced sedation with low doses of stimulants, and use high-potency neuroleptics for delirium.

STAFF ISSUES IN CARE OF DYING PATIENTS

Working with the dying patient produces a spectrum of painful emotions in the caregivers: helplessness, fear, guilt, anger, inadequacy, intolerance, vulnerability, overattachment, lack of control, ambivalence, and frustration (Barton 1977). These negative emotions are increased when the staff member experiences a personal loss, an illness, or a significant conflict or crisis. In one study, Kash and Holland (1990) found that the stress was buffered by three primary factors: a personal system of beliefs about life and death, a high level of peer support, and a supportive supervisor. Nurses and doctors who had the responsibility of taking care of patients dying of cancer and who considered themselves to be religious scored lower on the measures of burnout, suggesting that an existential perspective helped them to handle the stress of caring for many dying patients. The data also underscore the importance of social support derived from a cohesive staff with adequate supervision. A consultation-liaison psychiatrist is often able to identify problems that arise from poor cohesion and poor delineation of lines of authority.

The psychiatrist should monitor staff responses and be prepared to serve as a person with whom professional issues can be raised when the care of dying patients produces troublesome distress. Regular support meetings are helpful to promote the discussion of problems and interdisciplinary conflicts; a special meeting for staff should be arranged around a particularly difficult management problem or the death of a special patient. Providing support is draining, at times, for all caregivers. In evaluating a caregiver, the staff member's prior loss history should be obtained because overinvolvement or inappropriate underinvolvement most often reflects an unrecognized countertransference (Sourkes 1982). Teaching of medical and psychiatric team members should include admonitions to monitor self and colleagues for stress level. The value of sharing experiences with colleagues, including seeking psychiatric consultation, must be stressed.

SUMMARY

The patient who is dying presents a range of problems that the consultation-liaison psychiatrist is skilled at managing: the psychological aspects of the existential crisis; the management of comorbid psychiatric disorders such as anxiety, depression, and delirium; the management of pain; support of the patient in end-of-life decisions; advocacy for the patient; and teaching of medical staff about the psychological aspects of dying.

REFERENCES

Adams F, Quesada JR, Gutterman JU: Neuropsychiatric manifestations of human leukocyte interferon therapy in patients with cancer. JAMA 252:938–941, 1984

Barton D: The dying person, in Dying and Death: A Clinical Guide for Caregivers. Edited by Barton D. Baltimore, MD, Williams & Wilkins, 1977, pp 41–58

Bolund C: Suicide and cancer, II: medical and care factors in suicide by cancer patients in Sweden. Journal of Psychosocial Oncology 3: 17–30, 1985

Bottomley DM, Hanks GW: Subcutaneous midozolam infusion in palliative care. J Pain Symptom Manage 5:259–261, 1990

Boyer WF, Feighner JP: Side effects of the selective serotonin reuptake inhibitors, in Selective Serotonin Reuptake Inhibitors. Edited by Feighner JP, Boyer WF. Chichester, UK, Wiley, 1991

Breitbart W: Suicide in cancer patients. Oncology 1:49–53, 1987

Breitbart W: Psychiatric complications of cancer, in Current Therapy in Hematology, 3rd Edition. Edited by Brain MC, Carbone PP. Philadelphia, PA, Marcel Dekker, 1988, pp 268–274

Breitbart WB: Endocrine-related psychiatric disorders, in Handbook of Psychooncology: Psychological Care of the Patient With Cancer. Edited by Holland JC, Rowland JH. New York, Oxford University Press, 1989a, pp 356–366

Breitbart W: Cancer pain and suicide, in Advances in Pain Research and Therapy, Vol 16. Edited by Foley K, Bonica JJ, Ventafridda V, et al. New York, Raven, 1990, pp 399–412

Breitbart W, Mermelstein H: Pemoline: an alternative psychostimulant for the management of depressive disorders in cancer patients. Psychosomatics 33:352–356, 1992

Bruera E, Chadwick S, Brennels C, et al: Methylphenidate associated with narcotics for the treatment of cancer pain. Cancer Treatment Reports 71:67–70, 1987

Bruera E, MacMillan K, Kuchn N, et al: The cognitive effects of the administration of narcotics. Pain 39:13–16, 1989

Bukberg J, Holland JC: A prevalence study of depression in a cancer hospital population (abstract). Proceedings of the American Association for Cancer Research 21:382, 1980

Bukberg J, Penman D, Holland J: Depression in hospitalized cancer patients. Psychosom Med 46:199–212, 1984

Cassem NH: The dying patient, in Massachusetts General Hospital Handbook of General Hospital Psychiatry, 2nd Edition. Edited by Hackett TP, Cassem NH. Littleton, MA, PSG Publishing, 1987, pp 332–352

Chiarillo RY, Cole YO: The use of psychostimulants in general psychiatry. Arch Gen Psychiatry 44:286–295, 1987

Chochinov HM, Wilson KG, Enns M, et al: Prevalence of depression in the terminally ill: effects of diagnostic criteria and symptom threshold judgments. Am J Psychiatry 151:537–540, 1994

Cooper GL: The safety of fluoxetine: an update. Br J Psychiatry 153:77–86, 1988

Costa D, Mogos I, Toma T: Efficacy and safety of mianserin in the treatment of depression of women with cancer. Acta Psychiatr Scand 72 (suppl 320):85–92, 1985

Dean C: Psychiatric morbidity following mastectomy: preoperative predictors and types of illness. J Psychosom Res 31:385–392, 1987

DeAngelis LM, Delattre J, Posner JB: Radiation-induced dementia in patients cured of brain metastases. Neurology 39:789–796, 1989

Denicoff KD, Rubinow DR, Papa MZ, et al: The neuropsychiatric effects of treatment with interleukin-2 and lymphokine-activated killer cells. Ann Intern Med 107:293–300, 1987

Derogatis LR, Morrow GR, Fetting J, et al: The prevalence of psychiatric disorders among cancer patients. JAMA 249:751–757, 1983

DeSousa E, Jepson A: Midazolam in terminal care. Lancet 1:67–68, 1988

Elliott K, Foley KM: Pain syndromes. Journal of Psychosocial Oncology 8:11–45, 1990

Evans DL, McCartney CF, Nemeroff CB, et al: Depression in women treated for gynecological cancer: clinical and neuroendocrine assessment. Am J Psychiatry 143:447–452, 1986

Farberow NL, Schneidman ES, Leonard CV: Suicide Among General Medical and Surgical Hospital Patients With Malignant Neoplasms: Medical Bulletin 9. Washington, DC, U.S. Veterans Administration, 1963

Farberow NL, Ganzler S, Cuter F, et al: An eight-year survey of hospital suicides. Suicide Life Threat Behav 1:1984–2001, 1971

Feighner JP: The role of venlafaxine in national antidepressant therapy. J Clin Psychiatry 55:62–68, 1994

Fernandez F, Adams F, Holmes VF, et al: Methylphenidate for depressive disorders in cancer patients. Psychosomatics 28:455–461, 1987

Fernandez F, Adams F, Levy J, et al: Cognitive impairment due to AIDS related complex and its response to psychostimulants. Psychosomatics 29:38–46, 1988

Fisch R: Methylphenidate for medical inpatients. Int J Psychiatry Med 15:75–79, 1985–1986

Foley KM: The treatment of cancer pain. N Engl J Med 313:84–95, 1985

Fox BH, Stanek EJ, Boyd SC, et al: Suicide rates among cancer patients in Connecticut. Journal of Chronic Disease 35:89–100, 1982

Glassman AH: The newer antidepressant drugs and their cardiovascular effects. Psychopharmacol Bull 20:272–279, 1984

Hinton J: Psychiatric consultation in fatal illness. Proceedings of the Royal Society of Medicine 65:29–32, 1972

Holland JC: Anxiety and cancer: the patient and family. J Clin Psychiatry 50:20–25, 1989

Holland JC, Fasanello S, Ohnuma T: Psychiatric symptoms associated with L-asparaginase administration. J Psychiatr Res 10:105–113, 1974

Holland JC, Morrow G, Schmale A, et al: Reduction of anxiety and depression in cancer patients by alprazolam or by a behavioral technique (abstract). Proceedings of the American Society of Clinical Oncology 6:258, 1987

Kash KM, Holland JC: Reducing stress in medical oncology house officers: a preliminary report of a prospective intervention study, in Educating Competent and Humane Physicians. Edited by Hendrie HC, Lloyd C. Bloomington, IN, University Press, 1990, pp 183–195

Kathol RG, Mutgi A, Williams J, et al: Diagnosis of major depression in cancer patients according to four sets of criteria. Am J Psychiatry 147:1021–1024, 1990

Katon W, Raskind M: Treatment of depression in the medically ill elderly with methylphenidate. Am J Psychiatry 137:963–965, 1980

Kaufmann MW, Murray GB, Cassem NH: Use of psychostimulants in medically ill depressed patients. Psychosomatics 23:817–819, 1982

Khan A, Fabre LF, Rudolph R: Venlafaxine in depressed outpatients. Psychopharmacol Bull 27:141–144, 1991

Lansky SB, Lizt MA, Herrman CA, et al: Absence of major depressive disorder in female cancer patients. J Clin Oncol 3:1553–1560, 1985

Levine PM, Silberfarb PM, Lipowski ZJ: Mental disorders in cancer patients: a study of 100 psychiatric referrals. Cancer 42:1385–1391, 1978

Lieber L, Plumb MM, Gerstenzang ML, et al: The communication of affection between cancer patients and their spouses. Psychosom Med 38:379–389, 1976

Lipowski ZJ: Delirium (acute confusional states). JAMA 285:89–92, 1987

Louhivuori KA, Hakama J: Risk of suicide among cancer patients. Am J Epidemiol 109:59–65, 1979

Massie MJ: Anxiety, panic, phobias, in Handbook of Psychooncology: Psychological Care of the Patient With Cancer. Edited by Holland JC, Rowland JH. New York, Oxford University Press, 1989, pp 300–309

Massie MJ, Holland JC: The cancer patient with pain: psychiatric complications and their management. Med Clin North Am 71:243–248, 1987

Massie MJ, Holland JC: Depression and the cancer patient. J Clin Psychiatry 51:12–17, 1990

Massie MJ, Gorzynski JG, Mastrovito R, et al: The diagnosis of depression in hospitalized patients with cancer (abstract). Proceedings of the American Society of Clinical Oncology 20:432, 1979

Massie MJ, Holland JC, Glass E: Delirium in terminally ill cancer patients. Am J Psychiatry 140:1048–1050, 1983

Massie MJ, Holland JC, Straker N: Psychotherapeutic interventions, in Handbook of Psychooncology: Psychological Care of the Patient With Cancer. Edited by Holland JC, Rowland JH. New York, Oxford University Press, 1989, pp 455–469

Mastrovito R: Behavioral techniques: progressive relaxation and self regulatory therapies, in Handbook of Psychooncology: Psychological Care of the Patient With Cancer. Edited by Holland JC, Rowland JH. New York, Oxford University Press, 1989, pp 492–501

Mermelstein HT, Lesko L: Depression in patients with cancer. Psycho-oncology 1:199–215, 1992

Morton RP, Davies ADM, Baker J, et al: Quality of life in treated head and neck cancer patients: a preliminary report. Clin Otolaryngol 9:181–185, 1984

Patchell RA, Posner JB: Cancer and the nervous system, in Handbook of Psychooncology: Psychological Care of the Patient With Cancer. Edited by Holland JC, Rowland JH. New York, Oxford University Press, 1989, pp 327–341

Peck AW, Stern WC, Watkinson C: Incidence of seizures during treatment with tricyclic antidepressant drugs and bupropion. J Clin Psychiatry 44:197–201, 1983

Plumb MM, Holland JC: Comparative studies of psychological function in patients with advanced cancer, II: interviewer-rated current and past psychological symptoms. Psychosom Med 39:264–276, 1977

Popkin MK, Callies AL, MacKenzie TB: The outcome of antidepressant use in the medically ill. Arch Gen Psychiatry 42:1160–1163, 1985

Portenoy R, Foley KM: Management of cancer pain, in Handbook of Psychooncology: Psychological Care of the Patient With Cancer. Edited by Holland JC, Rowland JH. New York, Oxford University Press, 1989, pp 369–382

Posner JB: Nonmetastic effects of cancer on the nervous system, in Cecil's Textbook of Medicine, 8th Edition. Edited by Wyngaarden JB, Smith LH. Philadelphia, PA, WB Saunders, 1988, pp 1104–1107

Purohit DR, Nevlakha PL, Modi RS, et al: The role of antidepressants in hospitalized cancer patients. J Assoc Physicians India 26:245–248, 1978

Rifkin A, Reardon G, Siris S, et al: Trimipramine in physical illness with depression. J Clin Psychiatry 46 (sect 2):4–8, 1985

Satel SL, Nelson CJ: Stimulants in the treatment of depression: a critical overview. J Clin Psychiatry 50:241–249, 1989

Schachter S: Quality of life for families in the management of home care patients with advanced cancer. J Palliat Care 8:61–66, 1992

Sher M, Krieger JN, Juergen S: Trazodone and priapism. Am J Psychiatry 140:1362–1364, 1983

Shopsin B: Bupropion: a new clinical profile in the psychobiology of depression. J Clin Psychiatry 44:140–142, 1983

Sindrup SH, Gram LF, Brosen K, et al: The selective serotonin reuptake inhibitor paroxetine is effective in the treatment of diabetic neuropathy symptoms. Pain 42:135–144, 1990

Sourkes BM: The Deepening Shade: Psychological Aspects of Life Threatening Illness. Pittsburgh, PA, University of Pittsburgh Press, 1982

Spiegel D, Bloom JR: Group therapy and hypnosis reduce metastatic breast carcinoma pain. Psychosom Med 4:333–339, 1983

Spiegel D, Bloom JR, Yalom ID: Group support for patients with metastatic cancer: a randomized prospective outcome study. Arch Gen Psychiatry 38:527–533, 1981

Stein RS, Flexner JH, Graber SE: Lithium and granulocytopenia during induction therapy of acute myelogenous leukemia: update of an ongoing trial. Adv Exp Med Biol 127:1517–1519, 1980

Stiefel FC, Breitbart W, Holland JC: Corticosteroids in cancer: neuropsychiatric complications. Cancer Invest 7:479–491, 1989

Stiefel FC, Kornblith AB, Holland JC: Changes in the prescription patterns of psychotropic drugs for cancer patients during a 10 year period. Cancer 65:1048–1053, 1990

Stoudemire A, Fogel BS: Psychopharmacology in the medically ill, in Principles of Medical Psychiatry. Edited by Stoudemire A, Fogel BS. Orlando, FL, Grune & Stratton, 1987, pp 79–112

Twycross RG, Lack SA: Therapeutics in Terminal Disease. London, Pitman Brooks, 1984, pp 99–103

Weddington WW: Delirium and depression associated with amphotericin B. Psychosomatics 23:1076–1078, 1982

Weddington WW, Segraves KB, Simon MA: Current and lifetime incidence of psychiatric disorders among a group of extremity sarcoma survivors. J Psychosom Res 30:121–125, 1986

Weisman AD: On Dying and Denying: A Psychiatric Study of Terminality. New York, Behavioral Publications, 1972

Woods SW, Tesar GE, Murray GB, et al: Psychostimulant treatment of depressive disorders secondary to medical illness. J Clin Psychiatry 47:12–15, 1986

Young DF: Neurological complications of cancer chemotherapy, in Neurological Complications of Therapy: Selected Topics. Edited by Silverstein A. New York, Futura Publishing, 1982, pp 57–113

Chapter 26

HIV Disease/AIDS

Jonathan L. Worth, M.D.
Mark H. Halman, M.D., F.R.C.P.C.

The optimum psychiatric treatment of adult patients with human immunodeficiency virus/acquired immunodeficiency syndrome (HIV/AIDS[1]) requires that consultation-liaison psychiatrists understand 1) the transmission of HIV/AIDS; 2) the natural course of systemic HIV disease and general principles of its treatment; 3) HIV-1 central nervous system (CNS) infection and related neurological complications; 4) the diagnosis and management of psychiatric syndromes associated with HIV/AIDS; 5) aspects of pharmacotherapy that are unique to patients with HIV/AIDS; and 6) psychosocial factors that affect the illness course and implications for psychotherapeutic intervention.

◼ TRANSMISSION OF HIV

Effective media for the transmission of HIV-1 include blood and body fluids with visible blood, semen, vaginal secretions, breast milk, and cerebrospinal, synovial, pleural, peritoneal, pericardial, and amniotic fluids. In handling these media, universal safety precautions must be utilized. HIV-1 has not been shown to be transmissible through contact with nasal secretions, sputum, sweat, tears, urine, or vomitus, unless these fluids contain visible blood. There is no evidence of transmission by food, water, coughing, sneezing, mosquitoes, or insects. There is no clear evidence of HIV-1 transmission through close personal contact with an HIV-infected person at home, work, or school (Bartlett 1994).

Patients with major mental illness in urban areas with high AIDS prevalence appear to be at increased risk for HIV-1 infection. Studies from New York City demonstrate an estimated 6%–8% HIV-1 seroprevalence rate in this population, based on the serological testing of patients who were consecutively admitted to two public psychiatric hospitals (Cournos et al.

---

[1]HIV/AIDS applies to both HIV infection or persons with HIV infection and to full-blown AIDS or persons with AIDS.

1991) and a private, voluntary psychiatric hospital (Sacks et al. 1992), as well as a population of homeless, mentally ill patients committed to an inpatient psychiatric facility (Empfield et al. 1993). There were no racial or gender differences in seroprevalence rates in these studies. Schizophrenia or schizoaffective disorder was diagnosed in 54%–92% of these patients, with a majority of such patients engaged in frequent sexual activity involving high-risk behavior for HIV infection (Cournos et al. 1994).

THE VIRUS AND THE COURSE OF HIV DISEASE

HIV-1 is a ribonucleic acid (RNA) virus belonging to the cytopathic lentivirus family of retroviruses. Lentiviruses cause slowly progressive neurodegeneration, progressive immunodeficiency, or both. The HIV-1 viral particle is composed of an outer envelope and an inner core. The envelope is made up of 72 protruding, knoblike glycoproteins (gp120s), each of which is anchored on the lipid bilayer surface by glycoproteins known as gp41s. The viral core is a dense, cylindrical nucleoid containing core proteins, genomic RNA, and the reverse transcriptase enzyme, components that are necessary for the integration of the viral genome into the mammalian host's genome. Infection involves the attachment of the gp120 knobs to the CD4+ receptor sites on cells that bear the CD4 receptor on their surface, including T4+ (or helper) lymphocytes, as well as monocytes and macrophages. After binding, the virus enters the host cell and is uncoated. Viral RNA is transcribed into viral deoxyribonucleic acid (DNA) by the reverse transcriptase enzyme and is integrated into the host cell genome. HIV-1 replication occurs when the infected cell is activated and newly formed virions are released (Greene 1991; Ho et al. 1987).

The course of HIV-1 infection (Fauci 1993; Pantaleo et al. 1993) is characterized by asymptomatic primary infection and a prolonged period of clinical latency. Initial infection commonly produces no manifestations, although some patients will report a seroconversion syndrome involving fever, rash, myalgias, headache, photophobia, and stiff neck at some point in the first 12 weeks after infection. A detectable humoral and cellular immune response to the infection occurs 3–6 weeks thereafter. HIV-1 disease progresses during the period of asymptomatic infection, during which there is a gradual decline in markers of the cellular immune system. The progression of systemic HIV-1 disease parallels the decline in the host's immune system (see Figure 26–1).

After a mean interval of 7–11 years, AIDS-defining conditions—that is, opportunistic infections, neoplasms, and HIV-related neurological disorders—begin to occur (Brookmeyer 1991; Muñoz et al. 1989). The CD4+ lymphocyte count is the most useful marker of progression of immunological decline and predictor of disease progression (Fahey et al. 1990). At counts below 500 cells/mL, patients who are infected are at risk for developing symptomatic but non-AIDS-defining conditions. Below 200 cells/mL, patients are at increased risk for opportunistic infections; prophylactic treatment for *Pneumocystis carinii* pneumonia is recommended (Phair et al. 1990). At counts below 50 cells/mL, patients are at increased risk for fatal HIV-related illness (Yarchoan et al. 1991).

Treatment and management of systemic HIV-1 disease include the use of antiretroviral agents active against HIV-1 as well as aggressive treatment and prophylaxis against opportunistic infections and severe constitutional syndromes. The current mainstay of antiretroviral treatment relies on inhibiting viral reverse transcriptase (Connolly and Hammer 1992) with nucleoside analogues, including AZT, didanosine (also known as dideoxyinosine, or ddI), and zalcitabine (dideoxycytidine, or ddC). AZT has been shown to reduce morbidity and prolong life among patients with symptomatic HIV-1 disease, in-

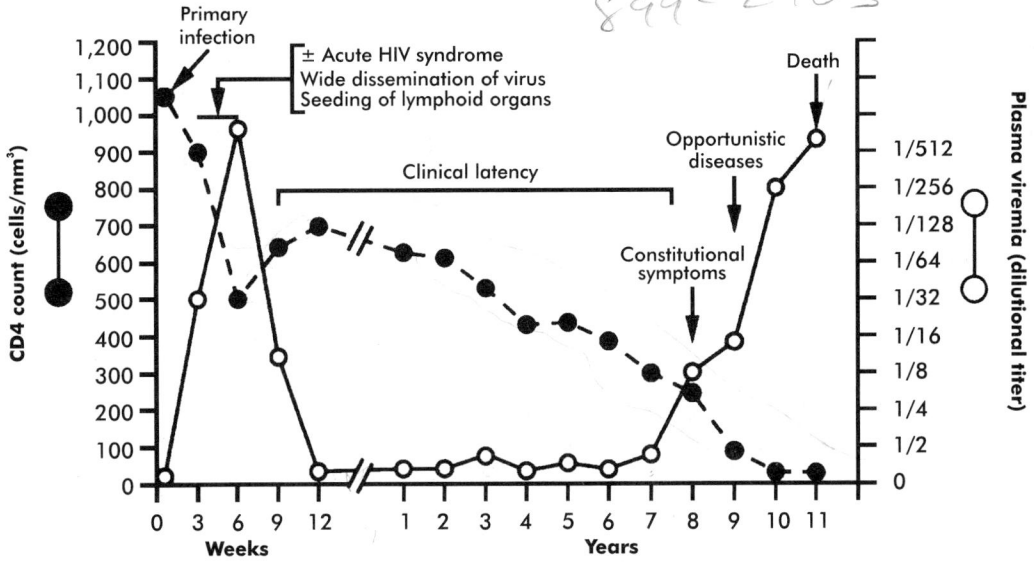

770.6219
899-2903

Figure 26–1. Typical course of HIV-1 infection. *Source.* Reprinted from Pantaleo G, Graziosi C, Fauci AS: "The Immunopathogenesis of Human Immunodeficiency Virus Infection." *New England Journal of Medicine* 328:327–335, 1993. Copyright 1993, Massachusetts Medical Society. All rights reserved. Used with permission.

cluding both those with AIDS and those with symptomatic non-AIDS-defining conditions (Fischl et al. 1987). It has also been shown to prevent HIV transmission from mother to newborn (Centers for Disease Control and Prevention 1994). Both ddI and ddC appear to be as effective as AZT and are approved for use in patients who are unresponsive to or intolerant of AZT and for use in combination with AZT. All of these nucleoside agents are associated with neuropsychiatric symptoms (see Table 26–1). For adequate absorption, ddI must be taken on an empty stomach, which can be logistically frustrating for patients who are taking many medications. ddC is associated with pancreatitis, which can severely limit its use in patients with a history of pancreatitis or alcohol abuse or dependence. These numerous side effects can add to the already considerable morbidity experienced by HIV/AIDS patients. The compromised quality of life can, on balance, outweigh the benefits of such medications (Gelber et al. 1992; Lenderking et al. 1994), leading patients to consider discontinuing treatment.

HIV/AIDS HEALTH CARE DELIVERY: CLINICAL AND SOCIAL CONTEXTS

The changes in HIV/AIDS epidemiology, the clinical course of HIV-1 infection, and the increasing efficacy of medical treatment and management of HIV/AIDS have all affected HIV-related health care services and their delivery in ways that influence psychiatric consultation on patients with HIV/AIDS. Decreased rates of hospitalization and lengths of stay have resulted from increased clinical expertise with HIV/AIDS care (Stone et al. 1992), a shift from patients dying in the hospital to their dying at home (Kelly et al. 1993), the development of dedicated, multidisciplinary HIV/AIDS outpatient clinics, and the advent of home infusion therapies for AIDS-related conditions. Consequently, psychiatric consultations on inpatients may occur less frequently but will increasingly involve more acutely ill patients, and outpatient consultations during clinic or home visits will probably increase.

Table 26–1.   Neuropsychiatric side effects of medications frequently used for HIV/AIDS

Drug	Side effect(s)	Drug	Side effect(s)
Acyclovir	Visual hallucinations	Methotrexate	Encephalopathy (high-dose)
	Depersonalization	Pentamidine	Hypoglycemia
	Tearfulness		Hypotension
	Confusion	Procarbazine	Mania
	Hyperesthesia		Loss of appetite
	Hyperacusia		Insomnia
	Thought insertion		Nightmares
	Insomnia		Confusion
	Agitation		Malaise
Amphotericin B	Delirium	Stavudine (d4T)	Mania
	Peripheral neuropathy	Steroids	Depression
	Diplopia		Euphoria
	Anorexia		Mania
Co-trimoxazole	Depression		Psychosis
	Loss of appetite	Thiabendazole	Hallucinations
	Insomnia		Olfactory disturbance
	Apathy	Vinblastine	Depression
	Headache		Anorexia
Didanosine (ddI)	Insomnia		Headache
	Peripheral neuropathy	Vincristine	Depression
	Mania		Hallucinations
Ganciclovir	Mania		Headache
	Psychosis		Ataxia
	Agitation		Sensory loss
	Delirium		Agitation
	Irritability	Zidovudine (AZT)	Headache
Interferon-α	Depression		Restlessness
	Weakness (dose-dependent)		Agitation
Isoniazid	Depression		Insomnia
	Agitation		Mania
	Hallucinations		Depression
	Paranoia		Irritability
	Impaired memory		

Note.   AIDS = acquired immunodeficiency syndrome; HIV = human immunodeficiency virus.

The breadth of the psychiatric consultation may extend beyond the patient to include the patient's care providers, who must not only care for severely ill young adults with a fatal illness but also face the social issues of HIV-related stigmatization. Clinically elevated levels of depression and anxiety have been observed in health care providers (Bellani et al. 1993) and community volunteers (Hawkins and Halprin 1992) who care for patients with AIDS, which has been referred to as "AIDS burnout." The consultation-liaison psychiatrist should refer such persons to community-based HIV/AIDS organizations that sponsor support groups for persons with AIDS burnout.

NEUROPSYCHIATRIC SYNDROMES

Because patients with HIV/AIDS are at high risk for secondary neuropsychiatric disorders, any change in mental status in a person with HIV infection must be considered to be secondary to a medical or toxic cause until proven otherwise. The neuropsychiatric differential diagnosis must broadly include the following causes: 1) HIV-1 CNS infection and associated disorders; 2) opportunistic infections and tumors; 3) metabolic consequences of systemic HIV-1 disease; 4) primary psychiatric disorders, including psychoactive substance-related disorders; 5) other neurological-medical complications of HIV-1 disease; and 6) medication side effects. The differential diagnosis of mental status changes in an individual with HIV infection is outlined in Table 26–2.

HIV-1 CENTRAL NERVOUS SYSTEM INFECTION AND NEUROLOGICAL DISEASE

HIV-1 is highly neuroinvasive and is thought to enter the CNS shortly after primary infection (Davis et al. 1992), being carried to the CNS via blood-borne infected macrophages (Peudenier et al. 1991). In addition, HIV-1 is highly neurotropic, infecting endothelial cells, the spinal cord (Ho et al. 1985), and the brain parenchyma, including glia, astrocytes, and oligodendrocytes, but sparing neurons (Wiley et al. 1986). HIV-1 is also neurovirulent, causing cell injury, dysfunction, and death (Navia et al. 1986b; Shaw et al. 1985).

The proposed pathophysiological mechanisms of AIDS dementia complex (ADC) suggest that CNS injury is due to direct and indirect effects of HIV-1 infection as well as the indirect consequences of the immune response mounted against it—early brain invasion and infection of nonneuronal cells by HIV-1 (e.g., microglia, astrocytes, macrophages) (Davis et al. 1992). This reservoir of HIV-1-infected cells and the production of viral products lead to activation of the cellular components of the immune system. These events alter the blood-brain barrier, with recruitment of additional immune components and further cytokine liberation. These several pathways ultimately lead to the production of excitoneurotoxins. The severity of ADC generally parallels the progression of systemic HIV-1 disease, with minimal to mild symptoms of ADC occurring during otherwise asymptomatic stages and more severe symptoms of ADC occurring during advanced stages of systemic HIV-1 disease. Systemic and CNS HIV-1 infection may lead to blood-brain barrier alterations and cytokine production and may enhance the production of neurotoxins and progression of ADC.

Neuropathology

In advanced cases of ADC, white matter and subcortical gray structures are primarily affected, with relative sparing of cortical gray matter. Pathological studies show diffuse white matter pallor, multifocal perivascular rarefaction, and focal vacuolation, with perivascular and parenchymal collections of macrophages, lymphocytes, and multinucleated giant cells, particularly in the centrum semiovale, basal ganglia, and pons (Navia et al. 1986b). The neuropathology of early stage ADC shows white matter myelin pallor and mild astrocytosis, without the inflammatory infiltrates, multinucleated giant cells, or brain atrophy of advanced-stage ADC (McArthur et al. 1989a, 1989b). The correlation of neuropathological (Budka et al. 1987) and clinical diagnostic criteria for ADC is poor, with an accuracy of only 50% (McArthur et al. 1992). Patients without clinical ADC can show all these neuropathological abnormalities.

Table 26–2. Differential diagnosis of HIV-1-related mental status changes

CNS opportunistic infections		Endocrinopathies and specific nutrient deficiencies
Fungi	*Cryptococcus, Histoplasma, Candida, Aspergillus*	Addison's disease (secondary to HIV-1, CMV, ketoconazole)
Parasites	*Toxoplasma,* ameba, others (endemic)	Hypothyroidism
Viruses	Creutzfeldt-Jakob papovavirus (progressive multifocal leukoencephalopathy), CMV,[a] herpes simplex, herpes zoster, human herpesvirus-6[b]	Overt low serum levels of zinc and vitamins B_6, B_{12}, A, and E in patients with asymptomatic infection;[f] B_{12} deficiency in up to 20% of patients who are referred for neurological evaluation[g]
Bacteria	*Mycobacterium avium-intracellulare, Mycobacterium tuberculosis,* gram-negative bacteria, *Treponema pallidum* (neurosyphilis found in 1.8% of patients infected with HIV-1 who are referred for neurological evaluation)[c]	Hypogonadism

CNS opportunistic infections

Neoplasms

Primary CNS non-Hodgkin's lymphoma: prevalence rate of 1.9% in patients with AIDS[d]

Metastatic Kaposi's sarcoma (? herpeslike virus)[e]

Burkitt's lymphoma

Others

Drug-related neurotoxicities

Endocrinopathies and specific nutrient deficiencies

Anemia

Metabolic abnormalities

Hypoxic encephalopathy

First-degree Axis I psychiatric disorders

Major depressive episode

Bipolar disorder

Schizophrenia

Psychoactive substance intoxication or withdrawal

Non-HIV-1-related medical or neurological illness

Alzheimer's disease in patients older than 65 years

Multi-infarct dementia in patients with hypertension

SLE in African American women of childbearing age: prevalence = 1/250

Note. AIDS = acquired immunodeficiency syndrome; CMV = cytomegalovirus; CNS = central nervous system; HIV = human immunodeficiency virus; SLE = systemic lupus erythematosus.
Source. [a]Wiley and Nelson 1988; [b]Knox and Carrigan 1995; [c]Berger 1991; [d]R. M. Levy and Bredesen 1988; [e]Chang et al. 1994; [f]Beach et al. 1992; [g]Kieburtz et al. 1991a.

AIDS DEMENTIA COMPLEX: CLINICAL SYNDROME, TREATMENT, AND MANAGEMENT

Nomenclature

The neurodegenerative disorder associated with HIV-1 infection has been variously termed *HIV-1 subacute encephalitis, HIV-1 encephalopathy* (Centers for Disease Control 1987), *ADC* (Navia et al. 1986a), and *HIV dementia* (McArthur et al. 1989a, 1989b). Dementia due

to HIV disease is the diagnosis in DSM-IV (American Psychiatric Association 1994), under the classification *cognitive impairment disorder,* that refers to this syndrome.

Prevalence

The clinical syndrome of ADC was initially characterized in 1986, before widespread use of AZT and the aggressive treatment and prophylaxis of opportunistic infections. At that time, ADC was estimated to affect up to two-thirds of AIDS patients (Navia et al. 1986a). Since the clinical introduction of AZT and improved prophylaxis against and treatment of opportunistic infections, some (Portegies et al. 1989), but not all (Bacellar et al. 1994), studies have demonstrated a decreased prevalence of ADC. Recent prevalence estimates for patients with ADC—that is, for patients at stage 2 or above according to the Memorial Sloan-Kettering (MSK) Clinical Staging System for ADC (see Table 26–3)—among those with advanced HIV-1 disease are 15%–19% (Janssen et al. 1992; McArthur et al. 1992), with an annual incidence of 3%–7% (Grant et al. 1993). Approximately 4% of patients with HIV-1 infection present with ADC as their AIDS-defining diagnosis. Risk factors for developing ADC include anemia, wasting syndrome, the number of constitutional symptoms that occur before

AIDS diagnosis, and older age (Janssen et al. 1992; McArthur et al. 1992).

The frequency of cognitive dysfunction secondary to HIV-1 infection appears to parallel the progression of systemic HIV-1 disease. Similar patterns of cognitive deficits in patients with symptomatic HIV-1 disease have been demonstrated among all major HIV/AIDS risk groups (Maj et al. 1994b) and in studies specifically involving gay and bisexual men (McArthur et al. 1989a, 1989b; Saykin et al. 1988; Tross et al. 1988) and users of injection drugs (Handelsman et al. 1992; Selnes et al. 1992).

Among ambulatory patients presenting for psychiatric treatment, the prevalence of ADC has been reported as 1%–12%, paralleling the stage of systemic disease (O'Dowd et al. 1993; Worth et al. 1993b). The percentage of inpa-

Table 26–3. Memorial Sloan-Kettering Clinical Staging System for ADC

ADC stage	Degree of severity	Characteristic
Stage 0	Normal	Normal mental and motor function.
Stage 0.5	Equivocal	Either minimal or equivocal symptoms of cognitive or motor dysfunction characteristic of HIV-1-associated cognitive/motor complex, or mild signs (snout response, slowed extremity movements), but without impairment of work or capacity to perform ADLs. Gait and strength are normal.
Stage 1	Mild	Unequivocal evidence (symptoms, signs, neuropsychological test performance) of functional intellectual or motor impairment characteristic of HIV-1-associated cognitive/motor complex, but able to perform all but the more demanding aspects of work or ADLs. Can walk without assistance.
Stage 2	Moderate	Cannot walk or maintain the more demanding ADLs, but able to perform basic ADLs of self-care. Ambulatory, but may require a single prop.
Stage 3	Severe	Major intellectual incapacity (cannot follow news or personal events, cannot sustain complex conversation, considerable slowing of all output) or motor disability (cannot walk unassisted, requiring walker or personal support, usually with slowing and clumsiness of arms as well).
Stage 4	End stage	Nearly vegetative. Intellectual and social comprehension and output are at a rudimentary level. Nearly or absolutely mute. Paraparetic or paraplegic with double incontinence (urinary and bowel).

Note. ADC = acquired immunodeficiency syndrome (AIDS) dementia complex; ADLs = activities of daily living.
Source. Adapted from Price and Brew 1992.

tients seen for psychiatric consultation who have ADC has been reported at 7%–25% (Buhrich and Cooper 1987; Dilley et al. 1985).

Clinical Characteristics

ADC is characterized by cognitive, affective, behavioral, and motor dysfunction. Cognitive deficits affect the neuropsychological domains of fine motor speed and control, concentration and attention, executive function, and visuospatial performance (Bornstein et al. 1993; Handelsman et al. 1992; Saykin et al. 1988; Stern et al. 1991; Tross et al. 1988). Patients describe short-term memory loss, word-finding difficulties, and difficulty with sequential tasks, and they state that activities that were once automatic now require effortful concentration for successful completion, suggesting impairment of implicit memory. Aphasia and agnosia are rare except in end-stage ADC.

Behaviorally, patients commonly report apathetic or depressed mood, abulia, social withdrawal, and decreased energy. Mania and hypomania are less common but have been reported (Halman et al. 1993a; Kieburtz et al. 1991) and are associated with advanced systemic HIV-1 disease (Lyketsos et al. 1993; Smith et al. 1992). New-onset psychosis, although rare, has also been reported as a consequence of ADC (Sewell et al. 1994) and is usually seen in patients with advanced ADC. Motorically, patients describe slowing of their movements, clumsiness, gait unsteadiness, and a decline in their handwriting.

Staging Systems and Diagnostic Criteria

The MSK Clinical Staging System for ADC (Price and Brew 1992) (see Table 26–3) is based on clinical history and neurological examination and designates stages of ADC according to the patient's level of functional impairment. Patients with minimal or mild ADC (MSK stages 0.5 or 1) experience cognitive and motor deficits that do not adversely affect basic activities of daily living and hence do not meet impairment criteria for "dementia." However, such patients are experiencing a neurological complication of HIV-1 infection.

Evaluation and Diagnosis

The diagnosis of ADC is based on a suggestive history and on neurological and psychiatric examination. Further evaluation should be performed to gather data both to support the diagnosis of ADC and to exclude other causes of CNS dysfunction. There is no single investigation, taken alone, on which the diagnosis of ADC can be made. The following are used to support the findings of clinical examination: neuropsychological testing, anatomical brain imaging, cerebrospinal fluid (CSF) examination, and blood tests, including hemoglobin, fasting glucose tolerance test, electrolytes, vitamin B_{12}, thyroid-stimulating hormone (TSH), and the rapid plasma reagent (RPR) or Venereal Disease Research Laboratory (VDRL) test for syphilis. We have observed that patients with ADC are cognitively highly sensitive to anemia.

Cerebral atrophy and ventricular enlargement may be found in ADC on both computed tomography (CT) and magnetic resonance imaging (MRI). MRI may also detect patchy T2-weighted white matter lesions (see Figure 26–2) (Jarvik et al. 1988; Kieburtz et al. 1990; Portegies et al. 1993; Post et al. 1991) and is more sensitive in detecting regional atrophic changes, such as those that may occur in the basal ganglia (Dal Pan et al. 1992). Both techniques are useful in detecting atrophy (see Figure 26–3), mass, or vascular lesions of *Toxoplasma* encephalitis, lymphoma, and stroke, all of which may complicate the course of HIV disease.

CSF examination may show pleocytosis, elevated levels of immunoglobulin G (IgG), oligoclonal bands, and increased levels of protein (McArthur et al. 1988), all of which are nonspecific findings and do not correlate well with clinical severity. The major use of the CSF ex-

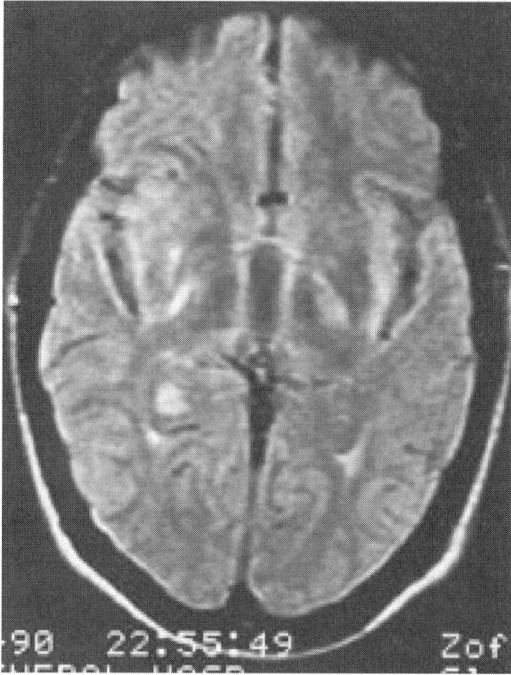

Figure 26–2. Brain magnetic resonance image (T2-weighted image) of a 39-year-old man with AIDS dementia complex and otherwise only non-AIDS-defining constitutional symptoms of HIV-1 infection.

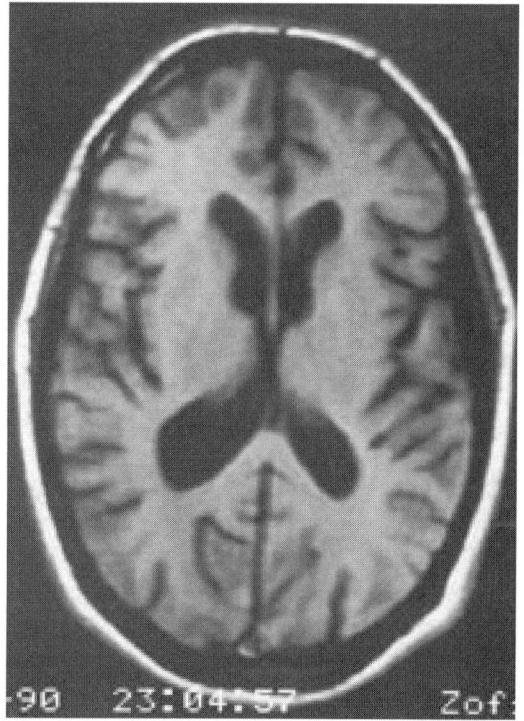

Figure 26–3. Brain magnetic resonance image (T1-weighted image) of the patient in Figure 26–2.

amination is to exclude other causes of mental status changes, including opportunistic infections, tumors, and syphilis.

Neuropsychological testing provides a means to objectively document cognitive deficits and to characterize cognitive function. Longitudinal follow-up testing provides a means to monitor for progression of cognitive dysfunction and to evaluate response to treatment interventions. Testing can also assist in planning cognitive rehabilitation or behavioral interventions used in treatment. Neuropsychological performance must be interpreted in the clinical context because confounding factors—including premorbid neuropsychiatric history, current medical illness(es), psychoactive substance use, and medication side effects—can affect the test results.

Tests of attention, memory, motor speed, and cognitive flexibility, which incorporate time pressure and problem solving, are sensi-

tive to HIV-related cognitive deficits. These tests include Trail Making Test (Trail Part A and B), Finger Tapping Test, Grooved Pegboard Test, Stroop Color/Word Interference Test, and the Digit Symbol and Digit Span portions of the Wechsler Adult Intelligence Scale—Revised (WAIS-R; Wechsler 1981).

Screening Tests

Screening tests, along with a clinical interview, may be useful to indicate which patients need a more extensive evaluation. We have evaluated four computer-based reaction time-screening measures developed by Miller et al. (1991) and found that two tests of complex reaction time—which assess divided attention, motor speed, and motor inhibition—achieved an 83%–88% positive predictive value in identifying patients with ADC (Worth et al. 1993a). The Mini-Mental State Exam (Folstein et al. 1975), relying on tests that measure cognitive functions that are rarely impaired until advanced stages of ADC, is not sensitive to mild dysfunction and alone is not useful as a screening test for ADC.

Treatment and Management

Pharmacotherapy. The antiretroviral agent AZT can improve cognitive function over the short term and may have a protective effect in delaying the progression of ADC, but its long-term effects on the course of ADC are largely unknown.

Theoretically, all nucleoside antiretrovirals may be effective in treating patients with ADC, but AZT may be the most effective because it demonstrates the greatest penetration of the blood-brain barrier, with a CSF-to-plasma ratio three times greater than that of ddI.

Symptomatic treatment with psychopharmacological medications is an important aspect of management. Cognitive symptoms—particularly poor concentration and attention, as well as dysphoria, apathy, and anergia—may improve with stimulants, either dextroamphetamine or methylphenidate (Fernandez et al. 1988). In our clinical experience, these agents are effective at low doses, are well tolerated, and can be used for months to years (see the subsection on pharmacotherapy in the section below, "Major Depressive Episode"). Specific syndromes, including delirium, psychosis, depression, and manic disorders, warrant specific evaluation and management, with attention paid to the possible direct contribution attributable to CNS HIV-1 infection, and we discuss these syndromes in subsequent sections in this chapter.

◼ DELIRIUM

Delirium is the neuropsychiatric complication that occurs most frequently in hospitalized patients with AIDS (Buhrich and Cooper 1987). Patients with advanced systemic disease and ADC are at high risk for delirium, the cause of

which is often multifactorial, as outlined in Table 26–4. A sudden change in mental status should not be ascribed to ADC alone and is more frequently the result of other "organic" causes superimposed on a brain vulnerable to insult because of CNS HIV-1 infection. In the management of delirium, the primary goal is identification and treatment of the underlying etiology. In patients who are in more advanced stages of immunosuppression, a high index of suspicion must be held for opportunistic infections, both systemic and intracranial, as well as metabolic derangements. The need for ancillary investigations, including anatomical brain imaging, electroencephalogram (EEG), CSF examination, and laboratory blood tests must be guided by clinical examination. (For a complete discussion of the treatment and management of delirium, please refer to Wise and Trzepacz, Chapter 7, in this volume.)

Symptomatic treatment with neuroleptics may be necessary to control agitation and assist in resolving confusion. Patients generally respond to daily doses of neuroleptic drugs equivalent to 0.5–5.0 mg of haloperidol. Patients with HIV-1 disease are at increased risk for neuroleptic-induced extrapyramidal side effects, hence the minimum neuroleptic dose necessary to control target symptoms should be used. Higher intravenous doses may be necessary for rapid tranquilization of the patient if this is dictated by the clinical situation. Intramuscular administration of medication should be avoided when the patient has reduced muscle mass or impaired coagulation or thrombocytopenia. Anticholinergic medications may worsen delirium and should be avoided. Benzodiazepines should not be used as a single agent in the treatment of patients with delirium. In a double-blind study comparing single-agent trials of haloperidol, chlorpromazine, and lorazepam for delirium in hospitalized patients with AIDS, Breitbart (1993) and his team found that low doses of neuroleptics were helpful in reducing symptoms of delirium, whereas lorazepam alone was not.

Table 26–4. Differential etiologies of delirium in the patient with HIV-1 infection

Anemia

Drug intoxication

Alcohol

Antibiotics

Anticholinergics, including antidepressants

Anticonvulsants

Antineoplastics

Cocaine

Opiates

Phencyclidine

Sedative-hypnotics

Endocrine disorders and vitamin deficiencies

Addison's disease

Thyroid disease

Vitamin B_{12} insufficiency

Head trauma

Hypoglycemia (of particular concern in patients receiving systemic pentamidine)

Hypotension

Infections

Systemic

Bacteremia

Disseminated herpes zoster, *Mycobacterium avium-intracellulare,* and candidiasis

Pneumonia

Septicemia

Subacute bacterial endocarditis

Intracranial

CMV encephalitis

Cryptococcal meningitis

Neurosyphilis

Progressive multifocal leukoencephalopathy (Creutzfeldt-Jakob papovavirus)

Toxoplasmosis

Tubercular meningitis

Intracranial neoplasms

Metastatic Kaposi's sarcoma (rarely)

Primary lymphoma

Metabolic encephalopathies

Acidosis

Alkalosis

Dehydration

Hepatic, renal, pulmonary, adrenal, and pancreatic insufficiency

Hypernatremia, hyponatremia

Hypocalcemia

Hypomagnesemia

Hypoxia

Water intoxication

Psychoactive substance withdrawal syndromes

Seizure disorder

In hospitalized patients with HIV/AIDS, 46% of new-onset seizures were due to HIV-1 CNS infection; of these, 10% were partial seizures, 30% were generalized.[a]

Note. AIDS = acquired immunodeficiency syndrome; CMV = cytomegalovirus; CNS = central nervous system; HIV = human immunodeficiency virus.
[a]Wong et al. 1990.

Lorazepam may be a useful adjunct to treatment with neuroleptics, particularly in very agitated patients in whom achieving sedation is desirable. Short-acting benzodiazepines with short-lived active metabolites are preferred. Because the symptoms of delirium can be frightening or disturbing for patients, their friends, and family, a brief clarifying explanation can be very reassuring to all parties.

PSYCHOTIC DISORDERS

Psychosis in patients with HIV-1 disease can occur when there is delirium, advanced ADC,

complex partial seizures, psychoactive substance-related disorders, and/or premorbid psychotic disorders, including schizophrenia and severe bipolar disorder. The accurate diagnosis of psychosis in patients with HIV disease is imperative because corresponding treatments for the clinical entities in the differential diagnosis are widely divergent. However, even after extensive evaluation, the consultation-liaison psychiatrist may often find himself or herself facing two to three likely etiological processes and suggesting two to three very different treatments.

HIV-1 seroprevalence rates of 6%–8%

among patients with chronic mental illnesses have been reported in metropolitan areas with a high prevalence of HIV-1. Studies have demonstrated substantial deficits in the practical understanding of AIDS and HIV-1 transmission and significant rates of high-risk behaviors among such patients (Carmen and Brady 1990; Kalichman et al. 1994). Treatment considerations with this patient population must include an assessment of HIV risk factors or risk markers. Patients with chronic psychosis who are infected with HIV frequently have difficulties in accessing adequate health care and in complying with the complex medical regimens used in the treatment of HIV/AIDS. Primary and secondary prevention programs (Carmen and Brady 1990) and health care delivery systems to meet the specific needs of patients with chronic mental illness and HIV-1 infection must be designed and implemented.

Patients with advanced HIV-1 disease are at high risk for seizures, including complex partial seizures, which may manifest as psychosis. Wong et al. (1990) found that among inpatients with HIV-1 infection and new-onset seizure disorders, 46% had seizures because of HIV-1 CNS infection alone, without evidence of other secondary opportunistic infections or tumors. Complex partial seizures in patients with ADC may present with new-onset, episodic symptoms, including formed visual hallucinations, visual perceptual distortions, panic attacks, and/or racing thoughts.

Pharmacotherapy

Neuroleptics remain the drugs of choice for HIV-related psychosis. Although the effects of HIV-1 infection on the pathophysiology of primary psychotic disorders are unknown, alterations to the subcortical structures and the blood-brain barrier in ADC suggest a theoretical interaction when the two disorders coexist. Both ADC and psychotic disorders appear to involve the striatum and subcortical gray matter. Clinically, patients with ADC who do not

have a history of chronic mental illness are known to have a higher-than-expected rate of extrapyramidal side effects with neuroleptic medications (Hriso et al. 1991). This observation may be partially explained by the apparently greater HIV-related atrophy noted in the basal ganglia versus other brain regions (Dal Pan et al. 1992). In addition, several cases of neuroleptic malignant syndrome have been reported (W. B. Bernstein and Scherokman 1986; Breitbart and Knight 1989; Halman et al. 1993a).

The use of clozapine in patients with HIV-1 infection has not been systematically studied, but theoretical concerns include an increased potential for myelosuppression when clozapine is used with antiretrovirals and other myelosuppressive agents and an increased risk of seizures in patients with CNS complications of HIV disease. More recently, we have found that low doses of risperidone can be effective and well tolerated. In patients with advanced ADC, we have observed a syndrome of near-delusional (nonspecific) fear or unbridled terror, which can often present as "insomnia." A short course of treatment with low-dose haloperidol or risperidone (e.g., 0.5–1.0 mg at bedtime for two to three nights) can completely resolve this highly disabling syndrome.

MOOD DISORDERS

Mania

An acute manic episode in a patient with HIV-1 infection may be the result of primary bipolar disorder, or it may be secondary to a toxic or metabolic insult or to a space-occupying lesion. Reported precipitants of HIV-related mania include ADC (Halman et al. 1993a; Kieburtz et al. 1991; Smith et al. 1992); CNS opportunistic infections such as toxoplasmosis cerebritis and cryptococcal meningitis; CNS opportunistic tumors from non-Hodgkin's lymphoma (Halman et al. 1993a; Johannessen and Wilson

- of Pemeron antichial
- Ritalin cognitive BBB
- ↓ LV
B12

1988); and medication side effects (see Table 26–1). Patients with mania and no personal or family history of a mood disorder tend to manifest manic symptoms at more advanced stages of systemic disease and comorbid ADC than do patients with a history of mood disorder (Lyketsos et al. 1993). A stress-diathesis model, incorporating both predisposing factors and organic insult resulting from HIV disease, may explain the etiopathogenesis of this disorder and the timing of its onset.

Evaluation and Diagnosis

The evaluation of mania in patients with early HIV disease usually presents little difficulty, but as HIV disease progresses, this can be challenging; the likelihood of secondary mania increases, as does treatment unresponsiveness. The temporal relations between the onset of manic symptoms and changes in HIV disease and medications must be carefully noted. New-onset mania in an HIV-1-infected patient should be considered secondary mania until proven otherwise, and the evaluation must include anatomical brain imaging and, in the otherwise immunosuppressed patient (CD4+ lymphocyte count ≤200 cells/mL), CSF examination. Mania resulting from covert use of steroids by patients should also be considered. We have treated secondary mania in patients who illicitly used steroids to regain muscle loss resulting from wasting syndrome. (For a complete discussion of mania, please refer to McDaniel et al., Chapter 10, in this volume.)

Treatment and Management

Standard pharmacotherapy with neuroleptics and lithium can be effective, but the usefulness of these agents may be restricted by the development of dose-limiting adverse side effects. We have observed that failure of response to standard pharmacotherapy with lithium and haloperidol was predicted by evidence of any abnormality on MRI, but all treatment-resistant or treatment-intolerant patients did respond to therapy with anticonvulsants (Halman et al. 1993a).

Volume shifts resulting from dehydration, diarrhea, and poor oral intake necessitate careful monitoring of lithium levels. However, lithium toxicity, including encephalopathy, may still develop despite normal therapeutic blood levels (Halman et al. 1993a). This hypersensitivity may be associated with HIV-related compromise of blood-brain barrier integrity, exposing the CNS to greater levels of lithium than is predicted by standard "therapeutic" serum levels.

Neuroleptics are often necessary in the acute treatment of patients with manic syndromes. Because patients with advanced HIV disease or evidence of brain pathology are sensitive to extrapyramidal side effects (Halman et al. 1993a; Hriso et al. 1991), low daily doses of high- to medium-potency neuroleptics should be used: haloperidol, 0.5–1.0 mg; perphenazine, 8–24 mg; or risperidone, 1–2 mg. The use of low-potency neuroleptics may subject patients to greater risks of other side effects, such as confusion and oversedation (Breitbart 1993).

Anticonvulsants are useful in patients with mania who have advanced HIV disease or abnormal anatomical brain imaging, particularly when standard agents are intolerable or dose-limiting side effects occur. Our drug of choice for treating patients with mania is valproic acid because we have found it to be generally effective and, if the enteric brand is used, well tolerated. A starting dose of 250 mg orally at bedtime is used; this dose is increased by 250 mg/day every 4–7 days until symptomatic control is achieved. A serum level > 50 µg/mL is recommended for seizure control, but often patients improve at lower levels. Liver function tests and hematological parameters, particularly platelet count, need to be monitored. Valproic acid has been used safely with antiretrovirals and is known to raise AZT levels with concomitant use (Lertora et al. 1992). Although carbamazepine can be effective for mania, its safe use in patients with HIV disease remains to be clarified because these patients are at increased risk for hematological and dermatological complications. Clonazepam, used either alone or in combination with other agents, has also been an effective alternative therapy (Halman et al. 1993a). We have also successfully used the calcium channel antagonist nimodipine in some patients with treatment-resistant HIV-related mania.

Major Depressive Episode

The stage of HIV disease is an important consideration when evaluating a patient for depression. As HIV-1 disease progresses, the clinician's index of suspicion for secondary mood disorders should increase. Many patients are at increased risk for major depression at various nodal points throughout their illness, but major depression is not a natural consequence of HIV disease. The consultation-liaison psychiatrist may frequently observe health care workers rationalizing depression as a reasonable response to developing a fatal illness, identifying with a patient's nihilism, and failing to accurately diagnose or to offer treatment. Withholding treatment only ensures a patient's suffering and emotional pain, adding to his or her often considerable burden.

Epidemiology

Major depression is diagnosed in 5%–15% of hospitalized patients with HIV/AIDS seen by consultation-liaison psychiatrists (Buhrich and Cooper 1987; Dilley et al. 1985) and in 8%–33% of ambulatory patients referred for psychiatric evaluation (Hintz et al. 1990; O'Dowd et al. 1993; Worth et al. 1993b). Community-based cohort studies in the United States showed rates of major depression at 4%–18% of gay/bisexual men at early stages of HIV-1 disease (Atkinson et al. 1988; Brown et al. 1992; Williams et al. 1991) and at 35% among HIV-infected patients who use injection drugs (Kosten 1993). Many studies based in the United States may underestimate the prevalence of major depression and other Axis I dis-

orders because they have been conducted on self-selected samples of well-educated, middle-class, primarily white men (Maj et al. 1994a). Some groups at high risk for HIV/AIDS also appear to have a high premorbid risk for major depression, including gay/bisexual men (Atkinson et al. 1988; Perkins et al. 1994; Williams et al. 1991) and individuals who use injection drugs (Kosten 1993).

Systemic HIV disease and its treatments, particularly as the disease progresses, may also contribute to major depression. Several medications used in the treatment of HIV disease may cause depression as a side effect (see Table 26–1). Several endocrinological and metabolic disturbances complicate advanced stages of HIV-1 disease and may also contribute to depressive symptomatology. These include 1) adrenocortical insufficiency, which occurs in up to 45% of patients with CD4+ cell counts <50 cells/mL (Abbott et al. 1993); 2) euthyroid sick syndrome (low free triiodothyronine [T_3] level with normal levels of TSH), which occurs during secondary infections and in association with wasting syndrome and elevated serum levels of tumor necrosis factor-α (Bélec et al. 1993; Grunfeld et al. 1993); 3) vitamin B_{12} deficiency, reported in 20% of patients with HIV-1 infection who have neuropsychiatric complications (Beach et al. 1992); 4) hypogonadism and hypotestosterone states (Grinspoon and Bilezikian 1992); and 5) protein and calorie malnutrition (Süttmann et al. 1993).

Diagnosis

The diagnosis of major depression in patients with early HIV-1 disease usually presents little difficulty. As HIV-1 disease progresses, however, the diagnosis can be challenging, with overlapping symptoms, including insomnia and poor appetite (Hintz et al. 1990; Williams et al. 1991), and complex treatment regimens. The effects of medications and HIV-1 disease must be carefully assessed. A careful history will enable the consultation-liaison psychiatrist to presumptively assign symptoms with cause.

The clinician should carefully note the temporal relations between the onset of depressed mood, specific neurovegetative symptoms, and changes in HIV-1 disease and medications. If the patient already has HIV-related symptoms that overlap with those of suspected major depression, the clinician should inquire if these symptoms have worsened or changed. If secondary mood disorder is high on the list of differential diagnoses, some patients with a premorbid history of major depression may be able to subjectively differentiate their current episode from prior episodes.

Treatment and Management

Pharmacotherapy. Pharmacotherapy is effective for most patients with HIV-related major depression and is well tolerated as long as certain principles are observed: start at low doses, increase doses slowly, choose agents to address the patient's specific neurovegetative symptoms, and avoid agents that are overly sedating, have anticholinergic effects, or are potent α-adrenergic antagonists. Short hospital admissions can limit the consultation-liaison psychiatrist's ability to complete a trial of antidepressants, which makes outpatient follow-up necessary.

Dosing schedules and side effects. Antidepressants are generally well tolerated and effective in patients with HIV-1 infection and depression, and they can be used safely in patients who are severely ill. Hintz et al. (1990) reported that treatment efficacy ratings of antidepressant response were similar in depressed patients who were HIV seropositive and in those who were HIV seronegative, although the efficacy ratings were higher for asymptomatic patients than for patients with AIDS-related complex (ARC) or AIDS. Rates of severe side effects paralleled the severity of HIV disease, ranging from 5% in the asymptomatic group to 25% in the AIDS group, and 9% in an HIV-seronegative control group.

Tricyclic antidepressants have been found to be effective in patients with HIV-1 infection. In a double-blind, placebo-controlled trial, Rabkin et al. (1994a) found a 74% response rate among patients with HIV-1 infection who received imipramine, compared with a response rate of 26% among placebo-treated control subjects. No adverse effects of imipramine were found on markers of immune function, including CD4+ and CD8+ lymphocyte counts (Rabkin et al. 1991).

Bupropion is effective (Fernandez and Levy 1991) and is particularly helpful for patients with significant fatigue. Dosing intervals of less than 4 hours are associated with generalized seizures. Because of impaired compliance with necessary dosing intervals, patients with ADC may be at increased risk for drug-induced seizures. The use of pillboxes with alarms may prevent these types of timing errors.

Selective serotonin reuptake inhibitors. The selective serotonin reuptake inhibitors (SSRIs) fluoxetine (Hintz et al. 1990; Levine et al. 1990), paroxetine, and sertraline (J. G. Rabkin, personal communication, May 1994) are all generally effective for HIV-related major depression and are well tolerated in patients with advanced HIV disease. In a 12-week, open-label trial, Rabkin et al. (1994b) found that fluoxetine was well tolerated and effective for HIV-related major depression, with an 83% response rate and no negative effect on immune status.

The dosing principle of starting low and increasing slowly applies with SSRIs. Fluoxetine or paroxetine should be started at dosages of 10 mg/day in patients with advanced disease, in whom drug interactions are most likely. The dosage of fluoxetine should be increased after 4–5 weeks, and the dosage of sertraline or paroxetine should be increased after 1–2 weeks; dosages for all SSRIs should be titrated against response and side effects. Decreased libido and difficulty maintaining an erection or achieving an orgasm are dose-dependent side effects of all SSRIs, which can be intolerable or dose-limiting for many. Gastrointestinal side effects, headache, and anxiety are also frequently reported; movement disorder side effects are less often reported. Because SSRIs are heavily protein-bound, they may raise the free level of other medications by displacing them from serum proteins. This interaction becomes particularly important in patients with HIV-1 infection who have coagulopathies and are being treated with warfarin.

Stimulants.   At low doses, both dextroamphetamine (Holmes et al. 1989) and methylphenidate can be effective for HIV-related major depression, as primary agents (Fernandez and Levy 1991; Holmes et al. 1989) or as adjuvant agents (Rabkin 1993); the response rate associated with these agents has been shown to be up to 80%. Stimulants are especially effective for anergia, apathy, and anorexia, but some patients also report improvement in mood, attention, and concentration. Stimulants are preferred to conventional antidepressants in patients with a predominance of apathy versus sadness and in patients who are unable to tolerate the side effects of conventional antidepressants.

The use of stimulants is guided by the fact that these drugs have a short half-life and a rapid onset of action. Only 1–2 days of treatment on any given dose is adequate to judge the efficacy and tolerance of that dose in an individual patient. The therapy trial should begin with a morning dose of 5 mg; that dose should be increased by 5-mg intervals every 1–2 days until a good response is achieved or until dose-limiting side effects occur. A second midday dose, usually half the morning dose, may be needed to sustain a clinical effect throughout the afternoon. For patients with ADC who have difficulty remembering to take their midday dose, sustained-release formulas of either dextroamphetamine or methylphenidate can be very useful. It is rare for single doses to be greater than 20 mg or daily dosages to be

greater than 30 mg. If a good response has not occurred at these levels, higher doses are unlikely to elicit a good response, and the incidence of adverse effects is higher. At low doses, stimulants are generally well tolerated and may stimulate appetite. Some patients experience a dose-dependent feeling of being "wired" or "nervous," and doses taken later than 1:00 P.M. may interfere with nighttime sleep.

Electroconvulsive therapy.   Schaerf et al. (1989) have reported successfully using electroconvulsive therapy (ECT) in four patients: three with asymptomatic HIV-1 infection and one with AIDS.

Psychotherapy.   Psychotherapy is useful for HIV-related major depression, but brief hospitalizations and severe medical illness limit its applicability for inpatients, with whom pharmacotherapy is often the treatment of choice. For ambulatory patients, the clinician should consider how long the patient can wait for symptom resolution, the chance of treatment interruption or discontinuation by intercurrent medical illness, and the presumed etiology and contributing factors of the major depressive episode (see also Rouchell et al, Chapter 9, and Lipsitt, Chapter 33, in this volume).

In a pilot study of short-term interpersonal psychotherapy in ambulatory patients with HIV disease and major depression or dysthymia, Markowitz et al. (1992) reported an 87% response rate as measured by patients' subjective reports and therapists' clinical global impressions. The approach included identification of problems from an interpersonal perspective, including grief, role transitions, interpersonal disputes and deficits, and exploration of options for changing dysfunctional behavior patterns. Unresolved grief resulting from multiple bereavements is a risk factor for patients with HIV-related major depression, and psychotherapy may be the treatment of choice when it occurs. Summers et al.

(1993) reported that short-term group psychotherapy was effective for major depression in association with unresolved grief and may be as effective as fluoxetine (J. Summers, personal communication, May 1994). In a randomized study of patients with asymptomatic HIV disease comparing short-term cognitive-behavior group therapy with fluoxetine or with placebo, Karasic and associates (1992) found similar reductions in levels of depression in both treatment groups.

Bereavement and Unresolved Grief

Many persons with HIV/AIDS—including gay men, individuals who use injection drugs, and persons from inner-city communities of racial and ethnic minorities—live in the socially circumscribed communities (Woodhouse et al. 1994) that have experienced high HIV/AIDS prevalence and as such have experienced multiple losses because of HIV disease. Repeated bereavement has psychiatric and social implications for patients with HIV disease and at-risk communities.

Multiple and frequent bereavements may not allow time for adequate grieving, and the risk for unresolved grief appears to be increasing among homosexual men with HIV disease. In a community-based study comparing infected and at-risk homosexual men, the rate of unresolved grief was higher among infected men (Sciolla et al. 1992). Compared with those with resolved grief, men with unresolved grief had a higher rate of major depression and panic disorder, higher levels of depression and anxiety, and lower levels of social support. Persons with multiple bereavement may experience the death of friends as "a normal event" and may be at risk for self-medicating their grief with psychoactive substances. Women may experience greater AIDS-related bereavement than do men (Summers et al. 1994). Adequate treatment, including short-term group (Summers et al. 1993) or individual psychotherapy, can be effective in reducing levels of depression and anxiety.

ADJUSTMENT DISORDERS

Maladaptive coping with HIV disease is a frequent complaint by and about hospitalized patients seen in consultation (Buhrich and Cooper 1987; Dilley et al. 1985). Between 29% and 69% of ambulatory patients referred for psychiatric evaluation have adjustment disorders (O'Dowd et al. 1993; Worth and Halman 1993). Issues that consistently precipitate referral for psychiatric evaluation include a patient's own illness, bereavement, disclosure of serological status, illness of a partner or relative, medication dilemmas, HIV serological testing, assault, and child-related problems. The presence of an Axis II disorder may increase the risk of poor psychological coping with HIV infection (Perkins et al. 1993) and place such patients at increased risk for adjustment disorder.

Assessment and Diagnosis

Most patients will be able to identify the important psychosocial stressors that have precipitated an adjustment disorder, although a thorough evaluation of the full range of psychological and psychosocial stressors may overtax the time and stamina of a hospitalized patient. As a bedside guide to assessing psychological coping and psychosocial stressors, we use a "running a marathon" model. We have also found it useful to relate this model to patients when reviewing with them our clinical impressions and suggestions for psychotherapy and psychosocial interventions. This model can be helpful for patients in conceptualizing psychosocial stressors and interventions. There are four basic components to successfully "running the HIV marathon":

1. *Training:* How well has the patient dealt with adversity in the past? What are his or her coping mechanisms?
2. *Personal team:* Who are the people, if any, who constitute the patient's support system? How supportive does the patient perceive those supports to be?

3. *Pit stops:* Can the patient take a respite or get away from HIV/AIDS (e.g., go away for a weekend, have a week without doctors' appointments, see a movie, stop nonvital medications) for a day?

4. *Corporate support:* Does the patient have an income source, health and/or disability insurance, a primary care doctor and hospital, and support from his or her workplace?

If each of these categories is not well represented, these relative deficits are likely problem areas for the patient with HIV-1 infection and should be areas of focus for the treatment and management plan.

Treatment

Psychotherapy

A wide range of psychotherapeutic interventions can be used in treating patients with HIV/AIDS. The goals of treatment will vary with the patient's psychosocial needs and stage of illness and often require that a flexible stance be held by the psychotherapist, who may need to be more "real" than in other clinical situations. Referral to appropriate community resources may help provide access to information, activities, and new social supports such as the "buddy" system (Velentgas et al. 1990). HIV disease will frequently restimulate old feelings of guilt, humiliation, and shame and prompt reexamination of old conflicts over identity and self-esteem. Similarly, the threat of a terminal illness might intensify the desire to resolve issues that have, to that point, been barriers to the formation of satisfactory intimate relationships. Intense affects of anger and sadness experienced over the course of the disease may be processed within the safety of a consistent, empathic, and trusting psychotherapeutic relationship and will help patients avoid "burning out" friends and family on whom they may feel that they are becoming a burden. Strengthening family support systems can effectively re-

duce distress and depression (Mayne and O'Leary 1993), and psychotherapy can help the patient examine the new roles in the family and in other significant relationships that have been brought about by his or her illness. Finally, psychotherapy may help to ease feelings of abandonment and isolation and help the patient to maintain a connection to the living, human world.

Group psychotherapies, particularly short-term modalities, have been extensively used psychotherapeutic techniques since the beginning of the AIDS epidemic. Some, but not all, investigators have reported that both short-term cognitive-behavioral and insight-oriented techniques are equally effective in diminishing psychosocial distress in gay men with HIV disease (Murphy et al. 1993). Rapid development of group cohesion appears to be achieved when the group is demographically homogeneous, particularly in exposure risk factor/marker and gender (Beckett and Rutan 1990). Universality, group cohesiveness, and instillation of hope have been rated as the most potent therapeutic factors in groups for HIV-infected women (Prager et al. 1992) and long-term-surviving gay men (Halman et al. 1993b). Countertransference issues can be marked (G. Bernstein and Klein 1995), and clinical supervision or consultation can be very helpful.

Family and caregiver psychotherapy. Psychosocial demands on the domestic caregivers of patients with HIV/AIDS can be significant and similar to those experienced by the patient, leading to "burnout" and depression (Folkman et al. 1994; van den Bloom and Gremmen 1992). Because this can strain or truncate social relationships that are important to the patient, family psychotherapy, as well as respite care, can be helpful. Family support systems can effectively reduce distress and depression in patients with HIV disease (Mayne and O'Leary 1993), and interventions must incorporate a range of caregivers, including male partners, mothers, and sisters (Stewart et al. 1993).

Family therapy interventions (Walker 1987) include 1) providing accurate information about HIV disease and about access to resource centers; 2) assisting families in processing a wide range of affects, including guilt, shame, fear, betrayal, anger, and sadness; 3) diminishing isolation by working through feelings of stigmatization, often through the use of peer support groups; 4) supporting healthy forms of self-protective denial and encouraging hopefulness when appropriate; and 5) grief work. Often, the crisis raised by the threat of imminent death will intensify the speed of psychotherapy and the depth of potential change, frequently allowing successful resolution of long-standing family conflicts.

Pharmacotherapy

Short-term trials of anxiolytics can be very helpful while the patient initially engages in psychotherapy and begins to reestablish his or her psychological equilibrium.

■ ANXIETY DISORDERS

Patients with HIV/AIDS can present with a range of anxiety syndromes, from short-term periods of anxious mood accompanying an adjustment disorder to more severe anxiety states such as panic disorder, acute stress disorder, posttraumatic stress disorder (PTSD), or obsessive-compulsive disorder. In outpatients, compared with hospitalized patients, anxiety disorders more frequently may underlie the chief complaint or the reason for referral to the consultation-liaison psychiatrist. Dilley et al. (1985) and Buhrich and Cooper (1987) reported anxiety disorders in only 8% of inpatient consultations, but anxiety disorders were reported at about twice that rate in outpatients referred to HIV/AIDS psychiatry clinics (O'Dowd et al. 1993; Worth and Halman 1993). Community studies showed the prevalence of anxiety disorders in HIV-1-infected individuals ranging from 2% (Williams et al. 1991) to 18% (Atkinson et al. 1988) in asymptomatic patients, to 38% in patients with symptomatic but non-AIDS-defining conditions (Atkinson et al. 1988), and to 27% in patients with AIDS (Atkinson et al. 1988). (A general discussion of anxiety disorders can be found in Colón and Popkin, Chapter 12, in this volume.)

Differential Diagnosis

Adjustment disorders with high levels of self-reported anxiety may occur in association with pivotal events in the course of HIV disease, including time of HIV-1 serological testing (S. Perry and Jacobsberg 1990; S. Perry et al. 1991), initiation of antiretroviral treatment, onset of constitutional but non-AIDS-defining symptoms (Atkinson et al. 1988; Chuang et al. 1989), diagnosis of first AIDS-defining condition, and first hospitalization. Many patients report that unpredictability around illness stage progression, declining CD4+ lymphocyte counts, uncertainty surrounding the investigations of new symptoms, and fears of isolation and abandonment provoke anxious feelings. Obsessive preoccupation with symptoms and compulsive checking of the body may occur, and the obsessional thought that one has HIV/AIDS can be the principal symptom of obsessive-compulsive disorder (Jenike and Patos 1986).

Acute stress disorder and PTSD syndromes are increasingly being reported in patients with HIV disease, who may describe a history of trauma and abuse as well as current multiple traumatic events. In one study (Zierler et al. 1991), men who reported a history of childhood sexual abuse had a twofold increase in prevalence of HIV infection compared with nonabused men. Women with HIV-1 infection who participate in sex-for-crack exchanges reported multiple traumatic events in their lives, including physical assault as an adult (87%), sexual assault as an adult (68%), and sexual assault as a child (77%) (Fullilove et al. 1992). Gay men who experience multiple losses over a brief period show increased feelings of isolation, depression, apathy, anger, and disbelief (Klein 1992).

Autonomic symptoms associated with anxiety disorders, including dyspnea, diarrhea, skin rashes, dizziness, nausea, sweating, and tremor, may overlap with symptoms of systemic HIV disease. In patients at more advanced stages of HIV disease, the consultation-liaison psychiatrist must include potential secondary causes in the differential diagnosis. Medications can cause side effects that include agitation, anxiety, or a number of somatic complaints that are sometimes diagnosed as anxiety (see Table 26–1). Metabolic disturbances, particularly anemia, hypoxia, and hypoglycemia secondary to pentamidine, can manifest as anxiety. Patients presenting with new-onset panic attacks may be experiencing complex partial seizures, which are not uncommon in patients infected with HIV-1.

Treatment and Management

Psychotherapy, including cognitive and behavioral therapies, is the therapeutic mainstay for adjustment disorders, acute stress disorder, and PTSD. Therapies such as biofeedback, self-relaxation techniques, and acupuncture can also be very useful. Brief pharmacotherapy trials with buspirone or judiciously determined dosages of high-potency benzodiazepines are helpful when used temporarily until the patient can regain his or her psychological equilibrium. Buspirone should be considered for use in patients with a history of psychoactive substance–related disorders. When using benzodiazepines, consider high-potency agents with short to intermediate half-lives at low daily dosages: lorazepam, 0.5–1 mg; temazepam, 15 mg; clonazepam, 0.5–1 mg; or oxazepam, 15 mg. Coadministration of benzodiazepines with AZT is safe and does not appear to affect the serum levels of either agent (Mole et al. 1992). Patients who take benzodiazepines at higher doses are at substantial risk for cognitive and motor side effects, particularly if they have coexistent ADC, intracranial lesions, or delirium (Breitbart 1993). Patients should be informed of the risk of tolerance to and dependence on benzodiazepines, and their use of these agents should be closely monitored. In patients with PTSD, tricyclic antidepressants and SSRIs are useful as adjuncts to psychotherapy and are very useful in the treatment of patients with panic disorder, especially among those with coexisting depression.

SUBSTANCE-RELATED DISORDERS

Prevalence

Substance-related disorders occur frequently in patients with HIV disease and must always be considered in the consultation-liaison psychiatrist's differential diagnosis of sleep complaints. (For a general discussion of this topic, please refer to Franklin and Frances, Chapter 13, in this volume.) The prevalence of substance-related disorders in ambulatory patients with HIV/AIDS who are referred for psychiatric evaluation has been reported to be 42%–45% (O'Dowd et al. 1993; Worth and Halman 1993). Among gay and bisexual men with HIV disease, estimates of the rates of current alcohol abuse and dependence are 2%–9% (Atkinson et al. 1988; Brown et al. 1992; Williams et al. 1991).

Noninjection psychoactive drugs impair the user's judgment and may lead to recidivism from behavior changes toward low-HIV-risk behaviors. Some (Hauth et al. 1993), but not all (M. J. Perry et al. 1994; Weatherburn et al. 1993), studies have shown such an effect associated with alcohol use. Crack cocaine use (Edlin et al. 1994, 1995; Susser and Valencia 1993) and inhalant abuse (Ostrow et al. 1990, 1993) are more consistently associated with high-HIV-risk behaviors.

A study of injection drug users at 59 drug treatment centers between April 1988 and December 1989 in 33 cities in the United States showed HIV seroprevalence rates ranging from 0% to 48%, with a mean rate of 5%. Seroprevalence rates among users of injection drugs were highest in cities in the Northeast and varied by race: 15.6% among blacks, 3.2% among Hispanics, 3.3% among whites (Allen et al. 1992).

Treatment and Management

The management of substance-related disorders and HIV disease follows the concept of "harm reduction" (Brettle 1991). This model is based on a pragmatic approach to social and individual problems associated with substance-related disorders, which recognizes that these disorders, by natural history, follow a chronic course characterized by relapses, and that for a program to be effective, it must provide not only information about HIV transmission but also access to drug abuse treatment programs and the means for behavior change in both drug use and sexual behavior. Harm reduction acknowledges that if drug use cannot be eliminated, then treatment should be aimed at minimizing the consequences of the drug use. This includes reducing HIV-transmission risk, minimizing social stigmatization, and helping the patient to increase accessibility to treatment and educational programs. The goals of harm reduction prevention programs for patients in this population include stopping all drug use, switching from injection drugs to other types, decreasing frequency of drug use, improving safer needle hygiene, decreasing needle sharing, and increasing safer sexual behavior. It is unclear whether prescribing oral forms of abused injection drugs has decreased HIV-1 seroconversion rates. This practice does not, however, promote recovery and may only introduce the problems of dependence on high doses of oral psychoactive substances (Ronald and Robertson 1993).

For hospitalized patients with a psychoactive substance–related disorder in remission,

maintenance of recovery is essential, but pain control should always be adequate (see the section below, "Pain Syndromes"). The use of opiate analgesia should not be withheld, but initiation of such a trial must involve the patient and his or her recovery program. Hospital visitation by a patient's 12-step program sponsor can be helpful. Some general hospitals have 12-step program meetings within the hospital facility that the patient may attend.

PAIN SYNDROMES

The evaluation of pain and adequate treatment and management for pain are essential in the care of patients with HIV/AIDS. Pain rather than death is often what patients fear most (Lenderking et al. 1994). Because it is known that pain afferent pathways pass through the limbic system (Talbot et al. 1991), it is understandable that pain can be amplified by anxiety, anger, depression, and psychological defenses. Pain syndromes, including neuropathy, myopathies, and headache, are common among patients with HIV/AIDS. The consultation-liaison psychiatrist may observe "psychopharmacological Calvinism" at the bedside of patients with HIV/AIDS, particularly in those with a history of psychoactive substance–related disorders. Staff members may inadequately treat a pain syndrome when they fail to distinguish between the management of the patient's "addiction" and the adequate treatment of his or her pain. Patients from racial and ethnic minority groups may also be subject to inadequate treatment of pain (Todd et al. 1993). (For a general discussion on pain treatment and management, please refer to Bouckoms, Chapter 31, in this volume.)

CONCLUSION

The consultation-liaison psychiatrist who is involved in the care of patients with HIV disease faces a highly satisfying challenge to his or her clinical abilities. Treatment and management considerations include assessment of both the biological consequences of CNS HIV-1 infection and the effects of systemic medical illness; a wide range of primary and secondary psychiatric disorders; and psychological and social issues, including stigmatization, repeated loss and bereavement, and variable accessibility to health services, that affect the patient's experience over the course of the illness. Multiple levels of therapeutic interventions are required over the spectrum of this disease, and the consultant has a clear opportunity to help patients who are affected by HIV disease.

References

Abbott M, Khoo SH, Wilkins EGL, et al: Adrenocortical deficiency common in late HIV. Scientific program and abstracts (PO-B01-0907), 9th International Conference on AIDS, Berlin, Germany, June 1993

Allen DM, Onorato IM, Green TA: HIV infection in intravenous drug users entering drug treatment, United States, 1988–1989. Am J Public Health 82:541–546, 1992

American Psychiatric Association: Diagnostic and Statistical Manual of Mental Disorders, 4th Edition. Washington, DC, American Psychiatric Association, 1994

Atkinson JH, Grant I, Kennedy CJ, et al: Prevalence of psychiatric disorders among men infected with human immunodeficiency virus. Arch Gen Psychiatry 45:859–864, 1988

Bacellar H, Muñoz A, Miller EN, et al: Temporal trends in the incidence of HIV-1-related neurologic diseases: Multicenter AIDS Cohort Study, 1985–1992. Neurology 44:1892–1900, 1994

Bartlett JG: Estimates and mechanisms of transmission of HIV in the US. Infectious Diseases in Clinical Practice 3:173–174, 1994

Beach RS, Mantero-Atienza E, Shor-Posner G, et al: Specific nutrient abnormalities in asymptomatic HIV-1 infection. AIDS 6:701–708, 1992

Beckett A, Rutan SJ: Treating persons with ARC and AIDS in group psychotherapy. Int J Group Psychother 40:19–29, 1990

Bélec L, Meillet D, Vohito MD, et al: High serum levels of TNF-α in HIV-1-infected patients with euthyroid sick syndrome. Scientific program and abstracts (PO-A13-0246), 9th International Conference on AIDS, Berlin, Germany, June 1993

Bellani ML, Trotti E, Pezzotta P, et al: Psychiatric disorders in health care personnel working in AIDS units. Scientific program and abstracts (PO-D21-4045), 9th International Conference on AIDS, Berlin, Germany, June 1993

Berger JR: Neurosyphilis in human immunodeficiency virus-type 1-seropositive individuals. Arch Neurol 48:700–702, 1991

Bernstein G, Klein R: Countertransference issues in group psychotherapy with HIV-positive and AIDS patients. Int J Group Psychother 45:91–99, 1995

Bernstein WB, Scherokman B: Neuroleptic malignant syndrome in a patient with acquired immunodeficiency syndrome. Acta Neurol Scand 73:636–637, 1986

Bornstein RA, Nasrallah HA, Para MF, et al: Neuropsychological performance in symptomatic and asymptomatic HIV infection. AIDS 7:519–524, 1993

Breitbart W: HIV-1 and delirium: psychopharmacology and HIV-1 infection. Presented at Clinical Challenges and Research Directions, National Institute of Mental Health, Washington, DC, April 27–28, 1993

Breitbart W, Knight RT: AIDS and neuroleptic malignant syndrome. Lancet 2:1488–1489, 1989

Brettle RP: HIV and harm reduction for injection drug users. AIDS 5:125–136, 1991

Brookmeyer R: Reconstruction and future trends of the AIDS epidemic in the United States. Science 253:37–42, 1991

Brown GR, Rundell JR, McManis SE, et al: Prevalence of psychiatric disorders in early stages of HIV infection. Psychosom Med 54:588–601, 1992

Budka H, Costanzi G, Cristina S, et al: Brain pathology induced by infection with the human immunodeficiency virus (HIV). Acta Neuropathol (Berl) 75:185–198, 1987

Buhrich N, Cooper DA: Requests for psychiatric consultation concerning 22 patients with AIDS and ARC. Aust N Z J Psychiatry 21:346–353, 1987

Carmen E, Brady SM: AIDS risk in the mentally ill: clinical strategies for prevention. Hosp Community Psychiatry 41:652–657, 1990

Centers for Disease Control: Revision of the CDC surveillance case definitions for acquired immunodeficiency syndrome. MMWR Morb Mortal Wkly Rep 36 (suppl 1):1S–15S, 1987

Centers for Disease Control and Prevention: Zidovudine for the prevention of HIV transmission from mother to infant. MMWR Morb Mortal Wkly Rep 43:285–286, 1994

Chang Y, Cesarman E, Pessin MS, et al: Identification of herpesvirus-like DNA sequences in AIDS-associated Kaposi's sarcoma. Science 266:1865–1869, 1994

Chuang HT, Devins GM, Hunsley J, et al: Psychosocial distress and well-being among gay and bisexual men with human immunodeficiency virus infection. Am J Psychiatry 146:876–880, 1989

Connolly KJ, Hammer SM: Antiretroviral therapy: reverse transcriptase inhibition. Antimicrob Agents Chemother 36:245–254, 1992

Cournos F, Empfield M, Horwath E, et al: HIV seroprevalence among patients admitted to two psychiatric hospitals. Am J Psychiatry 148:1225–1230, 1991

Cournos F, Guido JR, Coomaraswamy S, et al: Sexual activity and risk of HIV infection among patients with schizophrenia. Am J Psychiatry 151:228–232, 1994

Dal Pan GJ, McArthur JH, Aylward E, et al: Patterns of cerebral atrophy in HIV-1-infected individuals: results of a quantitative MRI analysis. Neurology 42:2125–2130, 1992

Davis LE, Hjelle BL, Miller VE, et al: Early viral brain invasion in iatrogenic human immunodeficiency virus infection. Neurology 42:1736–1739, 1992

Dilley JW, Ochitill HN, Perl M, et al: Findings in psychiatric consultations with patients with acquired immune deficiency syndrome. Am J Psychiatry 142:82–86, 1985

Edlin BR, Irwin KL, Faruque S, et al: Intersecting epidemics: crack cocaine use and HIV infection among inner-city young adults. N Engl J Med 331:1422–1427, 1994

Edlin BR, Word CO, McCoy CB, et al: HIV incidence among young urban street-recruited crack cocaine smokers. Program and abstracts, 2nd National Conference on Human Retroviruses, Washington, DC, January–February 1995

Empfield M, Cournos F, Meyer I, et al: HIV seroprevalence among homeless patients admitted to a psychiatric inpatient unit. Am J Psychiatry 150:47–52, 1993

Fahey JL, Taylor JM, Detels R, et al: The prognostic value of cellular and serologic markers in infection with human immunodeficiency virus, type 1. N Engl J Med 322:166–172, 1990

Fauci AS: Multifactorial nature of human immunodeficiency virus disease: implications for therapy. Science 262:1011–1018, 1993

Fernandez F, Levy JK: Psychopharmacotherapy of psychiatric syndromes in asymptomatic and symptomatic HIV infection. Psychiatr Med 9:377–394, 1991

Fernandez F, Adams F, Levy JK, et al: Cognitive impairment due to AIDS-related complex and its response to psychostimulants. Psychosomatics 29:38–46, 1988

Fischl MA, Richman DD, Grieco MH, et al: The efficacy of azidothymidine (AZT) in the treatment of patients with AIDS and AIDS-related complex: a double-blind, placebo-controlled trial. N Engl J Med 317:185–191, 1987

Folkman S, Chesney MA, Cooke M, et al: Caregiver burden in HIV-positive and HIV-negative partners of men with AIDS. J Consult Clin Psychol 62:746–756, 1994

Folstein MF, Folstein SE, McHugh PR: Mini-Mental State: a practical method for grading the cognitive state of patients for the clinician. J Psychiatr Res 12:189–198, 1975

Fullilove MT, Fullilove RE, Kennedy G, et al: Trauma, crack, and HIV risk. Scientific program and abstracts, 8th International Conference on AIDS, Amsterdam, The Netherlands, July 1992

Gelber RD, Lenderking WR, Cotton DJ, et al: Quality of life evaluation in a clinical trial of zidovudine therapy in patients with mildly symptomatic HIV infection. Ann Intern Med 116:961–966, 1992

Grant I, Heaton RK, Velin R, et al: Rates of cognitive impairment and prediction of neuropsychological decline in HIV+ persons: a 2-year follow up. Scientific program and abstracts, 9th International Conference on AIDS, Berlin, Germany, June 1993

Greene WC: The molecular biology of human immunodeficiency virus type 1 infection. N Engl J Med 324:308–317, 1991

Grinspoon S, Bilezikian J: AIDS and the endocrine system. N Engl J Med 327:1360–1365, 1992

Grunfeld C, Pang M, Doerrler W, et al: Indices of thyroid function and weight loss in HIV infection and AIDS. Metabolism 42:1270–1276, 1993

Halman MH, Worth JL, Sanders KM, et al: Anticonvulsant use in the treatment of manic syndromes in patients with HIV-1 infection. J Neuropsychiatry Clin Neurosci 5:430–434, 1993a

Halman MH, Sanders KM, Lenderking WR, et al: Short-term group psychotherapy for long-term AIDS survivors. Scientific program and abstracts, annual meeting of the Academy of Psychosomatic Medicine, New Orleans, LA, November 1993b

Handelsman L, Aronson M, Maurer G, et al: Neuropsychological and neurological manifestations of HIV-1 dementia in drug users. J Neuropsychiatry Clin Neurosci 4:21–28, 1992

Hauth AC, Perry MJ, Solomon LJ, et al: Alcohol use is strongly associated with continued risky sex among gay men: risk behavior patterns and alcohol-sex attributions. Scientific program and abstracts (PO-C23-3172), 9th International Conference on AIDS, Berlin, Germany, June 1993

Hawkins P, Halprin R: AIDS service provider burn-out: symptoms, prevention, and amelioration. Scientific program and abstracts (PO-B3432), 8th International Conference on AIDS, Amsterdam, The Netherlands, July 1992

Hintz S, Kuck J, Peterkin JJ, et al: Depression in the context of human immunodeficiency virus infection: implications for treatment. J Clin Psychiatry 51:497–501, 1990

Ho DD, Rota TR, Schooley RT, et al: Isolation of HTLV-III from cerebrospinal fluid and neural tissues in patients with neurologic syndromes related to the acquired immunodeficiency syndrome. N Engl J Med 313:1493–1497, 1985

Ho DD, Pomerantz RJ, Kaplan JC: Pathogenesis of infection with human immunodeficiency virus. N Engl J Med 317:278–286, 1987

Holmes VF, Fernandez F, Levy JK: Psychostimulant response in AIDS-related complex patients. J Clin Psychiatry 50:5–8, 1989

Hriso E, Kuhn T, Masdeu JC, et al: Extrapyramidal symptoms due to dopamine-blocking agents in patients with AIDS encephalopathy. Am J Psychiatry 148:1558–1561, 1991

Janssen RS, Nwanyanwu OC, Selik RM, et al: Epidemiology of human immunodeficiency virus encephalopathy in the United States. Neurology 42:1472–1476, 1992

Jarvik JG, Hesselink JR, Kennedy C, et al: Acquired immunodeficiency syndrome: magnetic resonance patterns of brain involvement with pathological correlation. Arch Neurol 45:731–736, 1988

Jenike MA, Patos C: Disabling fear of AIDS responsive to imipramine. Psychosomatics 27:143–144, 1986

Johannessen DJ, Wilson LG: Mania with cryptococcal meningitis in two AIDS patients. J Clin Psychiatry 49:200–201, 1988

Kalichman SC, Kelly JA, Johnson JR, et al: Factors associated with risk for HIV infection among chronic mentally ill adults. Am J Psychiatry 151:221–227, 1994

Karasic D, Targ E, Diefenbach P, et al: Structured group therapy and fluoxetine as treatment for mood disorder in HIV-seropositive individuals. Scientific program and abstracts, 8th International Conference on AIDS, Amsterdam, The Netherlands, July 1992

Kelly JJ, Chu SY, Buehler JW: AIDS deaths shift from hospital to home. Am J Public Health 83:1433–1437, 1993

Kieburtz KD, Ketonen L, Zettelmaier, et al: Magnetic resonance imaging findings in HIV cognitive impairment. Arch Neurol 47:643–645, 1990

Kieburtz K, Zettelmaier AE, Ketonen L, et al: Manic syndromes in AIDS. Am J Psychiatry 148:1068–1070, 1991

Klein SJ: AIDS related gay grief: an update including multiple loss syndrome. Scientific program and abstracts, 8th International Conference on AIDS, Amsterdam, The Netherlands, July 1992

Knox KK, Carrigan DR: Active human herpesvirus six infection of the CNS in patients with AIDS. Program and abstracts, 2nd National Conference on Human Retroviruses, Washington, DC, January–February 1995

Kosten T: Treatment of substance abusing AIDS patients: psychopharmacology and HIV-1 infection. Presented at Clinical Challenges and Research Directions, National Institute of Mental Health, Washington, DC, April 27–28, 1993

Lenderking WR, Gelber RD, Cotton DJ, et al: Evaluation of the quality of life associated with zidovudine treatment in asymptomatic human immunodeficiency virus infection. N Engl J Med 330:738–743, 1994

Lertora J, Akula S, Rege A, et al: Valproic acid inhibits zidovudine glucuronidation in patients with HIV infection. Scientific program and abstracts, 8th International Conference on AIDS, Amsterdam, The Netherlands, July 1992

Levine S, Anderson D, Bystritsky A, et al: A report of eight HIV-seropositive patients with major depression responding to fluoxetine. J Acquir Immune Defic Syndr 3:1074–1077, 1990

Levy RM, Bredesen DE: Central nervous system dysfunction in acquired immunodeficiency syndrome. J Acquir Immune Defic Syndr 1:41–64, 1988

Lyketsos CG, Hanson AL, Fishman M, et al: Manic syndrome early and late in the course of HIV. Am J Psychiatry 150:326–327, 1993

Maj M, Janssen R, Starace F, et al: WHO Neuropsychiatric AIDS Study, Cross-sectional Phase I: study design and psychiatric findings. Arch Gen Psychiatry 51:39–49, 1994a

Maj M, Satz P, Janssen R, et al: WHO Neuropsychiatric AIDS Study, Cross-sectional Phase II: neuropsychological and neurological findings. Arch Gen Psychiatry 51:51–61, 1994b

Markowitz JC, Klerman GL, Perry SW: Interpersonal psychotherapy of depressed HIV-positive outpatients. Hosp Community Psychiatry 43:73–78, 1992

Mayne T, O'Leary A: Family support is more important than friend or partner support in reducing distress among suburban and rural gay men. Scientific program and abstracts (WS-D17-4), 9th International Conference on AIDS, Berlin, Germany, June 1993

McArthur JC, Cohen BA, Farzedegan H, et al: Cerebrospinal fluid abnormalities in homosexual men with and without neuropsychiatric findings. Ann Neurol 23(suppl):S34-S37, 1988

McArthur JC, Cohen BA, Selnes OA, et al: Low prevalence of neurological and neuropsychological abnormalities in otherwise healthy HIV-1-infected individuals: results from the Multicenter AIDS Cohort Study. Ann Neurol 26:601–611, 1989a

McArthur JC, Becker PS, Parisi JE, et al: Neuropathological changes in early HIV-1 dementia. Ann Neurol 26:681–684, 1989b

McArthur JC, Hoover DR, Bacellar H, et al: Risk factors for the development of HIV dementia in homosexual men: report from the Multicenter AIDS Cohort Study. Program and abstracts, 8th International Conference on AIDS, Amsterdam, The Netherlands, July 1992

Miller EN, Satz P, Visscher B: Computerized and conventional neuropsychological assessment of HIV-1 infected homosexual men. Neurology 41:1608–1616, 1991

Mole LA, Israelski DM, Bubp JL, et al: The pharmacokinetics of zidovudine and oxazepam alone and in combination in the HIV-infected patient (ACTG 124). Scientific program and abstracts, 8th International Conference on AIDS, Amsterdam, The Netherlands, July 1992

Muñoz A, Phair J, Xu J, et al: Estimation of long term survivors under different models for the incubation period in homosexual men. Program and abstracts, 2nd National Conference on Human Retroviruses, Washington, DC, January–February 1995

Muñoz A, Wang MC, Bass S, et al: Acquired immunodeficiency syndrome (AIDS)-free time after human immunodeficiency virus type 1 (HIV-1) serocoversion in homosexual men. Am J Epidemiol 130:530–539, 1989

Murphy DA, Kelly JA, Bahr GR, et al: Comparison of cognitive-behavioral and social support group psychotherapies for HIV-infected persons. Scientific program and abstracts (PO-B35-2329), 9th International Conference on AIDS, Berlin, Germany, June 1993

Navia BA, Jordan BD, Price RW: The AIDS dementia complex, I: clinical features. Ann Neurol 19:517–524, 1986a

Navia BA, Cho ES, Petito CK, et al: The AIDS dementia complex, II: neuropathology. Ann Neurol 19:525–535, 1986b

O'Dowd MA, Biderman DJ, McKegney FP: Incidence of suicidality in AIDS and HIV-positive patients attending a psychiatry outpatient program. Psychosomatics 34:33–40, 1993

Ostrow DG, VanRaden MJ, Fox R, et al: Recreational drug use and sexual behavior change in a cohort of homosexual men. AIDS 4: 759–765, 1990

Ostrow DG, Beltran ED, Joseph JG, et al: Recreational drugs and sexual behavior in the Chicago MACS/CCS cohort of homosexually active men. J Subst Abuse 5:311–325, 1993

Pantaleo G, Graziosi C, Fauci AS: The immunopathogenesis of human immunodeficiency virus infection. N Engl J Med 328:327–335, 1993

Perkins DO, Davidson EJ, Leserman J, et al: Personality disorder in patients infected with HIV: a controlled study with implications for clinical care. Am J Psychiatry 150:309–315, 1993

Perkins DO, Stern RA, Golden RN, et al: Mood disorders in HIV infection: prevalence and risk factors in a nonepicenter of the AIDS epidemic. Am J Psychiatry 151:233–236, 1994

Perry MJ, Solomon LJ, Winett RA, et al: High risk sexual behavior and alcohol consumption among bar-going gay men. AIDS 8:1321–1324, 1994

Perry S, Jacobsberg R: Suicidal ideation and HIV testing. JAMA 263:679–682, 1990

Perry S, Fishman B, Jacobsberg L, et al: Effectiveness of psychoeducational interventions in reducing emotional distress after human immunodeficiency virus antibody testing. Arch Gen Psychiatry 48:143–147, 1991

Peudenier S, Hery C, Montagnier L, et al: Human microglial cells: characterization in cerebral tissue and in primary culture, and study of their susceptibility to HIV-1 infection. Ann Neurol 29:152–161, 1991

Phair J, Muñoz A, Detels R, et al: The risk of *Pneumocystis carinii* pneumonia among men infected with human immunodeficiency virus type 1. N Engl J Med 322:161–165, 1990

Portegies P, de Gans J, Lange JMA, et al: Declining incidence of AIDS dementia complex after introduction of zidovudine treatment. BMJ 299:819–821, 1989

Portegies P, Enting RH, de Gans J, et al: Presentation and course of AIDS dementia complex. AIDS 7:669–675, 1993

Post JM, Berger JR, Quencer RM: Asymptomatic and neurologically symptomatic HIV-seropositive individuals: prospective evaluation with cranial MR imaging. Radiology 178:131–139, 1991

Prager M, Nichols S, Schaffner B: Therapeutic factors in a support group for non-IVDU HIV(+) women. Scientific program and abstracts (PoB 3810), 8th International Conference on AIDS, Amsterdam, The Netherlands, July 1992

Price RW, Brew BJ: The AIDS dementia complex. J Infect Dis 158:1079–1083, 1992

Rabkin JG: Psychostimulant medication for depression and lethargy in HIV illness: a pilot study. Progress Notes 4:1–4, 1993

Rabkin JG, Williams JBW, Remien RH, et al: Depression, distress, lymphocyte subsets, and human immunodeficiency virus symptoms on two occasions in HIV-positive homosexual men. Arch Gen Psychiatry 48:111–119, 1991

Rabkin JG, Rabkin R, Wagner G: Effect of fluoxetine on mood and immune status in depressed patients with HIV illness. J Clin Psychiatry 55:92–97, 1994a

Rabkin JG, Rabkin R, Harrison W, et al: Effect of imipramine on mood and enumerative measures of immune status in depressed patients with HIV illness. Am J Psychiatry 151:516–523, 1994b

Ronald PJM, Robertson JR: Prescribing to drug misusers in the name of harm reduction. Scientific program and abstracts (PO-D18-3937), 9th International Conference on AIDS, Berlin, Germany, June 1993

Sacks M, Dermatis H, Looser-Ott S, et al: Seroprevalence of HIV and risk factors for AIDS in psychiatric inpatients. Hosp Community Psychiatry 43:736–737, 1992

Saykin AJ, Janssen RS, Sprehn GC, et al: Neuropsychological dysfunction in HIV infection: characterization in a lymphadenopathy cohort. International Journal of Clinical Neuropsychology 10:81–95, 1988

Schaerf FW, Miller RR, Lipsey JR, et al: ECT for major depression in four patients infected with human immunodeficiency virus. Am J Psychiatry 146:782–784, 1989

Sciolla A, Patterson T, Atkinson J, et al: Psychosocial characteristics of grief in HIV-infected men. Scientific program and abstracts, 8th International Conference on AIDS, Amsterdam, The Netherlands, July 1992

Selnes OA, McArthur JC, Royal W, et al: HIV-1 infection and intravenous drug use: longitudinal neuropsychological evaluation of asymptomatic subjects. Neurology 42:1924–1930, 1992

Sewell DD, Jeste DV, Atkinson JH, et al: HIV-associated psychosis: a study of 20 cases. Am J Psychiatry 151:237–242, 1994

Shaw GM, Harper ME, Hahn BH, et al: HTLV-III infection in brains of children and adults with AIDS encephalopathy. Science 227:180–182, 1985

Smith J, Craib KJB, Wales PW: Mood elevation/irritability in patients with AIDS dementia complex. Scientific program and abstracts, 4th International Conference, Neuroscience of HIV Infection, Amsterdam, The Netherlands, July 1992

Stern Y, Marder K, Bell K, et al: Multidisciplinary assessment of homosexual men with and without immunodeficiency virus infection, III: neurologic neuropsychological findings. Arch Gen Psychiatry 48:131–138, 1991

Stewart KE, Haley WE, Saag MA: Effects of caregiving tasks, social network, and patient functioning on informal caregivers of HIV-infected men. Scientific program and abstracts (PO-D22-4105), 9th International Conference on AIDS, Berlin, Germany, June 1993

Stone VE, Seage GR, Hertz T, et al: The relation between hospital experience and mortality for patients with AIDS. JAMA 268:2655–2661, 1992

Summers J, Robinson R, Zisook S, et al: The efficacy of short-term group therapy in men with unresolved grief at high risk for HIV. Scientific program and abstracts (PO-B35-2330), 9th International Conference on AIDS, Berlin, Germany, June 1993

Summers J, Sciolla A, Zisook S, et al: Gender differences in AIDS-related bereavement, in New Research Program and Abstracts: American Psychiatric Association 150th Annual Meeting, Philadelphia, PA, May 1994

Susser E, Valencia E: HIV risk behaviors among homeless mentally ill men. Scientific program and abstracts (PO-D04-3549), 9th International Conference on AIDS, Berlin, Germany, June 1993

Süuttmann U, Selberg O, Melzer A, et al: Nitrogen balance in HIV-infected patients during total parenteral nutrition. Scientific program and abstracts (WS-B34-4), 9th International Conference on AIDS, Berlin, Germany, June 1993

Talbot JD, Marrett S, Evans AC, et al: Multiple representations of pain in human cerebral cortex. Science 251:1355–1357, 1991

Todd KH, Samaroo N, Hoffman JR: Ethnicity as a risk factor for inadequate emergency department analgesia. JAMA 269:1537–1539, 1993

Tross S, Price RW, Navia BA, et al: Neuropsychological characterization of the AIDS dementia complex: a preliminary report. AIDS 2:81–88, 1988

van den Bloom F, Gremmen AW: AIDS and grief. Scientific program and abstracts (POB 3814), 8th International Conference on AIDS, Amsterdam, The Netherlands, July 1992

Velentgas P, Bynum C, Zierler S: The buddy volunteer commitment in AIDS care. Am J Public Health 80:1378–1380, 1990

Walker G: AIDS and family therapy. Family Therapy Today 26:1–7, 1987

Weatherburn P, Davies PM, Hickson FCI, et al: No connection between alcohol use and unsafe sex among gay and bisexual men. AIDS 7:115–119, 1993

Wechsler D: Wechsler Adult Intelligence Scale—Revised. San Antonio, TX, Psychological Corporation, 1981

Wiley CA, Nelson JA: Role of human immunodeficiency virus and cytomegalovirus in AIDS encephalitis. Am J Pathol 133:73–81, 1988

Wiley CA, Schrier RD, Nelson JA, et al: Cellular localization of HIV infection within the brains of AIDS patients. Proc Natl Acad Sci U S A 83:7089–7093, 1986

Williams JBW, Rabkin JG, Remien RH, et al: Multidisciplinary baseline assessment of homosexual men with and without human immunodeficiency virus infection. Arch Gen Psychiatry 48:124–130, 1991

Wong MC, Suite NDA, Labar DR: Seizures in human immunodeficiency virus infection. Arch Neurol 47:640–642, 1990

Woodhouse DE, Rothenberg RB, Potterat JJ, et al: Mapping a social network of heterosexuals at high risk for HIV infection. AIDS 8:1331–1336, 1994

Worth JL, Halman MH: Nine-month experience of an HIV/AIDS psychiatry clinic: demographics, diagnoses, and outcome. Poster presented at the 149th annual meeting of the American Psychiatric Association, San Francisco, CA, May 1993

Worth JL, Savage C, Baer L, et al: Computer-based screening for AIDS dementia complex. AIDS 7:677–681, 1993a

Worth JL, Renshaw PF, Johnson KA, et al: New onset depression in patients with AIDS dementia complex (ADC) is associated with frontal lobe perfusion defects on HM-PAO SPECT scan (abstract). Clin Neuropathol 12 (suppl 1):S28, 1993b

Yarchoan R, Venzon DJ, Pluda JM, et al: CD4 count and the risk for death in patients infected with HIV receiving antiretroviral therapy. Ann Intern Med 115:184–189, 1991

Zierler S, Feingold L, Laufer D, et al: Adult survivors of childhood sexual abuse and subsequent risk for HIV infection. Am J Public Health 81:572–575, 1991

Chapter 27

Geriatric Medicine

Gary W. Small, M.D.
Ibrahim Gunay, M.D.

Following decades of increasing medical subspecialization and a concurrent shrinkage of health care resources, we face a time when the United States' health care policy is moving toward primary care and away from subspecialty care. Despite this shift, advances in medical technology and growth of special patient populations argue in favor of not only subspecialization but additional narrowing foci within an established subspecialty. Such is the case when elderly medically ill patients require psychiatric care. Regardless of the eventual health care policy that the United States adopts, these patients have special needs that require expertise that is often unavailable in the primary care or general psychiatry settings.

NORMAL AGING AND QUALITY OF LIFE

The consultation-liaison psychiatrist must distinguish changes that are seen in normal aging from pathological changes, often a subtle distinction in elderly persons in the oldest age groups. Normal aging is defined as a decline in the number of active cells and overall reserve for biological systems. People older than 65 years were first considered "old" in the late nineteenth century, when Otto von Bismarck selected 65 years as the starting age for social welfare benefits. Increased illness survival rates have led to many more people living beyond age 65 years than during Bismarck's time. *Young-old* and *old-old* are newer terms that describe the population between ages 65 and 75 years and 75 years or older, respectively. The 75+ age group is sometimes further divided into *middle-old* (75–85 years) and *old-old* (85+ years).

Diagnosis is still complicated by normal age-associated changes. Although most people in their 60s and older complain of forgetfulness, the prognostic implications of such age-associated memory complaints remain a question for current research (Small et al. 1994, 1995). As people age, they sleep less. This normal age-related change must be distinguished from insomnia secondary to depression or anxiety or from primary sleep disorders such as apnea. Sensory deprivation from hearing and visual impairment can lead to social isolation and can exacerbate or cause psychotic symptoms.

Although people live longer, physical, psychological, and social losses may diminish the quality of life, especially during the sixth, seventh, and eighth decades. Improving functional independence, not just the length of life, is crucial. Social support and network characteristics that contribute to depression among patients in the geriatric population include loss of a spouse, inadequate emotional support, loss of a confidant, and fewer children making weekly visits (Oxman et al. 1992).

DEMOGRAPHIC TRENDS AND EPIDEMIOLOGY

Elderly persons constitute the fastest-growing segment of the population in the United States and, indeed, in all advanced industrial societies (Department of Health and Human Services 1990; World Health Organization 1992). In 1900, people age 65 and older made up only 4% of the total population; in 1988, the same group constituted more than 12% of the total population; by the year 2000, this group will represent 13%. The subgroup of elderly persons age 85 years or older is growing at an even faster pace, accounting for 10% of the 65+ age group in 1990 and a predicted 22% in 2050. This older group has the greatest frequency of chronic physical illnesses, dependency, and long-term care.

Large-scale epidemiological surveys designed to determine prevalence rates of mental disorders among medically ill elderly patients are unavailable. There are, however, some studies of psychiatric diagnostic rates among elderly patients receiving psychiatric consultations in general hospital settings. Most frequently, consultants diagnose mood disorder (17%–55%) or organic mental disorder (36%–46%). Older patients are more likely to have dementia or delirium but less likely to be diagnosed with personality disorders than are younger consultation-liaison patients. Younger and older groups in the general hospital, however, have similar rates of mood disorders.

PSYCHIATRIC CONSULTATION REQUESTS FOR GERIATRIC PATIENTS

Prevalence of mental disorders, especially cognitive and mood disorders, is higher among elderly general hospital inpatients than among elderly people in the community (Regier et al. 1988). Despite this high prevalence of psychiatric disorders among elderly hospitalized patients, psychiatric consultations are less frequently requested for such patients than for their younger counterparts (Rabins et al. 1983). Moreover, the referral rate for hospitalized inpatients age 65 or older is remarkably lower than the estimated prevalence of psychiatric problems in the same population (Folks and Ford 1985; Koenig et al. 1988b; Popkin et al. 1984). Ageism, prognostic pessimism, and the false assumption that mental impairment is a normal aspect of aging could contribute to this low referral rate.

Several research groups have examined psychiatric consultation request patterns for elderly patients in general hospitals (Grossberg et al. 1990; Levitte and Thornby 1989; Mainprize and Rodin 1987; Popkin et al. 1984; Ruskin 1985; Small and Fawzy 1988); 34%–78% of referrals are from medical services, and only 15%–25% are from surgical services. In general, evaluations for depression or cognitive impairment are the most frequent reasons for such requests. Other reasons for consultation requests include mental status evaluation, agitation, suicidal and other disturbing behaviors, and medication management.

CLINICAL SYNDROMES AND CONSULTATION ISSUES

Delirium

Structural brain disease, age-related central nervous system (CNS) changes, sensory deprivation, diminished hearing and vision, chronic medical illness, age-related changes in pharmacokinetics and pharmacodynamics, and decreased resistance to physical stress make elderly persons particularly vulnerable to delirium. If delirium is not recognized and treated promptly, 20%–80% of affected patients die (Lipowski 1989). A study (Francis and Kapoor 1992) of medical inpatients age 70 years and older showed a 2-year mortality of 39% for patients who had had an episode of delirium during hospitalization compared with 23% who had not developed delirium.

Early clinical features of delirium in elderly persons are similar to those in younger patients and include malaise, agitation, headache, sleep disturbance, irritability, disorientation, impaired short-term memory, perceptual disturbance, anxiety, and depression or decreased interests. As the illness progresses, disordered attention and concentration are prominent. Many medical illnesses can cause delirium, and medications are certainly an important cause in elderly patients.

Dementia

Both delirium and dementia are prevalent in medically ill elderly persons. It is difficult to determine whether a patient with delirium also has dementia, but it is not so difficult to determine whether a patient with dementia also has delirium. Patients with dementia are exceptionally vulnerable to acute insults to brain metabolism, which often result in a superimposed acute confusional state. Patients with dementia remain as medical inpatients significantly longer and require more daily nursing care than their counterparts without dementia (Erkinjuntti et al. 1986). Elderly patients with dementia may also have psychosis and agitation (Wragg and Jeste 1989), and the clinical picture in such patients can mimic that of delirium. Prominent fluctuations in the level of consciousness are not consistent with dementia.

Patients with progressive dementias and their relatives often deny the cognitive decline early in its course, and patients may first be seen by the physician when the illness is moderately severe. Psychosocial stresses (e.g., death of a spouse) also may cause an acute worsening and prompt recognition of the dementia by family members and clinicians.

Depression

Geriatric depression often presents differently from depression in young adults (Addonizio and Alexopoulos 1993; National Institutes of Health Consensus Development Panel on Depression in Late Life 1992; Small 1991); these features are compared in Table 27–1. For example, elderly depressed patients are less likely to express guilt feelings than are their younger counterparts (Small et al. 1986). In addition, elderly patients are known to minimize or even to deny their depressed mood and instead become preoccupied with somatic symptoms. Conwell et al. (1990) reported that six of one series of eight persons over age 65 who committed suicide had somatic delusions of having cancer and presented to their primary physicians with this concern before their deaths. Family members and even health care providers may also minimize the importance of geriatric depression and assume, incorrectly, that depression is the result of physical and social problems associated with "normal" aging. Symptoms such as loss of appetite, anhedonia, anergy, and insomnia are more prominent than depressed mood in elderly patients. The term *masked* is often used to describe the depressed condition of the patient who focuses on physical rather than affective complaints. Such patients frequently exhibit neutral affects but complain about constipation, back pain, or some other physical symptom.

Symptoms of depression and dementia frequently overlap in elderly patients, resulting in complex clinical syndromes (Small 1989). Some elderly patients with depression have cognitive complaints and present with a dementia syndrome of depression. The term *depressive pseudodementia* is no longer consid-

Table 27–1. Clinical features of geriatric depression

Compared with young adult depressed patients, geriatric patients who are clinically depressed are

More likely to

Minimize or deny depressed mood

Become preoccupied with somatic symptoms

Complain about memory

Less likely to

Express guilt

Seek help from a psychiatrist

Accept a psychological explanation for their illness

ered to be accurate by many clinicians because the cognitive dysfunction is real, albeit reversible. Such patients also are more likely to have an acute onset of symptoms and predominant affective complaints compared with patients with progressive dementias. Moreover, cognitive complaints usually improve with antidepressant treatment in the patient with depression.

To complicate the situation, patients with primary progressive dementias (e.g., Alzheimer's disease, multi-infarct dementia) frequently develop depression, especially when the dementia is of mild to moderate severity. Among such patients with chronic dementia, subsyndromal depressive symptoms are more common than depressive syndromes. Sometimes such depressive symptoms appear to be a psychological reaction to cognitive losses, but evidence also exists for an organic cause. Zubenko and Moosy (1988) found that a concurrent diagnosis of major depression and Alzheimer's disease was associated with greater loss of neurons in the locus coeruleus and substantia nigra than in patients without concurrent depressions.

Koenig et al. (1988a) found major depression in 12% and other depressive syndromes in 23% of 130 men age 70 and older who were hospitalized for medical illnesses. Studies of elderly patients attending medical outpatient

clinics have demonstrated rates of depression ranging from 10% to 20%. In general, health care providers are less likely to recognize major depression in hospitalized medically ill elderly patients than in younger hospitalized patients. In a study of 53 hospitalized elderly men with medical illness and major depression, 44% of the medical records contained no mention of depression (Koenig et al. 1992). The high frequency of affective symptoms in medically ill elderly patients and failure to recognize such symptoms present arguments in favor of routine screening in this patient population.

A significant public health problem related to depression is the high suicide rate, especially for elderly white men (Blazer et al. 1986; Rabins 1992). The suicide rate continues to be higher among men age 65 and older than among any other age group in the United States.

Anxiety

Hospitalized elderly patients often worry about medical illnesses and the accompanying pain, disability, and death. The loss of function and the possibility of death are difficult to deny and result in anxiety. Some elderly persons have an undiagnosed anxiety disorder, which is unmasked by the exacerbation of a physical illness, hospital admission, or surgery. A variety of physical and substance-related conditions can cause a secondary anxiety disorder; thyroid disease and medication effects are common causes of anxiety in elderly patients. Somatic anxiety symptoms, such as palpitations, dyspnea, and dizziness, can result from either underlying anxiety disorders or worsening physical illness, which complicates the differential diagnosis.

Phobic disorders are relatively common in old age, with 1-month prevalence rates ranging from 5% to 10% (Lindesay 1991; Regier et al. 1988). Agoraphobic fears in elderly persons are often precipitated by an episode of physical illness or other traumatic event (Lindesay 1991).

Late-Life Psychosis

An important change in DSM-IV (American Psychiatric Association 1994) is the absence of an age-at-onset criterion for the diagnosis of schizophrenia. Jeste et al. (1988), in their comparison of patients with early-onset and late-onset schizophrenia, described similarities in the degree of psychopathology and positive symptoms among the two groups. However, they reported a lower frequency of negative symptoms in the late-onset group.

Patients with dementias often develop psychotic symptoms. Patients with Alzheimer's disease often have simple persecutory delusions and visual hallucinations (Wragg and Jeste 1989). Zubenko and co-workers (1991) found associations between the presence of psychosis and densities of senile plaques and neurofibrillary tangles in the brains of patients with Alzheimer's disease. Jeste et al. (1992) reported that patients with Alzheimer's disease and psychosis show greater cognitive impairment than do their counterparts without psychosis.

Regardless of whether the psychiatric disorder is a dementia with psychotic symptoms or a primary psychosis, neuroleptic agents offer effective treatment (Lohr et al. 1992). Psychotic symptoms also occur in patients with delirium, and so careful diagnostic assessment is required.

Substance Dependence, Abuse, and Misuse

Elderly persons often underreport their alcohol consumption and related problems (Atkinson 1990), and clinicians fail to recognize alcohol-related problems in elderly patients (Curtis et al. 1989). In the absence of liver disease, hepatic metabolism of alcohol remains relatively unchanged with age. However, decreased lean body mass and total body water cause the total volume of distribution for alcohol to decline with age. Cognitive and cerebellar functions after a standard alcohol load worsen with age. Such effects make distinc-

tions between "heavy" and "problem" drinking less meaningful for elderly persons. After a standard alcohol load, an average 60-year-old man will have a peak blood alcohol level 20% higher than a man in his 30s (Vestal et al. 1977). In elderly patients, therefore, all heavy drinking is problem drinking.

Elderly persons sometimes abuse more than one substance at a time. Finlayson et al. (1988) reported that 14% of 216 alcoholic inpatients who were age 65 years or older were also abusing narcotic analgesics and anxiolytics. A useful and simple screen for alcohol consumption in elderly persons is the CAGE questionnaire (Buchsbaum et al. 1992). (The CAGE questionnaire is shown in Table 13–6 in Chapter 13; for more details on substance-related disorder in outpatient and inpatient consultation-liaison settings, see Franklin and Frances, Chapter 13, in this volume.)

Cohort Effects and Ageism

Elderly persons typically consider psychiatric intervention as a last resort for "crazy people." They are reluctant to accept psychiatric referral and sometimes have psychiatric disorders that are overlooked or are inadequately treated. Ageism or age-related prejudice also complicates intervention, clouds decision making, and can result in improper treatment. Psychiatrists are not immune to ageist attitudes, which may involve fears of death, the belief that psychiatric symptoms are somehow "appropriate" in the elderly, and the inaccurate belief that elderly people do not respond to treatment (Ford and Sbordone 1980).

Elder Abuse

Although both victims and perpetrators deny and minimize the frequency and severity of elder abuse, an estimated 10% of Americans over age 65 are abused (Council on Scientific Affairs 1987). The abuser is often a relative who lives with the victim; the abuse is generally recurring. Physical, sexual, or psychological abuse can take a variety of forms. A typical victim is a physically or mentally impaired 75-year-old widow whose limited finances force her to move in with a younger relative (Taler and Ansello 1985). Clinicians should consider the possibility of elder abuse when a caregiver 1) expresses frustration in providing care, 2) shows signs of psychological distress, 3) has a history of committing abuse or violence, or 4) has a history of alcohol or drug abuse.

■ DIAGNOSTIC EVALUATION

Clinical Examination

In consultation-liaison settings, attention to physical problems and the medical history is as important as obtaining detailed information about the patient's psychiatric history. This is even more crucial in evaluating geriatric patients, in whom the likelihood of multiple medical conditions is high and symptoms of medical and psychiatric disorders overlap. Obtaining the history and performing a mental status examination are sometimes tedious because of the many years patients have lived, complications from multiple illnesses, and brain dysfunction. A reliable collateral source can save time and contribute important clinical information; this is essential when the patient has cognitive impairment.

Physical Examination

Patients usually are examined by their primary physicians before the psychiatrist is consulted. The consultant should review the medical record to gather details of history, diagnosis, and management of the present illness. Sometimes the consultation-liaison psychiatrist must perform a limited physical examination, particularly a neurological examination. Consultants occasionally will discover a physical sign overlooked by the primary physician. For example, the patient who is agitated and disturbed (e.g.,

a frail elderly patient with psychosis) can make the primary physician anxious and thus cloud clinical assessment.

Mental Status Examination

Certain aspects of the mental status examination deserve special attention in elderly patients. Depressed elderly patients who minimize dysphoria may demonstrate it nonverbally through facial expressions and sighs. A careful investigation of suicidal thinking and intent is essential because of the lethal methods chosen by this age group. Cognitive assessment of geriatric patients is particularly important. A comprehensive cognitive examination usually includes examination of attention and concentration, language functions (e.g., spontaneous speech, comprehension, repetition, naming), orientation, memory functions, constructional ability, praxis, and frontal-lobe function. The Mini-Mental State Exam (MMSE; Folstein et al. 1975) provides a brief, yet reliable and valid, measure of cognition that includes tests of orientation, memory, concentration, language, and conceptual ability. Although the MMSE does not identify patients with subtle cognitive dysfunction and language items have low sensitivity, the memory item, attention-concentration items, and constructional item have adequate sensitivity and specificity in many clinical settings and correlate significantly with scores on neuropsychological tests (Feher et al. 1992).

Laboratory Findings

A clinical chemistry screen is routine for almost all hospital admissions and for most initial outpatient visits. Such screens are essential in diagnostic evaluations of patients with cognitive impairment. Abnormal sodium and chloride levels can warn of dehydration that may, if untreated, progress to delirium, lethargy, or convulsions. This screen will also detect respiratory or metabolic acidosis, which can lead to drowsiness and weakness that may be mistakenly diagnosed as depression.

Decreased protein intake and decreased muscle mass in older patients lead to an overestimate of renal function because blood urea nitrogen (BUN) and creatinine levels decrease. Therefore, normal serum levels for BUN and creatinine may indicate decreased renal function, and minor elevations may represent significant dysfunction. Liver function typically remains adequate throughout life, despite some decrease in the speed of drug metabolism.

The electrocardiogram (ECG) is most often used to screen for cardiovascular disease and to identify the presence of conduction defects that would complicate the use of tricyclic antidepressants or electroconvulsive therapy (ECT). It also reveals the presence of cardiovascular disease that can have psychiatric manifestations.

Brain Imaging Studies

Developed about 21 years ago, computed tomography (CT) is still widely used in geriatric psychiatry. Both abnormal anatomical and pathological structural alterations are revealed by CT scanning. Routine scans are often performed without contrast media; however, use of contrast media for scans in patients with suspected intracranial malignancy or bleeding may help to diagnose these conditions. Magnetic resonance imaging (MRI) was introduced a decade ago and offers greater resolution of structural images than does CT. The disadvantages of MRI include greater cost and greater discomfort (i.e., some patients become claustrophobic during the procedure).

■ TREATMENT AND MANAGEMENT

Treatment of Medical Problems

The treatment of medical problems in elderly patients is especially crucial. Most psychiatric problems in this population occur either because of or concurrently with medical illnesses. Although the attending physician controls the medical treatment, the consultant occasionally must suggest additional diagnostic evaluations or alternative medical treatments.

Psychopharmacological Treatment

Age-related pharmacokinetic and pharmacodynamic factors. Interactions of drugs with the brain and the rest of the body change with age (Abernethy 1992). Gastrointestinal (GI) function alterations include increased gastric pH, diminished splanchnic blood flow, and diminished intestinal motility, yet drug absorption generally does not diminish as people age. Most psychotropic medications are highly lipid-soluble and protein-bound. Aging causes a relative decrease in total body water, reduction in lean body mass, and increase in body fat. With the resultant larger volume of distribution, more time is required for drugs to reach steady-state levels, and plasma levels are lower at any given dose. Moreover, liver disease can impair protein synthesis, leading to decreased protein availability for binding to psychotropics in plasma. Thus, more unbound or active drug is present, causing greater clinical effect at any given plasma level. In addition, reduced hepatic blood flow and function diminish the metabolism of psychotropics (e.g., chlordiazepoxide, diazepam) that undergo phase I biotransformation (e.g., microsomal enzyme oxidation). Hepatic metabolism of cyclic antidepressants forms water-soluble hydroxy metabolites; such metabolites are cardiotoxic and depend on renal clearance. Renal function often decreases with age, and thus the risk of cardiotoxicity from such agents increases. Lithium also requires particularly careful monitoring in elderly patients because of predominant renal elimination and potentially serious toxicity.

Polypharmacy. The use of multiple drugs affects all pharmacokinetic processes. Because elderly persons are likely to use more than one medication, drug-drug interactions are a critical issue in management. The metabolism of psychotropic drugs is often complicated by chronic medical illnesses and medications that alter GI, hepatic, or renal functions. Educational programs that target health care providers reduce polypharmacy (Avorn et al. 1992). All psychotropic medications have been used to treat medically ill geriatric patients (Table 27–2). Unfortunately, however, the database from controlled studies in this patient population is limited. Thus, clinicians should use caution and conservative guidelines (see "Follow Conservative and Rational Pharmacological Guidelines," later in this chapter) when prescribing psychotropic drugs for elderly patients.

Mood-stabilizing medications.   More than two dozen double-blind, placebo-controlled antidepressant trials demonstrate that physically healthy depressed elderly patients respond to a variety of agents, including cyclic antidepressants and selective serotonin reuptake inhibitors (SSRIs) (Small 1991). Secondary amine tricyclic antidepressants (e.g., nortriptyline, desipramine) are also recommended in medically ill elderly patients because of their favorable side-effect profile compared with tertiary amines (e.g., amitriptyline, imipramine). Although fluoxetine is safe and effective for geriatric depression (Tollefson et al. 1995), newer SSRIs such as paroxetine and sertraline are also reasonable choices and offer the advantage of shorter elimination half-lives. The lack of anticholinergic and cardiac side effects with SSRIs offers a marked advantage for geriatric use.

The observation that monoamine oxidase activity increases with age (Bridge et al. 1985) suggests a place for monoamine oxidase inhibitors (MAOIs) in the treatment of geriatric depression. Initial reports indicate efficacy in patients with Alzheimer's disease and major depression (Jenike 1985). Unfortunately, the potential for MAOIs to produce orthostatic hypotension, especially in predisposed individuals, limits their usefulness for many geriatric patients.

Lithium is used safely and effectively in medically ill elderly patients, but some caution is needed (Foster 1992). In general, elderly patients require lower lithium doses and blood levels. Consultation-liaison psychiatrists must recognize and appreciate the potentially serious adverse interactions between lithium and other drugs such as diuretics, nonsteroidal anti-inflammatory drugs, cardiovascular drugs, anticonvulsants, antidepressants, and neuroleptics.

Limited data on psychostimulants suggest their usefulness in treating medically ill withdrawn elderly patients who cannot tolerate adverse effects (e.g., cardiac conduction abnormalities) that are associated with other antidepressants (Katon and Raskind 1980). Psychostimulants also have been used in combination with noradrenergic antidepressant drugs. The antidepressant effects of psychostimulants may result from catecholamine reuptake blockage that prolongs the effects of synaptically released norepinephrine (Chiarello and Cole 1987).

Benzodiazepines are recommended for anxiety and agitation, especially when the elderly patient's medical condition poses a risk of toxicity from other psychotropics (e.g., tricyclic antidepressants or antipsychotic drugs). Short-acting benzodiazepines are preferred. Alprazolam, for example, was found to be more effective than placebo in treating anxiety in depressed and anxious patients age 60 and older immediately following coronary bypass surgery (Freeman et al. 1986). Hart et al. (1991) found a relative absence of adverse cognitive and psychomotor effects with the use of alprazolam in healthy elderly persons; however, medically ill elderly patients may be more sensitive to such effects. Benzodiazepines with long elimination half-lives and active metabolites (e.g., diazepam) are likely to cause ataxia

Table 27–2.   Some psychotropic drugs and treatment recommendations in the elderly

Drug type	Recommended drug	Advantages	Disadvantages
Antidepressants			
Tricyclics	Desipramine	Less anticholinergic	Too activating for some patients
			Affects cardiac conduction
	Nortriptyline	Less orthostasis	Too sedating for a few patients
			Affects cardiac conduction
MAOIs	Tranylcypromine	Not anticholinergic	Diet restrictions
		No cardiotoxicity	Sedating for some/activating for others
			Hypertensive crisis
			Orthostasis
SSRIs	Fluoxetine	Few side effects	Long half-life
			Too activating for some patients
	Sertraline, paroxetine	Few side effects	Too activating for some patients
Other anti-depressants	Trazodone	Sedation	Orthostasis
		Not anticholinergic	Ventricular irritability
		No quinidine-like effects	Rare priapism
	Bupropion	Few side effects	Seizure risk
Benzodiazepines	Lorazepam	Conjugative metabolism less affected by aging	Cognitive impairment
	Oxazepam		Sedation
	Temazepam		Risk of falls
Neuroleptics	Haloperidol	Less anticholinergic	Extrapyramidal side effects
	Thiothixene	Less orthostasis	Tardive dyskinesia
			Requires careful dosing
Lithium		Effective in mania	Sensitive to renal function
		Possibly effective adjunct in unipolar depression	Increased receptor sensitivity

Note.   MAOI = monoamine oxidase inhibitor; SSRI = selective serotonin reuptake inhibitor.
Source.   Adapted from Wise MG, Tierney J: "Psychopharmacology in the Elderly." *Journal of the Louisiana State Medical Society* 144:471–476, 1992. Used with permission.

and confusion; they are best avoided in older patients.

Neuroleptic medications.   A limited number of studies indicates that neuroleptic medications are useful in treating psychotic symptoms in elderly patients with dementia, schizophrenia, psychotic depressions, or delirium. High-potency compounds such as halo-peridol are usually the agents of first choice because of fewer cardiovascular and anticholinergic effects. Side effects of concern include akathisia and tardive dyskinesia. Several studies documented the high vulnerability of elderly patients to tardive dyskinesia; incidences of 31% were reported after 43 weeks of neuroleptic treatment (Saltz et al. 1991; Yassa et al. 1992). Initial clinical experience with novel antipsychotic medications (e.g., risperidone, clozapine) suggests that they may have a place in treating some elderly patients with psychosis.

Electroconvulsive Therapy

ECT is generally the safest and most effective treatment for severely depressed elderly patients and is the treatment of choice for those with psychotic depression. Although patients with multiple medical problems and those over age 75 are at increased risk for adverse effects, modification of treatment can minimize risks. Although temporary effects on memory are common in elderly patients, overall cognitive dysfunction actually improves after ECT (Stoudemire et al. 1991).

Psychotherapy and Related Nonpharmacological Approaches

Psychotherapy is effective in the treatment of geriatric patients with depression, especially when a patient's cognitive impairment or severity of illness does not interfere with talk therapy (Thompson et al. 1987). Geriatric patients have been treated using individual psychodynamic, cognitive, and behavioral approaches, as well as group psychotherapy; most psychotherapy studies focus on geriatric depression (Weiss and Lazarus 1993). In a medical inpatient setting, psychotherapeutic interventions are often supportive and time-limited.

Many elderly patients receive care from spouses, adult children, and other relatives (Jarvik and Small 1990). Caregivers experience considerable stress and are prone to depression and health problems (Baumgarten et al. 1992). Psychological support for caregivers may lessen their emotional burden and, in the final analysis, benefit the older patient.

Environmental Management

Modifications of the environment help to minimize confusion of hospitalized elderly pa-

tients. Prominent clocks, night-lights, and personal items from home can assist orientation. Frequent visits from relatives and friends are also helpful.

STRATEGIES FOR PSYCHIATRIC CONSULTATION FOR GERIATRIC PATIENTS

Table 27–3 presents suggested strategies for psychiatric consultation for geriatric patients. These strategies are discussed in the following sections.

Collect Data From Multiple Sources

Many elderly patients rely on family members or other caregivers for assistance with activities of daily living (ADLs); thus, the consultant must obtain comprehensive histories from the caregivers and maintain close contact with them. For cognitively impaired patients, caregivers' and collateral histories are essential. The complexity and multiplicity of medical problems warrant careful review of previous medical records and detailed discussions with the patient's primary physicians and consultants.

Recognize Unique Clinical Presentations of Geriatric Syndromes

Geriatric depression often differs from depression in young adults. Physical and memory

Table 27–3. Suggested strategies for psychiatric consultation for geriatric patients

Collect data from multiple sources

Recognize unique clinical presentations of geriatric syndromes

Search for medical and toxic causes of psychiatric syndromes

Reduce polypharmacy

Follow conservative and rational pharmacological guidelines

Identify adverse drug effects sooner rather than later

Emphasize nonpharmacological interventions

complaints are more prominent in elderly patients.

Search for Medical and Toxic Causes of Psychiatric Syndromes

Although a psychiatric disorder may present with characteristic clinical features, the high prevalence of medical illness in elderly patients frequently requires an aggressive search for medical and toxic causes. A comprehensive history, physical examination, and laboratory tests usually identify underlying physical illnesses that cause psychiatric symptoms.

Reduce Polypharmacy

A relative should bring all medication bottles for initial evaluation. When possible, one medication at a time should be eliminated, especially drugs that are likely to cause adverse effects.

Follow Conservative and Rational Pharmacological Guidelines

"Start low and go slow" is the recommended strategy. Most elderly patients respond to low dosages; however, some will need the full adult dosage. Medications should be selected according to side-effect profile. For example, sedating antidepressants are best for patients with agitated depressions, and low-potency neuroleptics are appropriate for patients who are sensitive to extrapyramidal effects.

Identify Adverse Drug Effects Sooner Rather Than Later

Close monitoring of patients for side effects is crucial. For example, agitation in a patient with dementia may initially improve with a neuroleptic, then worsen after weeks of treatment (i.e., akathisia). Benzodiazepines with long elimination half-lives and active metabolites will accumulate over time and cause confusion and ataxia.

Emphasize Nonpharmacological Interventions

Physically ill geriatric patients are often sensitive to medication side effects and may not initially tolerate psychotropic medications. These situations call for nonpharmacological approaches. ECT, psychotherapy, phototherapy, and environmental interventions will help facilitate later pharmacological interventions, which can benefit the patient.

CONCLUSION

Providing expert evaluation and treatment for elderly medically ill patients can be both a challenging and rewarding experience for the consultation-liaison psychiatrist. A practical, systematic approach to diagnostic and treatment decision making is essential. The medical illnesses will, of course, often complicate accurate diagnosis, but the consultant must also consider complications from dementia syndromes, cohort effects, ageism, and heterogeneity of patient populations.

REFERENCES

Abernethy DR: Psychotropic drugs and the aging process: pharmacokinetics and pharmacodynamics, in Clinical Geriatric Psychopharmacology, 2nd Edition. Edited by Salzman C. Baltimore, MD, Williams & Wilkins, 1992, pp 61–76

Addonizio G, Alexopoulos GS: Affective disorders in the elderly. International Journal of Geriatric Psychiatry 8:41–47, 1993

American Psychiatric Association: Diagnostic and Statistical Manual of Mental Disorders, 4th Edition. Washington, DC, American Psychiatric Association, 1994

Atkinson RM: Aging and alcohol use disorders: diagnostic issues in the elderly. Int Psychogeriatr 2:55–70, 1990

Avorn J, Soumerai SB, Everitt DE, et al: A randomized trial of a program to reduce the use of psychoactive drugs in nursing homes. N Engl J Med 327:168–173, 1992

Baumgarten M, Battista RN, Infante-Rivard C, et al: The psychological and physical health of family members caring for an elderly person with dementia. J Clin Epidemiol 45:61–70, 1992

Blazer DG, Bachar JR, Manton KE: Suicide in late life: review and commentary. J Am Geriatr Soc 34:519–525, 1986

Bridge TP, Soldo BJ, Phelps BY, et al: Platelet monoamine oxidase activity: demographic characteristics contribute to enzyme activity variability. J Gerontol 40:23–28, 1985

Buchsbaum DG, Buchanan RG, Welsh J, et al: Screening for drinking disorders in the elderly using the CAGE questionnaire. J Am Geriatr Soc 40:662–665, 1992

Chiarello RJ, Cole JO: The use of psychostimulants in general psychiatry: a reconsideration. Arch Gen Psychiatry 44:286–296, 1987

Conwell Y, Caine ED, Olsen K: Suicide and cancer in late life. Hosp Community Psychiatry 41:1334–1339, 1990

Council on Scientific Affairs: Elder abuse and neglect. JAMA 257:966–971, 1987

Curtis JR, Geller G, Stokes EG, et al: Characteristics, diagnosis and treatment of alcoholism in elderly patients. J Am Geriatr Soc 37:310–316, 1989

Department of Health and Human Services, Public Health Service: Healthy People 2000: National Health Promotion and Disease Prevention Objectives. Washington, DC, Department of Health and Human Services, 1990

Erkinjuntti T, Wikstrom J, Palo J, et al: Dementia among medical inpatients: evaluation of 2000 consecutive admissions. Arch Intern Med 146:1923–1926, 1986

Feher EP, Mahurin RK, Doody RS, et al: Establishing the limits of the Mini-Mental State: examination of "subtests." Arch Neurol 49:87–92, 1992

Finlayson ER, Hurt RD, Davis LJ, et al: Alcoholism in elderly persons: a study of the psychiatric and psychosocial features of 216 inpatients. Mayo Clin Proc 63:761–768, 1988

Folks DG, Ford CV: Psychiatric disorders in geriatric medical/surgical patients, part I: report of 195 consecutive consultations. South Med J 78:239–241, 1985

Folstein MF, Folstein SE, McHugh PR: Mini-Mental State: a practical method for grading the cognitive state of patients for the clinician. J Psychiatr Res 12:189–198, 1975

Ford CV, Sbordone RJ: Attitudes of psychiatrists toward elderly patients. Am J Psychiatry 137:571–575, 1980

Foster JR: Use of lithium in elderly psychiatric patients: a review of the literature. Lithium 3:77–93, 1992

Francis J, Kapoor WN: Prognosis after hospital discharge of older medical patients with delirium. J Am Geriatr Soc 40:601–606, 1992

Freeman AM, Fleece L, Folks DG, et al: Alprazolam treatment of postcoronary bypass anxiety and depression. J Clin Psychopharmacol 6:39–41, 1986

Grossberg GT, Zimny GH, Nakra BRS: Geriatric psychiatry consultations in a university hospital. Int Psychogeriatr 2:161–168, 1990

Hart RP, Colenda CC, Hamer RM: Effects of buspirone and alprazolam on the cognitive performance of normal elderly subjects. Am J Psychiatry 148:73–77, 1991

Jarvik L, Small G: Parentcare. New York, Bantam, 1990

Jenike MA: MAO inhibitors as treatment for depressed patients with primary degenerative dementia (Alzheimer's disease). Am J Psychiatry 142:763–764, 1985

Jeste DV, Harris MJ, Pearlson GD, et al: Late-onset schizophrenia: studying clinical validity. Psychiatr Clin North Am 11:1–13, 1988

Jeste DV, Wragg RE, Salmon DP, et al: Cognitive deficits of Alzheimer's disease patients with and without delusions. Am J Psychiatry 149:184–189, 1992

Katon W, Raskind M: Treatment of depression in the medically ill elderly with methylphenidate. Am J Psychiatry 137:963–965, 1980

Koenig HG, Meador KG, Cohen HJ, et al: Depression in elderly hospitalized patients with medical illness. Arch Intern Med 148:1929–1936, 1988a

Koenig HG, Meador KG, Cohen HJ, et al: Detection and treatment of major depression in older medically ill hospitalized patients. Int J Psychiatry Med 18:17–31, 1988b

Koenig HG, Goli V, Shelp F, et al: Major depression in hospitalized medically ill older men: documentation, management, and outcome. International Journal of Geriatric Psychiatry 7: 255–334, 1992

Levitte SS, Thornby JI: Geriatric and non-geriatric psychiatry consultation: a comparison study. Gen Hosp Psychiatry 11:339–344, 1989

Lindesay J: Phobic disorders in the elderly. Br J Psychiatry 159:531–541, 1991

Lipowski ZJ: Delirium in the elderly patient. N Engl J Med 320:578–582, 1989

Lohr JB, Jeste DV, Harris MJ, et al: Treatment of disordered behavior, in Clinical Geriatric Psychopharmacology, 2nd Edition. Edited by Salzman C. Baltimore, MD, Williams & Wilkins, 1992, pp 79–113

Mainprize E, Rodin G: Geriatric referrals to a psychiatric consultation-liaison service. Can J Psychiatry 32:5–9, 1987

National Institutes of Health Consensus Development Panel on Depression in Late Life: Diagnosis and treatment of depression in late life. JAMA 268:1018–1024, 1992

Oxman TE, Berkman LF, Kasl S, et al: Social support and depressive symptoms in the elderly. Am J Epidemiol 135:356–368, 1992

Popkin MK, MacKenzie TB, Callies AL: Psychiatric consultation to geriatric medically ill inpatients in a university hospital. Arch Gen Psychiatry 41:703–707, 1984

Rabins PV: Prevention of mental disorder in the elderly: current perspectives and future prospects. J Am Geriatr Soc 40:727–733, 1992

Rabins P, Lucas MJ, Teitelbaum M, et al: Utilization of psychiatric consultation for elderly patients. J Am Geriatr Soc 31:581–584, 1983

Regier DA, Boyd JH, Burke JD, et al: One-month prevalence of mental disorders in the United States. Arch Gen Psychiatry 45:977–986, 1988

Ruskin PE: Geriatric consultation in a university hospital: a report on 67 referrals. Am J Psychiatry 142:333–336, 1985

Saltz BL, Woerner MG, Kane JM, et al: Prospective study of tardive dyskinesia incidence in the elderly. JAMA 266:2402–2406, 1991

Small GW: Behavioral disorders in Alzheimer disease: depression is common. Bull Clin Neurosci 54:2–7, 1989

Small GW: Recognition and treatment of depression in the elderly. J Clin Psychiatry 52(suppl): 11–22, 1991

Small GW, Fawzy FI: Psychiatric consultation for the medically ill elderly in the general hospital: need for a collaborative model of care. Psychosomatics 29:94–103, 1988

Small GW, Komanduri R, Gitlin M, et al: The influence of age on guilt expression in major depression. International Journal of Geriatric Psychiatry 1:121–126, 1986

Small GW, Okonek A, Mandelkern MA, et al: Subjective and objective age-associated memory loss: initial neuropsychological, family history, and brain metabolic findings of a longitudinal study. Int Psychogeriatr 6:23–44, 1994

Small GW, Mazziotta JC, Collins MT, et al: Apolipoprotein E type 4 allele and cerebral glucose metabolism in relatives at risk for familial Alzheimer disease. JAMA 273:942–947, 1995

Stoudemire A, Hill CD, Morris R, et al: Cognitive outcome following tricyclic and electroconvulsive treatment of major depression in the elderly. Am J Psychiatry 148:1336–1340, 1991

Taler G, Ansello EF: Elder abuse. Am Fam Physician 32:107–114, 1985

Thompson LW, Gallagher D, Breckenridge JS: Comparative effectiveness of psychotherapies for depressed elders. J Consult Clin Psychol 55:385–390, 1987

Tollefson GD, Bosomworth JC, Heiligenstein JH, et al: A double-blind placebo-controlled clinical trial of fluoxetine in geriatric patients with major depression. Int Psychogeriatr 7:89–104, 1995

Vestal RE, McGuire EA, Tobin JD, et al: Aging and ethanol metabolism. Clin Pharmacol Ther 21:343–354, 1977

Weiss LJ, Lazarus LW: Psychosocial treatment of the geropsychiatric patient. International Journal of Geriatric Psychiatry 8:95–100, 1993

Wise MG, Tierney J: Psychopharmacology in the elderly. J La State Med Soc 144:471–476, 1992

World Health Organization: World Health Statistics: Demographic Trends, Aging and Noncommunicable Disease. Geneva, Switzerland, World Health Organization, 1992

Wragg R, Jeste DV: Overview of depression and psychosis in Alzheimer's disease. Am J Psychiatry 146:577–587, 1989

Yassa R, Nastase C, Dupont D, et al: Tardive dyskinesia in elderly psychiatric patients: a 5-year study. Am J Psychiatry 149:1206–1211, 1992

Zubenko GS, Moosy J: Major depression in primary dementia. Arch Neurol 45:1182–1186, 1988

Zubenko GS, Moosy J, Martinez AJ, et al: Neuropathologic and neurochemical correlates of psychosis in primary dementia. Arch Neurol 48:619–624, 1991

Chapter 28

The Emergency Department

George E. Tesar, M.D.

PSYCHIATRIC CONSULTATION IN THE EMERGENCY DEPARTMENT

Smaller academic and nonacademic hospitals that are unable to sustain separate emergency psychiatric services continue to rely on consultation-liaison psychiatrists or on-call psychiatrists in the emergency department (ED). This is not an ideal approach because the request for an emergency consultation is typically added onto the schedule of a busy clinician. In addition, the consultant generally has little help with arrangement of the patient's disposition, which often must be carefully planned and orchestrated at the time the consultation is performed. Based on the paucity of available inpatient and outpatient psychiatric resources in most communities, disposition planning is often the most challenging part of an emergency psychiatric assessment.

Weapons Screening and Initial Management of Violent or Potentially Violent Patients

Contrary to what might be expected, it is not unusual for psychiatric patients to carry weap-

ons into the ED. In studies performed at the Langley Porter Psychiatric Institute Emergency Service in San Francisco, CA, 4%–8% of patients had weapons (McCulloch et al. 1986; McNiel and Binder 1987a). Traditionally, psychiatrists either underestimate the number of psychiatric patients who carry weapons or overestimate their ability to detect weapon-carrying patients. McNiel and Binder (1987a) found that only male gender and history of substance abuse distinguished patients who carried weapons from those who did not carry weapons among those who were seen in EDs for psychiatric evaluation or treatment.

The consulting psychiatrist must know the ED's policy toward weapons screening and patient violence (see section, "Patients Who Are Violent," later in this chapter). A written policy is mandatory. The policy should require either that patients are searched or that they wear a standard hospital gown. Violation of the psychiatric patient's civil liberties and unnecessary intrusiveness are potential arguments against such a policy. Admittedly, disrobing of patients is unnecessary in some instances, and a few patients may refuse to disrobe. Maintenance of safety, however, favors such a policy. Also, a physical examination is more likely to occur when a patient wears a hospital gown.

Requiring that the emergency psychiatric patient wear a hospital gown significantly reduces the risk of concealed weapons. It is essential to remember, however, that the ED is filled with potentially dangerous instruments (e.g., needles, scalpels, glass objects, razors, tourniquets)—patients' access to these objects must be restricted.

In the situation in which a patient produces a weapon, it is recommended that the clinician not take it directly; instead, the clinician should instruct the patient to place the weapon on a flat surface, and then the clinician should call security staff to confiscate it. Accepting the weapon directly poses a risk of accidental injury to either the clinician or the patient. Moreover, if there is any chance that the weapon was used to commit a crime, all hospital personnel should avoid touching it or handling it in a way that would contaminate what may be legal evidence.

Seclusion and Mechanical Restraint

All EDs must have a written policy for the seclusion and mechanical restraint of threatening, disruptive, or agitated patients. The policy must address 1) the indications for seclusion or mechanical restraint (e.g., the threat or occurrence of danger to oneself or others), 2) technical issues (e.g., the appropriate use and application of mechanical restraints, requirements for the monitoring and care of the restrained or secluded patient by both medical and nursing staff), and 3) facility requirements (e.g., a safe seclusion room that is adequately sound-proofed and that has an unbreakable window that offers a full view of the room).

An important feature of such policies is the standard of "least restrictive treatment." Caregivers must first attempt to calm a threatening or agitated patient by less restrictive means before seclusion or restraint is used (Soloff 1987).

The clinician should speak softly, move slowly, and behave deferentially during the evaluation procedure. An offer of food or liquids as a sign of the clinician's concern may encourage the patient's cooperation; medication may be offered to help the patient achieve control. A show of force by hospital security guards can demonstrate to the disruptive, provocative patient that adequate force is available to control unruly behavior if necessary. If these measures do not help the patient to achieve self-control, or if agitation is intense or rapidly escalating, then mechanical restraint is appropriate until the safety of both the patient and the staff is assured.

TRIAGE AND EVALUATION

Triage

The job of the triage nurse is challenging, especially in a busy, multispecialty urban ED. Rapid decisions are needed and are often made with little information. A patient's uncooperative, disagreeable, or inappropriate behavior not only interferes with obtaining important information but also is likely to alienate triage personnel. The patient's behavior can precipitate a cycle of animosity (e.g., the psychiatrist receives the nurse's displaced anger and frustration). It is helpful, therefore, for the consulting psychiatrist to know the triage personnel and to have a comfortable working relationship with each of them.

Psychiatric patients typically receive inadequate general medical evaluation (Weissberg 1979). For example, even basic vital sign measurements are sometimes not taken in an agitated or uncooperative psychiatric patient. Either the patient's behavior interferes with the performance of a physical examination or, once identified as "psychiatric," the patient's complaints and condition are taken less seriously. As a result, the quality of care is inadequate.

Patient Transfers

The consultant is occasionally asked to triage incoming telephone calls from a staff member at a hospital or an agency that wants to transfer a patient for psychiatric evaluation. Interhospital transfer has legal implications. The Consolidated Omnibus Budget Reconciliation Act of 1985 (COBRA) makes "patient dumping" a violation of federal law. The hospital that transfers a patient without first obtaining formal acceptance from the receiving institution is subject, as a result, to stiff penalties (Frew et al. 1988).

Several important questions must be addressed before the patient is transferred: 1) Is the proposed receiving facility the correct one? 2) Is the patient medically stable for transfer? and 3) Is the patient exhibiting transient symptoms that, if stabilized, could result in another disposition?

Federal law requires that all patients be medically stable before transfer from the ED (Frew et al. 1988). As noted previously, medical evaluation of psychiatric patients is often inadequate, particularly when patients are agitated or uncooperative. It is important, therefore, to inquire about vital sign measurements (including respiration), level of consciousness, results of physical examination, and results of specific laboratory studies that may have been performed (e.g., electrolyte levels, toxicology screen, and, in selected cases, electrocardiogram [ECG], chest X ray, and arterial blood gases). It is not appropriate to transfer a patient whose mental status changes are the result of a medical illness, alcohol withdrawal, or a life-threatening drug overdose that requires further monitoring or admission to a medical unit (e.g., tricyclic antidepressant, anticholinergic, aspirin, or acetaminophen overdose).

Interview and Mental Status Examination

Establishment of patient's request.   Successful consultation depends, among other things, on an understanding of the patient's request. The request is often different from the chief complaint. For example, the chief complaint may be "anxiety" or "trouble sleeping," and the request is for Xanax.

Investigations of the patient's request show that it is highly correlated with patient satisfaction and the negotiation of a treatment strategy. Unlike the chief complaint, the request is often concealed, and the patient may have more than one request; the most important request is often not revealed until later in the interview.

All requests neither can nor should be fulfilled, but their verbalization can open a process of negotiation that allows for an evaluation of their legitimacy (Lazare 1976; Lazare et al. 1975b). Lazare and colleagues (1975a) observed that the majority of walk-in patients had a very specific idea of what they wanted. Although the request did not always address the entire problem, it was often appropriate.

The involuntary patient generally has at least one demand or request: "Let me go!" or "Get me out of here!" Explicit demands are also subject to discussion and negotiation. For example, rather than ignoring the patient's demand to have restraints removed, it is often useful to address the demand directly and clarify, in an objective and nonpunitive manner, both the reason(s) for the use of mechanical restraints and the circumstances in which they will be removed.

Establishment of patient's reason for now seeking help.   It is important in the first encounter with any patient to determine the reason for his or her visit to the ED at this time. Many problems surface in the context of chronic illness or smoldering crisis. What has happened or what has changed to make the patient seek help now rather than last week, or yesterday, or next week? The answer often provides important information about the patient's baseline level of functioning and the precipitants of the current crisis. It can be productive to ask what the patient thinks would have happened had he or she not come for help now.

Mental status examination. The neuropsychiatric interview and mental status examination are discussed in detail in Wise and Strub, Chapter 2, in this volume. Given the rapid time frame of emergency evaluations, it is neither practical nor always necessary to perform every aspect of a complete neuropsychiatric examination. Several important components, however, warrant special emphasis in emergency psychiatric patients.

The spontaneity of ED presentation affords a unique view of the patient's appearance and behavior that is not usually evident once the patient is admitted to the hospital. The manner of dress (if street clothes are still being worn) and the level of hygiene often reveal useful information about the intensity and duration of illness.

The patient's speech and use of language must be examined carefully to avoid mistaking aphasic speech for the illogical, loosely connected thinking of a patient with acute psychosis or schizophrenia (Benson 1973).

In addition to the usual investigation for disordered thinking and perceptions, explicit inquiry about hopelessness, suicidal thinking, and command auditory hallucinations is essential. If the presentation suggests a psychotic or borderline disorder, the clinician must ask about auditory hallucinations that command the patient to harm either himself or herself or others.

Components of cognitive testing that are not specifically included in the Mini-Mental State Exam (Folstein et al. 1975) and that are often overlooked in routine clinical examination are tests of intention or executive function. Because frontal-lobe dysfunction can present without the usual focal, lateralizing findings elicited by routine neurological examination, it is easily overlooked. Although frontal-lobe dysfunction is not common, it probably occurs

more frequently in patients with chronic, diagnostically nonspecific psychoses and in those with a history of head injury or chronic alcoholism than in patients with other types of disorders. Clock drawing is a good screening test for global cortical dysfunction; evidence of improper placement or duplication of numbers around the face of the clock may be a clue to impaired executive functions and frontal-lobe damage or diffuse cortical dysfunction. Easily performed bedside maneuvers that more specifically check the integrity of the frontal lobes include visual pattern completion tests and Luria hand maneuvers (see Chapter 2 in this volume).

Physical examination. The practice of emergency psychiatry, perhaps more than any other discipline in psychiatry, mandates retention and continued use of one's medical skills. Not all ED patients receive a thorough medical evaluation before seeing the psychiatric consultant. Therefore, it is not necessarily prudent to rely on a general or emergency physician to detect underlying medical illnesses in psychiatric patients. Not only does the rush and pressure of the emergency setting increase the likelihood that subtle illnesses will be missed but, as Weissberg (1979) pointed out, "there is the all too common belief that alcoholics, drug abusers, and suicidal individuals create their own diseases and are therefore less entitled than others to sympathetic and thorough care" (p. 788). The psychiatric consultant must be able to integrate relevant physical findings into an overall understanding of the patient's problem.

Laboratory investigation. It is important to perform a battery of routine laboratory tests on the patient with an acute change in mental status or behavior. The battery should include a complete blood count, serum electrolytes, blood glucose, and a toxicology screen. A serum sample is necessary to obtain quantitative measures of medications and other chemical substances (e.g., antidepressants, sedative-hypnotic agents, alcohol), and a sample of the patient's urine is often required to detect rapidly metabolized agents that undergo renal clearance (e.g., cocaine and its metabolites, marijuana, phencyclidine [PCP], opiates) (Table 28–1). Other tests are optional and depend on the clinical circumstances.

Clinicians should consider imaging studies of the head (magnetic resonance imaging [MRI], computed tomography [CT] scan), as well as cerebrospinal fluid (CSF) analysis and electroencephalography (EEG), in cases in which a metabolic, traumatic, or infectious cause of an abnormal mental state is suspected or when other tests have not revealed a cause. Neurological literature suggests that scanning techniques have a low diagnostic yield in patients who lack focal neurological findings. However, it is probably prudent to regard an acute change of mental status as a "focal finding."

LIFE-ENDANGERING PSYCHIATRIC EMERGENCIES

Patients With Acute Psychosis

Acute psychosis, characterized by thought disorganization, delusions, hallucinations, and in-

Table 28–1. Approximate duration of detectability of drugs in urine

Drug	Retention time
Amphetamine and methamphetamine	48 hours
Barbiturates	
Short-acting (e.g., secobarbital, pentobarbital)	24 hours
Intermediate-acting (e.g., amobarbital, butalbital, butabarbital)	48–72 hours
Long-acting (e.g., phenobarbital)	2–3 weeks
Benzodiazepines (at therapeutic doses)	3 days
Cannabinoids	
Moderate smoker (4 times/week)	3 days
Daily smoker	10 days
Daily heavy smoker	3–4 weeks
Cocaine	6–8 hours
Cocaine metabolites	2–4 hours
Ethyl alcohol	7–12 hours
Methaqualone	7 days
Narcotics	
Codeine	48 hours
Heroin (as morphine)	36–72 hours
Hydrocodone	24 hours
Hydromorphone	48 hours
Methadone	3 days
Morphine	48–72 hours
Oxycodone	24 hours
Propoxyphene	6–48 hours
Phencyclidine (PCP)	8 days

Source. Reprinted from Hyman SE, Tesar GE (eds): *Manual of Psychiatric Emergencies,* 3rd Edition. Boston, MA, Little, Brown, 1994, p. 334. Copyright 1994, Little, Brown and Company. Used with permission.

appropriate or agitated behavior, is a medical-psychiatric emergency that requires careful evaluation, safety measures, and prompt treatment. Its causes are numerous, and failure to detect organic or substance-related etiologies can pose a significant medical risk to the patient. Acute psychosis also carries with it a significant risk of unlawful behavior, inadvertent injury to self or others, and suicide (Hyman 1994b).

The principles of treatment of patients with psychosis are similar to those for any acute change in mental status: the clinician must correct metabolic and systemic abnormalities (e.g., hypoglycemia, hypoxia, hypertensive encephalopathy), eliminate drug toxicity (e.g., alcohol, PCP, cocaine, or anticholinergic intoxication), treat drug withdrawal, and, if necessary, use tranquilizing medication.

The preferred route for administration of tranquilizing medication depends on the intensity of accompanying agitation (Hyman 1994a; Tesar 1993). Elixir preparations are indicated for patients who prefer them or for patients who are known to "cheek" tablets or capsules; peak clinical effectiveness with elixir preparations, however, is achieved no more rapidly than with pill forms (Dubin et al. 1985). Injection into the deltoid muscle ensures rapid absorption of benzodiazepine and neuroleptic agents (Greenblatt et al. 1983). Intravenous administration of haloperidol is also quite effective, achieves peak blood levels within 10–20 minutes (Tesar and Stern 1988), and is safe. Intravenous use of haloperidol, however, is not common in the ED, and intravenous administration of this drug is not approved by the U.S. Food and Drug Administration (FDA).

For rapid control of acute psychosis, concomitant intramuscular administration of 5 mg of haloperidol and 1 mg of lorazepam is superior to the use of either agent alone (Garza-Trevino et al. 1989; Mendoza et al. 1991). The combination can be injected from one syringe. One dose is adequate for most patients, but some patients require a second and, infrequently, a third injection. Although low- or intermediate-potency neuroleptic drugs (e.g., chlorpromazine, thioridazine, perphenazine) are indicated for certain patients, haloperidol is the preferred agent because it has little potential for anticholinergic toxicity and a low hypotensive effect. Lorazepam is the preferred benzodiazepine because its absorption after intramuscular injection is more reliable than that of other benzodiazepines.

When giving haloperidol alone or in combination with a benzodiazepine, coadministration of an anticholinergic agent is recommended to prevent acute dystonia (Arana et al. 1988; Goff et al. 1991). Benztropine mesylate, 1–2 mg orally or intramuscularly, is typically used. If neuroleptic medication is continued, the same dose of the anticholinergic agent is given twice daily, and this dosage is continued for at least 1 week, the period of greatest risk for acute dystonic reactions (Ayd 1961).

Patients at Risk for Suicide

A major priority of any emergency psychiatric service is the evaluation and disposition of patients who are at risk for suicide. Emergency psychiatric patients die by suicide at a significantly higher rate than do individuals in the general population (Hillard et al. 1983, 1985). However, studies by Hillard et al. (1983) and others (Browning et al. 1970; Stern et al. 1984) have demonstrated that eventual death by suicide does not occur immediately, or even within 2 weeks, after an ED visit. This may reflect the skill with which triage decisions are made or the value of emergency intervention in forestalling suicidal behavior. Ideally, before the consultant's evaluation, the patient should be kept in a safe place and monitored, and the risk of escape must be minimized. If a potentially suicidal patient threatens to leave the ED, then he or she should be detained until the evaluation is complete; this decision is carefully documented in the patient's record.

Suicidal patients reach the ED in a number

of different situations: 1) having just survived a suicide attempt; 2) complaining of suicidal thoughts or urges; 3) having other complaints, but admitting to suicidal thoughts during the evaluation; and 4) denying suicidal thoughts but behaving in ways that suggest potential for suicide. The consultant should consider these circumstances, as well as personal and demographic risk factors for suicide, when evaluating the patient who may be at risk for suicide.

Patients whose behavior is inconsistent with their denial of suicidal impulses are the most difficult to evaluate and treat. Some have a diagnosis of borderline personality disorder; their ambivalence about death and their manipulative behavior can make it impossible for the clinician to predict their ultimate actions. It is best to hospitalize patients when the clinician is uncertain about patients' safety and when an adequate plan for follow-up is not available. The rationale for involuntary hospitalization must be carefully documented in the hospital record.

Risk factors for suicide among emergency psychiatric patients are listed in Table 28–2 (see Bostwick and Rundell, Chapter 4, in this volume). Untreated depression is the most com-

Table 28–2. Risk factors for suicide

Major depression

Alcoholism

History of suicide attempts and threats

Male gender

Increasing age (peak incidence for men, age 75; peak incidence for women, ages 55–65)

Widowed or never married

Unemployed and unskilled

Chronic illness or chronic pain

Terminal illness

Guns in the home

Source. Reprinted from Hyman SE: "The Suicidal Patient," in *Manual of Psychiatric Emergencies,* 3rd Edition. Edited by Hyman SE, Tesar GE. Boston, MA, Little, Brown, 1994, pp. 21–27. Copyright 1994, Little, Brown and Company. Used with permission.

mon psychiatric diagnosis associated with suicide; the risk is even greater if the individual with depression also has features of psychosis or a family history of suicide. Alcohol use is highly associated with an increased risk of suicide. Acutely, alcohol may facilitate a suicide attempt by disinhibiting the patient who is feeling hopeless and depressed. In the ED, suicidal threats made by the alcoholic patient who is acutely intoxicated commonly prompt requests for immediate psychiatric consultation. All such threats must be regarded as serious while the patient remains intoxicated. However, most clinicians who have worked in the ED are quite familiar with the patient who vehemently threatens suicide while intoxicated only to deny suicidal intent and beg for discharge when he or she is again sober. The common practice is to discharge these patients once they have become sober, although presumably their long-term risk of suicide is great.

Patients Who Are Violent

When confronted by a patient who has committed or is contemplating a violent act, the psychiatrist has four obligations: 1) to ensure the safety of the patient and the staff; 2) to determine whether violent ideation or behavior stems from a specific psychiatric disorder; 3) to effect an appropriate treatment plan and disposition; and 4) to warn third parties if a serious threat of harm is present.

Safety is a priority whenever violence is a concern. In addition to the obvious benefits of a safe, protected environment, the clinician who feels safe and unafraid is more likely to be objective and nonthreatening. The measures taken to ensure safety will depend on the nature and severity of violence. If the patient retains adequate self-control, an interview in an office that permits adequate interpersonal distance and has no potential weapons (e.g., syringes, table lamps, ashtrays, pens, or pencils) is possible. The clinician and the patient should sit in a manner that allows both to have easy access to the door; in some instances, both the patient and the clinician may feel more comfortable if the door is left open. It is sometimes best to have one or more security guards stand by during the interview. In all instances, the clinician's behavior and interviewing style optimally should be nonthreatening, nonauthoritarian, and nonpunitive. It is always prudent to avoid frustrating the patient or, if necessary, to have adequate means of controlling the patient's behavior. It is important, particularly with patients who have paranoid delusions, to make intermittent eye contact and avoid staring with a deadpan expression, to position oneself at eye level with the patient, and to move slowly and predictably. The clinician should never turn his or her back to the patient and should always keep his or her hands open and visible. A helpful and understanding attitude without being judgmental or presumptive is best.

Available studies suggest that psychotic disorders (e.g., schizophrenia, mania, and paranoid states with or without command hallucinations ordering violence), drug abuse (especially PCP, cocaine, and other central nervous system [CNS] stimulants), and alcohol abuse are the most common psychiatric disorders in psychiatric emergency patients who become violent (Skodol and Karasu 1978; Stern et al. 1991). Stern and colleagues (1991) also emphasized the etiological role of organic brain syndromes. In several studies, a diagnosis of an organic brain syndrome was either considered or identified in 7%–28% of patients who were violent, hostile, angry, or agitated (Atkins 1967; Muller et al. 1967; Tischler 1966).

Most violent behavior that is manifested in the ED occurs in the context of family strife (Skodol and Karasu 1978). Psychiatric disorders may contribute directly to family violence, or family conflict may lead to intensified symptoms, resulting in violence. The ability to control violent impulses, as judged by clinicians, is the critical determinant of whether to hospitalize the patient who is violent (Mezzich

et al. 1984; Segal et al. 1988).

Crucial to accurate diagnosis, effective treatment, and safe disposition are thorough mental status and physical examinations of the violent patient. Assessment should include answers to the following questions (Simon 1988): Does the patient have a fever or exhibit evidence of autonomic arousal (e.g., hypertension, tachycardia, sweating, mydriasis, hyperreflexia), suggesting either drug or alcohol intoxication or withdrawal? Is there physical evidence of a violent lifestyle (e.g., tattoos, scars from bullet or knife wounds, bruised or disfigured knuckles)? Does the patient exhibit a thought disorder? If the patient has expressed violent fantasies, do these constitute a fear, a wish, or an intent? Is there a specific plan of action? And if the thoughts have achieved the level of intention, who is the object of the violent thoughts? When is the violent act to be carried out? Where will the violence occur? What is the motive? For how long have these thoughts been occurring? How imminent is the threat of violence? Does the patient have access to weapons?

For sedation, either diazepam (5–10 mg) or lorazepam (1–2 mg) should be given parenterally (either intramuscularly or intravenously). If the intravenous route is chosen, the benzodiazepine is administered slowly over 1–2 minutes to avoid respiratory depression; resuscitative equipment should always be immediately available. Haloperidol (2–5 mg), given intramuscularly or intravenously, may be used alone or may be given in combination with a benzodiazepine if the patient's agitation is intense and uncontrolled (Garza-Trevino et al. 1989).

Once the patient is stabilized, his or her attitude toward further violence should be assessed; the clinician should also evaluate the patient's social network and presence of external controls at this time. If there is no evidence of a psychiatric disorder and violent intentions persist, then the problem is best handled by legal authorities. In all cases, the final disposition is contingent on 1) evidence that emergency treatment has resulted in control of violent ideation and impulsivity, 2) the determination that the patient is not returning to circumstances that are likely to rekindle violent behavior, and 3) a commitment from the patient and/or family members to return to the ED immediately should the threat of violence recur. If these criteria cannot be met, then the patient should be hospitalized for protection, further evaluation, and treatment. Threatened parties must be notified if a patient's homicidal threats are judged to be significant (*Tarasoff v. Regents of the University of California* 1974). Although prediction of violence in the distant future is generally inaccurate (Monahan 1978), short-term predictions (i.e., within 72 hours of evaluation) made in the context of emergency civil commitment are distinctly more reliable (McNiel and Binder 1987b).

Patients With Substance-Related Emergencies

Patients who abuse substances come to the attention of the psychiatric consultant either because they have psychosis (or they are presumed to have psychosis when, actually, they have delirium) or because they are belligerent and disruptive, suicidal, or in denial of their substance abuse. Of paramount concern is the patient's immediate safety and the risks associated with further substance abuse. Patients should not be discharged from the ED while intoxicated.

Alcohol. As many as one-third of patients seen in general hospital EDs have alcoholism (Robins et al. 1977; Rund et al. 1981; Zimberg 1979). Alcohol use is linked with physical trauma, violent death, and psychiatric illness (Teplin et al. 1989). In a prospective study of the relation between blood alcohol level (BAL) and other variables associated with admission to the ED, Teplin et al. (1989) found that psychiatric patients had the highest mean BAL. This finding is consistent with epidemiological

data indicating a significant overlap of psychiatric illness and alcoholism (Schuckit 1983).

The patient should be evaluated for medical complications of alcoholism (e.g., hypoglycemia, subdural hematoma, other injuries, gastrointestinal [GI] bleeding), alcohol withdrawal, Wernicke's encephalopathy, alcohol amnestic disorder (Korsakoff's psychosis), and alcoholic dementia. All intoxicated patients with alcoholism should receive thiamine, 100 mg parenterally, because the signs of Wernicke's encephalopathy (e.g., listlessness or drowsiness, ophthalmoplegia, global confusion, ataxic stance or gait) are difficult to distinguish from the signs of intoxication itself; the classic triad (i.e., ophthalmoplegia, global confusion, and ataxia) is not typically present (Brew 1986; De Keyser et al. 1985). Patients with alcoholism who are agitated or belligerent should be calmed with lorazepam (1–2 mg, intramuscularly) or haloperidol (2–5 mg, intramuscularly). Low-potency neuroleptic drugs should not be used because of their tendency to lower blood pressure and the seizure threshold.

Alcohol withdrawal is potentially lethal if unrecognized and untreated. In general, a high index of suspicion is required because the clinical and laboratory manifestations are nonspecific, and the patient often conceals or is unable to provide the relevant history. The clinician should remember that the intoxicated alcoholic patient can develop early withdrawal as the BAL declines, even though it may be above 100 mg/dL, the legal limit for intoxication.

Early onset withdrawal, characterized by tachycardia, hypertension, sweating, tremor, fever, anxiety, irritability, and occasionally hallucinosis, often begins within 6–8 hours of a substantial decline in the BAL. Chlordiazepoxide, 25–100 mg orally every 6 hours, is indicated at the first sign of withdrawal, with the initial amount depending on the intensity of symptoms. Often, the appropriate initial dose can be ascertained by asking the patient how subjectively anxious he or she feels. Generalized tonic-clonic seizures occur usually within the first 24 hours of the last drink. Inpatient treatment is indicated in the presence of fever above 101°F, seizures, signs of Wernicke's encephalopathy, inability to hold fluids, or a serious underlying medical disorder (Hyman 1994c).

The most severe form of withdrawal, delirium tremens (DT), usually occurs after 24 hours and within 7 days of the last drink. Despite optimal treatment, the mortality associated with DT is still nearly 5% (Cushman 1987). DT is characterized by marked sympathetic overactivity, fever, hallucinosis, agitation, and delirium. DT requires treatment in the intensive care unit (ICU), including intravenous electrolyte and fluid therapy, acetaminophen and cooling blankets for significant hyperthermia, parenteral thiamine, monitoring for infection and cardiac arrhythmias, and parenteral benzodiazepines (diazepam, lorazepam, or midazolam). When DT commences in the ED, diazepam, 10 mg given intravenously, is recommended as the initial treatment. Diazepam is preferred because of its rapid onset of effect (Baldessarini 1985).

Cocaine and other psychostimulants. Approximately 22 million Americans have used cocaine, and nearly 5 million use it regularly (Rich and Singer 1991). Although casual use has declined, the number of hard-core users and the number of individuals seen in EDs for symptoms related to cocaine use have increased (Rich and Singer 1991). In a study of the frequency of cocaine-related medical, surgical, and psychiatric problems presenting in an urban, general hospital ED, psychiatric complaints accounted for most of the presentations (30.6%) (Rich and Singer 1991). Suicidal intent was the most common psychiatric problem. Polysubstance abuse was common; alcohol, opiates, and benzodiazepines were most commonly abused.

The immediate goals in the treatment of patients with stimulant toxicity are to reduce CNS excitation, sympathetic overactivity, and psychotic symptoms. A dual approach is recommended. Agents to acidify the urine should be used, and haloperidol should be administered to control agitation, delirium, or psychotic symptoms. Clonidine, 0.1–0.3 mg/day, helps to reduce craving and sympathetic arousal in some patients. Antidepressants have been used successfully to treat depression from cocaine abstinence (Gawin and Kleber 1984). Because cocaine and other psychostimulants are highly addictive, inpatient treatment is generally indicated to minimize the risk of further drug abuse.

Benzodiazepines and other sedative-hypnotics. Sedative-hypnotic drugs, which include benzodiazepines, barbiturates, meprobamate, chloral hydrate, ethchlorvynol, glutethimide, and methyprylon, are CNS depressants that inhibit central γ-aminobutyric acid (GABA) receptors. Drugs within this class Each of these nonbenzodiazepine sedative-hypnotic compounds is capable of producing dependence, tolerance, and potentially fatal toxicity and withdrawal. Familiarity with analgesic compounds that contain the short-lasting barbiturate butalbital is essential for consultation-liaison psychiatrists. Sudden discontinuation of these medications can result in a life-threatening barbiturate withdrawal syndrome.

Barbiturates have a high abuse potential because of their marked euphoriant effect, rapid induction of hepatic microsomal enzymes, and receptor adaptation (i.e., tolerance) (Rall 1990). Additionally, they are more dangerous than the benzodiazepines in overdose (resulting from greater cardiorespiratory and CNS depressant effects), and they have a far lower toxic-to-therapeutic ratio than the benzodiazepines (10 versus > 100). Tolerance to a barbiturate's hypnotic effect does not result in a proportional increase in the lethal dose. Sudden discontinuation of barbiturates and their analogues can cause a potentially fatal withdrawal syndrome.

Benzodiazepines are safer and are more widely prescribed than barbiturates. Patients with primary anxiety disorders tend to respond to relatively low, stable doses of high-potency benzodiazepines with little or no tolerance to the anxiolytic effects (Nagy et al. 1989; Pollack 1990). However, benzodiazepine dependence occurs almost universally, especially after 4 months of continuous use. Sudden withdrawal from therapeutic doses of a benzodiazepine may be followed by a fully developed, although nonlethal, physical withdrawal syndrome (Petursson and Lader 1981).

The psychiatric consultant must maintain a high index of suspicion for sedative-hypnotic abuse among patients who use emergency services. High-risk patients are likely to conceal substance abuse and to complain of anxiety symptoms instead (e.g., panic attacks). If a history or evidence of current substance abuse exists, benzodiazepines should not be prescribed except for patients in established outpatient treatment and then only with the approval of the outpatient psychiatrist. Characteristics of the patient who abuses substances include irritability, insistence, and impatience. The inability to recall the first attack by a patient who reports "panic attacks" or a history of "panic disorder" should trigger skepticism about the diagnosis. Substance abuse should be presumed until proven otherwise.

Withdrawal from sedative-hypnotics. Sedative-hypnotic withdrawal is a medical emergency. The symptoms of withdrawal from a sedative-hypnotic drug depend on the type of agent, its elimination half-life ($T_{1/2}$), and the duration of its use. In general, the presentation and course of withdrawal from barbiturates are similar to that of withdrawal from alcohol. Symptoms—including fever, autonomic arousal, sweating, neuromuscular irritability, paranoia, and frightening hallucinations—typically precede the onset of seizures, coma, and

death if adequate treatment is not given (Khantzian and McKenna 1979). Withdrawal from benzodiazepines is usually less intense than that from a barbiturate and rarely results in death.

The interval from drug discontinuation to the onset of withdrawal depends on the drug's elimination $T_{1/2}$. For example, withdrawal symptoms may not begin for up to 5 days after stopping diazepam because of the gradual elimination of the parent compound and its active metabolite, nordiazepam—$T_{1/2}$ = 100 hours and can be up to 200 hours in patients with hepatic dysfunction. In contrast, withdrawal occurs within hours of the last dose of a shorter-acting agent such as pentobarbital sodium ($T_{1/2}$ = 15–48 hours), butalbital, alprazolam ($T_{1/2}$ = 8–14 hours), or lorazepam ($T_{1/2}$ = 10–18 hours) (Baldessarini 1985; Rall 1990). Sudden discontinuation of a sedative-hypnotic drug is more likely to result in withdrawal after prolonged use (i.e., more than 4 months) (American Psychiatric Association 1990).

Successful treatment of a patient with sedative-hypnotic withdrawal syndrome depends on adequate replacement with the drug used or a cross-reactive substance (i.e., one that affects central GABA receptors). If the specific substance is known, resumption should be considered. If the substance is not known or cannot be given by the usual means, parenteral administration of a benzodiazepine or barbiturate is indicated. Adequate respiratory support is essential. Sodium amobarbital, 60–100 mg, or diazepam, 10 mg, given intramuscularly or intravenously, is indicated whenever a rapid response is desired (e.g., in the presence of delirium, intense agitation, or seizures). When the clinical situation permits, it is best to determine the patient's sedative-hypnotic requirement by using the pentobarbital tolerance test, switching to a long-lasting agent (e.g., phenobarbital), and then instituting a gradual taper (see Franklin and Frances, Chapter 13, in this volume).

Opioid dependence and abuse. Persons who are addicted to and abuse narcotics come to the ED for many reasons, including to request analgesics, because they have overdosed, because they are in a state of withdrawal, or because of a complication of substance abuse (e.g., acquired immunodeficiency syndrome [AIDS], endocarditis, hepatitis) (Weiss et al. 1994). Characteristically, the cloying, irritable, and demanding traits of persons addicted to opioids alienate emergency personnel. Because it is difficult to discern a legitimate request for analgesic medication from drug-seeking behavior, the ED may automatically prohibit prescribing or dispensing narcotic analgesics.

Opiate intoxication is indicated by a depressed level of consciousness, respiratory depression, and narrow pupils. The clinician should examine the patient for injection sites, needle tracks, and venous sclerosis, although these are not often prominent in the inexperienced user. Naloxone, a pure opioid antagonist, is administered intravenously in patients with suspected opioid overdose. The usual dose is 0.1 mg/kg, or one to two 0.4-mg ampules, depending on body size. Restraints should be placed before naloxone is given because excessive arousal or agitation can occur as intoxication is reversed ("precipitated withdrawal").

Opioid withdrawal is uncomfortable but not lethal. Typical symptoms include sweating, dilated pupils, gooseflesh, lacrimation, and hyperreflexia. In addition, the patient may experience muscle cramping, abdominal pain, and drug craving. The presence of physical findings indicative of opioid withdrawal helps to differentiate the drug seeker from a patient who is addicted, is withdrawing from opioids, and needs additional narcotics. The usual treatment of patients with narcotic dependence and withdrawal involves methadone maintenance supplemented, as necessary, by clonidine hydrochloride, a presynaptic α_2-adrenergic agonist.

Phencyclidine. PCP, also known as "dust" or "angel dust," is commonly used as a tranquilizer in veterinary medicine (Weiss et al. 1994). Users can experience depressant, stimulant, hallucinogenic, or analgesic effects, depending on the dose and mode of administration. Adverse reactions include delirium, psychosis, agitation, violence, and suicide. Although PCP is usually smoked, it is also taken orally, intranasally, or intravenously. Verification of PCP poisoning generally requires toxicological analysis of the urine, because the $T_{1/2}$ of PCP in serum is short (i.e., 45 minutes).

An overdose of PCP is usually accompanied by increased bronchial and salivary secretions, muscular incoordination, nystagmus, disconjugate gaze, and bizarre behavior (e.g., posturing, catatonia, and amnesia for the episode). In extreme cases, seizures, hypertensive crisis, respiratory depression, coma, or death occurs. The goals of treatment include protection of the patient and the staff while the drug effects subside, increasing the rate of the drug's elimination, and treatment of complications. Acidification of the urine helps to speed excretion of the drug. This may be accomplished with ammonium chloride, 2.75 mEq/kg in 60 mL of saline solution administered every 6 hours through a nasogastric tube, along with intravenous administration of ascorbic acid, 2 g in 500 mL of intravenous fluid every 6 hours. Diazepam, 10–30 mg, is the drug of choice for treating patients who are agitated or restless; however, a high-potency neuroleptic drug (e.g., haloperidol) and hospitalization are sometimes necessary for patients who have persistent psychotic reactions.

COMMON PSYCHIATRIC EMERGENCIES

Patients With Mood Disorders

Symptoms of mood disorders constitute one of the most frequent reasons that individuals seek emergency psychiatric intervention (Robins et al. 1977). In their study, Robins and colleagues (1977) found that the majority (28%) of diagnoses given to psychiatric emergency patients were affective disorders, as determined by Feighner's criteria (Feighner et al. 1972). Half of this group received only an affective disorder diagnosis (usually major depression), one-third received an additional diagnosis, and the rest received two or more additional diagnoses (e.g., mood disorder plus alcoholism, personality disorder, and schizophrenia). "Nervousness" was the most common complaint made by those with a diagnosis of mood disorder.

Traditionally, antidepressant medication was withheld until the patient underwent evaluation by a second physician, who would see the patient regularly. This was justified because of the potential for a life-endangering overdose of tricyclic antidepressant medication, the questionable validity of diagnoses made in the ED, and the delayed response to antidepressant medication. However, if the patient fulfills the diagnostic criteria for a major depression, the initiation of antidepressant medication is indicated as long as the clinician can provide follow-up. It is clinically indefensible to withhold treatment from a patient who is likely to benefit from it. Concerns about untoward effects of medication are less relevant with newer antidepressants (e.g., bupropion, fluoxetine, paroxetine, sertraline) or when a small supply of a tricyclic antidepressant is prescribed.

The patient with hypomania or mania who refuses treatment and is not a danger to himself or herself or to others presents a common and difficult management problem for the emergency psychiatric clinician. Caught between the competing responsibilities of protecting the patient's civil liberties and of providing appropriate medical care, the clinician must decide whether the patient's judgment is sufficiently impaired to warrant involuntary hospitalization and treatment. Frequently, the information provided by the patient is not reliable. Therefore, the history and the objective input of family members and associates are es-

sential. If there is either inadequate information at the clinician's disposal or insufficient social support to ensure the patient's safety, then involuntary commitment is indicated. The clinician's observations and rationale should be documented in the patient's hospital record.

Patients With Anxiety and Phobic Disorders

Data from the Epidemiologic Catchment Area (ECA) study indicate that anxiety and phobic disorders are the most prevalent form of psychiatric disturbance in the community (Barlow and Shear 1988); individuals with anxiety and phobias frequently use psychiatric, general medical, and emergency services (Markowitz et al. 1989). In one study, anxiety disorders constituted 36.1% of psychiatric diagnoses made in an ED (Fenichel and Murphy 1985). Only a minority of these patients received psychiatric consultation. Emergency physicians tend not to view anxiety as a disorder that requires specialized treatment and are likely to provide reassurance and small amounts of benzodiazepines or antihistamines to anxious patients who have an underlying medical illness (Schwartz et al. 1987).

Nearly half of the patients who come to primary care and emergency facilities with somatic complaints (e.g., chest pain, palpitations, choking sensation, respiratory distress, neurological symptoms, and GI disturbance) for which no organic basis is ultimately identified have panic disorder or depression (Bass and Wade 1984; Beitman et al. 1987, 1990; Lydiard et al. 1986; Rosenbaum 1987; Russell et al. 1991; Wulsin et al. 1991).

Patients who present acutely with a primary complaint of anxiety, nervousness, or panic attacks have a heterogeneous group of disorders, including mood, anxiety, adjustment, and substance-related disorders. Patients already in treatment for these disturbances often present to the ED in crisis or for medications. Requests for benzodiazepines should always arouse suspicion and require careful evaluation. In some instances of suspected drug-seeking, urine toxicology screening is helpful. When the patient complains of panic attacks, a helpful diagnostic maneuver is to ask for a description of the patient's first (herald) panic attack. Individuals with true panic disorder rarely forget the first attack, which is often the single most upsetting experience in his or her life. Inability to recall the first attack suggests another disorder, often substance abuse.

Given the high incidence of alcohol and substance abuse disorders in the emergency population, it is best to use nonbenzodiazepine medications (e.g., antidepressants) when possible to treat patients with panic disorder, obsessive-compulsive disorder, generalized anxiety disorder, and posttraumatic stress disorder.

Patients With Borderline and Antisocial Personality Disorders

Antisocial and borderline personality disorders—cluster B personality disorders, as classified in DSM-IV (American Psychiatric Association 1994), along with histrionic and narcissistic personality disorders—are the most common types of personality disorders seen among emergency psychiatric patients (Beresin et al. 1994; Robins et al. 1977). Because the ED is always open, it attracts individuals with an insatiable appetite for care and attention, as well as those who are impulsive, have a low tolerance for frustration, and have a low threshold for aggression. For some, dealing with unfamiliar caregivers enhances the opportunity for "scamming" an unwary practitioner. For others, the ED and its personnel become a surrogate extended family.

Vulnerable to either real or perceived abandonment, the patient with borderline personality disorder typically seeks urgent evaluation and care as a result of frustrated expectations or rupture of an important relationship. The patient may be angry and assaultive or helpless and vulnerable, frequently shifting back and forth, which makes it difficult for ED staff members to know how to respond. The patient may idealize certain members of the staff and respond spitefully or ungratefully to others (i.e., splitting).

Individuals who are vulnerable to frustration or antisocial (also referred to as psychopathic) often present with symptoms suggesting a mood or anxiety disorder (e.g., major depression or panic disorder). Typically, patients with antisocial personality disorder conceal a primary substance abuse disorder. Glib and charming, they ingratiate themselves with the staff, often with the intent of procuring narcotics, benzodiazepines, or an excuse from work or legal obligations.

In general, it is best to minimize waiting time and to employ a direct, problem-solving, and dispassionate approach with patients who have antisocial or borderline personality disorders. The clinician should avoid overreaction to helplessness, seduction, or intimidation. In particular, the clinician should ensure that the patient with borderline personality disorder appreciates the reality of the situation, the practitioner's limitations, and the patient's responsibility in collaborating to help solve the crisis (Beresin et al. 1994). Patients with antisocial personality disorder often lie about their symptoms or come to the ED to avoid incarceration or retaliation; thus, effective management requires a high index of suspicion and the examiner's willingness to spend time verifying questionable information. Because patients with antisocial or borderline personality disorders are often threatening or destructive, it is advisable to evaluate them in a safe setting and to ask security guards to stand by if the clinician feels threatened or unsafe. In some instances, security guards can escort uncooperative or inconsolable patients out of the hospital when the physician has determined that there is little risk of harm to either the patient or to others.

Homeless Patients

Homeless individuals present unique problems and challenges to emergency medical and psychiatric practitioners (Bierer and Tesar 1994). Diagnostic and management problems arise because homelessness produces changes suggestive of primary psychiatric disorders. Difficulty procuring food and trouble finding a safe place to sleep can be mistaken for symptoms of depression, guardedness and suspiciousness can be misconstrued as paranoia, and fighting or stealing may be misinterpreted as evidence of antisocial personality disorder. Comorbid substance abuse occurs in nearly 50% of homeless persons who are mentally ill. The absence of a stable social network complicates disposition planning and possibly contributes to a higher rate of psychiatric hospitalization of these individuals. Negative attitudes toward the homeless person often interfere with delivery of adequate care.

Effective emergency psychiatric evaluation and care of homeless individuals require attention to several special issues. Perhaps most important are the priorities of the homeless patient. Receiving adequate medical treatment for depression, for example, may not seem as crucial as obtaining food and adequate footwear. If these basic requirements are not addressed, the likelihood of compliance with antidepressant treatment diminishes. Foot care is a major priority in the clinical management of many homeless individuals because podiatric problems are common.

Special problems occur in the treatment and disposition of homeless people. In prescribing medications, the physician must consider the high prevalence of substance abuse, the special importance of remaining alert, the problem of finding a safe place to store medications, the likelihood of noncompliance, and the lack of money. The majority of homeless individuals are treated on an outpatient basis. However, the chaos of the homeless lifestyle, including its competing demands (e.g., the need to queue up daily for lunch or for a shelter bed, sometimes in distant parts of the city), makes it difficult to keep doctors' appointments and to adhere to a treatment regimen.

Moreover, effective coordination of outpatient psychiatric services often requires that the clinician communicate with area shelters, substance abuse treatment facilities, hospital social services, or one of the 110 federally funded Health Care for the Homeless programs in the United States (Bierer and Tesar 1994).

Psychiatric Emergency Repeaters

Repeat users of emergency services, often glibly referred to as "regulars" or "frequent flyers," constitute 7%–18% of emergency psychiatric patients and account for as many as one-half of total psychiatric emergency visits (Ellison et al. 1986, 1989). Overall, emergency psychiatric repeaters are a diverse group composed of 1) patients in treatment who periodically come to the ED for crisis intervention, 2) patients in need of treatment for a new or recurrent episode of illness, 3) patients not in regular treatment who frequent the ED during time-limited crises, and 4) patients who use the ED as part of their social network (Ellison et al. 1986; Tesar 1994).

Repeaters who have not successfully engaged in any sustained treatment are perhaps the most troublesome for crisis and emergency clinicians. Often, these individuals have a history of severe interpersonal difficulties, exhibit a pattern of self-destructive behavior (e.g., self-mutilation, low-risk suicide attempts, and chronic substance abuse), and were victims of early and severe abuse or deprivation (Bassuk and Gerson 1980). They are usually anxious, impulsive, help-rejecting, and prone to hostile interactions with caregivers, exhausting the caregivers'—and the clinicians'—welcome wherever they go.

Ironically, often little is known about these highly visible patients. Typically, the time spent with the patient is inversely proportional to the frequency of visits. Hesitant to gratify perceived neediness, the clinician is often unwilling to ask questions that engage the patient. The clinician may direct anger or hatred at the patient by arbitrarily limiting the duration of the clinical encounter. In some instances, compliance with a treatment protocol requires that the duration and frequency of visits are limited. Moreover, if multiple clinicians are seeing the patient during repeated visits, the responsibility for knowing and caring for the patient is gradually diffused. "Problem patient rounds" (Santy and Wehmeier 1984) is one way to pool the information of multiple clinicians, familiarizing them with what is and what is not known about the patient, and defusing uncomfortable and counterproductive negative reactions to the patient.

A treatment protocol that specifies the guidelines and limits of treatment is necessary to help shape and modify help-rejecting, abusive, or manipulative behavior. With this strategy, splitting of staff and fragmentation of care provided by multiple caregivers are less likely to occur. Timely definition and clarification of the type of treatment that the patient is to receive should also minimize disappointment and frustration (Tesar 1994).

When all available approaches, including hospitalization, treatment protocols, and therapeutic limit setting, have failed to control inappropriate or dangerous behavior, the repeater may have nowhere else to turn but the ED. Adopting an attitude of resignation and acceptance may help caregivers tolerate such patients and provide care for them. The ED is the de facto primary care facility for such individuals. Ironically, in some instances, acceptance of this role by the ED staff defuses the patient's anger and antagonism, resulting in greater compliance and a more comfortable working relationship.

DISPOSITION

The ultimate goal of all emergency work is to effect a safe and clinically sound disposition. Achieving this depends on the quality of the evaluation, attention to the clinically relevant

problem(s), and the effectiveness of treatment in the ED. If the evaluation is superficial and treatment is ineffective, then appropriate disposition is more difficult, roadblocks to discharge are more likely to be encountered, and the patient is apt to "bounce back."

The inevitable pressure of time (Gerson and Bassuk 1980), the complexity of the problem(s), and the paucity of clinical and psychosocial information available on most acute psychiatric patients often restrict the ability of the clinician to orchestrate an optimal disposition. An unfortunate tendency, especially in busy EDs, is for the consultant to focus disproportionately on disposition and to give comparatively little attention to evaluation and treatment.

Therefore, the consultant must create sufficient time not only to perform a thorough medical-psychiatric examination, but also to gather historical and psychosocial data that enhance understanding of the case and permit the development of an appropriate disposition.

Armed with sufficient clinical information, and having provided appropriate acute management, the consulting psychiatrist must then decide whether the patient requires hospital admission. Indeed, the decision to hospitalize is entertained from the moment evaluation begins.

Studies of the decision to hospitalize psychiatric patients from the ED consistently identify dangerousness as the single most significant criterion (Apsler and Bassuk 1983; Friedman et al. 1983; Gerson and Bassuk 1980; Segal et al. 1988; Tischler 1966). Other important criteria include severity of schizophrenic and psychotic symptoms (Friedman et al. 1983), the years of experience of the admitting clinician (Baxter et al. 1968; Mendel and Rapport 1969; Streiner et al. 1975), the presence of psychosocial supports (Mischler and Waxler 1963; Orleans-Rose et al. 1977), and whether the patient is expected to profit from treatment (Baxter et al. 1968; Orleans-Rose et al. 1977; Shader et al. 1969). Another important set of variables is the constraints imposed by health maintenance organizations and managed care programs on patient admission (Greenberg et al. 1989; Olfson 1989; Swift 1986).

Optimally, discharge from the hospital should include a plan that addresses both the patient's immediate and longer term needs. The clinician must assess the patient's ability to obtain food, shelter, and clothing and must also know about available outpatient mental health, substance abuse, and social service resources (Hillard 1990). Assuming that the patient's safety and basic needs are assured, the clinician then recommends follow-up with the patient's therapist, makes a referral for further evaluation and care at an appropriate facility (e.g., hospital outpatient clinic, a community mental health center, or an outpatient substance abuse service), or obtains the patient's agreement to return for follow-up evaluation in the ED.

SUMMARY

The most important goals of ED psychiatric consultation are to help the patient achieve self-control and to ensure the safety of the patient and others involved with him or her. Accomplishment of these goals requires constant vigilance for threatening behavior or loss of control, comprehensive medical-psychiatric evaluation, and the judicious use of the clinician's medical knowledge, judgment, and skills. The consultant must be prepared to help the ED staff to create circumstances that are safe and that permit thorough patient evaluation. Each evaluation must include a thorough mental status examination and relevant medical evaluation if the consultant suspects medical illness, CNS dysfunction, or substance abuse.

REFERENCES

American Psychiatric Association: Task Force Report of the American Psychiatric Association: Benzodiazepine Dependence, Toxicity, and Abuse. Washington, DC, American Psychiatric Press, 1990

American Psychiatric Association: Diagnostic and Statistical Manual of Mental Disorders, 4th Edition. Washington, DC, American Psychiatric Association, 1994

Apsler R, Bassuk E: Differences among clinicians in the decision to admit. Arch Gen Psychiatry 40:1133–1137, 1983

Arana GW, Goff DC, Baldessarini RJ, et al: Efficacy of anticholinergic prophylaxis for neuroleptic-induced acute dystonia. Am J Psychiatry 145:993–996, 1988

Atkins RE: Psychiatric emergency services. Arch Gen Psychiatry 17:176–182, 1967

Ayd FJ: A survey of drug-induced extrapyramidal reactions. JAMA 175:1054–1060, 1961

Baldessarini RJ: Chemotherapy in Psychiatry. Cambridge, MA, Harvard University Press, 1985

Barlow DH, Shear MK: Panic disorder, in American Psychiatric Press Review of Psychiatry, Vol 7. Edited by Frances AJ, Hales RE. Washington, DC, American Psychiatric Press, 1988, pp 5–9

Bass C, Wade C: Chest pain with normal coronary arteries: a comparative study of psychiatric and social morbidity. Psychosom Med 14:51–61, 1984

Bassuk E, Gerson S: Chronic crisis patients: a discrete clinical group. Am J Psychiatry 137:1513–1517, 1980

Baxter S, Chodorkoff B, Underhill R: Psychiatric emergencies: dispositional determinants and validity of the decision to admit. Am J Psychiatry 124:1542–1546, 1968

Beitman BD, Basha I, Flaker G, et al: Atypical or nonanginal chest pain: panic disorder or coronary artery disease. Arch Intern Med 147:1548–1552, 1987

Beitman BD, Kushner M, Lamberti JW, et al: Panic disorder without fear in patients with angiographically normal coronary arteries. J Nerv Ment Dis 178:307–312, 1990

Benson DF: Psychiatric aspects of aphasia. Br J Psychiatry 123:555–556, 1973

Beresin EV, Falk WE, Gordon C: Borderline and other personality disorders, in Manual of Psychiatric Emergencies, 3rd Edition. Edited by Hyman SE, Tesar GE. Boston, MA, Little, Brown, 1994, pp 178–193

Bierer M, Tesar GE: Homelessness and psychiatric emergencies, in Manual of Psychiatric Emergencies, 3rd Edition. Edited by Hyman SE, Tesar GE. Boston, MA, Little, Brown, 1994, pp 96–103

Brew BJ: Diagnosis of Wernicke's encephalopathy. Aust NZ J Med 16:676–678, 1986

Browning C, Tyson R, Miller J: A study of psychiatric emergencies, part II: suicide. Psychiatr Med 1:359–366, 1970

Cushman P: Delirium tremens: update on an old disorder. Postgrad Med 82(5):117–122, 1987

De Keyser J, Deleu D, Solheid C, et al: Coma as a presenting manifestation of Wernicke's encephalopathy. J Emerg Med 3:361–363, 1985

Dubin WR, Waxman HM, Weiss KJ, et al: Rapid tranquilization: the efficacy of oral concentrate. J Clin Psychiatry 46:475–478, 1985

Ellison JM, Blum N, Barsky AJ: Repeat visitors in the psychiatric emergency service: a critical review of the data. Hosp Community Psychiatry 37:37–41, 1986

Ellison JM, Blum N, Barsky AJ: Frequent repeaters in a psychiatric emergency service. Hosp Community Psychiatry 40:958–960, 1989

Feighner JP, Robins E, Guze SB, et al: Diagnostic criteria for use in psychiatric research. Arch Gen Psychiatry 26:57–63, 1972

Fenichel GS, Murphy JG: Factors that predict consultation in the emergency department. Med Care 23:258–265, 1985

Folstein MF, Folstein SE, McHugh PR: Mini-Mental State: a practical method for grading the cognitive state of patients for the clinician. J Psychiatr Res 12:189–198, 1975

Frew SA, Roush WR, LaGreca K: COBRA: implications for emergency medicine. Ann Emerg Med 17:835–837, 1988

Friedman S, Margolis R, David OJ, et al: Predicting psychiatric admission from an emergency room: psychiatric, psychosocial, and methodological factors. J Nerv Ment Dis 171:155–158, 1983

Garza-Trevino ES, Hollister LE, Overall JE, et al: Efficacy of combinations of intramuscular antipsychotics and sedative-hypnotics for control of psychotic agitation. Am J Psychiatry 146:1598–1601, 1989

Gawin FH, Kleber HD: Cocaine abuse and its treatment: open pilot treatment trial with desipramine and lithium carbonate. Arch Gen Psychiatry 41:903–909, 1984

Gerson S, Bassuk E: Psychiatric emergencies: an overview. Am J Psychiatry 137:1–11, 1980

Goff DC, Arana GW, Greenblatt DJ, et al: The effect of benztropine on haloperidol-induced dystonia, clinical efficacy and pharmacokinetics: a prospective trial. J Clin Psychopharmacol 11:106–112, 1991

Greenberg WM, Seide M, Scimeca MM: The hospitalizable patient as a commodity: selling in a bear market. Hosp Community Psychiatry 40:184–185, 1989

Greenblatt DJ, Shader RI, Abernathy DR: Current status of benzodiazepines (first of two parts). N Engl J Med 309:354–358, 1983

Hillard JR: Social treatment principles, in Manual of Clinical Emergency Psychiatry. Edited by Hillard JR. Washington, DC, American Psychiatric Press, 1990, pp 71–77

Hillard JR, Ramm D, Zung WWK, et al: Suicide in a psychiatric emergency room population. Am J Psychiatry 140:459–462, 1983

Hillard JR, Zung WWK, Ramm D, et al: Accidental and homicidal death in a psychiatric emergency room population. Hosp Community Psychiatry 36:640–643, 1985

Hyman SE: Acute psychoses and catatonia, in Manual of Psychiatric Emergencies, 3rd Edition. Edited by Hyman SE, Tesar GE. Boston, MA, Little, Brown, 1994a, pp 143–157

Hyman SE: The violent patient, in Manual of Psychiatric Emergencies, 3rd Edition. Edited by Hyman SE, Tesar GE. Boston, MA, Little, Brown, 1994b, pp 28–37

Hyman SE: Alcohol-related emergencies, in Manual of Psychiatric Emergencies, 3rd Edition. Edited by Hyman SE, Tesar GE. Boston, MA, Little, Brown, 1994c, pp 294–303

Khantzian EJ, McKenna GJ: Acute toxic and withdrawal reactions associated with drug use and abuse. Ann Intern Med 90:361–372, 1979

Lazare A: The psychiatric examination in the walk-in clinic: hypothesis generation and hypotheses testing. Arch Gen Psychiatry 33:96–102, 1976

Lazare A, Eisenthal S, Wasserman L: The customer approach to patienthood: attending to patient requests in a walk-in clinic. Arch Gen Psychiatry 32:553–558, 1975a

Lazare A, Eisenthal S, Wasserman L, et al: Patient requests in a walk-in clinic. Compr Psychiatry 16:467–477, 1975b

Lydiard RB, Laraia MT, Howell EF, et al: Can panic disorder present as irritable bowel syndrome? J Clin Psychiatry 47:470–473, 1986

Markowitz JS, Weissman MM, Ouellette R, et al: Quality of life in panic disorder. Arch Gen Psychiatry 46:984–992, 1989

McCulloch LE, McNiel DE, Binder RL, et al: Effects of a weapon screening procedure in a psychiatric emergency room. Hosp Community Psychiatry 37:837–838, 1986

McNiel DE, Binder RL: Patients who bring weapons to the psychiatry emergency room. J Clin Psychiatry 48:230–233, 1987a

McNiel DE, Binder RL: Predictive validity of judgments of dangerousness in emergency civil commitment. Am J Psychiatry 144:197–200, 1987b

Mendel WM, Rapport S: Determinants of the decision for psychiatric hospitalization. Arch Gen Psychiatry 20:321–328, 1969

Mendoza R, Battaglia J, Dubin W, et al: Rapid tranquilization of agitated psychotic patients in the emergency room. Paper presented at the annual meeting of the Association of General Hospital Psychiatrists, Cambridge, MA, November 1991

Mezzich JE, Evanczuk KJ, Mathias RJ, et al: Symptoms and hospitalization decision. Am J Psychiatry 141:764–769, 1984

Mischler EG, Waxler NE: Decision process in psychiatric hospitalization: patients referred, accepted and admitted to a psychiatry hospital. American Sociological Review 28:576–587, 1963

Monahan J: Prediction research and the emergency commitment of dangerous mentally ill persons: a reconsideration. Am J Psychiatry 135:198–201, 1978

Muller JJ, Chafetz ME, Blane HT: Acute psychiatric services in the general hospital, III: statistical survey. Am J Psychiatry 124:46–56, 1967

Nagy LM, Krystal JH, Woods SW, et al: Clinical and medication outcome after short-term alprazolam in behavioral group treatment of panic disorder. Arch Gen Psychiatry 46:993–999, 1989

Olfson M: Psychiatry emergency room dispositions of HMO enrollers. Hosp Community Psychiatry 40:639–641, 1989

Orleans-Rose S, Hawkins J, Apodaca L: Decision to admit: criteria for admission and readmission to a VA hospital. Arch Gen Psychiatry 34:418–421, 1977

Petursson H, Lader MH: Benzodiazepine dependence. British Journal of Addictions 76:133–145, 1981

Pollack MH: Long-term management of panic disorder. J Clin Psychiatry 51 (suppl 5):11–13, 1990

Rall TW: Hypnotics and sedatives; alcohol, in The Pharmacological Basis of Therapeutics, 8th Edition. Edited by Gilman GA, Rall TW, Nies AS, et al. New York, Pergamon, 1990, pp 359–383

Rich JA, Singer DE: Cocaine-related symptoms in patients presenting to an urban emergency department. Ann Emerg Med 20:616–621, 1991

Robins E, Gentry KA, Munoz RA, et al: A contrast of the three more common illnesses with the ten less common in a study and 18-month follow-up of 314 psychiatric emergency room patients, I: characteristics of the sample and methods of study. Arch Gen Psychiatry 34:259–265, 1977

Rosenbaum JF: Limited-symptom panic attacks. Psychosom Med 28:407–412, 1987

Rund DA, Summers WK, Levin M: Alcohol use and psychiatric illness in emergency patients. JAMA 245:1240–1241, 1981

Russell JL, Kushner MG, Beitman BD, et al: Nonfearful panic disorder in neurology patients validated by lactate challenge. Am J Psychiatry 148:361–364, 1991

Santy PA, Wehmeier PK: Using "problem patient" rounds to help emergency room staff manage difficult patients. Hosp Community Psychiatry 35:494–496, 1984

Schuckit MA: Alcoholism and other psychiatric disorders. Hosp Community Psychiatry 34:1022–1027, 1983

Schwartz GM, Braverman BG, Roth B: Anxiety disorders and psychiatric referral in the general medical emergency room. Gen Hosp Psychiatry 9:87–93, 1987

Segal SP, Watson MA, Goldfinger SM, et al: Civil commitment in the psychiatric emergency room: mental disorder indicators and three dangerousness criteria. Arch Gen Psychiatry 45:753–758, 1988

Shader RI, Binstock WA, Ohly JI, et al: Biasing factors in diagnosis and disposition. Compr Psychiatry 10:81–89, 1969

Simon RI: Clinical Psychiatry and the Law. Washington, DC, American Psychiatric Press, 1988

Skodol AE, Karasu TB: Emergency psychiatry and the assaultive patient. Am J Psychiatry 135:202–205, 1978

Soloff PH: Emergency management of violent patients, in Psychiatry Update: American Psychiatric Association Annual Review, Vol 6. Edited by Hales RE, Frances AJ. Washington, DC, American Psychiatric Press, 1987, pp 510–536

Stern TA, Mulley AG, Thibault GE: Life-threatening drug overdose: precipitants and prognosis. JAMA 251:1983–1985, 1984

Stern TA, Schwartz JH, Cremens MC, et al: The evaluation of homicidal patients by psychiatry residents in the emergency room: a pilot study. Psychiatr Q 62:333–343, 1991

Streiner DL, Goodman JT, Woodward CA: Correlates of hospitalization decisions: a replicative study. Can J Public Health 66:411–415, 1975

Swift RM: Negotiating psychiatric hospitalization within restrictive admissions criteria. Hosp Community Psychiatry 37:619–623, 1986

Tarasoff v Regents of the University of California, 118 Cal Rptr 129, 529 P2d 553 (1974)

Teplin LA, Abram K, Michaels SK: Blood alcohol level among emergency room patients: a multivariate analysis. J Stud Alcohol 50:441–447, 1989

Tesar GE: Emergency psychiatry: the agitated patient, part II: pharmacologic treatment. Hosp Community Psychiatry 44:627–629, 1993

Tesar GE: Psychiatric emergency repeaters, in Manual of Psychiatric Emergencies, 3rd Edition. Edited by Hyman SE, Tesar GE. Boston, MA, Little, Brown, 1994, pp 110–114

Tesar GE, Stern TA: Rapid tranquilization of the agitated intensive care unit patient. Journal of Intensive Care Medicine 3:195–201, 1988

Tischler GL: Decision-making process in the emergency room. Arch Gen Psychiatry 14:69–78, 1966

Weiss RD, Greenfield SF, Mirin SM: Intoxication and withdrawal syndromes, in Manual of Psychiatric Emergencies, 3rd Edition. Edited by Hyman SE, Tesar GE. Boston, MA, Little, Brown, 1994, pp 279–293

Weissberg MP: Emergency room medical clearance: an educational problem. Am J Psychiatry 136:787–790, 1979

Wulsin LR, Arnold LM, Hillard JR: Axis I disorders in ER patients with atypical chest pain. Int J Psychiatry Med 21:37–46, 1991

Zimberg S: Alcoholism: prevalence in general hospital emergency room and walk-in clinic. N Y State J Med 79:1533–1536, 1979

Chapter 29

The Consultation-Liaison Psychiatrist in the Primary Care Clinic

Gregory E. Simon, M.D., M.P.H.
Edward A. Walker, M.D.

One of the most striking changes in health care over the last decade has been the shift from inpatient to outpatient delivery of services. As health care costs have continued to increase, payers have attempted to control costs through prospective payment and aggressive concurrent utilization review. Technological advances have allowed many diagnostic and surgical procedures to move from inpatient wards to outpatient procedure centers. Together, these cost pressures and technological advances have led to dramatic decreases in hospitalization rates and length of stay. The emphasis of hospitalization has shifted toward rapid diagnosis and acute stabilization, with recovery and follow-up relegated to the outpatient clinic. This sometimes leads to deferral of psychiatric assessment and treatment until after hospital discharge.

Concern about rising health care costs has led to an increasing focus on the economic impact of psychiatric care. Arguments for increased funding of psychiatric services often hinge on the "cost-offset" effect of mental health treatment. The outpatient medical clinic is one of the principal sites where such an effect could be realized (Broadhead et al. 1990; Frasure-Smith et al. 1993; Morris et al. 1993; Simon 1992; Wells et al. 1989).

In addition, "gatekeeper" arrangements designed to manage specialty care costs are encouraging initial management of psychiatric conditions by primary care providers. A large portion of patients seen in outpatient psychiatric clinics will have been "filtered" through the primary care clinic. These changes in hospital utilization and outpatient referral patterns are shifting the focus of consultation-liaison psychiatry to the outpatient setting.

EPIDEMIOLOGY OF PSYCHIATRIC DISORDERS IN PRIMARY CARE

In community samples, fewer than 25% of patients with psychiatric disorders see specialty mental health providers; the majority of patients are seen in primary care settings (Regier et al. 1978, 1993; Shapiro et al. 1984). Epidemiological surveys in primary care typically show that 10%–15% of primary care patients have well-defined anxiety or depressive disorders (Eisenberg 1992). According to physician surveys, half of physician visits from patients with explicit psychiatric diagnoses occur in primary care clinics (Schurman et al. 1985); this proportion excludes primary care patients who present with physical symptoms. Primary care physicians write the majority of prescriptions for antidepressant (Simon and VonKorff 1993) and anxiolytic medication (Mellinger et al. 1984).

OUTPATIENT CONSULTATION-LIAISON PSYCHIATRY SETTINGS

Training Clinics

Training clinics for internal medicine or family medicine residents are probably the most common sites for outpatient consultation programs. In addition to providing consultation for specific patients, the consultant may also participate in seminars, didactic presentations, or case conferences as part of the residency training curriculum.

Primary Care Groups

As outpatient medical practice shifts more to large physician groups, more formal psychiatric consultation arrangements will probably become more common. A formal consultation-liaison relationship with a group of primary care physicians offers unique opportunities for teaching and true collaborative management.

Outpatient Medical Specialty Clinics

Some large medical specialty groups may have sufficient need for psychiatric consultation to

justify establishing a formal consultation program. Within tertiary care medical centers, medical and surgical specialists may continue to account for the bulk of providers and the bulk of referrals for outpatient consultation (Camara 1991). Some medical specialty populations involve unique clinical issues that are discussed in detail in other chapters of Section III in this volume.

STRUCTURE OF AN OUTPATIENT PSYCHIATRIC CONSULTATION-LIAISON PROGRAM

Location

Even when the psychiatric clinic is down the hall or up one floor, the psychological distance between the familiar primary care clinic and the often unfamiliar psychiatric clinic can be a real barrier. Patients who view their problems as "strictly medical" are less likely to resist a referral for psychiatric consultation when it occurs within the medical clinic.

For referring physicians, the presence of a consulting psychiatrist in the clinic, even part-time, significantly increases opportunities for communication and follow-up. Personal contact also greatly increases the ease of "curbside consultations" and informal discussions regarding patients who may not require a formal consultation. For consulting psychiatrists, work in the primary care clinic is an immersion in the culture of primary care. Consulting psychiatrists soon realize the personal understanding and therapeutic "leverage" that primary care physicians develop when the doctor-patient relationship extends over many years (and sometimes many family members).

Referral

Effective referral involves clear communication with both the patient and the consulting psychiatrist. Patients should understand the reason for psychiatric consultation, the questions to be addressed, and the anticipated plan for continued care. Without this preparation, some patients may misinterpret referral as rejection. Communication with the psychiatric consultant should summarize relevant history, state the question to be addressed by consultation, and indicate the primary care physician's expectations about subsequent management (e.g., will the consultation psychiatrist or the referring physician maintain primary responsibility for follow-up?). A written referral note is the basic requirement, but personal communication significantly increases the value of the consultation.

Consultation Visit

A consultation visit typically begins with clarification of goals and expectations. The consultant should ask about the patient's understanding of the reason for referral and the expected outcome of the consultation. Any clear conflict between the views of the patient and those of the referring physician should be explored. The consultant's role is not to resolve immediately such disagreements but to understand potential sources of difficulty.

In contrast with the "clean slate" of a more generic outpatient psychiatric evaluation, the psychiatric consultation requires that the psychiatrist step into an evaluation and treatment already in progress. The consultation assessment is often focused on a specific question. In some cases, the consultant may anticipate a relatively circumscribed role. Depending on the referring physician's request, the consultant may anticipate that only one or two visits will be necessary. The consultant must also consider, however, that the referring provider may have been unaware of important issues that will influence treatment. For example, the presence of a personality disorder may strongly influence the treatment of depression. A history of childhood abuse may influence a patient's ability to form a trusting alliance with both medical and psychiatric providers. These and other complicating issues may

necessitate a higher intensity of psychotherapeutic treatment.

Conjoint visits involving the patient, primary care physician, and consulting psychiatrist are sometimes quite useful. When consultation involves negotiation around conflict-laden issues (e.g., chronic use of pain medications), conjoint meetings may be essential. Coordination of both providers' schedules is a real logistical hurdle.

Follow-Up

Frequency and duration of psychiatric follow-up will vary widely, depending on patient needs. Many patients benefit from one or two consultation visits followed by management recommendations to the primary care physician. Some patients need a "trial period" of brief intervention, followed by either referral back to the primary care physician or transfer of care to the specialty mental health clinic (e.g., anxiety disorders clinic, geropsychiatry clinic). In some cases, the need for transfer to specialty mental health care may be apparent at the initial visit.

A period of shared follow-up with the primary care physician allows ongoing psychiatric follow-up while maintaining the involvement of the primary care physician. During the initial phases of treatment (e.g., beginning antidepressant therapy), alternating visits between psychiatrist and primary care physician for 4–6 weeks takes advantage of specialist expertise and the ongoing alliance with the referring physician. Some patients require chronic but infrequent psychiatric care. Patients with recurring or episodic psychiatric conditions (e.g., recurrent depression of moderate severity) may require brief psychiatric consultation during exacerbations of illness. These patients may return to the referring physician after initial evaluation and stabilization but return to the psychiatric consultant months or years later during another episode of illness.

The primary care clinic is rarely the best

setting for ongoing psychotherapy. Many factors that favor consultation in the primary care setting may conflict with a more traditional psychotherapeutic relationship: briefer visits, less strict confidentiality, and a less structured "treatment frame" with respect to scheduling. If ongoing psychotherapy is indicated, transfer to the specialty mental health clinic is usually preferable.

Communication Following Consultation

If possible, the consultant's assessment and recommendations should be communicated in person. A conversation about future management (whether face-to-face or over the telephone) is far more informative than a written report. Consultants must remember that the primary care outpatient record is a relatively "public" document. Notes about consultation visits are available not only to the referring primary care physician but also to other medical providers involved in the patient's care (including other medical specialists, nurses, and physical therapists). If confidential information is relevant to primary care management, the consultant may choose to discuss such issues with the referring physician directly. In some cases, psychiatric consultation records may be maintained separately from the general outpatient record.

Continuity

Much of the cumulative effect of clinic-based consultation comes from ongoing collaboration between the consulting psychiatrist and the referring primary care physician. A continuous collaborative relationship allows primary care physicians to refer patients with greater confidence. Over time, consulting psychiatrists develop a clearer understanding of the skills and interests of individual primary care physicians.

Service Planning

Typical consultation programs are designed to provide initial evaluation for all patients and brief treatment for many. Some programs may provide longer term care in the primary care clinic, whereas in others, patients who require longer term care will be referred to more traditional outpatient psychiatric settings. Staffing levels for an outpatient psychiatric consultation-liaison service that is directed at shorter term care should be adequate to provide initial consultation within 1 week of referral as well as an average of one to two follow-up visits for each patient referred. A typical primary care clinic of 10 physicians (15,000–20,000 patients) might generate at least two to three new consultation requests per week.

ROLES AND EXPECTATIONS

Consultant

The role of consultant differs significantly from that of sole provider. First, the consulting psychiatrist is expected to respond to the needs and requests of both the patient and the referring physician. Second, the consultant typically has narrow clinical responsibility.

A consultant's satisfaction with outpatient consultation work will be greatly enhanced by flexibility, an eclectic clinical approach, and a willingness to work with a wide range of patients and physicians. Referring physicians typically prefer a single referral destination for the wide range of problems presenting in outpatient clinics. Consultants should also expect that referring providers will differ widely in knowledge about and attitudes toward psychiatric problems.

Working effectively as a consultant in primary care often requires a shift away from the traditional psychiatric treatment paradigm. In the majority of cases, the consultant is less focused on developing a long-term therapeutic alliance with the patient than on bolstering his or her alliance with the primary care physician.

Effective consultants must translate the concepts of psychiatric diagnosis and treatment into language that is understandable and useful to the primary care provider.

Primary Care Physician

Effective collaborative management by the primary care provider and the consulting psychiatrist requires active participation from the referring physician. Unlike what occurs with the traditional referral to a medical or psychiatric specialist, the typical referral to a consultation-liaison psychiatrist in primary care involves the primary care physician sharing in the initial management of the patient's condition and the reassumption of full responsibility after brief involvement by the psychiatric consultant. For most primary care physicians, this higher level of involvement is a welcome change. Some primary care physicians, however, may view psychiatric treatment as too complex or may see psychological problems as lying outside the scope of primary care.

Patient

Most primary care patients are more accustomed to a medical treatment model than to a psychotherapeutic treatment model. Structured assessment followed by instruction and advice often fits well with these patients' experiences, desires, and expectations. Clarity about the time-limited nature of consultation will help avoid misunderstanding or disappointment. The initial visit should establish the goal of assessment and treatment recommendations for the referring physician. Patients who need or desire ongoing psychotherapy are often best served by referral or transfer to the psychiatric outpatient clinic.

LIAISON ACTIVITIES

Involvement in liaison activities will vary widely, depending on clinical setting and stage of development of the consultation program. Outside of training clinics, the initial stages of a consultation program typically focus on direct clinical service to patients. Broader involvement often comes with the development of collaborative relationships over time.

CLINICAL ISSUES

Functional Somatic Symptoms

Medically unexplained physical symptoms are a frequent reason for psychiatric consultation in outpatient clinics. In some cases, such symptoms may be indicators of a well-defined depressive or anxiety disorder. In other cases, however, unexplained physical symptoms are part of an overall pattern of repeated physical symptoms without medical explanation (Barsky 1992). Although most of these patients' conditions would not satisfy diagnostic criteria for somatization disorder, this syndrome of "subthreshold" somatization is associated with substantial morbidity and use of health services (Escobar et al. 1987).

Outpatient psychiatric consultation for the patient who somatizes should focus on reducing symptoms and restoring function. If a well-defined anxiety or depressive disorder is present, specific treatment is likely to relieve the associated physical symptoms. When physical symptoms accompany major life stresses, support and encouragement are often sufficient. The consulting psychiatrist must acknowledge and legitimize the presenting physical symptoms while gently shifting the agenda to precipitating stresses (Goldberg et al. 1989). For chronically symptom-sensitive patients, treatment includes attention to both physical symptoms and disease fears (Barsky et al. 1988). Relaxation training can both reduce anxiety-related symptoms and allow patients to divert attention away from bothersome physical sensations. Regular exercise can help to desensitize patients to somatic sensations by demonstrating that major physical changes (e.g., rapid heart rate, shortness of breath) are usually the result of benign or even desirable causes. Exploration of disease fears can help patients to identify and challenge exaggerated or catastrophic thoughts.

Depressive Disorders

The research literature suggests significant shortcomings in the current treatment of primary care patients with depression. Depression in patients who present in a primary care setting may go unrecognized (Ormel et al. 1990; Schulberg et al. 1985; Simon and VonKorff 1993; VonKorff et al. 1987). Compared with patients in psychiatric clinics, patients seen in primary care settings show less severe illness and may be more likely to present with physical symptoms (Blacker and Clare 1987). Primary care patients with depression are also older and are more likely to have comorbid medical conditions than are psychiatric outpatients with depression.

Research on treatment of primary care patients with depression reveals that antidepressant medications are often taken in low dosages and are discontinued after only a few days or weeks (D. A. W. Johnson 1974; Katon and Schulberg 1992; Simon et al. 1993). The available randomized trial data (from specialty psychiatric populations) clearly support more intensive treatment. Guidelines for the treatment of depression in primary care recently released by the Agency for Health Care Policy and Research (Depression Guideline Panel 1993) acknowledge the absence of clear data on primary care populations but clearly endorse more intensive treatment. We suggest, however, that consultants take care not to criticize the treatment practices of primary care colleagues. Such criticism will not foster collegial relationships and may be later proven incorrect.

Primary care-based treatment of depression usually emphasizes antidepressant medi-

cation over psychotherapy. Given the skills and training of primary care physicians and the time constraints of primary care practice, counseling during the primary care visit is limited to brief support and advice. Even brief visits with the psychiatric consultant, however, typically include limited psychotherapeutic intervention. Advice from the consulting psychiatrist will help primary care physicians to use their limited time more effectively. Brief, focused interventions by primary care providers may offer significant benefit (Klerman et al. 1987; Mynors-Wallis and Gath 1993).

Continued coordination with the primary care physician is critical. Primary care patients who begin treatment with antidepressant medication often discontinue treatment during the first few weeks. Given the significant risk for recurrence of depressive illness, the consultant must encourage the patient and the primary care physician to develop a plan for responding to signs of recurrence.

Anxiety Disorders

Symptoms of anxiety are easily mistaken for those of cardiac arrhythmia, asthma, coronary disease, vertigo, cerebrovascular disease, or an endocrine disorder. Consequently, patients with anxiety disorders are frequently referred for expensive and unnecessary examinations. The consulting psychiatrist can prevent this unnecessary medical utilization by increasing physicians' sensitivity to anxiety diagnoses.

Breathing control and relaxation training are often quite effective in relieving dyspnea, dizziness, or chest pains that often accompany both panic attacks and generalized anxiety. Cognitive interventions will often focus on the exaggerated disease fears that can accompany anxiety. Behavioral treatments should include efforts to reduce unnecessary health care use (e.g., emergency room visits) as a response to anxiety symptoms.

Substance Use Disorders

Alcohol is the most common drug of abuse among patients in most primary care settings. Epidemiological studies show current alcohol abuse among 5%–15% of primary care patients, with higher prevalence rates in urban clinics serving patients from lower socioeconomic groups (J. Johnson et al. 1993; Simon and VonKorff 1991). Psychiatric consultants must always consider alcohol abuse or dependence as a possible cause of anxiety or depressive symptoms. Effective treatment or referral of patients with alcoholism requires close collaboration between the consultant and the primary care physician. Both must clearly point out the medical, psychological, and social consequences of continued alcohol use.

SUMMARY

As the site of care shifts to the outpatient clinic, psychiatrists will increasingly be asked to provide consultative support to primary care and other outpatient medical providers. Consultation-liaison psychiatrists are ideally trained to assist in the evaluation of primary care patients and the development of integrated biopsychosocial treatment in outpatient medical clinics.

For many consultation-liaison psychiatrists, these effects will necessitate a major change in practice and employment of new skills. Lengthy diagnostic assessment will be supplanted by rapid, focused assessments. Psychiatric consultants will have to develop treatment plans that are brief and practical and that accommodate the limitations of primary care providers.

REFERENCES

Barsky A: Amplification, somatization, and the somatoform disorders. Psychosomatics 33: 28–34, 1992

Barsky A, Geringer E, Wool CA: A cognitive-educational treatment for hypochondriasis. Gen Hosp Psychiatry 10:322–327, 1988

Blacker C, Clare AW: Depressive disorders in primary care. Br J Psychiatry 150:737–751, 1987

Broadhead WE, Blazer DG, George LK, et al: Depression, disability days and days lost from work in a prospective epidemiologic survey. JAMA 264:2524–2528, 1990

Camara EG: A psychiatric outpatient consultation-liaison clinic. Psychosomatics 32:304–308, 1991

Depression Guideline Panel: Depression in Primary Care: Clinical Practice Guidelines (AHCPR Publ No 93–0550). Rockville, MD, U.S. Department of Health and Human Services, Public Health Service, Agency for Health Care Policy and Research, 1993

Eisenberg L: Treating depression and anxiety in primary care: closing the gap between knowledge and practice. N Engl J Med 326: 1080–1084, 1992

Escobar JI, Burnam MA, Karno M, et al: Somatization in the community. Arch Gen Psychiatry 44:713–718, 1987

Frasure-Smith N, Lesperance F, Talajic M: Depression following myocardial infarction: impact on 6-month survival. JAMA 270:1819–1825, 1993

Goldberg D, Gask L, O'Dowd T: The treatment of somatization: teaching techniques of reattribution. J Psychosom Res 33:689–695, 1989

Johnson DAW: A study of the use of antidepressant medication in general practice. Br J Psychiatry 125:186–192, 1974

Johnson J, Spitzer RL, Williams JBW, et al: Alcohol abuse/dependence diagnosed by primary care physicians: recognition rate, psychiatric comorbidity, and functional impairment. Paper presented at the seventh annual National Institute of Mental Health International Research Conference on Mental Health Problems in the General Health Care Sector, McLean, VA, September 1993

Katon W, Schulberg H: Epidemiology of depression in primary care. Gen Hosp Psychiatry 14: 237–247, 1992

Klerman G, Budman S, Berwick D, et al: Efficacy of a brief psychosocial intervention for symptoms of stress and distress among patients in primary care. Med Care 25:1078–1088, 1987

Mellinger G, Balter M, Uhlenhuth E: Prevalence and correlates of the long-term regular use of anxiolytics. JAMA 251:375–379, 1984

Morris P, Robinson RG, Samuels J: Depression, introversion, and mortality following stroke. Aust N Z J Psychiatry 24:443–449, 1993

Mynors-Wallis L, Gath DH: The treatment of major depression in primary care: a controlled clinical trial comparing problem-solving with amitriptyline and drug-attention placebo. Paper presented at the seventh annual National Institute of Mental Health International Research Conference on Mental Health Problems in the General Health Care Sector, McLean, VA, September 1993

Ormel J, vandenBrink W, Koeter MW, et al: Recognition, management, and outcome of psychological disorders in primary care: a naturalistic follow-up study. Psychol Med 20:909–923, 1990

Regier DA, Goldberg ID, Taube CA: The de facto US mental health services system: a public health perspective. Arch Gen Psychiatry 35:685–693, 1978

Regier D, Narrow WE, Rae DS, et al: The de facto US mental and addictive disorders service system: Epidemiologic Catchment Area prospective 1-year prevalence rates of disorders and services. Arch Gen Psychiatry 50:85–94, 1993

Schulberg HC, Saul M, McClelland M, et al: Assessing depression in primary medical and psychiatric practices. Arch Gen Psychiatry 42:1164–1170, 1985

Schurman RA, Kramer PD, Mitchell JB: The hidden mental health network: treatment of mental illness by nonpsychiatrist physicians. Arch Gen Psychiatry 42:89–94, 1985

Shapiro S, Skinner EA, Kessler LG, et al: Utilization of health and mental health services: three Epidemiologic Catchment Area sites. Arch Gen Psychiatry 41:971–978, 1984

Simon G: Psychiatric disorder and functional somatic symptoms as predictors of health care use. Psychiatr Med 10:49–60, 1992

Simon G, VonKorff M: Somatization and psychiatric disorder in the NIMH Epidemiologic Catchment Area Study. Am J Psychiatry 148:1494–1500, 1991

Simon G, VonKorff M: Management and outcomes of depression in primary care. Paper presented at the seventh annual National Institute of Mental Health International Research Conference on Mental Health Problems in the General Health Care Sector, McLean, VA, September 1993

Simon G, VonKorff M, Wagner EH, et al: Patterns of antidepressant use in community practice. Gen Hosp Psychiatry 15:399–408, 1993

VonKorff M, Shapiro S, Burke JD, et al: Anxiety and depression in a primary care clinic: comparison of Diagnostic Interview Schedule, General Health Questionnaire, and practitioner assessments. Arch Gen Psychiatry 44:152–156, 1987

Wells K, Stewart A, Hays R, et al: The functioning and well-being of depressed patients: results from the Medical Outcome Study. JAMA 262:914–919, 1989

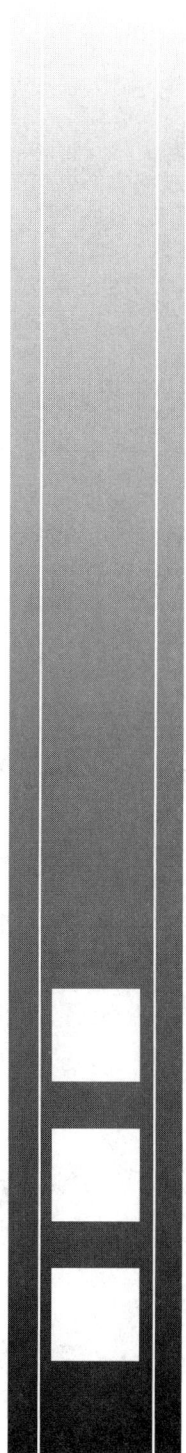

Section IV

Treatment

Chapter 30

Psychopharmacology

John S. Jachna, M.D.
Richard D. Lane, M.D.
Alan J. Gelenberg, M.D.

DRUG ACTIONS AND INTERACTIONS

Drug Absorption

A drug can be administered directly into the bloodstream (intravenous administration), by diffusion from a drug depot (intramuscular or subcutaneous administration), or across a mucosal surface such as the stomach, rectum, or sublingual area. Absorption rates differ among these routes, although absorption from different forms of oral medications (capsule, pill, liquid) is generally similar. Parenteral administration generally results in more rapid effects, although the erratic absorption of some drugs, such as diazepam, from intramuscular injection makes their clinical benefits less predictable and can paradoxically result in a slower onset. Special preparations, such as long-acting forms of both parenteral and oral drugs, change absorption further. Gastric absorption increases when the stomach is empty because more mucosal surfaces are available;

there is also more rapid emptying into the jejunum. Many psychotropic drugs are weak bases, which are better absorbed in the jejunum where the pH is higher. There is little overall change in oral absorption of drugs with aging, despite numerous individual changes, such as increases in gastric pH and decreases in surface villi, and changes in gastric motility, gastric emptying, and intestinal perfusion (Altman 1990; Ouslander 1981; Schmucker 1985; Siris and Rifkin 1981).

Drug Distribution

Most psychoactive drugs (except for lithium) are lipophilic and are absorbed preferentially into fatty tissue, including the brain. This means that psychotropic medications generally have large volumes of distribution. In addition, most psychiatric medications are bound to plasma proteins, such as albumin and glycoprotein. When medication is bound to proteins, it is not available to tissues such as the brain. Protein binding makes lowering of toxic levels of drugs more difficult. Other medications can alter the amount of protein binding. With aging and chronic medical illness, albumin decreases and the proportion of unbound drug generally increases. For lipid-soluble drugs, the volume of distribution increases with aging as a result of decreases in total body water and lean body mass, and as a result of increases in total body fat.

Drug Metabolism

Water-soluble drugs are readily excreted by the kidneys. Active lipid-soluble drugs tend to accumulate unless they are converted to more water-soluble compounds or they are metabolized by the liver to less active compounds. Lithium is a significant exception because it is not metabolized.

Because of the anatomical arrangement of blood flow from the gastrointestinal (GI) system, the absorbed drug passes through the liver before entering the systemic circulation. There, the drug may be metabolized before the rest of the body is exposed to it. The metabolites are sometimes active psychopharmacological agents, although the level of activity can vary significantly. This "first-pass effect" is sometimes very significant. This also helps explain why intramuscular preparations are often more potent than oral equivalents. For example, neuroleptic drugs given intramuscularly have about twice the potency of orally administered drugs, although this can vary widely from patient to patient.

Once in the liver, a drug is exposed to two main groups of metabolizing enzymes. This multistep catabolic process of drug elimination involves oxidation and conjugation of the oxidized metabolite. The oxidative process occurs via the monooxygenase or cytochrome P450 (CYP) enzyme system. Conjugation is usually the final catabolic enzymatic process, in which the drug or its metabolites are coupled with other compounds to form more easily excreted

(i.e., more hydrophilic) compounds. The rate of metabolism, especially the oxidative process, is affected by many factors (Table 30–1) and disease states.

Four CYP enzymes are especially important in the oxidation of medications: CYP2D6, CYP1A2, CYP2C, and CYP3A3/4. These enzymes are subject to inhibition and genetic mutations, and, in selective cases, induction (see Table 30–1). Medications usually have a high affinity for metabolism by a particular enzyme, can compete for metabolism with other substrates, and/or can inhibit an enzyme without being metabolized by it. These CYP-drug interactions are potentially harmful if the substrate has a low therapeutic index, as is the case with tricyclic antidepressants (DeVane 1994).

Drug Elimination

A drug and its metabolites can be excreted by the kidneys as well as into the bile or feces. Small amounts are also lost through sweat, saliva, or tears. Biological or elimination half-life is a measure of the amount of time needed to excrete half of the drug from the body. This is usually expressed as plasma half-life, which states how long it takes to remove half of the drug from the plasma. Frequency of drug administration is established by the length of its half-life. A "steady-state" drug level is generally achieved after four to five half-lives of a drug; it is at this point that accurate serum drug levels are obtained.

Because the pharmacokinetic properties of some drugs change with extended administration, a maintenance half-life is sometimes defined. For lipophilic, highly bound psychoactive drugs, the maintenance half-life is often much longer after long-term administration. Aging and renal disease also result in decreased renal blood flow and glomerular filtration, slowing the common renal route of elimination. Medical and surgical patients usually receive multiple medications; the medications

Table 30–1.   Cytochrome P450–drug interactions[a]

Substrates of P450 enzymes

1A2	2C (2C9/2C19)	2D6	3A3/4
Caffeine	Barbiturates	β-Blockers	Anticancer drugs
Clozapine	Demethylation of	Clozapine	Alprazolam
Demethylation of tertiary	tertiary TCAs	Codeine →Morphine	Calcium channel
TCAs	Diazepam	Haloperidol[b]	blockers
Phenacetin	NSAIDs	Paroxetine	Carbamazepine
Theophylline	Phenytoin	Phenothiazines	Cyclosporin
Warfarin	Propranolol	Risperidone	Erythromycin
	Tolbutamide	Secondary TCAs	Lidocaine
	Warfarin	Type 1C antiarrhythmics	Midazolam
		(flecainide, propafenone)	Nefazodone
		Venlafaxine	Quinidine
			Sertraline
			Terfenadine
			Demethylation of
			tertiary TCAs
			Triazolam
			Venlafaxine

Inhibitors of P450 enzymes

Fluvoxamine	Fluoxetine	Fluoxetine	Cimetidine
Grapefruit juice	Fluvoxamine	Fluphenazine	Erythromycin
	Sertraline	Norfluoxetine	Fluconazole
		Paroxetine	Fluoxetine
		Phenothiazines	Fluvoxamine
		Quinidine	Grapefruit juice
		Sertraline	Ketoconazole
		TCAs	Nefazodone
			Norfluoxetine
			Sertraline

Inducers

Cigarettes	Alcohol (?)	Not induced	Alcohol (?)
	Phenobarbital		Carbamazepine
	Phenytoin		

Note.   TCAs are metabolized by CYP2D6, CYP3A, CYP2C, and CYP1A2; (?) denotes incomplete or inconsistent data; CYP = cytochrome P450; NSAIDs = nonsteroidal antiinflammatory drugs; TCAs = tricyclic antidepressants.
[a]Includes both in vivo and in vitro data.
[b]Complex interaction.
Source.   Data compiled by M. G. Wise and L. Ereshefsky.

can interact to modify the pharmacokinetic properties of a given psychotropic drug.

Receptor Site Activity

Drug effects can occur at any of several points in the life of neurotransmitter chemicals. These points include synthesis of the neurotransmit-ter, transport in the presynaptic neuron, storage of the chemical in vesicles, extrusion of the vesicles' contents, effects on postsynaptic and presynaptic receptors, and disposal of the neurotransmitter through degradation, diffusion, or reuptake. Effects at the receptor depend on the chemical's affinity for the receptor, the amount of ligand available, and the presence of competing drugs. A drug's effect at the target receptor is usually mediated by a second messenger in the target cell.

ANTIDEPRESSANTS

Classes of Antidepressant Drugs

The structure of tricyclic antidepressants, which includes both tertiary and secondary amines, is similar to that of the phenothiazines. The tertiary tricyclics include imipramine, amitriptyline, trimipramine, doxepin, and clomipramine. Secondary tricyclics are formed as tertiary amines are metabolized; imipramine is demethylated to desipramine, and amitriptyline is demethylated to nortriptyline. Protriptyline is another secondary tricyclic. Although the structure of maprotiline is tetracyclic, its pharmacological profile is similar to that of the tricyclic antidepressants (see Table 30–2).

Newer antidepressants have distinct structures. Bupropion is a monocyclic phenylbutylamine of the aminoketone type. Trazodone is a triazolopyridine, and nefazodone is a synthetically derived phenylpiperazine. The dibenzoxazepine amoxapine is a metabolite of the neuroleptic loxapine. Venlafaxine, a structurally novel antidepressant, has a tricyclic configuration. Selective serotonin reuptake inhibitors (SSRIs) include fluoxetine (a straight-chain phenylpropylamine), paroxetine (a phenylpiperidine compound), sertraline (a naphthylamine derivative), and fluvoxamine (Table 30–3).

Mechanism of Action

The biogenic amine hypothesis holds that depression is associated with decreased levels of central nervous system (CNS) neurotransmitters norepinephrine (catecholamine) and/or serotonin (indoleamine). The various cyclic antidepressants were thought to work by blocking reuptake of these neurotransmitters into presynaptic neurons. Other antidepressants exist that do not have this property. In addition, because reuptake blockage occurs rapidly, it does not explain the delayed therapeutic action of antidepressants. Therefore, reuptake blockage alone does not account for the therapeutic effect of antidepressants. Although the specific mechanisms of action of these varied agents are still undefined, increased norepinephrine and serotonin neurotransmission likely plays some role.

Pharmacokinetics

The antidepressants are generally well absorbed orally and are highly protein-bound, except for venlafaxine. This means that low serum albumin or displacement of a drug from protein-binding sites by another medication can increase biological effects. Sertraline is more highly protein-bound than is fluoxetine or paroxetine.

There is a large variation in antidepressant steady-state levels. In addition, demethylation of tertiary tricyclic compounds produces active metabolites. Drug interactions also can occur. For example, most serotonin reuptake inhibitors inhibit CYP2D6. The comparative inhibition among SSRIs is currently debated, but paroxetine appears to be more strongly inhibitory compared with fluoxetine or sertraline (Crewe et al. 1992).

Dosage and Administration

Treatment with the tricyclic antidepressants is started at a low dose, and the dose is increased gradually every 3–4 days. The initial dose and rate of increase are usually described as "start lower, go slower" for elderly and medically ill patients. To take advantage of the natural hypnotic effect of most tricyclic antidepressants, these drugs are generally prescribed to be taken at bedtime. More activating medications, such as fluoxetine and other SSRIs, are an exception; these should be taken in the morning.

Table 30–2. Cyclic and related antidepressants

Generic name	Trade name	Class	Initial dose (mg)[a]	Usual therapeutic dose range (mg)[a]	Norepinephrine reuptake blockade	Serotonin reuptake blockade	Dopamine reuptake blockade	Acetylcholine blockade	Histamine blockade	Orthostatic blood pressure
Amitriptyline	Elavil, others	Tertiary TCA	25–75	150–300	1	2	1	4	3	3
Clomipramine	Anafranil	Tertiary TCA	25	100–250	2	4	1	2	0	2
Doxepin	Sinequan, others	Tertiary TCA	25–75	150–300	2	1	0	3	4	3
Imipramine	Tofranil, others	Tertiary TCA	25–75	150–300	2	2	0	3	2	3
Trimipramine	Surmontil	Tertiary TCA	25–75	75–300	1	2	0	3	4	3
Desipramine	Norpramin, others	Secondary TCA	25–75	75–200	4	0	0	2	1	2
Nortriptyline	Pamelor, others	Secondary TCA	20–40	50–200	3	1	0	2	2	1
Protriptyline	Vivactil	Secondary TCA	10–20	20–60	3	1	0	3	2	2
Maprotiline	Ludiomil	Tetracyclic TCA	25–75	75–300	4	0	1	2	3	2
Bupropion	Wellbutrin	Monocyclic phenylbutylamine	25–75 tid	300	1	0	2	1	1	1
Trazodone	Desyrel	Triazolopyridine	150	100–600	1	2	0	0	1	3
Amoxapine	Asendin	Dibenzoxazepine	50–150	100–600	3	1	1	1	2	2
Fluoxetine	Prozac	Straight-chain phenylpropylamine	20	20–60	1	3	1	1	0	1
Paroxetine	Paxil	Phenylpiperidine	20	20–50	1	4	1	2	0	1
Sertraline	Zoloft	Naphthylamine derivative	50	50–200	0	3	1	1	0	1
Venlafaxine	Effexor	Bicyclic cyclohexanol	25 tid	225–375	1	3	0	0	0	1
Nefazodone	Serzone	Phenylpiperazine	100 bid	300–600	2	2	1	0	0	2

Note. bid = twice a day; TCAs = tricyclic antidepressants; tid = three times a day; 0 = least effect; 4 = most effect.
[a]Doses for elderly and medically ill patients are often lower.

Table 30–3. Selective serotonin reuptake inhibitors

Generic name	Trade name	Plasma protein binding	Half-life
Fluoxetine	Prozac	High	1.9 days (norfluoxetine: 7 days)
Fluvoxamine	Luvox	Low	15 hours
Paroxetine	Paxil	High	15 hours
Sertraline	Zoloft	High	26 hours

Most tricyclic medications produce a response at doses of 150–300 mg in adult outpatients, but lower doses are often used in elderly or medically ill patients. Protriptyline, which has a very long half-life, and nortriptyline are more potent than the other tricyclics and require lower doses. For the SSRIs (see Table 30–3), dosing is also lower. For trazodone and nefazodone, dosing is higher (see Table 30–2).

Response

A substantial disadvantage with all antidepressants is the delay in onset of therapeutic action. At least 10 days to 2 weeks is required for initial response in patients with primary depression, and at least 6 weeks of an adequate dose should be maintained before abandoning a medication. A therapeutic response in elderly patients may take even longer to occur. Unlike some other psychotropic medications, in which variation in patients' responses generally refers only to side effects, there is significant interindividual variation in response to antidepressants and in the context of medical illness. For example, a patient's depression may not respond to one agent but then may respond well to another. If one medication does not improve the patient's condition, we recommend a trial with a drug that has a different neurotransmitter profile.

SSRIs are as effective as the tricyclics for mild and moderate depression in outpatients. Their effectiveness for the treatment of patients with severe depression is not as well established, and their relative efficacies in patients with secondary depression and in depression

in medical-surgical patients are largely unknown. Trazodone appears to achieve a somewhat lower rate of antidepressant response than most antidepressants, but this may be the result of undertreatment. Trazodone's side-effect profile offers some advantages in consultation-liaison settings, such as particular help for those with prominent sleep disturbance; the drug's disadvantages include priapism in men (and, rarely, persistent clitoral engorgement for women), hypotension, and possible exacerbation of myocardial instability. Nefazodone may have a good profile in patients who are medically ill because it has few, if any, sexual side effects, has little associated activation, and encourages sleep, although it may cause hypotension.

Side Effects

Tricyclic antidepressants. Frequent side effects of tricyclic antidepressants include anticholinergic effects, sedation, orthostatic hypotension, tachycardia, and weight gain. Cardiac effects (Jefferson 1989) include electrocardiographic (ECG) abnormalities (such as T-wave flattening or inversion and ST segment depression), conduction delays, and arrhythmias, despite the potency of the tricyclics as type IA antiarrhythmics. Other possible side effects are insomnia, confusion (especially in patients with preexisting CNS disease), psychosis, tremor, rash, sweating, and sexual dysfunction. All antidepressants can induce mania in certain individuals.

The anticholinergic effects are particularly

important, especially for medical-surgical and elderly patients. Frequent anticholinergic effects are dry mouth, blurred vision, constipation, and urinary retention; the side effect of urinary retention is sometimes used to advantage for treating patients with incontinence. Patients with prostate enlargement, which represents a majority of elderly men, are particularly susceptible to urinary retentive effects. Dry mouth, in addition to significant discomfort, can cause an increase in dental caries and gingivitis. In patients with untreated narrow-angle glaucoma, anticholinergic-induced pupillary dilation can cause an acute exacerbation. This is not a concern in patients with wide-angle glaucoma or following an iridectomy. Anticholinergic effects may contribute to the sexual dysfunctions that tricyclics can induce. Patients who are medically ill, elderly, or cognitively impaired are at particularly high risk for delirium from drugs with anticholinergic effects.

An increase in pulse rate is a frequent cardiac effect, which rarely interferes with using these drugs outside of the setting of the cardiac care unit (CCU). As noted above, tricyclics have an antiarrhythmic effect—specifically, a type IA quinidine-like effect on cardiac conduction. Therefore, for all hospitalized patients, the clinician should review the ECG before beginning treatment. Particular caution is required in patients with atrioventricular blocks, bundle-branch blocks, and bradyarrhythmias. Such preexisting cardiac abnormalities can warrant starting the antidepressant in a monitored environment. A cardiologist should be consulted concerning decisions about initiating tricyclic antidepressant treatment in such situations.

Tricyclic antidepressant treatment should not be started immediately after a patient has had a myocardial infarction (MI). The risk of inducing arrhythmias should be carefully evaluated against the need to treat the patient for depression. The Cardiac Arrhythmia Suppression Trial (CAST) demonstrated that antiarrhythmic drugs, including two class IC antiarrhythmics

(encainide and flecainide) and one class IA antiarrhythmic (moricizine), were associated with unexpectedly increased mortality rates in post-MI patients (Glassman et al. 1993; Roose and Glassman 1994). These results necessitate a reassessment of the potential hazards of tricyclic antidepressants in patients with organic heart disease. The authors suggest that, in some patients with heart disease, tricyclic antidepressants are potentially more hazardous than was previously believed because of the potential proarrhythmic effects of medications with quinidine-like properties.

Orthostatic hypotension is a serious side effect of tricyclic antidepressants, especially for elderly and medically ill patients who are at risk for falls (Thapa et al. 1995). Clinicians should always instruct patients who take tricyclic antidepressants to arise slowly from a lying or sitting to a standing position. Among the tricyclics, imipramine is associated with the highest risk of orthostasis, whereas nortriptyline is associated with the least risk and is preferred when hypotension is a particular concern.

In rare cases, tricyclics can impair cardiac muscle contractility and worsen congestive heart failure (CHF) (Warrington et al. 1989). This concern is based on individual case reports of reproducible worsening of CHF. The evidence for this adverse effect is not strong, however, and should not restrict the use of these medications, except possibly in patients with severely compromised cardiac output in whom a small change in cardiac output is clinically significant (e.g., patients who are candidates for heart transplants who have ejection fractions of 20% or less).

Other antidepressants. SSRIs have a different side-effect profile than do tricyclic antidepressants. SSRIs are generally considered "activating," although paroxetine seems less so and can actually cause sedation (Ayd 1993; Kiev 1992). Frequent side effects include nausea, headache, nervousness, insomnia, and anorgasmia. In contrast to the weight gain seen in patients taking tricyclic antidepressants, SSRIs can produce decreased appetite and weight loss and commonly cause nausea and gastric irritation. The anxiety-spectrum symptoms are less common with sertraline and paroxetine than with fluoxetine. SSRIs have minimal tendency to induce orthostatic hypotension, although adequate controlled studies comparing these drugs with tricyclics are not yet published. The effect of SSRIs on peripheral α_1 receptors in the context of serious medical illness has also not yet been evaluated in a systematic, conclusive way. SSRIs do not possess quinidine-like activity, so cardiac arrhythmias rarely occur. A few reports of SSRI-associated bradycardia exist (Hussein and Kaufman 1994). Gelenberg (1995, p. 41) states, "rare patients may develop severe bradycardia in association with SSRI antidepressants."

Additional SSRI side effects that are less frequent than with tricyclic antidepressants include somnolence, akathisia, rash, fever, arthralgia, alopecia, and elevations in aminotransferase levels. Even more rare are extrapyramidal symptoms (Leo et al. 1995) and seizures in patients with preexisting seizure disorder, leukocytosis, and respiratory distress. Hyponatremia is rarely seen with SSRIs. Fluoxetine toxicity, manifested by irritability and increased heart rates and respiratory rates, has been reported in neonates (Spencer 1993).

In the early 1990s, much attention was paid in the media to fluoxetine's purported tendency to produce suicidal ideation or violent behavior. Almost every physician and nurse on medical and surgical services has heard about this risk, even if they know little else about antidepressants; consultation-liaison psychiatrists are frequently questioned about these associations. For any antidepressant, a risk of suicide exists while the patient gains energy but still feels a subjective sense of depression. The tendency of SSRIs to produce nervousness or akathisia might add to this risk, although no clear association has been scientifically established.

Fluvoxamine, although only approved by the U.S. Food and Drug Administration (FDA) for the treatment of obsessive-compulsive disorder, may occasionally be prescribed as an antidepressant. It offers no benefits over the other SSRIs with similar half-lives (e.g., paroxetine or sertraline). It does inhibit CYP1A2, CYP3A3/4, and CYP2C but not CYP2D6.

Bupropion is stimulating and frequently produces anxiety, agitation, insomnia, and increased motor activity, along with tremor, nausea, and anorexia. It can also cause headache and rash. Like other cyclic antidepressants, bupropion is associated with a dose-related risk of seizures, especially in patients with bulimia. Compared with tricyclic antidepressants, bupropion may be associated with less risk of inducing mania and, therefore, may be especially useful in patients with mild bipolar disorder or rapid-cycling bipolar illness, although Fogelson and colleagues (1992) challenged this theory. Bupropion causes fewer anticholinergic effects than do the tricyclic antidepressants, little orthostatic hypotension, and few adverse sexual side effects. There are no significant cardiac effects associated with bupropion, although increases in blood pressure are occasionally seen. Bupropion is unique among the newer antidepressants because data are available on this drug in patients with depression and CHF, preexisting arrhythmias, and conduction delays; the drug was found to be safe in these patients (Roose et al. 1991). Weight gain or sedation has not been reported with bupropion. In overdose, bupropion lacks cardiovascular toxicity but does manifest significant neurological toxicity (Spiller et al. 1994).

Trazodone has significant α_1- and α_2-blocking activity and causes orthostatic hypotension as readily as do the tertiary amine tricyclic antidepressants (see Table 30–2). Rather than a quinidine-like slowing of conduction and suppression of premature ventricular contractions, trazodone at antidepressant doses is infrequently associated with an increase in premature ventricular contractions (Warrington et al. 1989). The sedating properties of trazodone are especially helpful for patients who have prominent sleep disturbance. Trazodone is associated with increased libido and has produced priapism in men (and, rarely, persistent clitoral engorgement for women). This effect is not dose-related and is likely caused by the combination of α_1 and α_2 blockade, as well as by the relative absence of anticholinergic effects.

Nefazodone has some characteristics in common with trazodone and some that are distinct. Nefazodone has multiple sites of action, including presynaptic reuptake blockade of serotonin and norepinephrine and antagonism of the 5-hydroxytryptamine$_2$ (5-HT$_2$) serotonin-postsynaptic receptor. It also blocks the α_1 receptor but not the α_2 receptor; no cases of priapism have been reported. Because of α_1 blockade, there is potential for orthostasis in frail, medically ill individuals. Nefazodone causes less activation (e.g., insomnia) than do SSRIs (except during rapid switch from SSRI to nefazodone), rapid decrease in anxiety, sexual dysfunction no greater than placebo, and no weight gain or loss.

Venlafaxine is a potent presynaptic reuptake blocker of norepinephrine and serotonin and is less potent for dopamine reuptake blockade. Venlafaxine's major side effects include activation, nausea, high rates of sexual dysfunction, and dose-related hypertension. No published research exists about the risk of hypertension in individuals with preexisting hypertension.

Withdrawal and Rebound

A withdrawal syndrome is associated with discontinuing tricyclic antidepressants, especially if it is done rapidly. Many symptoms of this syndrome are those associated with anticholinergic rebound, including GI upset, nausea, vomiting, diarrhea, salivation, increased perspiration, anxiety, restlessness, piloerec-

tion, and sometimes delirium (Dilsaver and Greden 1984). Dizziness, headache, malaise, and nightmares are also reported. Tricyclics should be tapered slowly (e.g., decreased by 25–50 mg every 2–3 days) after long-term use.

Pharmacologically active metabolites of fluoxetine can persist for 6 weeks or more. Therefore, the potential for drug interactions and the serotonin syndrome persists during this time. The elimination half-life is shorter for all other SSRIs and their metabolites (see Table 30–3).

Some case reports of paroxetine withdrawal have appeared (Barr et al. 1994; Keuthen et al. 1994). Symptoms included vertigo, dizziness, light-headedness, nausea, fainting, myalgia, and paresthesias. With all antidepressants, reemergence of original symptoms is a significant risk after drug discontinuation.

Drug Interactions

Inhibitors of the CYP system can increase antidepressant blood levels, whereas smoking and certain medications, such as barbiturates, can increase hepatic metabolism and reduce antidepressant levels (see Table 30–1). Adding an SSRI, especially fluoxetine, to a tricyclic antidepressant regimen can increase blood levels of the tricyclic (Preskorn et al. 1992).

Anticholinergic effects of tricyclic antidepressants add to the anticholinergic burden of other drugs, such as antiparkinsonian agents and low-potency neuroleptics. Sedation is increased when antidepressants are combined with benzodiazepines or alcohol. When given together, the levels and effects of antidepressants and neuroleptics are increased. Thiazide diuretics and acetazolamide can worsen an antidepressant's hypotensive effects. Using tricyclic antidepressants with medications that contain epinephrine, norepinephrine, or phenylephrine can produce hypertension or arrhythmias. Combining tricyclics with stimulants and sympathomimetic amines can also produce arrhythmias, particularly in predisposed patients. Tricyclic antidepressants prolong and magnify the effects of other type IA antiarrhythmic agents, such as quinidine and procainamide. Because tricyclic antidepressants block the uptake of guanethidine and guanadrel, the antihypertensive mechanism of the latter drugs is interrupted. Tricyclics can also block the effects of clonidine and methyldopa.

Concurrent use of monoamine oxidase inhibitors (MAOIs) and tricyclic antidepressants can produce the serotonin syndrome, with symptoms of mental status changes, restlessness, myoclonus, hyperreflexia, fever, diaphoresis, shivering, tremor, seizures, and death. If a treatment-resistant depression requires a trial of dual therapy with tricyclic antidepressants and an MAOI, the medications should be started simultaneously to decrease the chances of serotonin syndrome (Lader 1983; White and Simpson 1981). Fluoxetine should be stopped at least 6 weeks before treatment with an MAOI is started. After prolonged administration of fluoxetine, blood levels of fluoxetine and norfluoxetine should be obtained to ensure that levels are at zero before MAOI treatment is started (Coplan and Gorman 1993), especially in patients with hepatic disease or in elderly patients who are on multiple medications.

Monoamine Oxidase Inhibitors

Types. Because of the potential side effects associated with MAOIs, consultation-liaison psychiatrists rarely prescribe these drugs for patients who are medically ill. The available

MAOIs are the hydrazines phenelzine and isocarboxazid, and the nonhydrazine agent tranylcypromine (see Table 30–4). Brofaromine (Waldmeier et al. 1992) and moclobemide (Amrein et al. 1992) are experimental, short-acting, reversible MAOIs that may be useful in patients with social phobia and depression, respectively. Selegiline/L-deprenyl, at low doses, is a selective inhibitor of monoamine oxidase (MAO) type B. It is used for Parkinson's disease and may also have some antidepressant properties. At higher doses, selegiline is a nonspecific MAOI that can interact with SSRIs and other medications.

Mechanism of action. There are two forms of MAO: 1) MAO type A, which degrades serotonin, norepinephrine, and epinephrine; and 2) MAO type B, which degrades dopamine and phenylalanine. Tyramine, a potent pressor, is also degraded by the MAO type A system. The hydrazine MAOIs irreversibly bind to the mitochondrial enzymes MAO type A and MAO type B throughout the body and inactivate them. This effect continues for approximately 2 weeks, until the enzymes regenerate.

Pharmacokinetics. MAOIs are rapidly absorbed. They are hepatically inactivated and are excreted primarily via the intestinal tract. Patients who are "slow acetylators" may experience a prolonged drug effect.

Side effects. MAOIs are generally activating, and side effects frequently include CNS hyperactivity with restlessness, restless sleep, and insom-

Table 30–4. Monoamine oxidase inhibitors

Generic name	Trade name	Class	Initial dose (mg)[a]	Usual therapeutic dose range (mg)[a]
Phenelzine	Nardil	Hydrazine	45	45–90
Isocarboxazid	Marplan	Hydrazine	30	10–50
Tranylcypromine	Parnate	Nonhydrazine	20	10–60

[a]Doses for elderly and medically ill patients are often lower; caution is advised because of drug interactions.

nia. Daytime sleepiness and orthostatic hypotension also often occur (Teicher et al. 1988).

Drug interactions. Hypertensive crises are produced by the "cheese effect," when a patient consumes food containing tyramine or other pressors. Symptoms include headache, flushing, palpitations, nausea and vomiting, photophobia, and retro-orbital pain. Similar reactions are seen in patients on MAOIs with simultaneous use of a number of medications, including sympathomimetic amines and bronchodilators, psychostimulants, L-dopa, and buspirone.

Interaction with agents that enhance serotonergic transmission, such as SSRIs, can produce the serotonin syndrome. A potentially fatal hyperpyrexic reaction is also seen with meperidine. Dextromethorphan (found in antitussive medications) and some tricyclic antidepressants are also associated with this reaction. A serotonin syndrome–type reaction can be seen with tryptophan.

Patients who have been taking tricyclic antidepressants should have a 1-week drug-free period before beginning MAOI therapy; patients switching from an MAOI to a tricyclic should have a 2-week drug-free interval between medications. In patients with refractory depression in whom both drugs are to be used concomitantly, the medications should be started simultaneously. Because of its long-lasting metabolites, fluoxetine should be stopped for at least 6 weeks before MAOI therapy begins.

Psychostimulants

Types. The commonly used psychostimulants are methylphenidate, a piperidine deriva-

tive related to amphetamine; dextroamphetamine; and pemoline, which is similar in structure to methylphenidate (see Table 30–5).

Mechanism of action. Psychostimulant medications are structural analogues of catecholamines. They increase dopamine release and block its reuptake. They also increase norepinephrine's effect.

Pharmacokinetics. Psychostimulants are readily absorbed and are not tightly protein-bound. Excretion is essentially via the kidneys; acidification of the urine increases excretion. Pemoline has a longer half-life and more delayed onset than the most commonly used psychostimulants.

Indications. The use of psychostimulants has been limited because of real and perceived risks of abuse. In patients with primary depression, lack of clear scientific evidence of efficacy has reduced the use of these agents. Stimulant use for secondary depression (i.e., depression secondary to medical illness) appears more promising. The stimulant effects of these drugs provide specific advantages in patients who are medically ill (Kraus 1995; Wallace et al. 1995) with anergic depressions and may also aid some patients who are demoralized or apathetic (Satel and Nelson 1989). The psychostimulants are also used effectively in patients with acquired immunodeficiency syndrome (AIDS) either with or without cognitive impairment (Fernandez and Levy 1990). There is anecdotal evidence that psychostimulants are associated with increased appetite in some medically ill patients with depression.

Table 30–5. Psychostimulants

Generic name	Trade name	Starting dose range (mg)	Usual dose range (mg)
Dextroamphetamine	Dexedrine	5–10	5–30
Methylphenidate	Ritalin	5–10	5–40
Pemoline	Cylert	37.5	18.75–75

Dosage and administration. Dextroamphetamine is usually started at 5–10 mg/day, to be taken in the morning, and methylphenidate is usually started at a dosage of 2.5–5 mg twice daily (Frierson et al. 1991). To prevent insomnia, doses of these drugs are typically not given after 3:00 P.M. The usual maximum daily dosage of dextroamphetamine is 5–30 mg and of methylphenidate, 5–40 mg. Pemoline is usually started at 37.5 mg/day, to be taken in the morning; this is either reduced to 18.75 mg/day or increased to a maximum of 75 mg/day, depending on response and side effects.

Response. Response to an appropriate dosage of a psychostimulant usually appears within 1–2 days but can take longer, especially with pemoline. The rapid response of patients to psychostimulants has led to an evaluation of their effectiveness in predicting antidepressant response to tricyclics and other antidepressants. There is some evidence that dextroamphetamine predicts antidepressant efficacy (Little 1988) and that methylphenidate may predict efficacy of antidepressants with more noradrenergic properties (Gwirtsman and Guze 1989); however, the use of psychostimulants in this context is controversial (Joyce and Paykel 1989). Tolerance to the effects of psychostimulants may develop with extended use.

Side effects. Appetite suppression and insomnia can occur with psychostimulants, but anorexia caused by depression (along with other neurovegetative symptoms) is reversed by psychostimulants if an antidepressant effect occurs. Possible CNS side effects are activation, exacerbation of anxiety, and exacerbation of confusion. Other reported side effects are nausea, tremor, headache, exacerbation of spasticity, blurred vision, dry mouth, constipation, dizziness, and fatigue. Cardiovascular effects may include palpitations, dysrhythmias, tachycardia, and blood pressure changes. Dystonia is a rare occurrence. A delayed hepatic hypersensitivity reaction is reported

with pemoline use (Elitsur 1990; Patterson 1984; Pratt and Dubois 1990; Tolman et al. 1973). Side effects are infrequent at the relatively low dosages used to treat depression in patients who are medically ill.

Withdrawal. Abstinence symptoms following long-term use of psychostimulants may include drug craving, somnolence, rebound depression, and fatigue, as well as nausea, vomiting, hyperphagia, and tremor.

Drug interactions. Psychostimulants have additive effects with other drugs that produce CNS stimulation, such as caffeine. They also have additive cardioaccelatory effects with tricyclic antidepressants and interfere with the hypotensive effects of guanethidine and similar drugs (see Table 30–6).

MOOD-STABILIZING MEDICATIONS

Lithium

Mechanism of action. Postulates for lithium's mechanism of action are diverse. Hy-

Table 30–6. Reported drug interactions with psychostimulants

Medication	Interactive effect
Guanethidine	Decreased antihypertensive effect
Vasopressors	Increased pressor effect
Oral anticoagulants	Increased prothrombin time
Anticonvulsants	Increased levels of phenobarbital, primidone, phenytoin
Tricyclics	Increased blood levels of antidepressant
MAOIs	Hypertension

Note. MAOIs = monoamine oxidase inhibitors.
Source. Reprinted from Stoudemire A, Moran MG, Fogel BS: "Psychotropic Drug Use in the Medically Ill, Part II." *Psychosomatics* 32:38, 1991. Copyright 1991, Academy of Psychosomatic Medicine. Used with permission.

potheses include effects on neurotransmission, circadian rhythm slowing, inhibition of endocrine systems, membrane stabilization, and ion transmission changes. None of these hypotheses has proved satisfactory to date in clearly explaining the drug's effects.

Pharmacokinetics. Lithium is a natural element administered as a salt: in tablet or capsule form as lithium carbonate (an alternative extended-release form exists), or in liquid form as lithium citrate. The single-dose elimination half-life of lithium is 5–8 hours; at maintenance dosage levels, lithium's half-life is about 1 day. Its half-life is longer in patients with reduced renal clearance (e.g., patients with renal disease and most elderly patients). Steady state is achieved in 3–8 days.

Lithium is not metabolized but is directly eliminated via excretion from the kidneys. Lithium is reabsorbed in the proximal tubule, along with water and sodium, but is not further excreted in the distal nephron. In patients who have sodium deficiency, sodium retention causes more lithium reabsorption; this can produce toxicity. Conversely, high lithium levels can cause more sodium excretion. Lithium levels are also sensitive to the body's fluid balance. Dehydration will increase lithium concentration, especially if sodium intake is not maintained. However, when dehydration is induced by increases in ambient temperature accompanied by sweating, lithium concentration can decrease because sweat can contain high concentrations of lithium (Jefferson et al. 1982). Conversely, marked polydipsia, often induced by the lithium, can reduce lithium blood levels.

Dosage and administration. The therapeutic level of lithium is very close to toxic levels. Despite this, it is possible to reach and continue a stable maintenance level without major difficulty, even in hospitalized patients who are medically ill. Closely monitoring serum concentrations, especially when initiating lithium,

improves safety. Lithium levels should always be measured 10–12 hours after the last dose. The therapeutic level for patients with acute mania is 0.8–1.5 mEq/L. For long-term maintenance or prophylaxis in most patients with bipolar illness, the optimal therapeutic level is between 0.8 and 1.0 mEq/L (Gelenberg et al. 1989). Prophylactic levels are higher for some patients. As with all drug levels, certain patients require modification of guidelines. When lithium treatment is started, levels should be obtained weekly. Once a steady state is achieved, this frequency is reduced to monthly, and then quarterly. More frequent monitoring is often needed in patients who are at increased risk for toxicity, such as elderly patients, patients who are taking another medication that is known to interact with lithium, and patients with dementia or impaired renal function.

Response. An optimal therapeutic response in patients with acute mania may take 5–14 days. Before this response occurs, patients who are highly agitated or those who have psychosis usually require adjunctive treatment with benzodiazepines or neuroleptic medications.

Side effects. The most frequent side effects of lithium are gastric irritation, mild diarrhea, polydipsia, and polyuria (DasGupta and Jefferson 1990). Fine tremor often occurs and is often treated by reducing the lithium dose or by adding a β-blocking medication. Tremor is more likely to occur in patients with underlying CNS disorders. Nausea and fatigue usually resolve after the first weeks of lithium treatment but can reemerge and be accompanied by vomiting if blood levels climb abruptly. Weight gain and edema are sometimes persistent. Lithium may also cause mild leukocytosis; this side effect has been used to advantage in patients who have conditions with problematic leukopenia, such as in those with AIDS or in patients who have received bone marrow transplants. Other reported side effects include a metallic taste and a decreased sense of creativity.

A number of organs are potentially affected by lithium. Renal effects include tubular lesions, interstitial fibrosis, decreased creatinine clearance, nephrogenic diabetes insipidus, and renal tubular acidosis. A progressive decrease in renal function is rare, and acute renal failure is not clearly demonstrated (Fenves et al. 1984; Hwang and Tuason 1980; Ramsey and Cox 1982; Rose et al. 1988). Lithium depletes intracellular potassium, which can cause cardiac effects. ST and T-wave changes, such as T-wave flattening or inversion, are common. T-wave changes are potentially useful as an indirect indicator of compliance. Cardiac arrhythmias are rare; they include sick sinus syndrome, atrioventricular block, and ventricular premature contractions, especially in predisposed patients. Thyroid effects include goiter and hypothyroidism. Hyperthyroidism is unusual, as are other endocrine effects such as hypoglycemia and hyperparathyroidism. Dermatological side effects include severe acne, psoriasis, and folliculitis, as well as hair loss. In unusual cases, patients can experience persistent nausea and vomiting, parkinsonian symptoms, exophthalmos, Raynaud's phenomenon, and pseudotumor cerebri.

Because of side effects, lithium use demands special monitoring in elderly patients and in patients with dementia. Impaired renal function, cardiac disease, extracellular volume depletion, and use of potentially interacting medications increase the risk of toxicity. Caution is also needed in patients with impaired fluid balance, decreased sodium intake, or increased sodium loss. Problems can develop quickly among medically ill patients who are hospitalized, so close monitoring is important. Pretreatment screening should include an ECG, serum creatinine level, urinalysis, and thyroid function tests, including thyroid-stimulating hormone (TSH). In elderly patients or chronically ill medical patients, serum creatinine is often artificially low because of reduced muscle mass; 24-hour creatinine clearance for evaluation of kidney function is sometimes required in older patients and patients with renal dysfunction.

Lithium's use during pregnancy is risky. It can cause cardiovascular birth defects, especially Ebstein's anomaly. This defect consists of right ventricular hypoplasia, patent ductus arteriosus, and tricuspid valve insufficiency. Data from recent studies indicate that the risk for Ebstein's anomaly is not as high as was originally thought (Gelenberg 1992). Other birth defects have also been reported. Stopping pharmacological treatment or changing to a neuroleptic is recommended for pregnant women in the first trimester (L. S. Cohen et al. 1991). Pregnancy also increases glomerular filtration and can decrease lithium levels. Lithium is generally found in breast milk at a level one-third to one-half that of the mother's serum level.

Withdrawal.   Relapse in patients with bipolar disorder is the primary concern with lithium discontinuation. Patients with precarious fluid or electrolyte balance should be monitored closely following abrupt lithium discontinuation. Infrequently, patients who have stopped lithium will experience temporary anxiety or irritability.

Drug interactions.   Most diuretics, especially thiazides, decrease lithium clearance and increase the lithium level (see Table 30–7). However, furosemide, osmotic diuretics, and carbonic anhydrase inhibitors have the opposite effect. Nonsteroidal anti-inflammatory drugs (NSAIDs) reduce lithium clearance and increase levels. Spectinomycin and tetracycline also decrease lithium excretion, whereas aminophylline and theophylline increase it. Prolongation of succinylcholine's effects is also reported. Lithium has variable effects on glucose and insulin, so patients may require adjustment of insulin doses.

Concerns have been posed about the potential for neurotoxicity with concurrent use of

Table 30–7. Reported drug interactions with lithium

Medication	Interactive effect
Thiazide diuretics	Raise Li+ levels
Spironolactone	Raises Li+ levels
Triamterene	Raises Li+ levels
Enalapril	Raises Li+ levels
NSAIDs (e.g., indomethacin, ibuprofen, phenylbutazone, piroxicam)	Raise Li+ levels
Acetazolamide	Lowers Li+ levels
Theophylline	Lowers Li+ levels
Aminophylline	Lowers Li+ levels
Calcium channel blockers	May either raise or lower Li+ levels, effects not clear; verapamil may cause bradycardia when used with Li+
Metronidazole	May increase Li+ levels; may increase chances of nephrotoxicity
Tetracycline	Minor elevation of Li+ levels

Note. Li+ = lithium; NSAIDs = nonsteroidal antiinflammatory drugs.
Source. Reprinted from Stoudemire A, Moran MG, Fogel BS: "Psychotropic Drug Use in the Medically Ill, Part II." *Psychosomatics* 32:38, 1991. Copyright 1991, Academy of Psychosomatic Medicine. Used with permission.

lithium and neuroleptics (especially haloperidol) and the use of lithium in neurologically predisposed patients (W. Cohen and Cohen 1974). The cases that prompted these concerns probably represent variants of neuroleptic malignant syndrome (NMS). A number of case reports involving haloperidol and other neuroleptics have been published. It is important to monitor patients on neuroleptics and lithium for symptoms of NMS; however, there is no evidence of frequent, consistent, or predictable problems with this combination. Lithium's use with tricyclic antidepressants may worsen symptoms of lithium toxicity, especially tremor. Preexisting extrapyramidal symptoms from medications or movement disorder are sometimes exacerbated by lithium (Addonizio et al. 1988; Sachdev 1986). Increased sedation can occur with concurrent sedative use. Lithium neurotoxicity is also more likely with concurrent carbamazepine use (Chaudhry and Waters 1983; Shukla et al. 1984).

Anticonvulsants

Types. The use of anticonvulsants (see Table 30–8) is a recent pharmacological approach to mood stabilization. The primary anticonvulsant used is carbamazepine, a tricyclic medication; however, studies involving valproic acid, a branched-chain carboxylic acid, have produced data showing clear-cut efficacy (Bowden et al. 1994; Pope et al. 1991). Anticonvulsant medications are especially useful for patients who are resistant to treatment with lithium or have rapid-cycling bipolar disorder (more than four major mood swings in a 12-month period) (McElroy et al. 1989). Some consultation-liaison psychiatrists believe that an anticonvulsant is a better treatment than lithium for patients with secondary mania, although data beyond anecdotal reports are lacking. Anticonvulsants are also preferred when mania is associated with a seizure disorder, or in patients with atypical or mixed mania (commonly seen in consultation-liaison settings).

Mechanism of action. Carbamazepine is known to decrease noradrenergic release and reuptake. Valproic acid increases brain γ-aminobutyric acid (GABA) neurotransmission by increasing its synthesis, inhibiting breakdown, and enhancing its postsynaptic effects. The relationship of these effects to clinical efficacy is unknown.

Pharmacokinetics. Carbamazepine is well absorbed, but drug levels that produce therapeutic effects vary widely among individual

Table 30–8. Anticonvulsants

Generic name	Trade name	Starting dose (mg)[a]	Usual dose range (mg)[a]
Carbamazepine	Tegretol	200 bid	600–1,600
Valproic acid	Depakene, others	250 bid	625–3,800

Note. bid = twice a day.
[a]Doses for elderly and medically ill patients are often lower.

patients. It induces its own metabolism by hepatic enzymes as well as the metabolism of other medications; therefore, a predictable decrease in carbamazepine blood levels occurs about 3–4 weeks after initiation of treatment. Valproic acid is rapidly absorbed and is highly protein-bound. It is metabolized primarily by conjugation in the liver but does not induce its own metabolism and, in fact, may inhibit it.

Dosage and administration. Although the effective range of carbamazepine blood levels for patients with psychiatric disorders has not been established, suggested drug levels for treatment are from 6 to 12 mg/mL. This is usually achieved by starting with a dosage of 200 mg bid, then increasing to 200 mg tid in 3–5 days. The maintenance dosage of carbamazepine ranges from 600 to 1,600 mg/day, provided no complications associated with hepatic disease or multiple medications occur.

Valproic acid is usually started at 250 mg bid, then increased by 250 mg every 3–4 days. Maintenance dosages range from 600 to 3,800 mg/day, with an average of 1,200 mg/day. The target blood level is 50–100 mg/mL.

Response. As with lithium, there are usually delays ranging from 7 to 10 days in the therapeutic response from carbamazepine and valproic acid in patients with acute mania.

Side effects. Transient leukopenia is typically seen with initiation of carbamazepine treatment. The major concern with carbamazepine is aplastic anemia, a very rare and sometimes fatal hematological condition. Patients should be monitored for any sign of petechiae, infection, or anemia. A complete blood count is recommended weekly for 1 month, then every 3 months thereafter, although some clinicians have argued that only baseline hematological evaluation is needed in otherwise healthy and asymptomatic patients (Pellock and Willmore 1991). Medically ill patients may require more frequent monitoring. Carbamazepine produces a skin rash in 10%–15% of patients. The medication is stopped if the rash occurs. Rapid dosage increases can cause incoordination, ataxia, drowsiness, dizziness, and slurred speech. Asterixis and hyponatremia have also been reported. Safety in pregnancy is not established; although spina bifida has been reported in babies exposed to carbamazepine in utero, this association has not yet been established with certainty (Omtzigt et al. 1993; Rosa 1991).

Valproic acid's most common side effect is sedation. Also common are nausea, vomiting, and anorexia. Enteric coating, available with some preparations, helps to prevent these side effects. Valproic acid can cause an idiosyncratic, fatal hepatotoxicity (Brown 1989). Healthy patients can tolerate increases of up to two or, less comfortably, three times the normal levels of serum glutamic-oxaloacetic transaminase (SGOT) or serum glutamic-pyruvic transaminase (SGPT), but valproic acid treatment is usually discontinued if increased elevations persist or if higher elevations occur (Pellock and Willmore 1991; Stoudemire et al. 1991). Weight gain, hair thinning, and a fine hand tremor are also seen. A daily multivitamin containing 25 mg of selenium and 50 mg of zinc may prevent hair brittleness. Thrombocytopenia is a rare event. Neural tube defects have occurred with use during the first trimester of pregnancy.

Drug interactions. Carbamazepine's induction of hepatic enzymes produces several drug interactions (see Table 30–1). These interactions can decrease the effects of anticoagulants, neuroleptics, oral contraceptives (Rapport and Calabrese 1989), and theophylline. Also, carbamazepine toxicity is increased by medications that decrease hepatic metabolism, such as calcium antagonists and cimetidine. Conversely, carbamazepine's therapeutic effect is inhibited by medications that induce metabolism (see Table 30–1).

Valproic acid levels are also lowered by enzyme-inducing drugs, including carbamazepine, and are increased by inhibitors of hepatic metabolism. Valproic acid itself does not increase hepatic metabolism and actually appears to inhibit it.

NEUROLEPTICS

Types

The phenothiazines are tricyclic compounds; subtypes include aliphatic (such as chlorpromazine), piperidine (thioridazine), and piperazine (perphenazine) compounds. The thioxanthenes have aliphatic (chlorprothixene) and piperazine (thiothixene) subtypes. Haloperidol is a butyrophenone; pimozide is a member of the related diphenylbutylpiperidines. The dibenzoxazepines include loxapine, as well as the antidepressant amoxapine. The newer medication clozapine is a dibenzodiazepine. Molindone is one of the dihydroindolones. Risperidone belongs to a new chemical class, the benzisoxazole derivatives (see Table 30–9).

All neuroleptics have similar efficacy at equivalent doses, so the choice of a medication is based on side-effect profiles. The neuro-

leptics are ranked from low- to high-potency, a spectrum that helps to predict side effects. Their antipsychotic equivalencies are generally measured relative to chlorpromazine, the first antipsychotic that was developed and used.

Mechanism of Action

Neuroleptics block the postsynaptic dopamine receptor, particularly the D_2 subtype. Blockage occurs in the mesolimbic and mesocortical dopamine pathways, as well as in the nigrostriatal pathway that is the likely site of mediation of the parkinsonian side effects of these medications. The tuberoinfundibular dopamine system is also affected, elevating prolactin levels and producing neuroendocrine side effects. Neuroleptics, especially low-potency antipsychotics, also block α-noradrenergic receptors, producing hypotensive symptoms; neuroleptics also block muscarinic acetylcholine receptors, resulting in anticholinergic effects. In addition, some neuroleptics block histaminic and serotonin receptors. Clozapine is a unique medication that blocks dopamine at limbic sites but has substantially less effect on the extrapyramidal and neuroendocrine systems; however, it also antagonizes adrenergic, cholinergic, histaminergic, and serotonergic receptors. Risperidone's antipsychotic activity is mediated through a combination of D_2 and $5\text{-}HT_2$ antagonism.

Pharmacokinetics

Neuroleptics have variable oral absorption. They are highly lipophilic and protein-bound. Half-lives range from about 10 hours to 1 day. There are depot forms (two for fluphenazine and one for haloperidol), which are typically given every 1–4 weeks. In the brain, the duration of action after long-term administration can be months or even beyond a year with the decanoate forms.

Table 30–9. Neuroleptic agents

Generic name	Trade name	Class	Dose equivalent	Usual therapeutic range (mg)[a]	Parenteral form	Sedation	Extra-pyramidal symptoms	Anticho-linergic	Orthostatic blood pressure
Chlorpromazine	Thorazine	Phenothiazines, aliphatic	100	30–1,500	Yes	4	2	3	4
Thioridazine	Mellaril	Phenothiazines, piperidine	100	50–800	No	4	1	4	4
Chlorprothixene	Taractan	Thioxanthenes, aliphatic	100	30–600	Yes	3	2	3	3
Mesoridazine	Serentil	Phenothiazines, piperidine	50	25–400	Yes	3	1	3	2
Clozapine	Clozaril	Dibenzodiazepine	50	300–900	No	3	0	4	1
Triflupromazine	Vesprin	Phenothiazines, aliphatic	25	20–200	Yes	3	2	3	2
Acetophenazine	Tindal	Phenothiazines, piperazine	20	80–120	No	2	3	2	2
Prochlorperazine	Compazine	Phenothiazines, piperazine	15	50–150	Yes	3	2	2	3
Loxapine	Loxitane	Dibenzoxazepine	15	25–100	Yes	3	3	2	2
Perphenazine	Trilafon	Phenothiazines, piperazine	10	4–64	Yes	3	3	2	3
Molindone	Moban	Dihydroindolone	10	25–100	No	1	3	2	2
Trifluoperazine	Stelazine	Phenothiazines, piperazine	5	2–40	Yes	1	3	2	2
Thiothixene	Navane	Thioxanthenes, piperazine	4	6–60	Yes	2	4	2	2
Haloperidol	Haldol	Butyrophenone	2	5–40	Yes	1	4	1	1
Fluphenazine	Prolixin	Phenothiazines, piperazine	2	1–40	Yes	2	4	2	2
Risperidone	Risperdal	Benzisoxazole derivative	2	4–16	No	2	1	2	3
Pimozide	Orap	Diphenylbutyl-piperidine	1	1–10	No	3	4	2	3

Note. 0 = least effect; 4 = most effect.
[a]Doses for elderly and medically ill patients may be lower.

Dosage and Administration

Doses equivalent to 300–600 mg of chlorpromazine are generally adequate for an acute antipsychotic effect. Doses greater than 20 mg of haloperidol are thought to produce little additional benefit (and possibly less effect). Much higher doses are often used in treating patients with delirium. Patients who have neuropsychiatric syndromes associated with dementia generally show symptom relief with much lower doses, as low as 0.25–2.0 mg of haloperidol. Unlike the psychotic symptoms that are associated with schizophrenia, those that are associated with dementia and delirium often respond within hours to relatively low doses of neuroleptics.

One model used in treatment of patients with psychosis is *rapid neuroleptization*. This regimen consists of administering doses of a neuroleptic medication—for example, 5–10 mg of haloperidol—intramuscularly every 30–60 minutes until psychosis clears. Outcome studies of patients who were given rapid treatment show that they fared no better than patients who were treated with more conservative doses. Moreover, patients who are given rapid treatment are exposed to greater risk of extrapyramidal symptoms and, possibly, NMS. *Rapid tranquilization* is a related technique aimed at calming a patient with acute psychotic agitation rather than alleviating psychosis. Rapid tranquilization may be useful for some hospitalized patients, especially in ICUs. Rapid tranquilization with a neuroleptic is usually accomplished with haloperidol, 5–10 mg given orally, intramuscularly, or intravenously every 20–30 minutes until the patient is calm. Intravenous haloperidol is typically used in ICU settings at doses of 0.5–2 mg for patients with mild agitation, 5–10 mg for those with moderate agitation, and 10 mg or more for patients who are severely agitated (Tesar and Stern 1986). Much higher doses are used in some cases, but recent evidence links the risk of torsades de pointes ventricular tachycardia with very-high-dose

therapy (Metzger and Friedman 1993). Droperidol is also used for delirium-associated agitation (Frye et al. 1995). The benzodiazepine lorazepam (which, in contrast to diazepam and chlordiazepoxide, is effectively absorbed intramuscularly) is also used for rapid tranquilization, alone or in conjunction with neuroleptics, especially haloperidol.

Side Effects

Low- and high-potency neuroleptic medications have significantly different side-effect profiles. Low-potency medications, such as thioridazine, are more sedating and have more orthostatic effects. High-potency medications, such as haloperidol and piperazine phenothiazines, produce more extrapyramidal symptoms.

Extrapyramidal effects include dystonic reactions, parkinsonian symptoms, akathisia, and tardive phenomena. Dystonia usually appears within 1–5 days of the start of treatment. Dystonic symptoms include opisthotonos, torticollis, and oculogyric crises. Laryngeal and diaphragmatic dystonias occur, but these are rare. Young men, very ill patients, and patients with neurological disorders are particularly vulnerable. Acute treatment for dystonia requires benztropine, 1 or 2 mg given intramuscularly or intravenously, or diphenhydramine, 25–50 mg.

Parkinsonian signs are masked facies, cogwheel rigidity, tremor, and parkinsonian gait. Akinesia and bradykinesia are also seen. These extrapyramidal signs can appear from a few days to several weeks after initiating or increasing the dose of an antipsychotic. Anticholinergic medications are usually effective in counteracting these effects; these agents include benztropine, biperiden, procyclidine, and trihexyphenidyl. The antihistaminic medication diphenhydramine and the dopamine agonist amantadine are also used. A typical dosage of benztropine in general psychiatric settings is 0.5–2 mg tid, but lower doses (one-third to one-half) are typically used in patients in consultation-liaison settings in which the clinician is dealing with patients of advanced age or those who may be already using other medications with anticholinergic effects. Amantadine is excreted by the kidneys and can reach toxic levels in patients with impaired renal function. Arrhythmias and hypotension can occur in patients who experience amantadine overdose; 2 or 3 g of this drug can sometimes be fatal, an amount that a patient can obtain by filling a prescription for a 30-day supply of 100-mg capsules to be taken twice a day.

Akathisia is an internal sense of restlessness that is usually accompanied by outward restlessness, especially movements in the legs. Because akathisia can resemble psychotic agitation, the clinician's response to restlessness is sometimes to increase the dose of antipsychotic, further worsening the problem. Akathisia can also increase the risk of suicide in a suicide-prone patient. Akathisia does not abate with tolerance to neuroleptic medication, but lowering the dosage or changing to a neuroleptic with lower potency often reduces this side effect. Propranolol, 20–60 mg/day, can be helpful in reducing this symptom, as can benzodiazepines.

Sedation resulting from an antihistaminic effect can occur with all neuroleptics but is most prominent with the low-potency medications, such as chlorpromazine. Tolerance often develops to sedative effects. Anticholinergic effects occur most prominently with the lower-potency aliphatic and piperidine phenothiazines.

Orthostatic hypotension most frequently occurs with low-potency aliphatic and piperidine phenothiazines. Cardiac effects are rare but can include prolonged ventricular repolarization and quinidine-like effects, especially with the low-potency medications, particularly thioridazine. Torsades de pointes and other ventricular arrhythmias have occurred with thioridazine and high-dose intravenous haloperidol (Hunt and Stern 1995). ECG changes, including ST segment depression and prolonged T waves, are seen, especially with aliphatic and piperazine phenothiazines.

All neuroleptics, with the exception of clozapine, increase prolactin release and occasionally induce galactorrhea and menstrual changes. Impotence, decreased libido, and inhibition of ejaculation and orgasm can occur. The syndrome of inappropriate antidiuretic hormone (ADH) secretion has been reported in patients taking neuroleptics, but this syndrome also occurs among patients with psychosis in the absence of neuroleptic use. Low-potency phenothiazines can produce disturbed temperature regulation.

Any neuroleptic can lower the seizure threshold. Especially at higher doses, low-potency medications such as chlorpromazine have more tendency to do so. Neurotoxicity in patients with hyperthyroidism occurs on occasion with butyrophenone use. The phenothiazines can cause gastritis, nausea, and vomiting. Neuroleptics, especially chlorpromazine, can produce cholestatic jaundice. Low-potency medications have more tendency to cause cholestatic jaundice as well as hepatitis. Weight gain can occur with neuroleptic use, more often with phenothiazines than butyrophenones. Excessive salivation is more often seen with the high-potency medications. Clozapine, although it is a low-potency neuroleptic, is particularly problematic in this regard.

Skin abnormalities, which include rashes and photosensitivity, occur most often with low-potency medications. Skin pigmentation and blue-gray discoloration of the skin are rare reactions to low-potency phenothiazines. A lupuslike syndrome is a rare side effect of aliphatic phenothiazines. Anticholinergic effects include visual blurring and impaired memory. Aliphatic and piperazine phenothiazines can, in rare instances, produce lenticular deposits and opacities. The upper limit for thioridazine dosages, 800 mg/day, is based on the high incidence of pigmentary retinopathy at dosages above this level. All neuroleptics, but especially butyrophenones, occasionally cause blood dyscrasias. Agranulocytosis is rare, except with clozapine. It has not yet been established which neuroleptics are safest in patients with bone marrow suppression; clozapine is contraindicated in patients with myeloproliferative disorders.

Clozapine's more common side effects are sedation, excessive salivation, anticholinergic effects, and postural hypotension. Extrapyramidal symptoms are rare and can actually improve with this drug. Constipation, ECG changes, hypertension, increase in body temperature, priapism, pancreatitis, eosinophilia, and dose-dependent decreases in seizure threshold also occur. The most serious side effect is potentially fatal granulocytopenia or agranulocytosis, which is estimated to occur in about 1% of patients. Weekly blood counts are currently required to monitor for decreases in white blood cell count, although newer, less restrictive guidelines are expected soon.

Although neuroleptic use during pregnancy is weakly linked to fetal limb abnormalities, several large-scale studies have failed to show an increased risk of congenital malformations associated with exposure (L. S. Cohen et al. 1991). Effects related to prenatal exposure reported in neonates and infants are extrapyramidal symptoms, sedation, hyperbilirubinemia, neonatal jaundice, and induction of hepatic enzymes (Hauser 1985; Miller 1991; Robinson et al. 1986).

Tardive Phenomena

Tardive phenomena include tardive dystonia, tardive akathisia, and especially tardive dyskinesia. Tardive dyskinesia can occur with any neuroleptic. These involuntary buccolingual and choreoathetotic movements disappear during sleep. The Abnormal Involuntary Movement Scale (AIMS; Guy 1976; Lane et al. 1985) is used to rate these movements. Estimates of the prevalence of tardive dyskinesia vary widely, but the average estimate is 20%–30% of patients exposed to neuroleptics.

Tardive dyskinesia usually does not develop unless a patient is exposed to neuroleptics for at least 3 months (Glazer et al. 1993), but cases of tardive dyskinesia have been reported after shorter periods of exposure, particularly in elderly patients (Harris and Kingston 1992; Yassa et al. 1992). It has also been estimated that 5% of geriatric patients who have never been treated with neuroleptic medications have signs of tardive dyskinesia (Yassa et al. 1992). Increasing age, exposure to antipsychotics for 3 months or more, cumulative dose, concurrent presence of a mood disorder, and diabetes mellitus increase the risk of tardive dyskinesia.

Not surprisingly, tardive dyskinesia is a disorder that probably involves the dopamine system. A major etiological model for tardive dyskinesia postulates that it is an acquired dopamine supersensitivity. However, the lack of uniform response to pharmacological manipulation of the dopamine system suggests that this theory does not completely explain the phenomenon. Cholinergic, noradrenergic, and GABA involvement have all been suggested. Stopping the neuroleptic is the primary intervention. Symptoms are usually initially worse at the time of withdrawal and gradually improve in 3–6 months. If the symptoms do not remit in this time, the condition often is permanent. Treatment at that point has a very limited chance of success. Medications used to treat tardive dyskinesia include baclofen, benzodiazepines, reserpine, tetrabenazine, calcium channel blockers, and vitamin E (Szymanski et al. 1993).

Neuroleptic Malignant Syndrome

NMS is a rare but very serious and potentially fatal complication of treatment with neuroleptics. NMS has been reported in other situations, such as rapid discontinuation of carbidopa/levodopa (Wise and Rundell 1994) and combination treatment with amitriptyline/lithium (Fava and Galizia 1995). Awareness of this syndrome is especially important for the consulting psychiatrist who is treating patients on the medical service; in this patient population, the differential diagnosis includes many other medical and psychiatric disorders. The differential diagnosis of NMS is extensive: catatonia, lethal catatonia, heat stroke, malignant hyperthermia, serotonin syndrome, anticholinergic toxicity, meningitis, viral encephalitis, Parkinson's disease, Wilson's disease, collagen vascular diseases, cerebrovascular disease, head trauma, epilepsy, myotonia, akinetic mutism, general paresis, diabetic ketoacidosis, hepatic encephalopathy, acute intermittent porphyria, pellagra, hypocalcemia, tetanus, botulism, and the effects of strychnine, curare, phencyclidine, and sedative withdrawal.

The primary signs of NMS are hyperthermia, tremor, increased muscle tone (usually lead pipe rigidity), other extrapyramidal symptoms, altered consciousness (from confusion to coma), and autonomic instability. Autonomic instability usually manifests as changes in blood pressure and heart rate, dysrhythmias, diaphoresis, pallor, and sialorrhea. Patients may also have oculogyric crises, opisthotonos, trismus, Babinski sign, and seizures. Laboratory findings include dehydration; white blood cell count of 15,000–30,000, with or without a left shift; elevated levels of SGOT, SGPT, lactic dehydrogenase (LDH), and alkaline phosphatase; elevated creatine phosphokinase (CPK), possibly exceeding 16,000; and myoglobinuria. The increased CPK is believed to occur in 40%–50% of patients (Janicak et al. 1987). Electroencephalogram (EEG) and lumbar puncture findings are nonspecific.

NMS generally develops over a 1- to 3-day period and lasts for 5–10 days after a nondepot neuroleptic is stopped. Mortality is high, most often quoted as 20%–30% (Gelenberg et al. 1988). Mortality is higher if rhabdomyolysis develops. It is estimated that about 0.1% of patients exposed to neuroleptics develop NMS (Gelenberg et al. 1988). It can occur at any age, but most often occurs in patients younger than 40 years and may occur more frequently in

men. Patients who receive neuroleptics for any disorder or condition can develop NMS. In consultation-liaison settings, the possible contribution of metoclopramide and prochlorperazine should not be overlooked. Case reports suggest that a similar disorder can develop in patients who have received medications other than neuroleptics—essentially, a "neuroleptic malignant disorder" without the neuroleptic (Gelenberg et al. 1988). NMS has occurred in patients who have discontinued using anticholinergic medications and dopamine agonists such as amantadine and L-dopa. "NMS-like" reactions have also been reported with tricyclics, MAOIs, and the combination of lithium and haloperidol.

The main intervention is to stop the neuroleptic. All other treatment follows that basic action. Once patients become severely ill or comatose, they require attendant supportive care, such as respiratory support and cooling the body core. Medication interventions include dopaminergic medications to decrease effects of dopamine receptor blockade, β-adrenergic blockers to decrease heart rate, and calcium channel blockers or muscle relaxants to decrease rigidity.

Bromocriptine is a dopamine agonist that is used in dosages of 2.5–10 mg tid orally. Amantadine, another dopamine agonist, is used in dosages of 100 mg orally bid to qid. Dantrolene acts as a direct muscle relaxant; daily dosages are 8–10 mg/kg body weight intravenously or 50–200 mg orally. The use of dantrolene is limited by hepatic toxicity. Other interventions used include antiparkinsonian medications, L-dopa, lorazepam, propranolol, curare, and electroconvulsive therapy (ECT). Rechallenge of patients who still require neuroleptic treatment after NMS is a controversial topic. It is estimated that the recurrence rate is 30% with rechallenge (Rosebush et al. 1989). At least 2 weeks should elapse before neuroleptic treatment is restarted; then a different, low-potency medication should be used. The dosage should be increased slowly, and the patient should be carefully monitored for changes in body temperature or mental status, the occurrence of muscle rigidity or cog-wheeling, and increases in CPK levels.

Withdrawal

Sudden discontinuation of high doses of neuroleptics can cause a short-lived flulike syndrome and withdrawal-related dyskinesias. Of course, relapse is the most worrisome consequence of stopping neuroleptics. The time delay before the return of psychotic symptoms is quite variable. Premature discontinuation of haloperidol in patients who are being treated for delirium can lead to rapid relapse. (For further details on the management of delirium, please refer to Wise and Trzepacz, Chapter 7, in this volume.)

Drug Interactions

Additive anticholinergic effects are especially problematic with neuroleptics. Alcohol causes additive sedative effects. The use of low-potency neuroleptics with tricyclic antidepressants or type IA antiarrhythmic medications (e.g., quinidine) can delay cardiac conduction and precipitate arrhythmias. When used concomitantly with neuroleptics, NSAIDs can cause extreme drowsiness, especially the combination of haloperidol and indomethacin. β-Blockers worsen the orthostatic side effects of neuroleptic drugs. Anesthetics can produce severe hypotension in patients taking phenothiazines. Chlorpromazine, thioridazine, and mesoridazine are potent α-adrenergic blockers and can induce hypotension in combination with vasodilators. Haloperidol has virtually no α-adrenergic-blocking properties. A decreased antihypertensive effect can occur, however, with guanethidine and related drugs. Because of its mixed α and β effects, epinephrine can lower the blood pressure of persons taking phenothiazines, so Neo-Synephrine or levarterenol is used to treat marked hypotension in these patients.

As hepatically degraded drugs, the neuroleptics are susceptible to decreased effects resulting from concomitant use of medications such as anticonvulsants, which increase metabolism. Antacids can delay absorption. Because of the ability of neuroleptics to block dopamine receptors, antiparkinsonian medications are antagonized. Neurotoxic interactions with lithium have been reported. The initial report of severe reactions with haloperidol and lithium (Turpin and Schuller 1978) has been debated, but case reports continue, including interactions with thioridazine (Spring 1979) and clozapine (Blake et al. 1992; McElroy et al. 1991).

ANTIANXIETY AND SEDATIVE MEDICATIONS

Benzodiazepines

Types. Benzodiazepines (Table 30–10) are divided into several groups. The 2-ketobenzodiazepines include diazepam and chlordiazepoxide. Oxazepam, lorazepam, and temazepam are the 3-hydroxybenzodiazepines. Alprazolam and triazolam are triazolobenzodiazepines. Clonazepam is a 7-nitrobenzodiazepine. Midazolam is an imidazobenzodiazepine derivative.

Mechanism of action. Benzodiazepines induce binding of GABA, an inhibiting neurotransmitter.

Pharmacokinetics. The benzodiazepines are rapidly absorbed in the GI tract. Intramuscular absorption is quite variable, except for lorazepam and midazolam. The absorption of diazepam and chlordiazepoxide administered intramuscularly is particularly erratic. There are significant differences in the half-lives and kinetics among the benzodiazepines. In general, benzodiazepines are lipophilic and have rapid onset of action. Most are degraded by hepatic oxidation, and some have several active metab-

Table 30–10.   Benzodiazepines

Generic name	Trade name	Onset	Duration of action	Usual therapeutic dose range (mg)[a]	Approximately equivalent antianxiety dose (mg)	Approximately equivalent hypnotic dose (mg)
Flurazepam	Dalmane	Rapid–intermediate	Long	15–30	—	30
Clorazepate	Tranxene	Rapid	Long	15–60	7.5	15
Diazepam	Valium	Rapid	Long	5–40	5	10
Prazepam	Centrax	Slow	Long	20–60	10	20
Chlordiazepoxide	Librium	Intermediate	Long	15–150	10	25
Lorazepam	Ativan	Intermediate	Intermediate	1–6	1	2
Oxazepam	Serax	Intermediate–slow	Intermediate	30–120	15	30
Temazepam	Restoril	Intermediate–slow	Short	15–30	15	30
Midazolam	Versed	Rapid	Very short	0.1 mg/kg body weight	2	2
Clonazepam	Klonopin	Intermediate	Short	1–3	1	1
Alprazolam	Xanax	Intermediate	Short	2–8	0.5	1
Estazolam	ProSom	Rapid	Intermediate	1–2	—	1
Triazolam	Halcion	Intermediate	Short	0.125–0.5	—	0.5
Quazepam	Doral	Rapid	Long	7.5–15	—	15

[a]Doses for elderly and medically ill patients are often lower.

olites. Benzodiazepine metabolism slows with age, medication interactions, and hepatic insults, such as cirrhosis. Lorazepam, oxazepam, and temazepam are degraded primarily by glucuronide conjugation and are without active metabolites; for these reasons, these three benzodiazepines have a distinct advantage in patients who are older or who are seriously ill.

Dosage and administration. Benzodiazepines are given in as-needed or regularly scheduled doses. A daily maximum of 40 mg of diazepam or its equivalent is usually sufficient, although higher doses are occasionally needed in patients who are undergoing detoxification. The dosage of alprazolam for the treatment of patients with panic disorder in some patients is 2–8 mg/day; most patients require 4–8 mg (see Table 30–10).

Response. The onset of the effects of benzodiazepines is usually rapid. Maximum benefit is usually reached by 6 weeks (Rickels and Schweizer 1987).

Side effects. Sedation and drowsiness are the most common acute adverse effects of the benzodiazepines. These effects are often more pronounced in elderly patients and in patients who are medically ill. Other cognitive effects include transient anterograde amnesia. Some patients who are treated for anxiety or insomnia experience an inability to recall events for a few hours after taking a benzodiazepine, but these drugs are used regularly, with good effects, in patients who are undergoing surgical procedures and in those being treated in ICUs. There are occasional problems with confusion, impaired attention, impaired psychomotor skills, and dizziness. Ataxia also occurs frequently. Some patients have behavioral disinhibition (Kales et al. 1987), which can lead to aggressive behavior. Paradoxical excitement, paradoxical rage reactions, and paradoxical anxiety are occasionally reported (Lion et al. 1975). Depression can also occur. Although

the benzodiazepines provide a hypnotic effect, they also decrease sleep latency and the amount of delta sleep. Benzodiazepines are contraindicated in patients with sleep apnea because the decrease in central respiratory response to elevated CO_2 levels caused by benzodiazepines is potentially fatal (Dolly and Block 1982).

Dependence develops with chronic benzodiazepine use. This includes both psychological and physical dependence (e.g., tolerance and withdrawal symptoms). Because benzodiazepines are used for "recreational" purposes, the clinician must weigh the risks of dependence against the substantial benefits accrued from treatment of a patient with a primary or secondary anxiety disorder.

Benzodiazepines have a respiratory depressant effect that is dangerous in patients with compromised respiration. In hospitals, flumazenil is available as an antidote in cases of intentional, accidental, or iatrogenic toxicity. Benzodiazepines suppress the respiratory response to hypoxia, so they are contraindicated in patients who retain CO_2.

Withdrawal. Benzodiazepines cause a clinically important withdrawal syndrome. The likelihood of symptoms increases with dosage, duration of treatment, and speed of discontinuance. Benzodiazepine withdrawal symptoms include dizziness, sweating, shakiness, headache, blurred vision, and tinnitus. Also possible are hypotension, nausea and vomiting, twitching, muscle cramps, paresthesias, and irritability. Hallucinations can and do occur. The most serious withdrawal effect is seizure. In addition to return of pretreatment anxiety, some patients develop rebound withdrawal anxiety or insomnia. The withdrawal syndrome is worse with benzodiazepines that have short half-lives; the gradual clearance of benzodiazepines that have a long half-life results in a gradual tapering, although withdrawal symptoms from drugs such as diazepam do occur. Clinicians report that withdrawal is especially difficult with alprazolam (Albeck 1987; Risse et al. 1990). The occurrence of seizures has been documented in patients who have withdrawn from alprazolam, even though they received other benzodiazepines that are normally considered adequate for cross-coverage (Browne and Hauge 1986; Warner et al. 1990). Although this is not clearly documented, it suggests that clinicians must use at least an equivalent dose of other benzodiazepines during withdrawal (see Table 30–10 and Chapter 13 in this volume).

Drug interactions. There is an additive effect when alcohol is combined with other CNS depressants (see Table 30–11). Prolonged neuromuscular blockade with succinylcholine can occur with concomitant benzodiazepine use. Benzodiazepines can induce digoxin toxicity by reducing its excretion (Castillo-Fernando et al. 1980; Guven et al. 1993; Tollefson et al. 1984). As with other drugs that are metabolized by oxidation, the long-acting benzodiazepines are vulnerable to medications that inhibit hepatic enzymes (e.g., cimetidine).

Table 30–11.   Reported drug interactions with benzodiazepines

Medication	Interactive effect
Cimetidine Disulfiram Ethanol Isoniazid	May elevate serum levels of benzodiazepines metabolized predominantly by oxidation
Estrogens Cigarettes Methylxanthine derivatives Rifampin	Tend to lower benzodiazepine levels

Source.   Reprinted from Stoudemire A, Moran MG, Fogel BS: "Psychotropic Drug Use in the Medically Ill, Part II." *Psychosomatics* 32:38, 1991. Copyright 1991, Academy of Psychosomatic Medicine. Used with permission.

Buspirone

Mechanism of action.   Buspirone is an azaspirodecanedione. Buspirone has moderate affinity for dopamine D_2 receptors and appears to have mixed agonist/antagonist activity for serotonin 5-HT_{1A} receptors but no significant antipsychotic effect. It does not affect benzodiazepine or GABA receptors to any significant degree (Sussman 1994).

Pharmacokinetics.   Buspirone is a lipophilic drug that is well absorbed, but much of the drug is lost to the first-pass effect. It is metabolized by hepatic oxidation and has a half-life of 211 hours.

Indications.   Buspirone has a number of clinical advantages, especially in consultation-liaison settings. It does not cause the sedation or functional impairment that occurs with the benzodiazepines. It does not change the seizure threshold, so withdrawal convulsions are not a problem. Buspirone has no known abuse potential. It is associated with fewer drug interactions than are the benzodiazepines. In particular, it does not interact with alcohol. Because of these features, buspirone is recommended for treatment of patients with chronic anxiety, particularly those who are older, those who are sicker, and those in whom substance abuse or dependence is a potential complication. Because it stimulates respiration in animals and is not known to suppress respiration in humans, buspirone is particularly useful in patients with anxiety whose respiratory status is compromised. In acute medical treatment settings, buspirone has a disadvantage: it can take 1–2 weeks or more for its anxiolytic properties to take effect. In addition, buspirone is sometimes less effective—or may be seemingly ineffective—in patients who were previously treated with a benzodiazepine.

Dosage and administration.   An initial buspirone dosage is 5 mg tid, which can be increased by 5 mg/day every 3 or 4 days. Symptoms usually resolve at a dosage of 15–45 mg daily, given in divided doses.

Response. There is usually a delay of 1–2 weeks, or sometimes longer, before an anxiolytic effect is seen.

Side effects. Buspirone's most frequent side effects are dizziness and headache. Less frequent are nausea, diarrhea, nervousness, and paresthesias.

Withdrawal. Following rapid or abrupt discontinuation of buspirone, some patients experience drowsiness, insomnia, nervousness, dizziness, headache, or GI upset.

Drug interactions. Buspirone can produce a hyperpyrexic interaction when combined with MAOIs. It also can displace less firmly protein-bound drugs such as digoxin.

■ MANAGING SIDE EFFECTS

In general, when the psychiatric disorder permits, the dosage of a problematic medication should be reduced. When dose reduction is impossible, side effects are often controlled by adding counteracting medications.

Anticholinergic effects are usually very uncomfortable for patients. Dry mouth is helped by periodically drinking water or by the use of unsweetened hard candy or artificial saliva. Blurred vision is sometimes treated with pilocarpine drops. Bethanechol is used to relieve urinary retention. Adequate dietary balance, laxatives, and stool softeners can relieve constipation.

Patients with orthostatic hypotension should be instructed to arise slowly from their beds. Support hose is also occasionally helpful. Medications that are reportedly effective for managing orthostasis are salt tablets, 600–1,800 mg bid; triiodothyronine, 25 mg/day; thyrox-

ine, 0.1–0.2 mg/day; methylphenidate, 10–15 mg/day; dextroamphetamine, 5–20 mg/day; or 9α-fluorohydrocortisone (fludrocortisone acetate), 25–50 mg 1–2 times daily.

Sexual side effects of psychoactive drugs include decreased libido, impaired erection, and inhibited orgasm or ejaculation (Gitlin 1995; Segraves 1989, 1992). All patients who are seen in outpatient consultation-liaison clinics should be asked about sexual function. There is no clear treatment for decreased libido, although there is a report that neostigmine might help. Impaired erection is sometimes helped by switching to less anticholinergic/antiadrenergic drugs or adding yohimbine, 5.4 mg, or bethanechol, 30 mg, 1–2 hours before sexual activity. Neostigmine, 7.5–15 mg taken 30 minutes before sexual activity, can help patients with impaired ejaculation. Serotonergic mechanisms are involved in anorgasmia. Treatments for anorgasmia include bethanechol, 10–20 mg 1–2 hours before sexual activity; yohimbine, 5.4 mg tid or 10 mg 1 hour before sexual activity; or cyproheptadine, 4–12 mg 1–2 hours before sexual activity.

For obvious reasons, controlled studies that examine the effects of psychotropic medications in pregnancy are lacking. If at all possible, drugs should be avoided and alternative means of controlling symptoms should be used. The potential teratogenic and other effects are described in the sections on individual drugs in this chapter.

■ SUMMARY

Many psychotropic medications are available for use in medically ill patients who have psychiatric symptoms. With careful diagnosis, target symptom identification, and the use of other treatment modalities, these medications can relieve the psychic suffering of patients and improve the chances that their physical illnesses will heal. Further research is needed to help define the causes of secondary psychiatric disorders. Further knowledge about mechanisms of action of psychotropic medications, especially in patients who are medically ill, will facilitate the development of new drugs that are more effective and safer. Meanwhile, education about the current psychiatric pharmacopoeia and the psychoactive effects of nonpsychiatric medications will help the consultation-liaison psychiatrist to improve treatment. Consultation-liaison psychiatrists must also educate patients so that, in partnership with them, the principles outlined in this chapter can be used to tailor treatment to individual patient needs.

REFERENCES

Addonizio G, Roth SD, Stokes PE, et al: Increased extrapyramidal symptoms with addition of lithium to neuroleptics. J Nerv Ment Dis 176:682–685, 1988

Albeck JH: Withdrawal and detoxification from benzodiazepine dependence: a potential role for clonazepam. J Clin Psychiatry 48(suppl): 43–49, 1987

Altman DF: Changes in gastrointestinal, pancreatic, biliary, and hepatic function with aging. Gastroenterol Clin North Am 19:227–234, 1990

Amrein R, Hetzel W, Stabl M, et al: RIMA: a safe concept in the treatment of depression with moclobemide. Can J Psychiatry 37 (suppl 1): 7–11, 1992

Ayd FJ (ed): Paroxetine, a new selective serotonin reuptake inhibitor. International Drug Therapy Newsletter 28:5–12, 1993

Barr LC, Goodman WK, Price LH: Physical symptoms associated with paroxetine discontinuation (letter). Am J Psychiatry 151:289, 1994

Blake LM, Marks RC, Luchins DJ: Reversible neurologic symptoms with clozapine and lithium. Clin Psychopharmacol 12:297–299, 1992

Bowden CL, Brugger AM, Swann AC, et al: Efficacy of divalproex vs lithium and placebo in the treatment of mania: the Depakote Mania Study Group. JAMA 271:918–924, 1994

Brown R: U.S. experience with valproate in manic depressive illness: a multicenter trial. J Clin Psychiatry 50:13–16, 1989

Browne JL, Hauge KJ: A review of alprazolam withdrawal. Drug Intelligence and Clinical Pharmacy 20:837–841, 1986

Castillo-Fernando JR, Garcia M, Carmona J, et al: Digoxin levels and diazepam (letter). Lancet 2:368, 1980

Chaudhry RP, Waters BG: Lithium and carbamazepine interaction: possible neurotoxicity. J Clin Psychiatry 44:30–31, 1983

Cohen LS, Rosenbaum JF, Heller VL: Psychotropic drug use in pregnancy, in The Practitioner's Guide to Psychoactive Drugs, 3rd Edition. Edited by Gelenberg AJ, Bassuk EL, Schoonover SC. New York, Plenum, 1991, pp 389–405

Cohen W, Cohen N: Lithium carbonate, haloperidol and irreversible brain damage. JAMA 230: 1283–1287, 1974

Coplan JD, Gorman JM: Detectable levels of fluoxetine metabolites after discontinuation: an unexpected serotonin syndrome (letter). Am J Psychiatry 150:837, 1993

Crewe HK, Lennard MS, Tucker GT, et al: The effect of selective serotonin re-uptake inhibitors on cytochrome P4502D6 (CYP2D6) activity in human liver microsomes. Br J Clin Pharmacol 34:262–265, 1992

DasGupta K, Jefferson JW: The use of lithium in the medically ill. Gen Hosp Psychiatry 12:83–97, 1990

DeVane CL: Pharmacogenetics and drug metabolism of newer antidepressant agents. J Clin Psychiatry 55 (suppl 12):38–45, 1994

Dilsaver SC, Greden JF: Antidepressant withdrawal phenomena. Biol Psychiatry 19:237–256, 1984

Dolly FR, Block AJ: Effect of flurazepam on sleep-disordered breathing and nocturnal oxygen desaturation in asymptomatic subjects. Am J Med 73:239–243, 1982

Elitsur Y: Pemoline (Cylert)-induced hepatotoxicity. J Pediatr Gastroenterol Nutr 11:143–144, 1990

Fava S, Galizia AC: Neuroleptic malignant syndrome and lithium carbonate. J Psychiatry Neurosci 20:305–306, 1995

Fenves AZ, Emmett M, White MG: Lithium intoxication associated with acute renal failure. South Med J 77:1472–1474, 1984

Fernandez F, Levy JK: Psychiatric diagnosis and pharmacotherapy of patients with HIV infection, in American Psychiatric Press Review of Psychiatry, Vol 9. Edited by Tasman A, Goldfinger SM, Kaufmann CA. Washington, DC, American Psychiatric Press, 1990, pp 614–630

Fogelson DL, Bystritsky A, Pasnau R: Bupropion in the treatment of bipolar disorders: the same old story? J Clin Psychiatry 53:443–446, 1992

Frierson RL, Wey JJ, Tabler JB: Psychostimulants for depression in the medically ill. Am Fam Physician 43:163–170, 1991

Frye MA, Coudreaut MF, Hakeman SM, et al: Continuous droperidol infusion for management of agitated delirium in an intensive care unit. Psychosomatics 36:301–305, 1995

Gelenberg AJ: Lithium teratogenesis revisited. Biological Therapies in Psychiatry 15:25–26, 1992

Gelenberg AJ: Fluoxetine and bradycardia. Biological Therapies in Psychiatry 18:41, 1995

Gelenberg AJ, Bellinghausen B, Wojcik JD, et al: A prospective survey of neuroleptic malignant syndrome in a short-term psychiatric hospital. Am J Psychiatry 145:517–518, 1988

Gelenberg AJ, Kane JM, Keller MB, et al: Comparison of standard and low serum levels of lithium for maintenance treatment of bipolar disorder. N Engl J Med 321:1489–1493, 1989

Gitlin MJ: Effects of depression and antidepressants on sexual functioning. Bull Menninger Clin 59:232–248, 1995

Glassman AH, Roose SP, Bigger JT: The safety of tricyclic antidepressants in cardiac patients. JAMA 269:2673–2675, 1993

Glazer WM, Morgenstern H, Doucette JT: Predicting the long-term risk of tardive dyskinesia in outpatients maintained on neuroleptic medications. J Clin Psychiatry 54:133–139, 1993

Guven H, Tuncok Y, Guneri S, et al: Age-related digoxin-alprazolam interaction. Clin Pharmacol Ther 54:42–44, 1993

Guy W: ECDEU Assessment Manual for Psychopharmacology, Revised 1976. Washington, DC, United States Department of Health, Education and Welfare, 1976

Gwirtsman HE, Guze BH: Amphetamine, but not methylphenidate, predicts antidepressant response. J Clin Psychopharmacol 9:453–454, 1989

Harris CR, Kingston R: Gastrointestinal decontamination: which method is best? Postgrad Med 92:116–122, 125, 128, 1992

Hauser LA: Pregnancy and psychiatric drugs. Hosp Community Psychiatry 36:817–818, 1985

Hunt N, Stern TA: The association between intravenous haloperidol and torsades de pointes. Psychosomatics 36:541–549, 1995

Hussein S, Kaufman BM: Bradycardia associated with fluoxetine in an elderly patient with sick sinus syndrome (letter). Postgrad Med J 70: 819, 1994

Hwang S, Tuason VB: Long-term maintenance lithium therapy: possible irreversible renal damage. J Clin Psychiatry 41:11–19, 1980

Janicak PG, Bresnahan DB, Comaty JE: The neuroleptic malignant syndrome: a clinical update. Psychiatric Annals 17:551–555, 1987

Jefferson JW: Cardiovascular effects and toxicity of anxiolytics and antidepressants. J Clin Psychiatry 50:368–378, 1989

Jefferson JW, Greist JH, Clagnaz PJ, et al: Effect of strenuous exercise on serum lithium level in man. Am J Psychiatry 139:1593–1595, 1982

Joyce PR, Paykel ES: Predictors of drug response in depression. Arch Gen Psychiatry 46:89–99, 1989

Kales A, Bixler EO, Vela-Bueno A, et al: Alprazolam: effects on sleep and withdrawal phenomena. J Clin Pharmacol 27:508–515, 1987

Keuthen NJ, Cyr P, Ricciarot JA, et al: Medication withdrawal symptoms in obsessive-compulsive disorder patients treated with paroxetine (letter). J Clin Psychopharmacol 14:206–207, 1994

Kiev A: A double-blind, placebo-controlled study of paroxetine in depressed outpatients. J Clin Psychiatry 52(suppl):27–29, 1992

Kraus MF: Neuropsychiatric sequelae of stroke and traumatic brain injury: the role of psychostimulants. Int J Psychiatry Med 25:39–51, 1995

Lader M: Combined use of tricyclic antidepressants and monoamine oxidase inhibitors. J Clin Psychiatry 44 (part 2):20–24, 1983

Lane R, Glazer W, Hansen T, et al: Assessment of tardive dyskinesia using the abnormal involuntary movement scale. J Nerv Ment Dis 173:353–357, 1985

Leo RJ, David GL, Hershey LA: Parkinsonism associated with fluoxetine and cimetidine: a case report. J Geriatr Psychiatry Neurol 8:231–233, 1995

Lion JR, Azcarate CL, Koepke HH: Paradoxical rage reactions during psychotropic medication. Diseases of the Nervous System 36:557–558, 1975

Little KY: Amphetamine, but not methylphenidate, predicts antidepressant efficacy. J Clin Psychopharmacol 8:177–183, 1988

McElroy SL, Keck PE Jr, Pope HG Jr, et al: Valproate in psychiatric disorders: literature review and clinical guidelines. J Clin Psychiatry 50(suppl):23–29, 1989

McElroy SL, Dessain EC, Pope HG, et al: Clozapine in the treatment of psychotic mood disorders, schizoaffective disorder, and schizophrenia. J Clin Psychiatry 52:411–414, 1991

Metzger E, Friedman R: Prolongation of the corrected QT and torsades de pointes cardiac arrhythmia associated with intravenous haloperidol in the medically ill. J Clin Psychopharmacol 13:128–132, 1993

Miller LF: Clinical strategies for the use of psychotropic drugs during pregnancy. Psychiatr Med 9:275–298, 1991

Omtzigt JGC, Los FJ, Meijer JW, et al: The 10,11-epoxide-10,11-diol pathway of carbamazepine in early pregnancy in maternal serum, urine, and amniotic fluid: effect of dose, comedication and relation to outcome of pregnancy. Ther Drug Monit 15:1–10, 1993

Ouslander JG: Drug therapy in the elderly. Ann Intern Med 95:711–722, 1981

Patterson JF: Hepatitis associated with pemoline (letter). South Med J 77:938, 1984

Pellock JM, Willmore LJ: A rational guide to routine blood monitoring in patients receiving antiepileptic drugs. Neurology 41:961–964, 1991

Pope HG, McElroy SL, Keck PE Jr, et al: A placebo-controlled study of valproate in mania. Arch Gen Psychiatry 48:62–68, 1991

Pratt DS, Dubois RS: Hepatotoxicity due to pemoline (Cylert): a report of two cases. J Pediatr Gastroenterol Nutr 10:239–241, 1990

Preskorn SH, Alderman J, Kaufman BM, et al: Desipramine levels after sertraline or fluoxetine. Poster presented at the annual meeting of the American Psychiatric Association, Washington, DC, May 1992

Ramsey TA, Cox M: Lithium and the kidney: a review. Am J Psychiatry 139:443–449, 1982

Rapport DJ, Calabrese JR: Interactions between carbamazepine and birth control pills. Psychosomatics 30:462–464, 1989

Rickels K, Schweizer EE: Current pharmacotherapy of anxiety and panic, in Psychopharmacology: The Third Generation of Progress. Edited by Meltzer HY. New York, Raven, 1987, pp 1193–1203

Risse SC, Whitters A, Burke J, et al: Severe withdrawal symptoms after discontinuation of alprazolam in eight patients with combat-induced posttraumatic stress disorder. J Clin Psychiatry 51:206–209, 1990

Robinson GE, Stewart DE, Flak E: The rational use of psychotropic drugs in pregnancy and postpartum. Can J Psychiatry 31:183–190, 1986

Roose SP, Glassman AH: Antidepressant choice in the patient with cardiac disease: lessons from the cardiac arrhythmia suppression trial (CAST) studies. J Clin Psychiatry 55:83–100, 1994

Roose SP, Dalack GW, Glassman AH, et al: Cardiovascular effects of bupropion in depressed patients with heart disease. Am J Psychiatry 148:512–516, 1991

Rosa FW: Spina bifida in infants of women treated with carbamazepine during pregnancy. N Engl J Med 324:674–677, 1991

Rose SR, Klein-Schwartz W, Oderda GM, et al: Lithium intoxication with acute renal failure and death. Drug Intelligence and Clinical Pharmacy 22:691–694, 1988

Rosebush PI, Stewart TD, Gelenberg AJ: Twenty neuroleptic rechallenges after neuroleptic malignant syndrome in 15 patients. J Clin Psychiatry 50:295–298, 1989

Sachdev PS: Lithium potentiation of neuroleptic-related extrapyramidal side effects (letter). Am J Psychiatry 143:942, 1986

Satel SL, Nelson, JC: Stimulants in the treatment of depression: a critical overview. J Clin Psychiatry 50:241–249, 1989

Schmucker DL: Aging and drug disposition: an update. Pharmacol Rev 37:133–148, 1985

Segraves RT: Effects of psychotropic drugs on human erection and ejaculation. Arch Gen Psychiatry 46:275–284, 1989

Segraves RT: Overview of sexual dysfunction complicating the treatment of depression. J Clin Psychiatry Monograph 10:4–10, 1992

Shukla S, Godwin CD, Long LE, et al: Lithium-carbamazepine neurotoxicity and risk factors. Am J Psychiatry 141:1604–1606, 1984

Siris SG, Rifkin A: The problem of psychopharmacotherapy in the medically ill. Psychiatr Clin North Am 4:379–390, 1981

Spencer MJ: Fluoxetine hydrochloride (Prozac) toxicity in a neonate. Pediatrics 92:721–722, 1993

Spiller HA, Ramoska EA, Krenzelok EP, et al: Bupropion overdose: a 3-year multi-center retrospective analysis. Am J Emerg Med 12:43–45, 1994

Spring GK: Neurotoxicity with combined use of lithium and thioridazine. J Clin Psychiatry 40:135–138, 1979

Stoudemire A, Moran MG, Fogel BS: Psychotropic drug use in the medically ill, part II. Psychosomatics 32:34–46, 1991

Sussman N: The uses of buspirone in psychiatry. J Clin Psychiatry Monograph 129:3–19, 1994

Szymanski S, Munne R, Safferman A, et al: A selective review of recent advances in the management of tardive dyskinesia. Psychiatric Annals 23:209–215, 1993

Teicher MH, Cohen BM, Baldessarini RJ, et al: Severe daytime somnolence in patients treated with an MAOI. Am J Psychiatry 145:1552–1556, 1988

Tesar GE, Stern TA: Evaluation and treatment of agitation in the intensive care unit. Journal of Intensive Care Medicine 1:137–148, 1986

Thapa PB, Gideon P, Fought RL, et al: Psychotropic drugs and risk of recurrent falls in ambulatory nursing home residents. Am J Epidemiol 142:202–211, 1995

Tollefson G, Lesar T, Grothe D, et al: Alprazolam-related digoxin toxicity. Am J Psychiatry 141:1612–1613, 1984

Tolman KG, Freston JW, Berenson MM, et al: Hepatotoxicity due to pemoline: report of two cases. Digestion 9:532–539, 1973

Turpin JP, Schuller AB: Lithium and haloperidol incompatibility reviewed. Psychiatric Journal of the University of Ottawa 3:245–251, 1978

Waldmeier PC, Feldtrauer JJ, Graf T, et al: Brofaromine, a drug inhibiting MAO-A and 5-HT uptake. Clin Neuropharmacol 15 (suppl 1, part A):341A–342A, 1992

Wallace A, Kofoed LL, West AN: Double-blind, placebo-controlled trial of methylphenidate in older, depressed, medically ill patients. Am J Psychiatry 152:929–931, 1995

Warner MD, Peabody CA, Boutros NN, et al: Alprazolam and withdrawal seizures. J Nerv Ment Dis 178:208–209, 1990

Warrington SJ, Padgham C, Lader M: The cardiovascular effects of antidepressants. Psychol Med Monogr Suppl 16:1–40, 1989

White K, Simpson G: Combined MAOI-tricyclic antidepressant treatment: a reevaluation. J Clin Psychopharmacol 1:264–282, 1981

Wise MG, Rundell JR: Concise Guide to Consultation Psychiatry, 2nd Edition. Washington, DC, American Psychiatric Press, 1994, pp 151–166

Yassa R, Nastase C, DuPont D, et al: Tardive dyskinesia in elderly psychiatric patients: a 5-year study. Am J Psychiatry 149:1206–1211, 1992

Chapter 31

Chronic Pain: Neuropsychopharmacology and Adjunctive Psychiatric Treatment

Anthony J. Bouckoms, M.D.

Pain is often a symptom of illness, but it is also an illness in its own right. Cancer, trauma, and sickle cell crises are examples of illnesses in which pain is a symptom. Phantom pain, reflex sympathetic dystrophy, and anesthesia dolorosa are examples of disorders in which pain is the illness. Pain is best thought of as an illness with diagnostic features, an epidemiology, as well as chemical and neurological pathologies.

Pain has both mental and physical components. To divide pain into the categories of exclusively mental ("It's all in your head") or exclusively physical ("real") pain confuses clinicians and patients and derails treatment efforts. Pain is always in one's head and is almost always real, except in the malingerer.

PAIN TERMINOLOGY

- *Pain* is an unpleasant sensory and emotional experience that is associated with actual or potential tissue damage or is described as such.
- *Nociceptive* refers to a noxious peripheral stimulus, as in a traumatic injury.
- *Acute pain* is a term that is used for a nociceptive stimulus, acute in onset, waxing and waning in intensity, but resolving within days to 6 weeks. Nonsteroidal anti-inflammatory drugs (NSAIDs), narcotics, and rest are usually helpful.
- *Chronic pain* refers to pain that is prolonged beyond 6 weeks. It subsumes chronic nociceptive pain (e.g., osteomy-

elitis), central pain, sympathetically maintained pain (SMP), chronic pain syndrome (a behavioral syndrome), and intractable pain (e.g., cancer pain). Rehabilitation therapies, complex neuropsychopharmacology, and psychiatric therapies beyond simple antinociceptive measures are often required.

- *Allachesthesia* is a condition in which a sensation is referred to a site distant from which the stimulus is applied.
- *Allodynia* is pain caused by a nonnoxious stimulus, such as cold, vibration, or light mechanical touch (i.e., brushing against skin hairs).
- *Hypoesthesia* is a decreased sensitivity to any stimulation. Diminished sensitivity to noxious stimulation is called *hypoalgesia,* which is a subtype of hypoesthesia.
- *Hyperalgesia* is an increased sensitivity to noxious stimulation.
- *Hyperesthesia* is an increased sensitivity to noxious or nonnociceptive stimuli, such as touch or temperature. It includes hyperalgesia and allodynia.
- *Hyperpathia* is a form of hyperesthesia that is typically delayed after the offending stimulus is removed, continues to worsen for minutes or hours, and is sometimes felt at a site distant from the original stimulus (allachesthesia).
- *Central pain* is caused by deafferentation nerve injury or dysfunction in the central nervous system (CNS). Central pain is often independent of peripheral nociception and is the result of abnormal excitation/inhibition in the CNS. A central pain syndrome is recognized clinically by a delayed onset, decreased sensory threshold, increased sensitivity to nonnoxious stimuli (allodynia), and a limited response to narcotics (Arner and Meyerson 1988).
- *Reflex sympathetic dystrophy* (RSD) is a burning pain with allodynia, vasomotor symptoms, sweating, and late trophic changes in which muscles and bones waste, producing a swollen, painful, discolored, and dysfunctional organ. Sympathetic blockade that relieves the pain is the defining characteristic. Janig (1991) defined three types of RSD: 1) algodystrophy (the full syndrome); 2) sympathetic dystrophy (RSD without pain); and 3) SMP, in which pain is the only obvious manifestation of RSD.

- *Placebo effect* is a combination of expectation and neurochemical and conditioned responses that transforms an anticipated effect into a real effect. The placebo effect can positively or negatively affect pain, swelling, that patient's mental state, and the side effects of treatment. Placebo effect and "true" effects are not independent, consistent within an individual, or related to personality. Prior conditioning, active versus inactive placebo, and expectation can all vary the placebo response within and among individuals. Unfortunately, the placebo effect is often tested in a patient with pain by surreptitious substitution of a dose of saline for a strong analgesic. The intention is to test the patient by deceiving him or her. This is not helpful, and it potentially destroys the doctor-patient relationship by establishing the physician as an agent of deception. A positive placebo response (i.e., analgesia with saline) does not prove that the pain is not real, that the person is an addict or malingerer, or that the patient is not benefiting from an active medication. Healthy individuals have placebo responses because everyone is subject to conditioning and expectation. The more effective the previous medication, the more effective a subsequent placebo is likely to be; this is an expected, typical conditioned response. Placebo trials should only be performed with the cooperation of informed patients (Wall 1992).

EPIDEMIOLOGY OF CHRONIC PAIN

Chronic pain is common and costly, in terms of both dollars and suffering. Pain causes Americans to miss 550 million workdays each year. Pain can exhaust the chronic sufferer, impair the immune system, promote tumor growth, impair respiratory function and mobility, and encourage drug and alcohol overuse (Liebeskind 1991). Back pain adds about $1,000 to the cost of each American car sold because of pain-related medical disability payments (Taylor and Curran 1985).

A definitive physical diagnosis is reached in only 5%–10% of individuals with low back pain, which is the most common reason for disability (Osterweis et al. 1987). A population survey (Taylor and Curran 1985) showed that 9% of the population had back or joint pain for more than 100 days during the last 5 months. Muscle pain from fibromyalgia afflicts as many as 6 million people in the United States and accounts for 5% of people coming to a general medical clinic.

Posttraumatic pain has a complex mechanism illustrated by three puzzling facts: 1) up to 40% of injured patients admitted to hospitals initially have no pain complaints; 2) 90% of patients with brachial plexus root avulsions have pain, even though afferent pain fibers are absent; and 3) hyperalgesia at the site of injury is associated with an increased flexion withdrawal reflex, even after a local anesthetic is used to numb the site of tissue injury. Apparently, posttraumatic pain is associated with excitability in the spinal cord even without afferent input (Sweet 1984; Tverskoy et al. 1990).

A significant minority of people with chronic pain have a psychiatric disorder—that is, 20%–30% have an Axis I diagnosis (Reich et al. 1983). The link between pain and emotional disturbance may involve early developmental attachments to significant others, as well as biological psychiatric disorders (Barsky et al. 1994). Psychiatric problems can complicate chronic pain through behavioral, interper-

sonal, and affective mechanisms (Gamsa 1990; Kohler and Kosnaic 1992). Despite the psychiatric morbidity associated with chronic pain, emotional symptoms are more often a consequence rather than an antecedent to pain. Even so, the cause-and-effect relation between comorbid physical pain and psychiatric disorders is often unresolvable. Part of the role of the consultation-liaison psychiatrist is to ensure that both physical and psychiatric aspects of pain are evaluated and treated.

PATHOPHYSIOLOGY OF CHRONIC PAIN

Why is nonnoxious sensory input from the periphery sometimes perceived as "pain"? How does the CNS allow pain to persist, increase, and become chronic? What are the mechanisms for hyperalgesia, and what are the central changes in sensory processing that make pain intractable? The general answers to these questions may lie in overlapping pathophysiologies wherein firing thresholds for pain cells are lowered, allowing pain to be triggered more easily. There is recruitment of wide dynamic range (WDR) cells, so that touch or movement causes pain. Other explanations include general mechanisms such as convergence of cutaneous, vascular, muscle, and joint inputs (i.e., one tissue refers pain to another) and/or ephaptic interneuronal connections (i.e., electrical short circuits between the sympathetic and sensory nerves, producing causalgia).

CNS Neuroplasticity

Pain is a perception of the CNS, and nociceptor input is only one factor in pain threshold, intensity, quality, time course, and location. Although a relation between nociception and perception exists, it is not direct or linear (Wall 1988). One explanation for neuroplasticity is that acute pain from nerve trauma results in a rewiring of cortical and subcortical neurons. Within days of the injury, disconnected nerve cells receive input from other parts of the body. For example, cells previously responsive to the pinprick of a finger may now respond to light touch of a hair on the forehead. Consequently, touching a hair may trigger a burst of pain at a site distant from the injury (allodynia and allachesthesia). Prevention of chronic pain from this neuroplastic response to trauma includes early aggressive treatment of acute pain. A major goal for research is to better understand the pathophysiology of neuroplasticity so that preventing the transition from acute to chronic pain is possible (Baringa 1992; Coderre et al. 1993; Fields 1992).

Sensitization of Touch, Movement, Pressure (Wide Dynamic Range) Cells

When WDR cells are activated by low-threshold mechanoreceptors, nonpainful stimuli can invoke pain. Unlike nociceptive pain, the resultant pain from WDR cell activation is not neatly defined in dermatomes. Rather, the painful areas move, changing shape and size. Pain can be triggered by touch, joint movement, vibration, or visceral stretch. Pain becomes a CNS phenomenon that exists apart from peripheral nerve endings. Sensitization is probably produced by N-methyl-D-aspartate (NMDA), calcitonin gene-related peptide, or substance P. The clinical implication is that early treatment of pain is very important to prevention or minimization of sensitization. Multimodal treatments for acute, myofascial, vascular, and central pain, as well as psychological contributors to pain, are important in decreasing the sensitization of WDR cells. For example, the early use of anticonvulsants or other membrane-stabilizing agents can sometimes prevent the sensitization that occurs following nerve damage. Preventing the sensitization of WDR cells in RSD syndromes may involve early physical therapy, treatment of acute pain, and α-blockade.

NMDA-GABA Receptors and Chronic Pain

One mechanism that produces rapid sensitization of spinal cord pain cells is the excitatory amino acid glutamate. NMDA receptors, responsive to glutamate, sensitize the pain receptors in the spinal cord, which creates hyperalgesia (Baringa 1992; Dubner 1991). Drugs that inhibit NMDA receptors inhibit hyperalgesia, although the sensation of pain remains intact. Hyperalgesia is also reversed by opiates (Aanonsen and Wilcox 1987; Mao et al. 1992). Acute, short-lived pain does not stimulate NMDA receptors; chronic pain stimulation does. The second component in the development of hyperalgesia involves γ-aminobutyric acid (GABA). GABA normally inhibits incoming nonpainful stimuli to the thalamus (i.e., inhibits light touch and muscle and joint movement) but not painful stimuli. If non-nociceptive stimuli are not inhibited by GABA, chronic pain might occur. Touch or the movement of a muscle or joint then becomes painful. The clinical implications of these two mechanisms are as follows: 1) NMDA antagonists may be useful for treating chronic pain when hyperexcitability of peripheral and central cells has occurred (Woolf and Thompson 1991), and 2) GABA agonists might decrease pain when central hyperalgesia is the mechanism for intractability or chronicity.

Neurotoxins

A neurotoxic etiology for chronic pain is seen with neuropathic pain related to acquired immunodeficiency syndrome (AIDS). Patients with AIDS produce cerebrospinal quinolinic acid levels 10 to 1,000 times greater than normal. For AIDS-related neuropathic pain, serotonergic agents possibly shift metabolism away from the potentially neurotoxic kynurenine-quinolinic pathway to the pain-relieving serotonin (5-hydroxytryptamine [5-HT]) pathway.

The Opioid Paradox

Increased sensitivity to pain (hyperalgesia) caused by narcotics presents an apparent paradox. Nevertheless, clinicians have described patients who experience more pain on rather than off narcotics. For this reason, a trial off narcotics should be considered, not because of fear of addiction but because pain sometimes decreases without narcotics.

Sympathetically Maintained Pain

SMP is found not only in classic cases of RSD but can be present when pain is the only symptom. Regional guanethidine (Bonelli et al. 1983) or intravenous phentolamine blocks (Arner 1991) sometimes offers pain relief when other pain treatments fail. α-Receptors also modulate spinal opiate receptors. Given this information, the consultation-liaison psychiatrist should consider the early use of sympathetic blockade in any patient with chronic pain syndrome with features of sympathetic dysfunction. Even pain syndromes associated with trauma, facial pain, herpetic infections, and arthritis, not usually identified as sympathetically maintained, sometimes respond to sympathetic blockage. Therefore, α-blocking drugs have a role in the pharmacotherapy of pain, with and without opiates. Phentolamine (intravenous block), α-blocking antidepressants (e.g., doxepin, 150 mg), and clonidine (0.1 mg tid) are all potentially useful in some patients who have chronic pain. β-Blockers are not useful for SMP, except in patients with migraine headache.

Myofascial Pain

Myofascial trigger points, hypertonic muscles, and limited joint movement can produce a chronic pain syndrome known as fibromyalgia (Fricton and Awad 1990). Chronicity ensues because of the concurrence of muscle trigger points, hypersensitive skin, subjective sense of swelling and numbness, anxiety, and deficient

stage 4 sleep (Moldofsky et al. 1975).

In 1990, the American College of Rheumatology stated that the diagnosis of fibromyalgia required tenderness where muscles join their tendons in 11 of 18 specific trigger points, plus widespread pain without other obvious causes. Despite efforts toward greater specificity, the relation between fibromyalgia, depression, chronic fatigue syndrome, and sleep disruption is not clear (Campbell et al. 1983; Osterweis et al. 1987; Wolfe and Cathay 1985; Yunus et al. 1981).

Fibromyalgia muscle pain is best treated as a specific diagnosis with physical therapies and, in certain cases, appropriate trigger point analgesia. Physical conditioning, especially with behavioral modification of bad sleep habits, and proper diet are important adjunctive therapies. Partial protection from sleep disruption may be obtained through aerobic conditioning. It is also important to identify and treat depression that may underlie the sleep–muscle tension syndrome. The simultaneous treatment of concomitant pain, such as vascular pain or SMP, can turn treatment resistance into success.

Monoaminergic Influence on Pain

Serotonin, norepinephrine, and dopamine are found in pain-modulating pathways from the periphery to the CNS periaqueductal-frontal pathways. These monoamines often comodulate pain peptides as well.

Serotonin function must be intact for pain inhibition. In the spinal cord, the dorsolateral funiculus is a serotonergic inhibitory descending spinal pain pathway that modulates 80% of receptor spinal analgesic effect of opiates (Anderson and Proudfit 1981). Human spinal receptors are probably $5-HT_2$ and $5-HT_1$ subtypes, explaining why antidepressants have direct spinal inhibitory effects on pain. In the periphery, the early inflammatory sensitization of peripheral nociceptors depends on $5-HT_3$ receptors; $5-HT_3$-receptor antagonists block the hyperalgesia of inflammation (Eschalier et

al. 1989). Another type of peripheral serotonin receptor, 5-HT$_{1D}$, is found in cerebral blood vessels. Sumatriptan, a selective 5-HT$_{1D}$ antagonist, acts to produce vasconstriction and migraine headache relief. The raphe and meso-limbic structures are important sites of sub-cortical serotonin receptors; these are mainly types 5-HT$_{1A}$, 5-HT$_{2A}$, and 5-HT$_{2B}$. These receptors modulate pain and mood.

Despite the importance of serotonin in pain, there are exceptions to the simplistic notion that increasing serotonin decreases pain (Lance 1991). Serotonin is just one part of a complex picture.

Norepinephrine is important in pain modulation, which is demonstrated by a variety of neurophysiological acute pain experiments. It is known that α-adrenergic receptors comodulate opiate receptors in the spinal cord. Clinical studies of norepinephrine-modulating drugs suggest that they have value in treating patients with chronic pain. Desipramine (average 200 mg/day) relieved pain in patients with diabetic neuropathy, both in those who had depression and those who did not have depression (Max et al. 1992). Desipramine also relieves postherpetic neuralgia (Kishore-Kumar et al. 1990). This emphasizes the importance of norepinephrine in the treatment of patients with chronic pain, not alone but in tandem with opiates, serotonin, and peptides.

Dopamine is associated with both clinical and experimental pain. Clinically, dopamine agonists (e.g., stimulants) augment narcotic analgesia. Methylphenidate and pergolide help to relieve the suffering aspect of pain. It is known that antidepressants such as tricyclics and selective serotonin reuptake inhibitors (SSRIs) can upregulate mesolimbic dopamine. Experimentally, dopamine comodulates opiate and substance P receptors in the CNS. Painful dysesthesias sometimes occur in patients with Parkinson's disease. Low levels of dopamine and its metabolite homovanillic acid (HVA) were found in the cerebrospinal fluid (CSF) of patients with chronic pain (Bouckoms et al. 1991). Although dopa-

mine is important in the modulation of pain, it is not known how to combine dopamine agonists and other medications.

PSYCHIATRIC EXAMINATION AND DIFFERENTIAL DIAGNOSIS

When a psychiatric diagnosis is made in a patient who has chronic pain, the patient's interpretation is, "They believe it's all in my head." Even when the psychiatrist and patient agree on the psychiatric diagnosis (i.e., the pain is "real" and there is also a complicating psychiatric diagnosis), many others—the insurance companies, managed care organizations, disability providers, legal and social agencies, and some physicians—may not. Precision in diagnosis is particularly important because of its long-term implications (see Table 31–1).

Depression

Depression is present in 20%–30% of patients who have chronic pain (Reich et al. 1983). In many patients, the depression predates the pain. Denial, masking of depressive symptoms with narcotics or benzodiazepines, and other comorbid psychiatric diagnoses can all obscure depression in patients who have chronic pain (Bouckoms et al. 1985; Holmes et al. 1986). When asking a patient with chronic pain about neurovegetative symptoms, the clinician should focus on the following questions: "If you awaken at night, do you have difficulty returning to sleep?" "Are there still things that give you joy and pleasure?" "How much sadness do you feel with the pain?" Regardless of the skill of the interviewer, denial, rationalization, anger, and fear can interfere with truthful answers to those questions. Four useful diagnostic aids are

1. Patient-rated visual analogue scales, scored from best-to-worst mood and most-to-least pain
2. The Minnesota Multiphasic Personality Inventory (MMPI; Hathaway and McKin-

Table 31–1. Fifteen psychiatric conditions that can coexist with, cause, or exacerbate pain

Psychiatric diagnosis	Key diagnostic features in patient with pain
Depression	Anhedonia; sadness; and early-morning awakening
Anxiety disorders	Panic or generalized anxiety not fully relieved by analgesics
Somatoform disorders (six disorders)	Physical complaints unexplained by physical diagnoses that are associated with psychological factors
Factitious disorder with physical symptoms	Deception of the physician in order to maintain a sick role
Malingering	**W**ithholds information deliberately
	Antisocial
	Somatic findings are changeable
	Treatment compliance is erratic
	External gains
Dissociative states	Amnesia (partial); anxiety; nightmares; flashbacks; conflicted avoidance of close relationships
Chronic pain syndrome	Physical disability is emphasized, while the importance of interpersonal factors in the suffering is both demonstrated and denied
Sexual pain disorders	Dyspareunia or vaginismus
Psychosis	Bizarre, illogical thought; disordered attributions of cause and effect
Personality disorders	Diminished ability to cope with pain

ley 1943)—the clinician should be alert for high depression scores on the subtle and overt scales

3. Sleep electroencephalogram (EEG), with special attention to any observation of shortened rapid eye movement (REM) latency (less than 90 minutes)

4. Serial examinations of affect, behavior, and emotional reactivity

Pharmacological treatment of patients with depression who have chronic pain is not unique. The clinician should ensure that adequate doses of antidepressants are used. Depression, even subthreshold cases, should be treated. Depression is never an "appropriate" response to chronic pain.

Anxiety Disorders

Anxiety symptoms sufficient to meet DSM-IV (American Psychiatric Association 1994) criteria for an anxiety disorder (usually generalized anxiety or panic disorder) occur in approximately 30% of patients with intractable pain. More than half of patients with anxiety disorders have comorbid psychiatric disorder; major depression and substance-related disorders are the most common (Bouckoms and Hackett 1991). Treatment of these comorbid conditions often reduces anxiety and pain complaints.

Other causes of anxiety in patients with pain include disruptions in normal relationships, bodily functions, and sense of self. These narcissistic injuries complicate physical and emotional rehabilitation and require treatment. Existential issues increase because the person must reorient his or her expectations and views of life. This is particularly common in cancer-associated pain. The patient's existential anxiety can often be reduced when the clinician spends time and has discussions with the individual. Anger is another source of anxiety;

the anger is typically denied by the patient and is often expressed in psychosomatic symptoms (Antczak-Bouckoms and Bouckoms 1985). Mild organic brain syndromes can also present with anxiety, as a result of frustration. Cognitive deficits are present in 5%–10% of patients with pain.

Somatoform Disorders

Somatoform disorders are a group of disorders in which physical symptoms are a manifestation of psychological pathology. Somatization disorder is the flagship somatoform disorder, derived historically from Briquet's syndrome; it is quite specific and reliably predicts an individual's future behavior. Unfortunately, most people with physical complaints without physical etiologies do not fit into this neatly defined diagnosis. The other somatoform disorders have less stringent criteria. Diagnosis of these disorders in patients with chronic pain requires the exercise of a great deal of clinical judgment and knowledge about the psychology of illness. Five problems are

1. Central pain may mimic somatoform disorders.
2. An unrecognized medical condition can lead the clinician to diagnose the pain as "psychiatric," by exclusion.
3. Judgment whether pain is "excessive" for a particular individual or medical condition is usually impossible.
4. Pain can decrease with psychotropic drugs or psychological techniques without the presence of psychiatric diagnosis.
5. Deciding whether psychological factors are causes or effects is often impossible in a patient with chronic pain.

Patients with somatoform disorders often exhibit exaggerated physical complaints and irrational fears and anxiety about physical illness. Weintraub's (1992) study of 210 patients with chronic pain involved in litigation found

that 63% had "psychogenic symptoms," meaning nonanatomical or nonphysiological sensory and motor examination findings—ipso facto, somatoform. Weintraub stated that strict reliance on subjective complaints of pain is often misleading and is potentially harmful. Unfortunately, objective findings do not always reflect pain-producing pathology, either. For example, 20%–30% of patients who have myelograms for reasons other than pain have disk bulges (Deyo et al. 1992). Although 20%–80% of all pain complaints to physicians do not have well-defined etiologies, these complaints do not always warrant a somatoform or psychiatric diagnosis. Prevalence studies of somatoform disorders report a rate of 5%–15% among patients treated for chronic pain (Bouckoms and Hackett 1991). However, comorbidity and variation within population samples make these studies of somatoform disorders in patients with chronic pain problematic.

Four pragmatic tactics may help to resolve the clinician's confusion. First, a physical examination should be performed. The physical examination will often unmask illness behavior and decrease the patient's antipsychiatry bias. It also allows a neurological examination for central pain and myofascial pain. Second, the clinician should search for positive criteria for a psychiatric illness so that somatization is not diagnosed by default. Third, the clinician should look for additional Axis I disorders using DSM-IV criteria. The two most common comorbid conditions with somatoform disorders are major depression and anxiety disorder. If a somatoform diagnosis is present, the odds are 3:1 that the patient also has depression; the odds are similarly high for anxiety disorder. Fourth, objective tests should be performed to reduce reliance on subjective impressions. For example, computerized motion analysis can be used to reliably and reproducibly compare degrees of flexion, extension, and torque with national statistics.

Conversion Disorder

The diagnosis of conversion disorder requires one or more symptoms or deficits affecting voluntary motor or sensory function that suggest a neurological or medical condition. The symptoms must cause significant distress or must impair function. If pain or sexual dysfunction is the only complaint, a diagnosis of conversion disorder is not made; the correct diagnosis is *pain disorder* or *sexual pain disorder,* respectively. If the symptom is initiated, exacerbated, or preceded by conflicts or other stressors, psychological factors are judged to be associated with the symptom. The diagnosis requires that the symptom cannot be fully explained by a neurological or medical condition. From a study of patients seen in a pain clinic, Weintraub (1988) observed that the triad of pain, numbness, and weakness represents a common conversion syndrome. The presence of primary gain increases diagnostic certainty, whereas la belle indifférence and histrionic personality traits do not. A "conversion" V on the MMPI denotes hypochondriacal traits and a relative absence of depression. This pattern is consistent with conversion disorder. Electromyogram (EMG), EEG, and repeated physical examination often help to identify the approximately 50% of patients who actually have a medical disorder but were erroneously diagnosed as "hysterical" (Reed 1975).

Hypochondriasis

Hypochondriasis is preoccupation (that persists for longer than 6 months) with fears of having, or the idea that one has, a serious disease based on the misinterpretation of bodily symptoms. Head and orofacial pains, cardiac pain, dyspeptic pain, or tingling, burning, numb pains are common foci of hypochondriacal concern. "Yes, Doctor, but . . . ," is a statement that typifies the defiant and help-rejecting complaints of the hypochondriac. No test, reassurance, discussion, or explanation is enough. The person interprets every physical sensation as evidence of physical illness, is significantly distressed or impaired by the symptoms, and yet is not delusional, nor does he or she have an anxiety disorder or major depression. The patient with pain who has hypochondriasis frequently sees nonpsychiatrists because these patients firmly believe that "the pain is not in my head." The consultation-liaison psychiatrist must also be aware of the patient with pseudohypochondriasis, in whom the perception of illness foretells an early cancer, multiple sclerosis, or central pain syndrome. Transient hypochondriasis is not uncommon in elderly patients. Separation of hypochondriasis from psychosis, major depression, somatic symptoms of panic disorder or generalized anxiety disorder, obsessive-compulsive disorder, and somatization disorder is important because the treatments for these various entities are quite different. Severe hypochondriasis often masks major depression or psychosis.

Pain Disorder

Pain disorder is defined in DSM-IV as a syndrome in which pain is the focus of clinical presentation. Physical pathology, if present, does not adequately explain the pain. The diagnostic criteria require that pain causes either significant impairment in occupational or social functioning or that it results in marked distress. Three diagnostic subtypes are defined, although only the first and third are formally diagnosed on DSM-IV Axis I; they are pain disorder 1) associated with psychological factors, 2) associated with a general medical condition (i.e., not a psychiatric disorder), and 3) associated with both psychological factors and a general medical condition.

The psychological factors must have an important role in the onset, severity, exacerbation, or maintenance of the pain. Clues in the past history are physical abuse, counter-dependent personal relationships, family history of alcoholism, and personal developmental history of attachment deficits. Pain disorder due to a general medical condition is diagnosed when a nonpsychiatric medical condition accounts for the onset, severity, exacerbation, or maintenance of pain. If psychological factors are present, they play only a minor role in accounting for the pain. The medical disorder is listed on Axis III.

Factitious Disorder With Physical Symptoms

An intentional production or feigning of pain to achieve the sick role is diagnosed as a factitious disorder. Three subtypes are listed in DSM-IV: 1) with predominantly physical signs and symptoms, 2) with predominantly psychological signs and symptoms, and 3) with combined psychological and physical signs and symptoms. Renal colic, orofacial pains, and abdominal pain are three commonly feigned pain complaints. These individuals do not have psychosis despite the vague, meandering nature of their stories. The onset of factitious disorder is usually in early adulthood, and a lifelong pattern of repeated hospitalizations is typical. Pain is often reported in such elaborate, exaggerated detail that it intrigues the listener (e.g., pseudologia phantastica). Assiduous, detailed inquiry into the exact circumstances of previous admissions and discharges will often lead to a sudden demand for discharge from the hospital. (For a discussion of individuals with factitious disorders, please refer to Ford and Feldman, Chapter 16, in this volume.)

Malingering

The patient who is malingering intentionally produces false physical or psychological symptoms and is motivated by avoiding work, obtaining financial compensation, evading criminal prosecution, or obtaining drugs. In order to obtain a reward, the patient who is malingering consciously fakes a complaint. Lack of this external gain or evidence of an intrapsychic need to maintain a sick role suggests factitious disorder rather than malingering. A clever patient who is malingering can skew an MMPI toward normality, evade accountability (such as old medical records), and defeat the goals of uncovering data via an Amytal interview or hypnosis. The WASTE mnemonic to screen for malingering is described in Table 31–1.

One type of pseudomalingering with dissociative features is Ganser's syndrome. Sensory and motor symptoms are typically seen; Ganser's syndrome presents a puzzling diagnostic challenge because there is not only malingering but also an underlying, additional psychiatric illness. This syndrome leads to diagnoses such as conversion disorder, dissociative disorder, or factitious disorder. (Further information about malingering can be found Chapter 16 in this volume.)

Dissociative States

According to DSM-IV, dissociation is a disturbance or alteration in the normally integrative functions of identity, memory, or consciousness. Dissociative disorders are important because a history of childhood abuse is quite common in individuals who develop chronic pain; abused children are prone to dissociative disorders. Pelvic pain, sexual pain disorders, headache, and abdominal pain are the most common pain complaints in developmentally traumatized individuals (Barsky et al. 1994). Walker and colleagues (1992) noted that in 22 women with chronic pelvic pain, 18 reported childhood abuse. Of the 21 women selected as control subjects (i.e., women who had no pelvic pain), 9 reported childhood abuse ($P < .0005$). Disconnection from important events, emotionally or by amnesia, is characteristic of patients with dissociative disorders.

Chronic Pain Syndrome

Chronic pain syndrome is characterized by pain behaviors and interpersonal and affective features that merge into a pattern that emphasizes physical disability, suffering, and attention from others. It is more broadly defined than pain disorder but is not easily distinguished from it. Treatment typically addresses self-defeating, behavioral patterns, as well as the affective dysfunction and psychodynamic conflicts inherent in the behavior (described in Table 31–2).

Personality Disorders

No single personality type or pathology is uniquely associated with chronic pain. Even in individuals who experience migraine headaches, who are often fastidious and have obsessive traits, no characterological differences were found between patients who had migraines and control subjects (Kohler and Kosnaic 1992). However, clinicians who work with patients longitudinally might disagree. The patient's attachments to others, such as doctors and family, are problematic. Typically, the psychodynamics are a mixture of regression, ambivalence over care and getting well, shame, and reexperiencing old conflicts about nurturance.

Psychosis

Pain as part of a psychosis is easy to recognize when it occurs in the context of active schizophrenic symptoms, a delusional idea of persecution, a depressive illness, substance-induced psychosis, or dementia. However, when pain is a singular complaint, denial is prominent, and some physical findings are present, teasing out a psychotic process is not easy. The following tactics are helpful. The patient should be asked to draw a picture of the pain in his or her body. This exercise can illustrate a thought disorder that is otherwise obscured by denial and rationalization. The clinician should perform a physical examination. Failure to examine patients with psychosis is the reason that acute abdomens, ischemic heart disease, and traumatic injuries are often overlooked in psychiatric hospitals.

PHYSICAL EXAMINATION OF THE PATIENT WITH CHRONIC PAIN

Physical examination of the patient who has chronic pain is essential to a correct diagnosis (Deyo et al. 1992). Psychiatrists who believe they should not touch patients during an evaluation cannot properly treat patients with pain. The physical examination involves a traditional neurological examination, during which the clinician looks for abnormal pain behavior, inconsistencies, and vague or changeable findings. A physical examination should also include examination for features of central pain (Table 31–3).

Table 31–2. Characteristics of chronic pain syndrome

Behavior[a]	Interpersonal[b]	Affective features[c]
Physical display of disability maximized	"Nothing helps"	Sour, angry, resentment for others
Suffering emphasized (verbally)	Authenticity of complaint emphasized	Sweet, endearing, denying, passive
Suffering dramatized (nonverbally)	High anxiety expressed and denied	Strong moods, dysphoria, irritability
Disability prolonged by avoidance and noncompliance	"Only you can help; I can't do anything"	Weak, low self-esteem, counterdependent

Source. [a]Fordyce 1976; [b]Bouckoms and Hackett 1991; [c]Bouckoms 1989.

Table 31–3. Physical examination for central pain

Clinical feature	Examination finding
Nondermatomal distribution of pain	Pinprick or light touch examination of the distribution of pain is nondermatomal
Increased sensory threshold	Pinprick is not felt as sharp, but rather as light touch
Decreased pain threshold; patient perceives pain from nonnoxious stimulation	Allodynia is present (i.e., painful response to vibration, minimal movement of a few body hairs, or contact with a cold metallic object or ice cube)
Hyperpathia	Delay, summation, and prolonged after sensation to nonnoxious stimulation; allachesthesia may be present
Paroxysmal attacks of pain	Pain is paroxysmal, either occurring spontaneously or induced by light touch

PHARMACOTHERAPY AND ADJUNCTIVE TREATMENTS FOR CHRONIC PAIN

Nonsteroidal Anti-Inflammatory Drugs

NSAIDs are useful for acute and chronic pain; for problems such as inflammation, muscle pain, vascular pain, and posttraumatic pain; or for cases in which a potent, nonnarcotic analgesic is indicated. NSAIDs are generally equal in efficacy and side effects. They can all cause bronchospasm in aspirin-sensitive patients, cause gastric ulcers, interact with angiotensin-converting enzyme (ACE) inhibitors to cause renal failure, precipitate lithium toxicity, and, with long-term use, impair renal function. However, certain NSAIDs have special features that make them preferable over others in particular treatment situations; these are outlined elsewhere (Bouckoms 1994).

Risk of gastric ulcers. The patient who is at risk for gastric ulcers but who requires a sustained course of an NSAID can receive misoprostol, 100–200 μg four times daily. The course of therapy should start with 100 μg because the lower dose is better tolerated and is only slightly less effective than the 200-μg dose. Misoprostol is effective in preventing NSAID- or aspirin-induced gastric ulcers, whereas histamine H_2-receptor antagonists and sucralfate are not.

Cancer pain. NSAIDs have been shown to be useful for some cancer-related pain, especially bone pain, but not neurogenic pain. Ibuprofen also works well as a narcotic adjunct. Naproxen has a good clinical track record as a narcotic adjuvant, although flurbiprofen does not.

WHO analgesic ladder. NSAIDs are the first step on the World Health Organization's (1990) three-step guideline for pain treatment (Table 31–4). The WHO ladder was created for patients with cancer pain. It has a reported efficacy of 90% in cancer patients. It is also a useful template for other kinds of pain.

Opiates

Opiates benefit some patients who have chronic cancer and noncancer pain. Cancer pain is the most common reason for prescription of maintenance narcotics (Ventafridda et al. 1987). Acute pain, when severe and unremitting, also requires narcotics treatment (Table 31–4).

Narcotic use in patients with nonmalignant pain. Narcotics are often the only effective treatment for patients experiencing nonmalignant chronic pain (Portenoy and Foley 1986). For example, in one study (Bouckoms et al. 1992), long-term oral narcotics were shown to provide effective pain relief

Table 31–4. World Health Organization analgesic ladder

Step	Pain intensity	Drugs
1	Mild to moderate	Aspirin, acetaminophen, or NSAIDs
2	Moderate to severe	Add codeine or hydrocodeine to the NSAID; consider other adjuvant medications
3	Severe to very severe	Morphine, methadone, hydromorphone, fentanyl, or levorphanol (parenterally in many cases); adjuvant medications frequently used

Note. NSAID = nonsteroidal antiinflammatory drug.
Source. Adapted from World Health Organization 1990.

in about two-thirds of patients with nonmalignant chronic pain; however, even when patients were carefully selected (i.e., lack of previous substance dependency or gross personality disorder), one-third developed abuse, tolerance, or dependency over a 3-year period. Nociceptive pain, absence of depression, and absence of drug abuse were all significantly associated with long-term narcotic treatment efficacy. However, patients with neuropathic pain and major depression did particularly poorly—minimal or no pain relief was four times more likely to occur in these patients than was marked to complete pain relief.

The following eight recommendations can be applied to maintenance therapy with narcotic analgesics in patients with chronic pain:

1. Do not prescribe narcotics for patients who previously used, abused, or were addicted to illicit drugs unless there is a new major medical illness with severe pain (e.g., cancer, trauma). In such cases, a second opinion from another physician is suggested for narcotics prescribed longer than 1 month.

2. Do not place pregnant opiate users at risk for withdrawal. Therefore, any pregnant woman with opiate dependency should receive methadone, about 20 mg/day, to prevent withdrawal effects in the fetus (Allen 1991).

3. Consider maintenance narcotics only after other methods of pain control fail.

Other methods typically include nonsteroidal drugs, epidural opiates and nonopiates, membrane-stabilizing drugs, monoaminergic agents, nerve blocks and nerve stimulation, and physical therapy.

4. Obtain a second opinion from a physician who is familiar with pain management if narcotics are prescribed for longer than 3 months and a follow-up consultation at least once a year if narcotics are continued.

5. Designate one pharmacy and one prescriber as the "exclusive" agent for opiate treatment.

6. Define narcotic dosage and consequences if deviations occur. For example, the development of abuse should lead to rapid tapering of the drug and a detoxification program, if necessary. Leave the patient with no doubt that you will stop the drug if use becomes inappropriate.

7. Document informed consent to include the rationale for use, risks, benefits, and alternative treatments.

8. Document the treatment course to include response to treatment; changes in the disease process; medication efficacy, abuse, and tolerance; or the appearance of addictive behaviors.

Antihistamines

Antihistamines may have an analgesic effect. This effect is best documented for diphenhydramine and hydroxyzine. For example, hydroxyzine, 100 mg given intramuscularly, may increase narcotic efficacy by 50%. Mechanisms of antihistamine analgesia include both peripheral effects (anti-inflammatory, antispasmolytic, local anesthetic) and central effects (i.e., antihistamines may facilitate opioid binding; may inhibit serotonin, norepinephrine, and dopamine reuptake; and may inhibit substance P release). Antihistamines can also decrease morphine clearance (Rumore and Schlichting 1986).

Steroids

Steroids are used orally and intravenously for the pain associated with bone metastases, brain swelling, and spinal cord compression. They may also help with anorexia associated with pain, even at doses as low as 15–25 mg/day of prednisone. Pain from sickle cell crises may respond to two boluses of methylprednisolone, 15 mg/kg to a maximum of 1 g/bolus, repeated after 24 hours. This drug lessens the amount and duration of narcotics required during the crisis (Griffen et al. 1994).

Anticonvulsants and Benzodiazepines

Carbamazepine, clonazepam, and phenytoin are three agents used to treat central or neuropathic pain. The physiological mechanism for analgesia is suppression of the hyperexcitability of low-threshold mechanoreceptive neurons in the brain. Phenobarbital does not have this effect and is not useful for pain (Fromm 1993).

Carbamazepine is generally superior to phenytoin for pain; a dosage of 200–1,400 mg/day of carbamazepine is effective for trigeminal neuralgia, postherpetic pain, postsympathetic pain, diabetic neuropathy, multiple sclerosis, and assorted neuralgias (Maciewicz et al. 1985). Blood levels have not been reported in most studies, but when they are reported, higher levels (8–12 µg/L) were necessary for optimal efficacy. Phenytoin is ef-

fective in various neuropathies—in particular, trigeminal, diabetic, and poststroke pain. Sharp, "shooting," lancinating pain responds to phenytoin. Phenytoin is less effective than carbamazepine; this makes it a second choice for analgesia.

Valproate was effective in the treatment of migraine pain in two double-blind placebo-controlled trials (Hering and Kuritzky 1992; Silberstein et al. 1993). Valproate given in combination with amitriptyline has been shown to decrease postherpetic neuralgia, episodic and chronic cluster headaches, postoperative pain, and various neuralgias (Bowsher 1992; Hering and Kuritzky 1989; Martin et al. 1988). These studies demonstrate the efficacy of valproate in the treatment of pain, in addition to its place in the treatment of bipolar disorder.

Clonazepam, in oral doses from 1 to 4 mg, is particularly useful because it has few side effects, decreases allodynia, and is compatible with other agents, such as antidepressants or opioids. Combinations of benzodiazepines with antidepressants or opiates are clinically useful. Intravenous lorazepam was shown to be superior to morphine, Xylocaine, and placebo in a single-blind study of neuropathic pain (Bouckoms 1987). Clonazepam is the oral drug of choice. It binds more to central than to peripheral benzodiazepine receptors and it is synergistic with serotonergic pain mechanisms, which distinguishes it from other benzodiazepines. There are at least 11 publications citing the value of clonazepam in neuralgias (Bouckoms and Litman 1985). A useful diagnostic test for benzodiazepine-sensitive pain is to administer lorazepam, in a 2-mg intravenous bolus, in a single-blind manner with the response evaluated by visual analogue scale monitoring. Positive results (a visual analogue scale decrease > 3 cm) signify relief of ongoing pain. If positive results are achieved, the pain cycle in patients with severe pain may be broken with sequential intravenous doses of lorazepam or oral clonazepam, 1 mg twice a day and 2–4 mg at bedtime.

Membrane-Stabilizing Agents

Tocainide, mexiletine, and lidocaine are also used to treat neuropathic pain; the first two agents are given orally, and the latter, intravenously. Lidocaine-sensitive pain is best diagnosed by giving a bolus dose of 100 mg of lidocaine intravenously or 4 mg/kg over 30 minutes. The analgesic effect is monitored with the use of a visual analogue scale. Diabetic neuropathy and other deafferentation neuralgias also often respond to lidocaine (Bouckoms 1987; Marchettini et al. 1992). Mexiletine is the oral agent of choice because serious anemia was reported with tocainide (Dejgard et al. 1988).

α-Blockers and Sympathetically Maintained Pain

Intrathecally, epidurally, and systemically administered clonidine produces analgesia (Coombs et al. 1986). Clonidine is often useful in patients who have developed tolerance to opiates and in those with some types of vascular or neuropathic pain. Transdermal clonidine (0.3 mg/day) is sometimes useful in neuropathy, although results are mixed (K. D. Davis et al. 1991).

The ischemic arm block (Hannington-Kiff block) is one of the most useful methods for treating SMP. Guanethidine, bretylium, reserpine, or phentolamine may be used to produce a chemical sympathectomy. Phenoxybenzamine was once considered a useful oral agent but is probably less useful than the Hannington-Kiff block.

Peptides

Calcitonin. Calcitonin is a well-established treatment for the bone pain associated with Paget's disease. Cancer pain from bone metastasis was also eliminated in seven out of eight patients treated with intrathecal calcitonin. Twice-daily systemic administration for 4 days relieved metastatic bone pain caused by multi-

ple myeloma (Allan 1983). Phantom limb pain, treated during the early postoperative period, was relieved by salmon calcitonin infusion during a double-blind placebo-controlled study (Jaeger and Maier 1992).

Somatostatin. The value of somatostatin is its ability to inhibit the release of substance P. Somatostatin, 25 μg/minute administered intravenously for 20 minutes, helped some patients who had cluster headache. Somatostatin was superior to placebo and ergotamine in this study (Sicuteri et al. 1984). Somatostatin can inhibit pain but can also cause vasculopathy and neurotoxicity. However, Penn and colleagues (1992) reported the safe and effective use of a somatostatin analogue, octreotide, in six cases of morphine tolerance—in two cases the effect lasted for longer than 1 year. The annual cost of several thousand dollars precludes the use of octreotide (Penn et al. 1992).

Substance P. Substance P enhances pain transmission through the spinal cord by activation of NMDA. Comodulators of substance P include HVA and NMDA (Mjellem-Joly et al. 1992). By depleting substance P, capsaicin (cream, 0.025%) can desensitize peripheral nociceptive terminals to pain. It is used for relief of pain associated with cluster headache (Sicuteri et al. 1990), hyperalgesia (Simone et al. 1989), herpetic neuralgia, diabetic neuropathic pain, postmastectomy pain, and arthritis (Watson and Evans 1992). In a double-blind, randomized, placebo-controlled trial of capsaicin in 101 patients, pain was reduced by 33% in patients with osteoarthritis and by 57% in patients with rheumatoid arthritis (Genderm Corporation 1993).

Antidepressants

The mechanism for an antidepressant's action as an analgesic is best thought of as monoaminergic rather than as antidepressant (Garattini and Samanin 1988). The pain relief obtained from antidepressants is often independent of effects on mood or the alleviation of major depression (Feinmann 1985; Godefroy et al. 1986; Goodkin and Gulion 1989). Potential pain-relieving effects of antidepressants include local anesthetic membrane-stabilizing effects, antihistaminic effects, peptide synergy, and binding to brain opiate receptors. The greatest response to antidepressants in patients with headaches often occurs among those who do not have depression (Max et al. 1987).

Efficacy. There are several reviews of antidepressants used in pain syndromes. Each author describes a wide range of generally positive but poorly designed studies (Feinmann 1985; Getto et al. 1987). It seems that although some patients' pain may respond to low doses of antidepressants, a complete trial of an antidepressant in pain requires a full-dose regimen.

In an effort to extract meaning from the pain-antidepressant data, Onghena and Van Houdenhove (1992) conducted a meta-analysis of 39 controlled trials of antidepressants for nonmalignant pain. Of these, 28 studies showed a statistically significant difference between drug and placebo. Overall, the average patient with chronic pain who received an antidepressant had less pain than 74% of those who received placebo.

Conclusions about antidepressants and pain. Analgesic effects are at least partly independent of antidepressant effects. The degree of the analgesic effect is not significantly different in the presence or absence of depression. Therefore, a trial of antidepressant medication in any chronic pain condition is warranted regardless of whether the patient is depressed.

Serotonin reuptake blockade is not essential to pain relief. There is doubt about the efficacy of purely serotonergic drugs for neuropathic pain (i.e., fluoxetine, zimelidine, and trazodone) (Gourlay et al. 1986; Max 1992; Watson and Evans 1985). No singular biochemical profile or type of antidepressant is clearly superior for pain control. Monoamine oxidase inhibitors (MAOIs) are probably as useful as tricyclics or SSRIs for pain, especially in patients with atypical facial pain, myofascial pain, atypical depression, or depression that has not responded to other antidepressants.

Stimulants

Stimulants, namely methylphenidate and amphetamine, are effective analgesic adjuncts. They decrease pain as well as sedation produced by opiates. These benefits occur rapidly (6–48 hours), tolerance is not usually a problem, and side effects quickly disappear when the drug is stopped or decreased. Patients with postoperative pain and pediatric patients with cancer respond well to analgesic-stimulant combinations. One of the most quoted studies is Forrest and associates' (1977) double-blind administration of 5–10 mg of intramuscular dextroamphetamine with morphine. The combination doubled the acute postoperative pain relief achieved by morphine alone, while it also improved cognition and lessened sedation.

Methylphenidate has a 2- to 7-hour half-life, compared with dextroamphetamine's unpredictable 4- to 21-hour half-life (Frierson et al. 1991). This finding may explain the clinical perception that methylphenidate is better tolerated (Katon and Roskind 1980).

Neuroleptics

Neuroleptics are usually not thought of as analgesics. However, analgesic effects are reported for some neuroleptics, such as haloperidol. The most interesting potential explanation for this analgesic effect is that haloperidol binds to sigma opiate receptors. Levomepromazine (15 mg) compared favorably to morphine (10 mg) in a double-blind study by Bloomfield and colleagues (1964). Phenothiazines and butyrophenones all have some pain-relieving effects

(Farber and Burks 1974; Nathan 1978).

The genesis of clinical interest in neuroleptics as analgesics came from the finding that a combination of amitriptyline and prolixin relieved one of the most resistant pain syndromes, postherpetic neuralgia (Taub 1973). Diabetic neuropathy also responded to the amitriptyline-prolixin combination (J. L. Davis et al. 1977). It is common clinical lore, unproven by rigorous study, that a neuroleptic combined with an antidepressant is more potent for pain relief than either medication used alone (Zitman et al. 1991).

◼ REHABILITATION

Rehabilitation of patients who have chronic pain syndromes typically combines the disciplines of physiatry, physical therapy, psychiatry, behavioral psychology, and neurology. Successful rehabilitation requires an integrated approach to mind-body issues. A consultation-liaison psychiatrist is in a good position to help with this integration, both with imparting knowledge and with coordinating pain therapy. Psychiatrists can prescribe neuropsychopharmacological agents, transcutaneous electrical nerve stimulation (TENS), behavioral therapies, and psychotherapy.

Transcutaneous Electrical Nerve Stimulation

Although TENS is no panacea, it has received nonspecific criticism as a pain treatment. This criticism is partially the result of errors in the use of TENS. A common mistake made with TENS is using continuous, or nonintermittent, nonpulsed stimulation, which leads to rapid tolerance. Burst intermittent stimulation is generally more helpful. The second error is using TENS for central pain disorders, which it can exacerbate. Neuralgia without a central component responds quite well, however. The third error is excessively strong stimulation, which leads to muscle contraction that exacerbates the pain. TENS should be a subsensory-threshold stimulus. Used judiciously, it can be quite effective. When used appropriately, half of long-term TENS users have their pain reduced by more than one-half. TENS can help restore a sense of self-control and avoids medication side effects.

Cognitive and Behavioral Therapies

Fernandez and Turk (1989) performed a meta-analysis on the use of cognitive strategies for the alteration of pain perception. Imagery methods were the most effective, whereas positive expectancy was equivalent to no treatment. The reality is that patients often use cognitive imagery methods themselves, typically in combination with other methods of pain control. Combined therapies are in wide use but have not been assiduously studied. In their extensive review, Turner and Chapman (1982a, 1982b) examined relaxation training, biofeedback, operant conditioning, hypnosis, and cognitive-behavior therapy and concluded that biofeedback and relaxation training were probably equally effective for headache and that evidence for the efficacy of the other therapies was inconclusive. Data necessary for evaluation of long-term benefits do not exist in the published literature.

Psychotherapy

Coping is a euphemism to describe the sum of many things, such as attachment behavior and intrapsychic defenses (Jensen and Romano 1991). Coping is also context-dependent, which means that coping skills are most effective when the focus includes the patient and his or her partner or family (Manne and Zautra 1990). Therefore, efforts to improve a patient's ability to cope must include more than education and counseling. The psychological aspects of coping involve conflicts over autonomy and care. To help the patient to cope, the psychiatrist must be a teacher, doctor, soothsayer, and wise friend with the right mixture of palliative care, hope, denial, catharsis, family counseling, relaxation, exercise, physical rehabilitation, pharmacotherapy, and sensitivity to the unconscious.

Multidisciplinary Pain Clinics

In one study, comprehensive multidisciplinary treatment returned 48% of 42 patients to work and an additional 28% to vocational rehabilitation. None of the 15 control subjects improved (Deardorff et al. 1991). Aranoff's (1985) review of follow-up studies of pain clinics suggested that at least 50% of patients achieved some benefit from this multidisciplinary approach. Multidisciplinary pain clinics are successful because they work at the interface of psychiatry, neurology, psychology, and physical therapy. Recognition and treatment of psychiatric illness in patients with chronic pain are also very cost-effective. For example, proper treatment of hypochondriasis reduces dollar costs by 53%; recognition and treatment of somatization disorder save an average of $5,000 per year per patient (Bouckoms and Hackett 1991; Smith et al. 1986). Multidisciplinary pain clinics are useful for some patients with chronic pain (Gach 1983; Manniche et al. 1991; Schatz 1991).

There is danger in overemphasizing behavioral explanations for chronic pain because most pain is driven not by behavioral maladaptation but rather by intransigent physical pathology. There is also a danger in claiming that behavioral methods relieve pain. Behavioral treatments are not intended primarily to relieve pain but rather to extinguish the behaviors associated with it (Fordyce 1985).

The following are recommendations for determining which patients should be referred to a multidisciplinary pain clinic:

■ Diagnosis of the physical and psychiatric pathology is already complete or is so obscure that intensive observation is necessary (e.g., malingering suspected).
■ Consultation from an independent physi-

cian, who is an expert in the treatment of chronic pain, confirms that no single modality of outpatient treatment is likely to work.
■ Patient has gotten maximum benefit from outpatient treatment (e.g., nonsteroidal drugs, nerve blocks, antidepressants, simple physical and behavioral rehabilitation).
■ Intensive daily interventions are required, usually with multiple concurrent types of therapy, such as nerve blocks, physical therapy, and behavior modification.
■ If behavior modification is the focus of the clinic, then the patient must exhibit abnormal pain behavior.
■ Medications for the pain are so complex or compliance management so difficult that direct supervision of medical therapy is necessary (e.g., high-dose narcotics or drug abuse).
■ A medication contract is mutually acceptable for patient and doctor (Bouckoms 1994).

CONCLUSION

The consultation-liaison psychiatrist is a key person in the evaluation, management, and treatment of the patient with chronic pain because no physician from any other specialty is as prepared to examine the patient psychiatrically and physically; to prescribe neuropsychopharmacological, psychological, and adjunctive therapies; and to integrate these therapies into a rehabilitation program for the patient (Bouckoms 1988). The psychiatrist can assume all these responsibilities as a pain expert or can provide consultation to a team of caregivers.

The complexity of issues surrounding the diagnosis and treatment of patients with chronic pain syndromes is increasing as we learn more about CNS dysfunction in pain while attempting to manage patients' conditions using the least costly treatments. Effective pain therapies in the future will rest on the judicious selection of medical, psychiatric, and rehabilitation modalities that are tailored to an individual's needs.

◼ REFERENCES

Aanonsen LM, Wilcox GL: Nociceptive action of excitatory amino acids in the mouse: effects of spinally administered opioids, phencyclidine and sigma agonists. J Pharmacol Exp Ther 243:9–19, 1987

Allan E: Calcitonin in the treatment of intractable pain from advanced malignancy. Pharmatherapeutica 3:482–486, 1983

Allen MH: Detoxification considerations in the medical management of substance abuse in pregnancy. Bulletin of the New York Academy of Medicine 67:270–276, 1991

American Psychiatric Association: Diagnostic and Statistical Manual of Mental Disorders, 4th Edition. Washington, DC, American Psychiatric Association, 1994

Anderson EG, Proudfit HK: The functional role of the bulbospinal serotonergic system, in Serotonin Neurotransmission and Behavior. Edited by Jacobs BL, Gelperin A. Cambridge, MA, MIT Press, 1981, pp 307–338

Antczak-Bouckoms AA, Bouckoms AJ: Affective disturbance and denial of problems in dental patients with pain. International Journal of Psychosomatics 32:9–11, 1985

Aranoff GM: Evaluation and Treatment of Chronic Pain. Baltimore, MD, Urban & Schwarzenberg, 1985

Arner S: Intravenous phentolamine test: diagnostic and prognostic use in reflex sympathetic dystrophy. Pain 48:17–22, 1991

Arner S, Meyerson BA: Lack of analgesic effect of opioids on neuropathic and idiopathic forms of pain. Pain 33:11–23, 1988

Baringa M: The brain remaps its own contours. Science 258:216–218, 1992

Barsky A, Wool C, Barnett M, et al: Histories of childhood trauma in adult hypochondriacal patients. Am J Psychiatry 151:397–401, 1994

Bloomfield S, Simard-Savoie S, Bernier J, et al: Comparative analgesic activity of levopromazine and morphine in patients with chronic pain. Can Med Assoc J 90:1156–1159, 1964

Bonelli S, Conoscente F, Movilia FG, et al: Regional intravenous guanethidine vs. stellate ganglion block in reflex sympathetic dystrophies: a randomized trial. Pain 16:297–307, 1983

Bouckoms AJ: Intravenous lorazepam for pain relief of intractable neuralgia. Pain 32 (suppl 4):S347–S472, 1987

Bouckoms AJ: Pharmacological treatment of severe pain and suffering in the critically ill. Problems in Critical Care 2:47–62, 1988

Bouckoms AJ: Pain Outpatient Psychiatry, Diagnosis and Treatment, 2nd Edition. Baltimore, MD, Williams & Wilkins, 1989, pp 301–303

Bouckoms AJ: Chronic pain: neuropsychopharmacology and adjunctive psychiatric treatment, in American Psychiatric Press Textbook of Consultation-Liaison Psychiatry. Edited by Rundell JR, Wise MG. Washington, DC, American Psychiatric Press, 1994, pp 1007–1036

Bouckoms AJ, Hackett TP: The pain patient: evaluation and treatment, in Massachusetts General Hospital Handbook of General Hospital Psychiatry, 3rd Edition. Edited by Cassem NH. St Louis, MO, CV Mosby, 1991, pp 39–68

Bouckoms AJ, Litman RE: Clonazepam in the treatment of neuralgic pain syndromes. Psychosomatics 26:933–936, 1985

Bouckoms AJ, Litman RE, Baer L: Denial in the depressive and pain-prone disorders of chronic pain. Clin J Pain 1:165–169, 1985

Bouckoms AJ, Poletti CH, Sweet WH, et al: Trigeminal facial pain: a model of peptides and monoamines in intracerebral cerebrospinal fluid. Agressologie 32:271–274, 1991

Bouckoms AJ, Masand PS, Murray GB, et al: Non-malignant pain treated with long term oral narcotics. Ann Clin Psychiatry 4:185–192, 1992

Bowsher D: Acute herpes zoster and postherpetic neuralgia: effects of acyclovir and outcome of treatment with amitriptyline. Br J Gen Pract 42(359):244–246, 1992

Campbell SM, Clark S, Tindall EA, et al: Clinical characteristics of fibrositis, I: a "blinded" controlled study of symptoms and tender points. Arthritis Rheum 26:817–824, 1983

Coderre TJ, Katz J, Vaccarino AL, et al: Contribution of central neuroplasticity to pathological pain: review of clinical and experimental evidence. Pain 52:259–285, 1993

Coombs DW, Saunders RL, Fratkin JD, et al: Continuous intrathecal hydromorphone and clonidine for intractable cancer pain. J Neurosurg 64:890–894, 1986

Davis JL, Gerich JE, Schultz TA: Peripheral diabetic neuropathy treated with amitriptyline and fluphenazine. JAMA 238:2291–2292, 1977

Davis KD, Treede RD, Raja SN, et al: Topical application of clonidine relieves hyperalgesia in patients with sympathetically maintained pain. Pain 47:309–317, 1991

Deardorff W, Rubin H, Scott D: Comprehensive multidisciplinary treatment of chronic pain: a follow-up study of treated and non-treated groups. Pain 45:35–44, 1991

Dejgard A, Petersen P, Kastrup J: Mexiletine for treatment of chronic painful diabetic neuropathy. Lancet 1:9–11, 1988

Deyo RA, Rainville J, Kent DL: What can the history and physical examination tell us about low back pain? JAMA 268:760–765, 1992

Dubner R: Pain and hyperalgesia following tissue injury: new mechanisms and new treatments. Pain 44:213–214, 1991

Eschalier A, Kayser V, Guilbaud G: Influence of a specific 5-HT3 antagonist on carrageenan-induced hyperalgesia in rats. Pain 36:249–255, 1989

Farber GA, Burks JW: Chlorprothixene therapy for herpes zoster neuralgia. South Med J 67:808–812, 1974

Feinmann C: Pain relief by antidepressants. Pain 23:1–8, 1985

Fernandez E, Turk DC: The utility of cognitive coping strategies for altering pain perception: a meta-analysis. Pain 38:123–135, 1989

Fields HL: Editorial comment. Pain 49:161–162, 1992

Fordyce WE: Behavioral Methods for Chronic Pain and Illness. St Louis, MO, CV Mosby, 1976

Fordyce W: The behavioral management of chronic pain: a response to critics. Pain 22:113–125, 1985

Forrest W, Brown B, Brown C: Dextroamphetamine with morphine for treatment of postoperative pain. N Engl J Med 296:712–715, 1977

Fricton J, Awad E: Advances in Pain Research and Therapy. New York, Raven, 1990

Frierson RL, Wey JJ, Tabler JB: Psychostimulants for depression in the medically ill. Am Fam Physician 43:163–170, 1991

Fromm GH: Physiological rationale for the treatment of neuropathic pain. American Pain Society Journal 2(1):1–7, 1993

Gach MR: The Bum Back Book. Berkeley, CA, Acu Press, 1983

Gamsa A: Is emotional disturbance a precipitator or a consequence of chronic pain? Pain 42:183–195, 1990

Garattini S, Samanin R: Biochemical hypotheses on antidepressant drugs: a guide for clinicians or a toy for pharmacologists? Psychol Med 18:287–304, 1988

Genderm Corporation: Enhanced pain control in patients with osteoarthritis and rheumatoid arthritis following treatment with topical capsaicin (Study Report No 87–04). Genderm Corporation, 1993

Getto CJ, Sorkness CA, Howell T: Antidepressants and chronic nonmalignant pain: a review. J Pain Symptom Manage 2:9–18, 1987

Godefroy F, Butler SH, Weil-Fugazza J, et al: Do acute or chronic tricyclic antidepressants modify morphine antinociception in arthritic rats? Pain 25:233–244, 1986

Goodkin G, Gulion CM: Antidepressants for the relief of chronic pain: do they work? Ann Behav Med 11:83–101, 1989

Gourlay GK, Cherry DA, Cousins MJ, et al: A controlled study of a serotonin reuptake blocker, zimelidine, in the treatment of chronic pain. Pain 25:35–52, 1986

Griffen T, McIntire D, Buchanan G: High dose intravenous methylprednisolone therapy for pain in children and adolescents with sickle cell disease. N Engl J Med 330:733–737, 1994

Hathaway SR, McKinley JC: Minnesota Multiphasic Personality Inventory. Minneapolis, MN, University of Minnesota, 1943

Hering R, Kuritzky A: Sodium valproate in the treatment of cluster headache: an open clinical trial. Cephalalgia 9:195–198, 1989

Hering R, Kuritzky A: Sodium valproate in the prophylactic treatment of migraine: a double blind study versus placebo. Cephalalgia 12:81–84, 1992

Holmes V, Rafuls W, Bouckoms AJ: Covert psychopathology in chronic pain. Clinical Diagnosis 2(2):79–85, 1986

Jaeger H, Maier C: Calcitonin in phantom limb pain: a double blind study. Pain 48:21–27, 1992

Janig W: Experimental approach to reflex sympathetic dystrophy and related symptoms. Pain 47:241–245, 1991

Jensen MP, Romano JA: Coping with chronic pain: a critical review of the literature. Pain 47:249–283, 1991

Katon W, Roskind M: Treatment of depression in medically ill elderly with methylphenidate. Am J Psychology 137:963–965, 1980

Kishore-Kumar R, Max MB, Schafer SC: Desipramine relieves postherpetic neuralgia. Clin Pharmacol Ther 47:305–312, 1990

Kohler T, Kosnaic S: Are persons with migraine characterized by a high degree of ambition, orderliness, and rigidity? Pain 48:321–323, 1992

Lance JW: 5-Hydroxytryptamine and its role in migraine. Eur Neurol 31:278–281, 1991

Liebeskind JC: Pain can kill. Pain 44:3–4, 1991

Maciewicz R, Bouckoms AJ, Martin J: Drug therapy of neuropathic pain. Clin J Pain 1:39–49, 1985

Manne SL, Zautra AJ: Couples coping with chronic illness: women with rheumatoid arthritis and their healthy husbands. J Behav Med 13:327–342, 1990

Manniche C, Lundberg E, Christensen I, et al: Intensive dynamic back exercises for chronic low back pain: a clinical trial. Pain 47:53–63, 1991

Mao J, Price DO, Hayes RL, et al: MK 801, an NMDA antagonist and peripheral nerve block synergistically reduce painful symptoms in a rat model of mononeuropathy. Brain 51:254–262, 1992

Marchettini P, Lacerenza M, Marangoni C, et al: Lidocaine test in neuralgia. Pain 48:377–382, 1992

Martin C, Martin A, Rud C, et al: Experimental data has shown that sodium valproate has analgesic properties in animals, probably by way of the increase in cerebral and spinal gamma amino-butyric acid (GABA) it induces. Ann Fr Anesth Reanim 7:387–392, 1988

Max MB: Improving outcomes of analgesic treatment: is education enough? International Association for the Study of Pain Newsletter, November–December, 1992, pp 2–6

Max MB, Culnane M, Schafer SC: Amitriptyline relieves diabetic neuropathy pain in patients with normal or depressed mood. Neurology 37:589–596, 1987

Max MB, Lynch SA, Muir J, et al: Effects of desipramine, amitriptyline, and fluoxetine on pain in diabetic neuropathy. N Engl J Med 326:1250–1288, 1992

Mjellem-Joly N, Lund A, Odd-Geir B, et al: Intrathecal co-administration of substance P and NMDA augments nociceptive responses in the formalin test. Pain 51:195–198, 1992

Moldofsky H, Scarisbrick P, England R: Musculoskeletal symptoms and non-REM sleep disturbances in patients with "fibrositic" syndromes and healthy subjects. Psychosom Med 37:341–351, 1975

Nathan PW: Chlorprothixene (taractan) in postherpetic neuralgia and other severe chronic pains. Pain 5:367–371, 1978

Onghena P, Van Houdenhove B: Antidepressant-induced analgesia in chronic non-malignant pain: a meta-analysis of 39 placebo-controlled studies. Pain 49:205–219, 1992

Osterweis M, Kleinman A, Mechanic D: Institute of Medicine's Committee on Pain, Disability, and Chronic Illness Behavior. Washington, DC, National Academy Press, 1987

Penn R, Paice J, Kroin J: Octreotide: a new non-opiate analgesic for intrathecal infusion. Pain 49:13–19, 1992

Portenoy RK, Foley KM: Chronic use of opioid analgesics in non-malignant pain: report of 38 cases. Pain 25:171–186, 1986

Reed JL: Hysteria. British Journal of Psychiatry Special Publication No 9, 1975, pp 141–149

Reich J, Tupin J, Abramowitz S: Psychiatric diagnosis of chronic pain patients. Am J Psychiatry 140:1495–1498, 1983

Rumore MM, Schlichting DA: Clinical efficacy of antihistamines as analgesics. Pain 25:7–22, 1986

Schatz MP: Back Care Basics. Berkeley, CA, Rodmell Press, 1991

Sicuteri F, Geppetti P, Marabini S, et al: Pain relief by somatostatin in attacks of cluster headache. Pain 18:359–365, 1984

Sicuteri F, Fanciullaci M, Nicolodi M, et al: Substance P theory: a unique focus on the painful and painless phenomena of cluster headache. Headache 30:69–79, 1990

Silberstein S, Saper J, Mathew NT: The safety and efficacy of divalproex sodium in the prophylaxis of migraine headache: a multicenter, double blind, placebo-controlled trial (abstract). American Association for the Study of Headache, San Francisco, CA, June 1993

Simone DA, Baumann TK, LaMotte RH: Dose-dependent pain and mechanical hyperalgesia in humans after intradermal injection of capsaicin. Pain 38:99–107, 1989

Smith JR, Monson RA, Ray DC: Psychiatric consultation in somatization disorder. N Engl J Med 314:1407–1413, 1986

Sweet WH: Deafferentation pain after posterior rhizotomy, trauma to a limb, and herpes zoster. Neurosurgery 15:928–932, 1984

Taub A: Relief of postherpetic neuralgia with psychotropic drugs. J Neurosurg 39:235–239, 1973

Taylor H, Curran NM (eds): Nuprin Pain Report. New York, Louis Harris and Associates, September 1985

Turner JA, Chapman CR: Psychological interventions for chronic pain: a critical review, I: relaxation training and biofeedback. Pain 12:1–21, 1982a

Turner JA, Chapman CR: Psychological interventions for chronic pain: a critical review, II: operant conditioning, hypnosis, and cognitive behavioral therapy. Pain 12:23–46, 1982b

Tverskoy M, Cozavoc C, Ayache M, et al: Postoperative pain after inguinal herniorrhaphy with different types of anesthesia. Anesth Analg 70:29–35, 1990

Ventafridda V, Tamburini M, Caraceni A, et al: A validation study of the WHO method of cancer pain relief. Cancer 59:850–856, 1987

Walker EA, Katon WJ, Neraas K, et al: Dissociation in woman with chronic pelvic pain. Am J Psychiatry 149:534–536, 1992

Wall PD: The prevention of postoperative pain (editorial). Pain 33:289–290, 1988

Wall PD: The placebo effect: an unpopular topic. Pain 51:1–3, 1992

Watson CPN, Evans RJ: A comparative trial of amitriptyline and zimelidine in postherpetic neuralgia. Pain 23:387–394, 1985

Watson CPN, Evans RJ: The postmastectomy pain syndrome and topical capsaicin: a randomized trial. Pain 51:375–379, 1992

Weintraub MI: Regional pain is usually hysterical. Arch Neurol 45:914–915, 1988

Weintraub MI: Litigation chronic pain syndrome—a distinct entity: analysis of 210 cases. American Journal of Pain Management 2:198–204, 1992

Wolfe F, Cathay M: The epidemiology of tender points: a prospective study of 1520 patients. J Rheumatol 12:1164–1168, 1985

Woolf CJ, Thompson SWN: The induction and maintenance of central sensitization is dependent on N-methyl-d-aspartic acid receptor activation; implications for the treatment of post-injury pain hypersensitivity states. Pain 44:293–299, 1991

World Health Organization: 1990 Cancer pain relief and palliative care. Geneva, World Health Organization, 1990

Yunus M, Masi AT, Calbro JJ, et al: Primary fibromyalgia (fibrositis): clinical study of 50 patients with matched normal controls. Semin Arthritis Rheum 11:151–171, 1981

Zitman FG, Linseen ACG, Edelbroek PM, et al: Does addition of low-dose flupentixol enhance the analgesic effects of low-dose amitriptyline in somatoform pain disorder? Pain 47:25–30, 1991

Chapter 32

Electroconvulsive Therapy: An Overview

Mark D. Beale, M.D.
Charles H. Kellner, M.D.

E lectroconvulsive therapy (ECT) has been in continuous use as a treatment for patients with severe psychiatric illness since its introduction in 1938 (Cerletti and Bini 1938). ECT is now, more than ever, an integral and effective part of the psychiatric armamentarium. In this chapter, we review those aspects of ECT that are most relevant to the consultation-liaison psychiatrist. Additional information on the application of ECT to medically ill patients is available in other references (e.g., Abrams 1992; Knos and Sung 1993; Weiner and Coffey 1993).

■ INDICATIONS

ECT is most commonly used in cases of severe depression, both bipolar and unipolar. It is also used for patients who are in the manic phase of bipolar illness and in mixed affective states (American Psychiatric Association Task Force on Electroconvulsive Therapy 1990). Addi-

tionally, ECT is indicated for schizoaffective disorder, for schizophrenia with catatonic or prominent affective features, or when there is a history of favorable response to ECT (American Psychiatric Association Task Force on Electroconvulsive Therapy 1990) (Table 32–1).

ECT is typically prescribed only after a patient fails to respond adequately to psychotropic medications; however, it is used as a first-line treatment in several specific instances

Table 32–1. Indications for electroconvulsive therapy

Major depressive episode (unipolar and bipolar)
Mania
Mixed affective state
Catatonia
Schizophrenia with prominent affective symptoms
Schizoaffective disorder

Source. American Psychiatric Association Task Force on Electroconvulsive Therapy 1990.

(Table 32–2), including the following: 1) when there is a need for rapid improvement in depression for medical or psychiatric reasons (e.g., malnutrition, catatonia, or suicidality); 2) when the risks of other treatments outweigh the risks of ECT; 3) when the patient has a history of favorable response to ECT; or 4) when the patient prefers to proceed directly to ECT (American Psychiatric Association Task Force on Electroconvulsive Therapy 1990). ECT is also indicated when a patient cannot tolerate the side effects of psychotropic medications or when his or her condition deteriorates to the point at which a more rapid and definitive treatment is required.

SITUATIONS OF INCREASED RISK

There are no absolute contraindications and few relative contraindications to ECT. The psychiatrist will sometimes choose to treat a patient with ECT despite the presence of medical risk factors. Situations that increase risk are listed in Table 32–3.

CONSENT AND PRETREATMENT EVALUATION

Informed consent should be obtained from the patient and, if possible, from the patient's family before ECT is begun. In cases in which informed consent cannot be given by the patient,

it should be obtained from whoever is legally responsible for the patient's care. Information about ECT should be presented in such a way that it does not frighten the patient. Depressed patients often have difficulty processing new information and making decisions, and the psychiatrist should be sensitive to this during the consent process.

The pretreatment evaluation (Table 32–4) must include a medical history, physical examination, psychiatric history, mental status examination, complete blood count (CBC), electrolyte measurements, and electrocardiogram (ECG). Computed tomography (CT) or magnetic resonance imaging (MRI) of the brain is sometimes necessary for patients in consultation-liaison settings to rule out space-occupying lesions and/or increased intracranial pressure (ICP). If no brain image is obtained, particular attention should be paid to the funduscopic examination to rule out papilledema. An electroencephalogram (EEG) may be helpful in detecting previously undiagnosed organic brain disease (e.g., delirium or toxic-metabolic encephalopathy). Anesthesia consultation is an important part of the evaluation before ECT. Other consultations may be obtained (e.g., neurology, cardiology) if history, physical examination, or laboratory findings suggest the need for further evaluation.

Because no additive benefit has been demonstrated, we advise tapering and discontinuation of most psychotropic medications before a course of ECT. Neuroleptics may be given dur-

Table 32–2. Indications for electroconvulsive therapy as a first-line treatment

When there is a need for rapid improvement
  Suicidality
  Malnutrition
  Catatonia
  Severe psychosis with agitation
When other treatments are considered more risky
  Elderly patients
  Pregnancy
When the patient prefers electroconvulsive therapy

Table 32–3. Situations of increased risk

Space-occupying cerebral lesion
Increased intracranial pressure
Recent myocardial infarction
Recent hemorrhagic cerebrovascular accident
Unstable aneurysm
Retinal detachment
Pheochromocytoma

Source. Adapted from American Psychiatric Association Task Force on Electroconvulsive Therapy 1990.

Table 32–4. Evaluation before electroconvulsive therapy

Medical and psychiatric history
Physical examination
Mental status examination
Complete blood count
Serum electrolytes
Liver function tests
Electrocardiogram
Anesthesia consultation
Consider
  Computed tomography or magnetic resonance imaging of the head
  Electroencephalogram
  Chest X ray

ing ECT, with the dosage decreased as the patient's agitation and psychosis subside over the course of several ECT treatments. It is especially important to discontinue lithium because delirium has been reported in patients given ECT and lithium (Weiner et al. 1980). Other possible adverse interactions include a risk of prolonged seizures and status epilepticus in patients with high serum theophylline levels, a risk of cardiac arrhythmias in patients taking antidepressants (McCracken and Kosanin 1984), impaired efficacy in patients taking benzodiazepines (Pettinati et al. 1990), and increased seizure threshold in patients taking anticonvulsants (including benzodiazepines).

ELECTROCONVULSIVE THERAPY TECHNIQUE

A typical treatment sequence is described in Tables 32–5 and 32–6. Before ECT, the patient should receive nothing by mouth for 6–8 hours other than cardiac drugs and medications for gastric reflux. An intravenous catheter is placed in the patient's arm, and the patient is given either intravenous atropine, 0.4–1.0 mg, or intravenous glycopyrrolate, 0.2–0.4 mg, to reduce the risk of vagally mediated bradyarrhythmias (American Psychiatric Association Task Force on Electroconvulsive Therapy 1990). Light general anesthesia is then induced with intrave-

nous methohexital, 0.75–1.0 mg/kg (American Psychiatric Association Task Force on Electroconvulsive Therapy 1990). Intravenous succinylcholine, 0.5–1.0 mg/kg, is administered to produce muscle relaxation (American Psychiatric Association Task Force on Electroconvulsive Therapy 1990). A blood pressure cuff is inflated on the right ankle before injection of the succinylcholine ("cuffed limb" method). This is done so that the clinician can observe motor activity associated with the seizure. While the patient is unconscious, 100% oxygen is administered by Ambu bag and mask.

Stimulus electrodes are placed on the head, and once neuromuscular block is complete (Beale et al. 1994a), the electrical stimulus is delivered and the seizure, measured by both motor and EEG evidence, is timed and recorded. If a seizure does not occur, or if motor

Table 32–5. Orders before electroconvulsive therapy

Patient should take nothing by mouth after midnight
Patient should void before transport to electroconvulsive therapy session
If cardiac drugs or medications for gastric reflux are prescribed, these should be taken with a sip of water about 2 hours before treatment

Table 32–6. Electroconvulsive therapy technique

Place intravenous catheter
Give glycopyrrolate (0.2–0.4 mg intravenously)
Give methohexital (0.75–1.0 mg/kg intravenously)
Inflate blood pressure cuff on right ankle
Give succinylcholine (0.5–1.0 mg/kg intravenously)
Ventilate with 100% oxygen by Ambu bag and mask
Deliver stimulus when muscle relaxation is achieved and bite block is in place

activity lasts for less than 20 seconds, restimulation is performed at a higher stimulus intensity. A seizure is terminated if it lasts longer than 3 minutes (American Psychiatric Association Task Force on Electroconvulsive Therapy 1990). Commonly, seizures are terminated by administration of 50%–100% of the original dose of methohexital. If this drug does not terminate the seizure, intravenous diazepam, 5–15 mg, or intravenous midazolam, 1–3 mg, may be used (Abrams 1992).

Electrode Placement

Two types of stimulus electrode placement are commonly used in ECT—*bilateral* (bifrontotemporal) and *nondominant-unilateral* (d'Elia 1970). Bilateral electrode placement is associated with a more robust and rapid therapeutic response, but it also causes more cognitive impairment (Abrams 1992). Nondominant-unilateral ECT causes less cognitive impairment, but some patients may not respond to it and may need to be switched to bilateral treatments after several sessions (Abrams 1992). We recommend that the choice of electrode placement be based on severity of illness. Patients with severe illness, those who are suicidal, or those with psychosis should receive bilateral ECT; patients without psychosis who are less severely ill should initially receive nondominant-unilateral ECT. In addition, the clinician may change electrode placement during a course of treatment, depending on the patient's response.

Currently available ECT devices (e.g., MECTA and THYMATRON) deliver a constant-current, brief-pulse, square-wave stimulus. This type of stimulus, when compared with the sine-wave current generated by older ECT machines, causes less cognitive impairment (Weiner et al. 1986).

Stimulus Dosing

Several methods for selecting the stimulus dose in ECT have been proposed. For example, it

has been recommended that the dose be selected based on the patient's age (e.g., 50 years equals 50% stimulus intensity on the THYMATRON DGX machine) (Swartz and Abrams 1994). Others estimate the dose based on a combination of patient characteristics (e.g., age, gender) (MECTA 1986). A third method is the administration of a relatively high, fixed dose to all patients (Abrams et al. 1991).

Although seizure threshold estimates may be valid in some cases, the inherent variability of this individual characteristic may lead to excessively high doses being administered to patients whose seizure threshold does not fall within the estimated range (Beale et al. 1994b). It has been demonstrated that excessively high stimulus doses contribute to cognitive impairment in patients receiving ECT (Ottoson 1960; Weiner et al. 1986). Therefore, we recommend "tailoring" the stimulus dose to individual patients using the technique of stimulus dose titration first reported by Sackeim and colleagues (1987). This involves giving successive, incremental stimuli at the first session until a seizure is produced. The seizure threshold is then estimated to be the midpoint between the stimulus producing a seizure and the previous stimulus that did not cause a seizure. At the second treatment, the patient is given a stimulus dose slightly above seizure threshold for bilateral ECT and about 2.5 times threshold for nondominant-unilateral ECT (Sackeim et al. 1987). Other variations of the dose titration method are published (Sackeim et al. 1987), and the practitioner should consult the instruction manual that accompanies his or her ECT device.

Treatments are usually given three times per week on alternate days in a course of 6–12 treatments. Treatments are usually discontinued when the patient has reached his or her best achievable baseline. The Mini-Mental State Exam (Folstein et al. 1975) and the Hamilton Rating Scale for Depression (Hamilton 1960) are used to monitor cognitive effects and clinical improvement, respectively.

ADVERSE EFFECTS

The most bothersome, commonly observed effect of ECT is transient cognitive impairment, usually in verbal memory (American Psychiatric Association Task Force on Electroconvulsive Therapy 1990). If a patient experiences significant cognitive impairment during a course of ECT, the physician should review medications, spacing of treatments, and ECT technique (i.e., laterality of electrode placement, stimulus dosing) (American Psychiatric Association Task Force on Electroconvulsive Therapy 1990) (Table 32–7). If bilateral electrode placement is being used, switching to nondominant-unilateral placement minimizes cognitive effects and may allow continuation of the ECT course. If treatments are being administered thrice weekly, reducing the frequency to twice or once weekly should be considered. The physician should also consider decreasing the stimulus dose, especially if bilateral electrode placement is used. If modifications in technique do not solve the problem, interruption or discontinuation of ECT should be considered. In the vast majority of cases, severe cognitive impairment does not occur and, in fact, improved cognitive functioning is often observed as the patient's psychiatric condition improves (Abrams 1992). There are rare reports of patients claiming extensive, permanent memory loss after ECT.

Other complications, including unusually prolonged apnea, persistent cardiovascular dysfunction, and between-treatment seizure activity, are rare. Transient cardiac arrhythmias

Table 32–7. Measures to take if severe cognitive dysfunction develops

Switch from bilateral to unilateral electrode placement

Decrease treatment frequency (from thrice to twice or once weekly)

Decrease stimulus dose

Review concurrent medications for contribution to cognitive dysfunction

frequently occur during and immediately following the seizure but usually do not require any intervention. Myalgias, headache, and nausea are common reactions, are usually self-limited, and respond to symptomatic treatment.

ELECTROCONVULSIVE THERAPY IN PATIENTS WITH MEDICAL ILLNESS

Because the consultation-liaison psychiatrist treats many patients with concurrent, serious medical illnesses, he or she may sometimes need to make modifications in ECT technique.

Central Nervous System Diseases

Parkinson's disease. It has been estimated that up to 40%–60% of patients with Parkinson's disease experience major depression (Brown and Wilson 1972; Oh et al. 1992). ECT is effective in such patients not only for the psychiatric illness but also for the motor symptoms of Parkinson's disease. ECT may be indicated as a primary treatment for patients with Parkinson's disease who have become refractory to antiparkinsonian medications or who cannot tolerate their side effects (Kellner et al. 1994). The mechanism of action is probably related to ECT's dopamine-enhancing effects (Fochtmann 1988).

Dementia. When cognitive impairment is the result of depression (i.e., dementia syndrome of depression or "pseudodementia"), it is likely to improve as the depression improves. When dementia coexists with depression, cognitive function may improve as depression remits (Weiner and Coffey 1987). When patients with dementia experience cognitive worsening with ECT, the treatment frequency should be decreased from thrice to once or twice weekly and, if bilateral electrode placement is being used, a change to nondominant-unilateral placement should be considered (American Psychiatric Association Task Force on Electroconvulsive Therapy 1990).

Central nervous system tumor.   ECT causes a transient increase in ICP, probably the result of increased cerebral blood flow during the seizure (Weiner and Coffey 1987). Increased ICP puts patients with space-occupying lesions at risk for brain herniation during ECT (Savitsky and Kavlinger 1953). However, modifications in technique can allow such patients to receive ECT successfully. These modifications include the use of anti-hypertensives, steroids, osmotic diuretics (e.g., mannitol), and hyperventilation (Abrams 1992; Zwil et al 1990). Not all brain tumors present the same risk. Small, slow-growing or calcified tumors are less dangerous than large malignant tumors of more recent onset (Abrams 1992). For example, small meningiomas probably pose relatively little risk (Goldstein and Richardson 1988; Hsiao and Evans 1984; Kellner et al. 1991a). Thus, once considered an absolute contraindication to ECT, the presence of a brain tumor no longer automatically precludes a patient from receiving ECT (Abrams 1992), but the presence of a brain tumor remains one of the most serious risks (Maltbie et al. 1980).

Subdural hematoma.   A subdural hematoma is also a potential cause of increased ICP and, whenever possible, should be evacuated before ECT. There is at least one report of the successful use of ECT in a patient with a chronic subdural hematoma (Malek-Ahmadi et al. 1990).

Cerebrovascular accident.   There are no specific guidelines regarding how long one should delay ECT in a patient with a recent cerebrovascular accident (CVA) (American Psychiatric Association Task Force on Electroconvulsive Therapy 1990). Generally, waiting weeks to months following a CVA is recommended before proceeding with ECT. The waiting period is particularly important following a hemorrhagic stroke because such patients are at risk for recurrent bleeding during the seizure (Weiner and Coffey 1993). However, if the waiting period is believed to be dangerous itself (because of the severity of the psychiatric illness), ECT may be carried out sooner (Weiner and Coffey 1993). Longer waiting periods are advised if the CVA is large or is associated with significant edema or increased ICP (American Psychiatric Association Task Force on Electroconvulsive Therapy 1990).

ECT has been used safely in patients with cerebrovascular aneurysms, with attention to strict blood pressure control (Husum et al. 1983).

Epilepsy.   Patients with concurrent psychiatric illness and epilepsy can be safely treated with ECT. It is recommended that patients with epilepsy continue to receive their anticonvulsant medications during a course of ECT, although higher stimulus settings are typically necessary to produce adequate seizures (Abrams 1992).

Brain injury or craniotomy.   In patients with a skull fracture or craniotomy, the practitioner should not place ECT stimulus electrodes directly over a skull defect. Patients with recent brain trauma can have prolonged and/or spontaneous seizures and may need treatment with anticonvulsants (e.g., carbamazepine) while receiving ECT.

Intraventricular shunts.   Patients with intraventricular shunts may be treated safely; however, shunt patency must be established before beginning ECT, as shunt blockage may lead to increased ICP (Coffey et al. 1987). Patients should undergo brain imaging and funduscopic examination to rule out increased ICP before ECT begins.

Chronic pain. ECT may be of some benefit in patients with chronic pain, possibly through endorphin release (Mandel 1975). It is not yet clear whether ECT is beneficial only in patients with chronic pain and concomitant depression or if ECT is useful as a treatment for chronic pain alone.

Cardiovascular Disease

Myocardial infarction and ischemic heart disease. Serious cardiac complications are rare in patients who receive ECT; however, such complications represent the most common cause of death associated with ECT (American Psychiatric Association Task Force on Electroconvulsive Therapy 1990). In patients who have had a recent myocardial infarction (MI), it is prudent to wait as long as possible (e.g., 1 month) before beginning ECT. In order to decrease the risk of cardiac ischemia, nitrates, intravenous administration of β-blockers, and careful attention to maximal oxygenation are all important measures. We recommend use of labetalol (5–20 mg iv) or esmolol (5–60 mg iv) in patients with hypertension and/or tachycardia, and nitroglycerine paste or sublingual aerosol in patients with coronary artery disease. Also, regularly prescribed cardiac medications (e.g., antihypertensives or digoxin) should be given with a small sip of water the morning of each ECT.

Arrhythmias. Patients at risk for bradycardia (including those receiving sympathetic blocking agents) should receive an anticholinergic medication (glycopyrrolate or atropine) before each ECT session to protect against worsening bradycardia or asystole (American Psychiatric Association Task Force on Electroconvulsive Therapy 1990). Some practitioners recommend routine use of anticholinergics for all patients receiving ECT, particularly if the stimulus dose titration method is used at the first treatment (Beale et al. 1994a). Patients with tachyarrhythmias (as well as those with hypertension) may be treated with intravenous β-blockers. However, it is common for transient, inconsequential arrhythmias, tachycardia, and hypertension to persist for several minutes after ECT and to resolve spontaneously (Weiner and Coffey 1993). Therefore, unless life-threatening arrhythmias occur, it may be prudent to adopt a "do no harm" approach during the immediate postictal period. Patients who have other arrhythmias present before ECT may need further evaluation by a cardiologist, who can provide recommendations for optimal hemodynamic management during ECT.

Other Medical Conditions

Pulmonary disease. Patients with chronic obstructive pulmonary disease (COPD) or asthma should have these conditions medically optimized before ECT. This may involve obtaining pulmonary function tests and consultation with an internist or pulmonary specialist (Knos and Sung 1993). In patients with reactive airway disease, inhalant bronchodilators (e.g., albuterol, 2 puffs) are recommended before each ECT session (Knos and Sung 1993). Theophylline (and aminophylline) should be avoided or kept in the low therapeutic range (e.g., < 15 µg/mL) to prevent prolonged seizures and/or status epilepticus (Weiner and Coffey 1993).

Cancer. Limited data exist on the use of ECT in depressed cancer patients. In 1967, Goldfarb et al. reported on three patients with advanced carcinomatosis and depression who responded well to cancer chemotherapy and ECT. These authors and others have hypothesized that ECT may have some beneficial effect on immune function, thereby working synergistically with cancer chemotherapy. As previously mentioned, patients with intracranial tumors who require emergent treatment may receive ECT successfully, after careful consideration of the risk-benefit ratio.

Human immunodeficiency virus disease and acquired immunodeficiency syndrome. Depressive syndromes are common among patients with human immunodeficiency virus (HIV) disease and acquired immunodeficiency syndrome (AIDS) (Dilley et al. 1985; Frierson and Lippman 1987; Perry and Tross 1984). Schaerf and associates (1989) reported successful treatment of depression using ECT in three HIV-seropositive men and one man with AIDS. None of the four patients described had signs of increased ICP at the time of ECT. Kessing et al. (1994) reported the successful treatment of HIV-related catatonia with ECT.

Catatonia. Catatonia, a motor syndrome associated with both schizophrenia and mood disorders (Abrams and Taylor 1976), is a life-threatening neuropsychiatric condition. It is often refractory to pharmacotherapy but is dramatically responsive to bilateral ECT (Francis and Fink 1992; Mann et al. 1990; Pataki et al. 1992). Catatonia may also be associated with systemic medical disorders, and ECT is very effective in these instances (Pataki et al. 1992). ECT may be used as a first-line treatment in patients with catatonia and should be considered a treatment of choice once the diagnosis of catatonia is made (American Psychiatric Association Task Force on Electroconvulsive Therapy 1990).

Pregnancy. ECT has been used during all trimesters of pregnancy without adverse effects (Weiner and Coffey 1987). In fact, ECT may be preferred over pharmacotherapy during pregnancy and the nursing period because of concerns of teratogenicity from psychotropic medications (Abrams 1992). Fetal monitoring during ECT is recommended only in cases of high-risk pregnancy (Abrams 1992; Weiner and Coffey 1987). It is clinically prudent to have an obstetric consultant readily available when a pregnant woman undergoes ECT.

Organ transplantation. Very few data exist regarding organ transplantation and ECT.

Kellner et al. (1991b) and Block et al. (1992) each reported successful use of ECT without special modifications in a patient with depression who had undergone cardiac transplantation. Showalter et al. (1993) reported similar experience with a patient with depression who had had a liver transplant. Although we know of no reported cases of ECT in patients with renal or lung transplants, ECT would likely be useful in appropriately selected cases.

Neuroleptic malignant syndrome. ECT is an effective treatment for patients with neuroleptic malignant syndrome (NMS) (Casey 1987; Greenberg and Gujavarty 1985; Pearlman 1990). Davis et al. (1991) reported that 60% of patients with NMS respond, and the mortality rate is reduced by about one-half. Abrams (1992) condemned the concurrent use of ECT and neuroleptics in the presence of NMS because this combination has resulted in death from cardiac arrest (Davis et al. 1991; Hughes 1986; Regestein et al. 1971). In our opinion, ECT is indicated as a treatment for NMS when patients do not respond to pharmacological treatment.

Elderly Patients

Increasing age has been associated with a favorable response to ECT (Carney et al. 1965; Mendels 1965; Roberts 1959). Abrams (1992) stated that ". . . some of the most rewarding results with convulsive therapy are obtained in elderly, debilitated patients whose primary affective disorder masquerades as senile dementia" (p. 105). Modification in technique should include careful attention to cardiovascular status. Also, in patients with osteoporosis, avoidance of the "cuffed limb" method is advised (Abrams 1992).

CONCLUSION

ECT is a safe and effective treatment for a limited number of severe psychiatric conditions.

As we learn more about the mechanisms of action of ECT and as ECT becomes further refined, consultation-liaison psychiatrists will be increasingly able to provide this treatment to patients with concomitant serious medical and psychiatric illness.

REFERENCES

Abrams R: Electroconvulsive Therapy, 2nd Edition. New York, Oxford University Press, 1992

Abrams R, Taylor MA: Catatonia: a prospective study. Arch Gen Psychiatry 33:579–581, 1976

Abrams R, Swartz CM, Vedak C: Antidepressant effects of high-dose right unilateral electroconvulsive therapy. Arch Gen Psychiatry 48: 746–748, 1991

American Psychiatric Association Task Force on Electroconvulsive Therapy: The Practice of Electroconvulsive Therapy: Recommendations for Treatment, Training, and Privileging. Washington, DC, American Psychiatric Association, 1990

Beale MD, Kellner CH, Lemert R, et al: Skeletal muscle relaxation in patients undergoing electroconvulsive therapy (letter). Anesthesiology 80:957, 1994a

Beale MD, Kellner CH, Pritchett JT, et al: Stimulus dose-titration in ECT: a 2-year clinical experience. Convulsive Therapy 10:171–176, 1994b

Block M, Admon D, Bonne O, et al: Electroconvulsive therapy in a depressed heart transplant patient. Convulsive Therapy 8:290–293, 1992

Brown GL, Wilson WP: Parkinsonism and depression. South Med J 65:540–545, 1972

Carney MWP, Roth M, Garside RF: The diagnosis of depressive syndromes and the prediction of ECT response. Br J Psychiatry 111:659–674, 1965

Casey DA: Electroconvulsive therapy in the neuroleptic malignant syndrome. Convulsive Therapy 3:278–283, 1987

Cerletti U, Bini L: Un nuevo metodo di shock-terapie "L'elettroshock" [A new method of shock therapy]. Bollettino Accademia Medica Roma 64:136–138, 1938

Coffey CE, Hoffman G, Weiner RD: Electroconvulsive therapy in a depressed patient with a functioning ventriculo-atrial shunt. Convulsive Therapy 3:302–306, 1987

Davis JM, Janicak PG, Sakkus P, et al: Electroconvulsive therapy in the treatment of the neuroleptic malignant syndrome. Convulsive Therapy 7:111–120, 1991

d'Elia G: Comparison of electroconvulsive therapy with unilateral and bilateral stimulation, II: therapeutic efficiency in endogenous depression. Acta Psychiatr Scand Suppl 215:30–43, 1970

Dilley JW, Ochitill HN, Perl M, et al: Findings in psychiatric consultations with patients with acquired immune deficiency syndrome. Am J Psychiatry 142:82–86, 1985

Fochtmann L: A mechanism for the efficacy of ECT in Parkinson's disease. Convulsive Therapy 4:321–327, 1988

Folstein MF, Folstein SE, McHugh PR: Mini-Mental State: a practical method for grading the cognitive state of patients for the clinician. J Psychiatr Res 12:189–198, 1975

Francis A, Fink M: ECT response in catatonia (letter). Am J Psychiatry 149:581–582, 1992

Frierson RL, Lippman SB: Psychological implications of AIDS. Am Fam Physician 35:109–116, 1987

Goldfarb C, Driesen J, Cole D: Psychophysiologic aspects of malignancy. Am J Psychiatry 123:1545–1552, 1967

Goldstein MZ, Richardson C: Meningioma with depression: ECT risk or benefit? Psychosomatics 29:349–351, 1988

Greenberg LB, Gujavarty K: The neuroleptic malignant syndrome: review and report of three cases. Compr Psychiatry 26:63–70, 1985

Hamilton M: A rating scale for depression. J Neurol Neurosurg Psychiatry 23:56–62, 1960

Hsiao JK, Evans DL: ECT in a depressed patient after craniotomy. Am J Psychiatry 141:442–444, 1984

Hughes JR: ECT during and after the neuroleptic malignant syndrome: case report. J Clin Psychiatry 47:42–43, 1986

Husum B, Vester-Andersen T, Buchmann G, et al: Electroconvulsive therapy and intracranial aneurysm: prevention of blood pressure elevation in a normotensive patient by hydralazine and propranolol. Anesthesia 38:1205–1207, 1983

Kellner CH, Burns CM, Bernstein JH, et al: Safe administration of ECT in a patient with a calcified frontal mass (letter). J Neuropsychiatry Clin Neurosci 3:353–354, 1991a

Kellner CH, Monroe RR, Burns CM, et al: Electroconvulsive therapy in a patient with a heart transplant (letter). N Engl J Med 325:669, 1991b

Kellner CH, Beale MD, Pritchett JT, et al: Parkinson's disease and ECT: the case for further study. Psychopharmacol Bull 30:495–500, 1994

Kessing L, LaBianca JH, Bolwig TG: HIV-induced stupor treated with ECT. Convulsive Therapy 10:232–235, 1994

Knos GB, Sung YF: ECT anesthesia strategies in the high risk medical patient, in Psychiatric Care of the Medical Patient, 2nd Edition. Edited by Stoudemire A, Fogel B. New York, Oxford University Press, 1993, pp 225–240

Malek-Ahmadi P, Beceiro JR, McNeil BW, et al: Electroconvulsive therapy and chronic subdural hematoma. Convulsive Therapy 6:38–41, 1990

Maltbie AA, Wingfield MS, Volow MR, et al: Electroconvulsive therapy in the presence of brain tumor: case reports and an evaluation risk. J Nerv Ment Dis 168:400–405, 1980

Mandel MR: Electroconvulsive therapy for chronic pain associated with depression. Am J Psychiatry 132:632–636, 1975

Mann SC, Caroff SN, Bleier HR, et al: Electroconvulsive therapy of the lethal catatonia syndrome. Convulsive Therapy 6:239–247, 1990

McCracken J, Kosanin R: Trazodone administration during ECT associated with cardiac conduction abnormality. Am J Psychiatry 141:1488–1489, 1984

MECTA Corporation: Instruction Manual, SR and JR Models. Portland, OR, 1986

Mendels J: Electroconvulsive therapy and depression, I: the prognostic significance of clinical factors. Br J Psychiatry 111:675–681, 1965

Oh JJ, Rummans TA, O'Conner MK, et al: Cognitive impairment after ECT in patients with Parkinson's disease and psychiatric illness (letter). Am J Psychiatry 149:271, 1992

Ottoson JO: Experimental studies of the mode of action of electroconvulsive therapy. Acta Psychiatr Scand Suppl 145:1–141, 1960

Pataki J, Zervas I, Jandorf L: Catatonia in a university inpatient service (1985–1990). Convulsive Therapy 8:167–173, 1992

Pearlman C: Neuroleptic malignant syndrome and electroconvulsive therapy. Convulsive Therapy 6:251–254, 1990

Perry SW, Tross S: Psychiatric problems of AIDS inpatients at the New York Hospital: preliminary report. Public Health Rep 99:200–205, 1984

Pettinati HM, Stephens SM, Willie KM, et al: Evidence for less improvement in depression in patients taking benzodiazepines during unilateral ECT. Am J Psychiatry 147:1029–1036, 1990

Regestein QR, Kahn CB, Siegel AJ, et al: A case of catatonia occurring simultaneously with severe urinary retention. J Nerv Ment Dis 152:432–435, 1971

Roberts JM: Prognostic factors in the electroshock treatment of depressive states, I: clinical features from history and examination. Journal of Mental Science 105:693–702, 1959

Sackeim H, Decina P, Prohovnik I, et al: Seizure threshold in electroconvulsive therapy. Arch Gen Psychiatry 44:355–360, 1987

Savitsky N, Kavlinger W: Electroshock in the presence of organic disease of the nervous system. Journal of Hillside Hospital 2:3–22, 1953

Schaerf FW, Miller RR, Lipsey JR, et al: ECT for major depression in four patients infected with human immunodeficiency virus. Am J Psychiatry 146:782–784, 1989

Showalter PE, Young SA, Bilello JF, et al: Electroconvulsive therapy for depression in a liver transplant patient (letter). Psychosomatics 34:537, 1993

Swartz CM, Abrams R: ECT Instruction Manual, 5th Edition. Lake Bluff, IL, Somatics, 1994

Weiner RD, Coffey CE: Electroconvulsive therapy in the medically ill, in Principles of Medical Psychiatry. Edited by Stoudemire A, Fogel BS. New York, Grune & Stratton, 1987, pp 113–134

Weiner RD, Coffey CE: Electroconvulsive therapy in the medical and neurologic patient, in Psychiatric Care of the Medical Patient, 2nd Edition. Edited by Stoudemire A, Fogel BS. New York, Oxford University Press, 1993, pp 207–224

Weiner RD, Whanger AB, Erwin CW, et al: Prolonged confusional state and EEG seizure activity following concurrent ECT and lithium use. Am J Psychiatry 137:1452–1453, 1980

Weiner RD, Rogers HJ, Davidson JR, et al: Effects of stimulus parameters on cognitive side effects. Ann N Y Acad Sci 462:315–325, 1986

Zwil AS, Bowring MA, Price TRP, et al: Prospective electroconvulsive therapy in the presence of intracranial tumor. Convulsive Therapy 6:299–307, 1990

Chapter 33

Psychotherapy

Don R. Lipsitt, M.D.

Surprisingly little has been written or researched on psychotherapy in patients who are medically ill. Systematic application of early findings has occurred only in the past 50 or 60 years (Lipowski 1986). Attempts to understand the "mysterious leap from the mind to the body" (Deutsch 1959, p. 101) generated hypotheses about mind-body interrelations that could be studied systematically in medical settings. These endeavors coincided with the evolution of general hospital psychiatry, which burgeoned during and after World War II.

From these early foundations, a variety of psychotherapeutic approaches to the broad spectrum of illness and disease encountered in medical settings today has emerged.

This chapter 1) defines "medical" psychotherapy as it is similar to and differs from psychoanalytic and psychodynamic interventions; 2) describes the unique aspects of psychotherapy in the general hospital and the specialized skills and tasks of the consultation-liaison psychiatrist; 3) enumerates and describes varieties of psychotherapy used in the medical setting; 4) illustrates psychotherapeutic applications of consultation-liaison psychiatry; and 5) demonstrates a specialized model of outpatient medical psychotherapy.

DEFINITION OF MEDICAL PSYCHOTHERAPY

Psychotherapeutic intervention is defined here as that which is intentionally (as contrasted with coincidentally) exercised on patients with medical illness by physicians with psychiatric training.

As Marmor (1979a) stated, "The very fact that the patient is able to discuss a personal problem in an ambience of hope and positive expectancy is the beginning of a therapeutic experience" (p. 523). Indeed, the initial interview, skillfully negotiated, is "a therapeutic transaction, although neither the physician nor the patient may consciously regard it as such" (p. 523).

The author gratefully acknowledges the technical assistance of Ann Marie Sullivan.

Nonpsychiatrist physicians who have honed their interview and counseling skills to a high degree of sophistication generally are not capable of practicing medical psychotherapy without the intense case supervision and special training of the psychiatrist (Balint 1964; Greenhill 1981).

Practitioners of medical psychotherapy as herein defined are psychiatrists who identify themselves as consultation-liaison practitioners and who apply the principles of that special domain of psychiatry and medicine to a great spectrum of situations, conditions, systems, and settings related to the general practice of medicine. This definition exempts psychiatrists who—by choice or chance—have excluded patients with significant "medical disease" from their practices.

Commonalities in Psychotherapies

Some investigators now believe that there are at least 400 forms of "psychotherapy" (Waldinger 1990, p. 512). Whatever the theoretical underpinnings and psychotherapeutic techniques, however, most psychotherapies are believed to share some commonalities.

So plentiful are the variables that influence the outcome of illness that a single satisfactory definition of psychotherapy is untenable.

Whatever the differences, all psychotherapeutic interventions rely on some form of communication and a sharing of interest and expectation on the part of patient and therapist. Polatin (1966, p. 41) suggested that "psychotherapy is a form of treatment in psychiatry relying essentially on the verbal communication between therapist and patient and on the interaction between the personalities of therapist and patient in a dynamic interpersonal relationship, whereby maladaptive behavior is altered toward a more effective adaptation, relief of symptoms occurs, and insights are developed."

Bibring (1954) suggested that virtually all psychotherapies made use of five major psychotherapeutic principles: suggestion, abreaction, manipulation (related to furthering the aims of effective therapy), clarification, and interpretation. The unique aspects of psychotherapy in the general hospital lend themselves more to techniques other than interpretation, although opportunities for use of this technique are not entirely absent.

Psychoanalytic Foundations

The developmental aspects of psychoanalytic theory are relevant to all of medicine; they help the physician to understand time-related changes in each individual's life cycle, thus permitting illness to be viewed in relation to normal growth. Because of the importance of the phase in the life cycle, all case presentations in medicine begin with the age of the patient as a backdrop for all else about the individual. Opportunities abound in inpatient medical situations to recognize "management problems" that are caused by maladaptive transferences, by unconscious meanings of symptoms or procedures, and by fantasies or complications related to neuropsychiatric syndromes.

Derivatives of psychoanalysis that are relevant to consultation-liaison psychiatry include "working through," "grief work," and "object identification." Furthermore, the psychoanalytic model of depression as anger directed inward is widely subscribed to in treating medical-surgical patients with all varieties and degrees of depression (Klerman et al. 1984). Many interpretive leaps made in the medical setting by consultation-liaison psychiatrists are based on much cumulative psychoanalytic wisdom even when sufficient time for "working through" is unavailable.

Psychoanalytic knowledge has also contributed greatly to the need to recognize the uniqueness of each individual in personality structure, in specific patterns of response to stress, in use of defense mechanisms, and in production of memories, fantasies, wishes, dreams, thoughts, and feelings.

Psychodynamic Foundations

Psychodynamic psychotherapy focuses more on the patient's life situation and environmental circumstances in the therapeutic relationship, whereas psychoanalysis puts a higher premium on intrapsychic conflict and the transference neurosis. By lifting repression and making the unconscious conscious, it aims to alleviate symptoms in the context of a corrective experience.

Many authors suggest that a psychodynamic orientation is the sine qua non of consultation-liaison psychiatry on which foundation other psychotherapeutic interventions rest (Gabbard 1990; Green 1993; Greenhill 1981; Hackett and Weisman 1960; Horowitz and Kaltreider 1979; Luborsky 1990; Ursano and Hales 1986). According to Gabbard (1990),

> dynamic psychiatry . . . provides a coherent conceptual framework within which all treatments are prescribed. Regardless of whether the treatment is dynamic psychotherapy, behavior therapy, or pharmacotherapy, it is *dynamically informed* . . . a crucial component of the dynamic psychiatrist's expertise is knowing when to avoid exploratory psychotherapy in favor of treatments that do not threaten the patient's psychic equilibrium. (p. 4)

■ UNIQUE ASPECTS OF PSYCHOTHERAPY WITH MEDICALLY ILL PATIENTS

Variations From Traditional Psychotherapy

Standard definitions of psychotherapy do not fully represent the interaction between the psychiatrist and the patient who is medically ill. Psychotherapeutic intervention in the consultation-liaison context relies on a potpourri of eclecticism required to understand patients and their often unspoken problems, the relationships of staff to patients and to each other, the dynamics of interviewing (both medical and psychiatric), and systems structure of the hospital setting. To date there is no systematized theory of consultation-liaison intervention that parallels that of psychotherapy as traditionally defined (Greenhill 1981).

Referral.   Patients referred to the consultation-liaison psychiatrist differ significantly from those seen in an outpatient psychiatric setting.

The consultation-liaison psychiatrist usually goes to the patient rather than having the patient seek him or her out. The psychiatrist's patients usually have not identified a particular problem of an emotional nature for which they seek help; it is more often the attending physician, house officer, or nurse who requests consultation. Patients in the consultation-liaison setting, therefore, seldom have the "motivation" for or "receptivity" to psychotherapy in its "purer" sense; some would consider this orientation as a dilution or "alloying" of the more refined definition of psychotherapy.

Setting.   The consulting psychiatrist in the medical setting is called on to provide assistance in circumstances covering the spectrum from an immediate crisis (e.g., in emergent situations wherever they occur in the hospital) to a chronic condition requiring protracted outpatient follow-up. Outpatient treatment may be brief, extended, or, as will be described, "attenuated." In each instance, assessment follows evaluation of the "situation," whether patient-, staff-, or system-centered. Whatever the setting and focus, appraisal includes a psychodynamic assessment in addition to a review of reasons (medical or surgical) for the patient's illness and reactions and reasons for the consulter's concerns. The latter may range from the primary physician's puzzlement over a diagnostic dilemma to the concerns of a patient with schizophrenia about major surgery. In order to be of maximal assistance to the consulter, the psychiatrist must understand the medical circumstances of the case, know the medication regimens and their effects, and glean as much as possible from the patient's chart. Early in the encounter, a decision is made whether active crisis intervention or a more extended and methodical approach is indicated. Ultimately, a plan will derive from a "formulation" of the case. The setting of the medical psychotherapist is often the bedside, a hospital conference room, an intensive care unit (ICU), or—in special circumstances—even a hallway, not a well-furnished consulting office. Hospitalized patients wear hospital garb and are accustomed to an extraordinary lack of privacy. The stereotypical 50-minute hour is nowhere more challenged than in these environs.

Patients are often ill-prepared for receiving the psychiatrist, and in this atypical patient assessment context, it is impressive that medically hospitalized patients are so frequently receptive to psychiatric attention. An alliance often develops within minutes, and effective psychotherapeutic intervention can be achieved during a single bedside visit (Lipsitt 1985). With such brief contacts, the consultation-liaison psychiatrist is frequently called on to diagnose and treat a variety of anxiety reactions and depressive disorders, acute grief, delirium, conversion, adjustment disorders, psychosis, and atypical pain reactions to acute physical illness. These interventions, tailored to individual personality styles and defenses, selectively involve the psychotherapeutic principles mentioned in Table 33–1 (Bibring 1954) to alleviate symptoms, clarify distortions, and minimize the negative effects of the patient's dysfunctional relationships with staff that may compromise medical care.

Psychotherapeutic Range and Limitations

An essential skill of the consultation-liaison psychiatrist in the consultative role is the ability to apply a variety of brief psychotherapeutic techniques (Groves and Kucharski 1991), from "brief" (Budman and Stone 1983; Horowitz and Kaltreider 1979; Marmor 1979b; Sifneos 1972; Strupp and Binder 1984), to "very brief" (Liberzon et al. 1992), to "single session" (Bloom 1981), to "briefest" (Blacher 1984), and to crisis intervention as practiced during wartime and other emergencies.

Psychotherapies are characterized according to the therapist's stance as interpretive, suggestive, persuasive, or educative. Furthermore, depending on the depth of psychic exploration, they may be superficial or deep. The duration varies from brief to prolonged, and psychotherapy may be applied to an individual, a group, or a family. It is rare that the more exploratory techniques are used in the hospital setting.

Treatment in groups has been found to be very useful by consultation-liaison psychiatrists and liaison teams for patients who tend to express affects through somatic representation. Such groups may be psychoeducational, supportive, expressive, homogeneous or heterogeneous (regarding illness), closed- or open-ended, and inpatient or outpatient, although reduced hospital stays have made the former less practical.

Table 33–1. Common psychotherapeutic principles

Principle	Description	Use in type of therapy	
		Expressive	Supportive
Suggestion	Induction of mental processes by therapist	+	+++
Abreaction	Emotional discharge, catharsis	+	++
Manipulation	Use of patient's existing emotional systems to achieve therapeutic change	+	++++
Clarification	Helping patient "to see more clearly"	+++	+
Interpretation	Attempt to change attitudes by explaining unconscious thoughts	++++	+

Note. + = least use; ++++ = most use.
Source. Bibring 1954.

Patients who are sometimes thought to have alexithymia (Sifneos 1973) are found to become more communicative in group settings and to relinquish denial that has previously hampered relationships with others.

The consultation-liaison therapist's orientation is, of necessity, one of brevity. Many patients in the general hospital have illnesses that have compromised their ability to maintain attention, concentration, and orientation (e.g., brain disorders such as delirium or dementia, toxicities, severe pain). For these and other reasons, the consultation-liaison psychiatrist's therapeutic interventions more often consist of shoring up rather than challenging intact defenses. Many patients who would not otherwise seek psychiatric attention on an outpatient basis will accept and benefit from such attention in the hospital. Evidence of ego strength is almost always possible to find in most patients, even if only in their capacity to cope more or less successfully with the stressful and sometimes strange experience of hospitalization. Sometimes the patient's distraction by physical illness or discomfort is inappropriately perceived by staff as a willful failure of the patient to communicate.

The requirement of versatility in the consultation-liaison psychiatrist determines that his or her therapeutic interventions will fall typically between uncomplicated consultation/evaluation and more formal psychotherapy. Knowledge, if not unmodified use, of the varieties of psychotherapy is an essential part of the consultation-liaison psychiatrist's armamentarium. Some psychotherapies from which the consultation-liaison psychiatrist may choose are listed in Table 33–2.

TASKS OF THE CONSULTATION-LIAISON PSYCHIATRIST

According to Greenhill (1981), a major task of the consultation-liaison psychiatrist is dealing with psychosocial influences in medical illness. The tasks required to make a psychiatric con-

sultation therapeutic are delineated in Table 33–3. All of these tasks culminate in selection of an appropriate psychotherapeutic approach based on formulation of the case (Hackett and Weisman 1960).

Establishing the Alliance

As I have written elsewhere (Lipsitt 1985), "the psychiatric consultant makes use of all the principles of good psychotherapy, although they are often modified to accommodate the realities of the hospital setting and the unusual way in which psychiatrist and patient are brought together" (p. 8).

Although transferential reactions can occur in any setting, that which accompanies the alliance in the medical setting is not addressed as it would be in extended psychodynamic therapies. Rather, it is referred to in terms of empathic understanding, reassurance, supportive interaction, and meaningful communication. The psychiatrist in the medical setting does not undertake reconstructive therapy of long-standing problems, although awareness of their existence permits them to be utilized in the "manipulative" aspects of psychotherapeutic interventions (Bibring 1954) in even the briefest encounters. Blacher (1984), for example, described how to use the principles of psychotherapy effectively in a single session to treat patients in medical crises that "evoke old conflicts and problems about the self and family relationships" (p. 226). Although the therapeutic alliance does not exist in the psychoanalytic sense, the acceptance by the patient of the psychiatrist's investment creates a "holding environment" in which the clinical improvement occurs, often without adjunctive psychopharmacological treatment.

Making a "Personality Diagnosis"

A useful foundation for consultation-liaison work has been the personality typology developed by Kahana and Bibring (1964) for application in the general hospital setting. "Person-

Table 33–2. Types and characteristics of psychotherapies

Characterized by	Description	Consultation-liaison example	Reference
Time			
Brief	Limited (< 12–20) sessions Focus on specific problem Exploratory or supportive Stringent selection criteria Motivated or receptive patient	Unresolved grief exacerbating physical disease	Davanloo 1978 Malan 1963 Mann 1973 Marmor 1979b Sifneos 1972
		Single-session evaluation of depressive response to illness	Bloom 1981
		"Briefest"—acute postsurgical reactions "Attenuated" treatment of somatization disorder in outpatient setting	Blacher 1984 Lipsitt 1964
Extensive	Protracted treatment Exploratory Reconstructive Deals with transference and development of insight	Only in cases in which initial brief intervention leads to discovery of long-standing conflicts amenable to treatment	Gabbard 1990 Gitelson 1973
Format			
Individual	Patient seen alone Others usually (but not always) not involved	Patient with unremitting abdominal pain with no physical findings	Harrison and Carek 1966 Ursano and Hales 1986
Couples	Usually for interpersonal problems between two related people (not necessarily married)	Young married executive with myocardial infarction who "aggravates" and frightens wife by denying seriousness of illness; she requests appointment	Melges 1985
Family	Related groups with usually one "identified patient" Explores family dynamics as contributor to "problem"	20-year-old woman with anorexia seen with family to explore stresses	Jacobs 1993
Group	Heterogeneous or homogeneous assembly of 8–10 patients with sense of shared stress, symptoms, interests, conflicts Provides modeling, sharing, learning Time-limited or open	Group of women with breast cancer; also, Alcoholics Anonymous groups	Spira and Spiegel 1993 Stein and Weiner 1978 Yalom 1975

Goals

	Strengthen defenses and coping skills to reduce anxiety and to enhance well-being and social function "Here and now" orientation	Patient with asthma who is afraid to return home because of spouse who has cardiac disease and smokes	Green 1993 Hackett and Weisman 1960 Viederman 1984
Reconstructive	Bring about changes in adaptation, behavior, and personality to alter lifelong patterns Intensive, insight-oriented; deals with transference neurosis, early developmental problems Psychoanalysis, dynamic psychotherapy	After nearly dying in automobile accident, college professor decides to examine his life, relationships, and goals	Gitelson 1973
Reeducational	Remove symptoms by direct intervention, guidance, persuasion, and relearning Correct misperceptions and misattributions "Here and now" orientation No exploration of early events, no transference or insight Behavioral and cognitive approaches Symptom removal is goal	Patient becomes acutely anxious in magnetic resonance imaging machine; responds to systematic desensitization	Hamburg and Adams 1967 Horowitz et al. 1984

Techniques

Suppressive	Reassure, support strengths, bolster ego-syntonic defenses Use suggestion, clarification, and manipulation to enhance self-control	"Management" of patient with labile hypertension who has "difficulty" in following diet and taking medications	Green 1993 Viederman 1984, 1985
Exploratory	Encourage self-discovery and insight through interpretation of behavior, conflict, and transference Make unconscious conscious Examine early life	Help patient to understand persistent smoking in face of recently diagnosed pulmonary disease	Davanloo 1978 Malan 1963 Mann 1973 Sifneos 1972, 1973
Directive	Retrain or reframe ways of thinking, feeling, and behaving through direct intervention, guidance, and persuasion	Redirect thinking of patient with diabetes who feels guilt and depression about difficulty in controlling brittle diabetes	Hersen and Bellack 1982 Klerman et al. 1984 Zeiss et al. 1979

Table 33–3.   Psychotherapeutic tasks of the consultation-liaison psychiatrist

Identify most relevant problem as expressed by primary care physician

Establish alliance with patient

Take history through associative interviewing

Assess personality structure and defenses

Understand, empathize, translate, inform, communicate, and educate, based on historical data

Derive psychodynamic formulation

Enhance self-esteem of patient

Selectively gratify transference wishes

Decrease intensity of painful affects

"Normalize" (universalize) reactions

Enhance healing environment

Propose practical management plan

Define psychiatrist's and other staff's participation

ality diagnosis" is based on normal character development and is not to be misconstrued as personality disorder or other psychopathology. Based on the psychoanalytic theory of character structure and development, it facilitates description of the meaning of illness to patients of different personality types, permitting some degree of matching of therapeutic interventions with more or less predictable patient responses. To delineate nonpathological behaviors as they are influenced by developmental differences in individuals, Kahana and Bibring identified seven types (Table 33–4).

Defensive and adaptive coping approaches that are fairly characteristic of each personality type are called into play in the face of threatening situations such as medical illness, surgery, or hospitalization. (For further discussion about the relation between personality and response to illness, see Ursano et al., Chapter 3, in this volume.)

Personality diagnosis is, by itself, insufficient to serve psychotherapeutic purposes but is a valuable adjunct to all medical psychotherapy. It must also be kept in mind that an individual's personality may be altered in appearance, either transiently or more permanently, under conditions of marked emotional stress or physical disease.

ESSENTIAL SKILLS OF THE CONSULTATION-LIAISON PSYCHIATRIST

In company with other skills and knowledge, psychodynamic thinking offers the eclecticism and flexibility required of an effective psychiatrist in outpatient or inpatient general medical settings. The repertoire of the consultation-liaison psychiatrist calls on psychiatry's roots in psychoanalysis, psychosomatic medicine, stress theory about the relevance of critical life events and trauma, biopsychosocial concepts of illness and illness behavior, as well as general medicine, neurology, and psychopharmacology.

Versatility

The activities of the consultation-liaison psychiatrist are always potentially psychotherapeutic. They range from behavioral therapy to insight-oriented psychotherapy. The skills of the consultation-liaison psychiatrist are those of the most proficient full-time psychotherapist, with perhaps a greater versatility born of necessity. Consultation-liaison psychiatrists who interact on a daily basis with patients who are medically ill and their caretakers should be adept at the skills listed in Table 33–5.

Associative Anamnesis

One interview technique especially suited to consultation-liaison work is that described as associative anamnesis (Deutsch 1939; Deutsch and Murphy 1955), derived in part from the psychoanalytic free associative process. Deutsch and Murphy noted that the patient "drifts into a communication in which he inattentively mixes emotional and symptom material" (p. 20). In this way, they said, "it is possible to observe the somatic and the psychic components more nearly simultaneously" (p. 19). Em-

Table 33–4. Personality types in medical management

Personality type	Psychodynamic descriptor	Illness behavior	Treatment approach
Dependent, overdemanding	Oral, needy	Urgent requests	Show signs of caring, but with clear limit setting
Orderly, controlled	Compulsive	Self-disciplined	Use "scientific" approach; share information
Dramatizing, emotional	Hysterical	Flighty, teasing	Calm "professional" approach
Long-suffering, self-sacrificing	Masochistic	Help-rejecting	Avoid excessive reassurance; acknowledge pain
Guarded, querulous	Paranoid	Suspicious, wary	Acknowledge, but do not reinforce, perceptions; do not argue or withhold information
Superior, grandiose	Narcissistic	Exaggerated self-confidence	Do not challenge patient's "expert" status
Uninvolved, aloof	Schizoid	Seeks isolation	Accept "unsociability," but avoid complete withdrawal

Source. Originally adapted from Kahana RJ, Bibring GL: "Personality Types in Medical Management," in *Psychiatry and Medical Practice in a General Hospital.* Edited by Zinberg NE. New York, International Universities Press, 1964, pp. 108–123. Reprinted from Waldinger RJ: *Psychiatry for Medical Students,* 2nd Edition. Washington, DC, American Psychiatric Press, 1990. Used with permission.

pathic concern for the patient's physical distress strengthened the alliance, while "the patient is stimulated to give the needed information . . . without being made aware of a psychological background in his illness" (p. 20).

This process of data gathering informs the interviewer of the patient's personality structure, salient defenses, style of interacting with others (including the patient's physician), patterns of adapting to and coping with stresses, personal and family psychodynamics, physical symptoms, and social skills. Viederman's (1984) "active dynamic interview" has characteristics similar to the associative anamnesis.

"Preassessment"

Before any psychotherapeutic intervention can begin, the consultation-liaison psychiatrist sizes up the situation. This may include as much exploration as necessary to grasp the precipitating reason for the consultation request. The attending physician's perception of the need for psychiatric assessment, a fairly detailed review of the patient's medical record, and the primary care nurse's impressions of the patient usually constitute the desirable minimum. This systemic appraisal before face-to-face interaction with the patient facilitates a focused approach to the core problem during the actual interview with the patient and may well enter into the subsequent formulation of the problem.

Therapeutic Examination

The examination or interview itself can carry a high psychotherapeutic valence. Unlike the interview of the self-referred patient that might take place in an outpatient setting, the interview of the hospitalized patient must avoid testing for motivation or heightening anxiety through uncovering techniques. Questions that too quickly attempt to assay "feelings" or even details of interpersonal relationships often bring forth only quizzical expressions from the patient (Lipsitt 1977). The consultant's exploration is usually limited initially to only

Table 33–5. Psychotherapeutic skills of the consultation-liaison psychiatrist

Knowing about psychoanalytic/psychodynamic concepts, biopsychosocial approach, stress theory, general medicine, neurology, and psychopharmacology

Knowing how to conduct medical-psychiatric interviewing (e.g., associative anamnesis)

Knowing how to extrapolate meaning from casual talk and empathic listening

Knowing when and how to "confront" a patient's "worries"

Knowing how and when to "neutralize" negative emotional conflicts with psychopharmacological agents[a]

Knowing how to create a supportive "holding environment"

Knowing how to select and apply a "tailored" psychotherapeutic approach

Knowing how and when to appropriately use interventions such as reassurance, support, limit setting, guidance, and management

Knowing how to relate comfortably to nonpsychiatrist professionals and to work with liaison team members

Knowing how to curb inappropriate therapeutic zeal, especially outside one's field of expertise

Knowing how to combine psychotherapy and psychopharmacotherapy

[a]After Fenichel 1954.

those aspects of the history that are absolutely necessary to address the question posed by the primary physician.

Special Considerations in the General Hospital Setting

The consultation-liaison psychiatrist must be able to adapt to the realities of the general hospital environment. Because of time limitations, consultation-liaison psychiatrists will sometimes have to be comfortable with some degree of incompleteness of the anamnesis as well as with the tendency of many patients to want to sustain a medical or physical focus during much of the interview.

Successful alliance and therapeutic effectiveness depend on the consultation-liaison psychiatrist's capacity for empathic resonance to "where the patient lives" at any particular moment, whether during a mental status examination or associatively following self-disclosures considered by the patient to be relevant to the "problem." Positive alliances (Lipsitt 1985) can develop very quickly, even in patients who are initially refractory to psychiatric assessment, and can allow the patient to comfortably disclose abundant personal data in a very short time.

When patients enter a hospital for medical or surgical treatment, they often experience some degree of regression. In this predicament, professional contact that provides comfort, compassion, honesty, and empathy fosters a high degree of receptivity in the patient, with alliance following soon after engagement (Nadelson 1980). The consultation-liaison psychiatrist often finds it necessary to deal tactfully with the patient's occasional iatrogenesis.

Defenses that are weakened by the experience of sickness and hospitalization must not only be respected but bolstered because they are often useful in adapting to the current "crisis." Part of the consultation-liaison psychiatrist's task is to assess personality and defense structure during the first examination. The patient's adaptation to illness will confirm the "old time" medical dictum that "it is as important to know what kind of patient has the disease as to know what disease the patient has," as illustrated by that important aspect of medical psychotherapy that addresses personality diagnosis in the patient (Kahana and Bibring 1964), as described earlier in this chapter.

Formulation

The formulation, more than the diagnostic label, remains the road map to further intervention. Based on the data obtained from the patient and other sources, the formulation includes features listed in Table 33–6. Such for-

Table 33–6. Elements of formulation

Character structure ("personality diagnosis")

Presenting problem (reason for request of consultation)

Patient's narrative ("life story"), including perceptions and attributions of current illness

Identified life event(s) or crisis that precipitated response

Defenses used by patient to negotiate stresses of medical illness, surgery, and hospitalization

Patterns of engagement from past as predictors of patient's response to caregivers and treatment interventions

Leads to guidelines for
Psychotherapeutic intervention
Physicians and other staff about
  • Doctor-patient relationship
  • Relevance of patient's behavior to current illness
  • Consultation-liaison psychiatrist's role in care of the patient

mulation, although it need not include all of these elements in every case, can lead quite naturally to recommendations for treatment.

Selecting and Implementing Treatment

After arriving at a formulation, the consultation-liaison psychiatrist has a range of psychotherapeutic interventions to choose from. The consultant applies these techniques when indicated in commonly encountered situations in the general hospital calling for psychotherapeutic intervention (see Table 33–7).

Viederman's (1985) "life narrative" approach elicits the patient's personal fears and the meanings of symptoms, simplifies the patient's response to illness, and describes it to him or her as a disturbance that is a natural product of his or her personal psychology. This technique lessens the emotional disequilibrium that has been aroused by the crisis of illness by giving it a "rational" foundation.

This technique is intended to help the patient place the physical illness "in the context of the patient's life trajectory" and acknowledges

the threats and fears of the person confronted with serious physical disease, as described by Strain and Grossman (1975, p. 26) (see Table 33–8).

According to Viederman (1985), this approach is applicable at the bedside even in relatively brief contacts. The choice of psychotherapy often determines which member(s) of the consultation-liaison team will most actively work with the patient and, as appropriate, with his or her family. The psychiatric examination by the consultation-liaison psychiatrist may itself constitute a psychotherapeutic intervention, and follow-up visit(s) may be utilized to consolidate the benefits of the intervention or to assess its durability. At other times, as, for example, in helping a patient work through acute or delayed grief, a psychiatric nurse, social worker, or psychologist on the team may undertake the therapeutic work while the psychiatrist provides a bridge with staff involved with the patient's care. In still other instances, the consultation-liaison psychiatrist may provide psychopharmacological oversight while psychotherapy is administered by another mem-

Table 33–7. Common psychotherapeutic activities of the consultation-liaison psychiatrist in the general hospital

Helping patients endure or overcome pain, fear, and denial

Helping patients' families cope with disruption by illness

Facilitating medical-surgical treatment

Helping patients grieve losses or face dying and death

Enhancing the capacity to bear dependency, isolation, rumination, sleep disturbance, and other perturbations of illness

Helping patients adapt to the sick role

Helping patients to effect changes in self-representation, object representation, and ideal self-representation[a,b]

Helping caretaking staff to recognize and utilize psychosocial factors in patient care planning

Source. [a]Mohl and Burstein 1982; [b]Viederman 1985.

Table 33–8.   Threats and fears that accompany illness

Threat to narcissistic integrity and the sources of self-esteem

Regressive fear of strangers on whom patient must rely

Separation anxiety, reflecting regressive activation of childhood fears of loss of nurturing and protective objects

Regressive activation of fears of loss of love and approval

Regressive fears of loss of control of developmentally acquired functions (e.g., bowel and bladder control, motor functions, speech, emotional regulation)

Guilt and fear of retaliation, reflecting unconscious view that illness is a punishment for past unacceptable behavior

Source.   Strain and Grossman 1975.

ber of the team. It is not uncommon for the recommendation to be "no intervention at all" (Frances and Clarkin 1981, p. 925). At other times, behavioral or cognitive approaches, including hypnosis, stress reduction, or other interventions, are used. Some programs are able to provide brief inpatient group experiences.

The consultation-liaison psychiatrist selects that approach—or, more commonly, the combination of approaches—that most parsimoniously addresses the patient's conditions or symptoms. Consideration of many factors will determine whether the approach will be primarily supportive or exploratory in its application (Table 33–9).

In those instances that pose a problem for the patient beyond discharge from inpatient status, therapeutic maintenance will require outpatient follow-up that is acceptable to the reluctant patient. Modification in therapeutic expectation and treatment setting may be required.

Which psychotherapeutic approach is selected depends not only on the needs of the patient but also on the training and theoretical predilection of the therapist. Efficacy of the treatment relies heavily on a combination of the therapist's skill and the patient's expectant faith in the treatment. For most consultation-liaison psychiatrists, theoretical orthodoxy does not pose a significant problem. The ultimate aim of medical psychotherapy is to systematically apply biopsychosocial interventions toward psychotherapeutic change.

The magnitude of this challenge is heightened in the medical setting, where the psychiatrist often encounters a prominent mind-body dualism that is so detrimental to effective health care. Maintaining a biopsychosocial mind-set is further compromised by the current trend to abbreviate hospital stays and to focus strictly on symptom amelioration. It is not uncommon, for example, for a patient complaining of chest pain to be medically discharged immediately after ruling out myocardial infarction, even though other emotional reasons for chest pain (e.g., somatization) have not been fully explored.

The consultation-liaison psychiatrist who consults on patients in the hospital may continue work begun there in the outpatient setting. Making this bridge requires assessment of the patient's motivation to continue and some therapeutic sensitivity and skill in helping the patient to make this transition successfully.

ILLUSTRATION OF PSYCHOTHERAPEUTIC APPLICATIONS IN CONSULTATION-LIAISON PSYCHIATRY

Treatment strategies include engaging and shoring up successful defenses that bolster self-esteem; promoting restoration of adaptive strategies and patterns that have been effective under previous stress; and facilitating effective medical management by reducing dysphoric affects. A case example will more fully illustrate these strategies and the process of psychotherapeutic intervention by a consultation-liaison psychiatrist.

Utilizing the skills of the consultation-liaison psychiatrist enumerated in Table 33–5,

Table 33–9. Factors determining selection of therapeutic approach

	Supportive	Exploratory
Level of cognitive function	Low	High
Psychosis	Yes	No
Suicidality	Yes	No
Life-threatening behavior	Yes	No
Time available for consultation-liaison care	Short	Long
Level of sexual development	Low	High
Setting	Inpatient	Outpatient
Educational level	Low, variable	High, variable
Interpersonal patterns (ability to interact with others)	Uneasy	Comfortable
Degree of autonomy	Low	High
Ability to assume responsibility	Low	High
Ability to tolerate affect	Low	High
Ability to express feelings	Low	High
Level of motivation to change	Low	High
Ability to maintain focus on conflict	Low	High
Capacity for insight	Low	High
Ability to trust	Low	High
Ability to identify "stressors"	Low	High
External "support system"	Poor	Good

the clinical encounter with each patient produces a "portrait" of the patient. This emerges not in a standardized sequential manner, but in the style of the artist who puts a dab here and another there to round out the picture. The portrait is complete when it has made use of only those ingredients—no more or less—that are essential to the total picture in each instance. Each encounter is a unique production in a special setting. All elements of the consultation are seamlessly interwoven.

Case Example

An urgent call for psychiatric consultation was received from the ICU when a 76-year-old man climbed over his bed rails, removed his intravenous pole, and smashed an outer window, threatening to jump. This stocky, robust man, described as psychotic by the ICU staff, was restrained in bed and given a mild sedative. The staff reported that the patient underwent open heart surgery for replacement of a

defective valve and that, under rather heavy sedation, he appeared to be progressing very well. However, shortly after extubation and lightening of sedation, he became quite agitated and hypervigilant. He repeatedly asked nurses for water and was repeatedly (and increasingly emphatically) told that he was not allowed to have liquids. Shortly thereafter, he climbed over his bed rails.

The relative calm of the patient when the psychiatrist arrived permitted a review of the chart. The chart contained detailed notes about the patient's surgery and anesthesia, but little personal, social, or family history. When approached by the consultation-liaison psychiatrist, the patient was lying quietly in bed with a cold cloth across his forehead and a Posey restraint on his torso. He was quite receptive, rational, and cooperative. There was no evidence of psychosis, poor reality-testing, or suicidal intent. He recounted what happened with bewilderment and shame. He gave a chronological account of his physical condition that had warranted surgery and was forthcoming about his early personal history.

He was a Polish immigrant to the United States shortly after World War II, who had lived through the experience of labor camps where he and his future wife were forced to toil for 10–11 hours a day without water. He recalled that experience as he became more alert following surgery; he cried as he recounted it. He described a life in which he had adapted to cruel behavior, many losses, impoverished circumstances, and other hardships. He expressed his gratitude at being able to live in the United States, to own his own home, to have a good and steady job in a bakery, and to raise a son who was now in a United States medical school. Again with tears, he expressed puzzlement that "anything like this" could occur because it would seem that he had "everything to live for," especially with the success of his surgery.

Formulation, after one consultation visit, was that this man, who had evidence of considerable ego strength and good patterns of adaptation to stress in the past, was compromised by medications and the physiological stress of the surgery (with possible mild cerebral hypoxia). In this twilight zone of perception, he reexperienced the labor camps of his youth, which he had survived without impulsive self-defeating behavior. Now, at age 76, while confused, he experienced panic—most likely triggered by the refusal of water—and was overcome with the "need to escape."

Recommendations included the use of ice chips in acceptable moderation; avoidance of sedating drugs, although small doses of haloperidol were recommended in the face of further psychotic behavior; transport of the patient to a less hectic and stressful environment as soon as appropriate to normalize behavior; avoidance of the exploration of early history at this time; an increase in communication with patient; and assignment of tasks that could be performed in bed to instill a greater sense of activity, freedom, and mastery.

On follow-up visits, the consultation-liaison psychiatrist found that no further episodes occurred and the patient was soon moved to a ward bed; he continued to recover from surgery without medical, surgical, or psychiatric complications. He did express feelings of depression, intense shame, and embarrassment over his experience in the ICU. Visits from the ICU head nurse, who explained her understanding and acceptance of the event, did much to allay his concerns. The patient was seen in follow-up after discharge when he returned to the hospital for postsurgical evaluation. At that time, he requested continued outpatient visits with the consultation-liaison psychiatrist because of difficulty sleeping, poor appetite, and anxiety. Monthly visits and small doses of thioridazine continued until his dysphoria improved.

ATTENUATED "BRIEF" PSYCHOTHERAPY: A MODEL OF OUTPATIENT PSYCHOTHERAPY

Although in this chapter I deal primarily with medical psychotherapy as applied to medical inpatients in the general hospital, I call the reader's attention to an approach referred to here as brief, intermittent, attenuated therapy (BIAT). Length of visits is no more than 30 minutes, and the interval between visits is almost always monthly. This translates to fewer than 12 sessions (6 hours per year), less total time than most models of brief psychotherapy. Because none of the classical models of brief psychotherapy were derived from experience in a medical setting, this summary is offered to shed light on the special requirements of an outpatient medical population. Indeed, the selection criteria in Mann's (1973) model specifically exclude patients with psychosomatic disorders who do not tolerate loss well.

BIAT was found to be appropriate and effective for patients referred to a special ("integration") clinic (Lipsitt 1964) that evaluated and managed patients with chronic medical diseases who used somatization as a major defense. Earliest referrals were in response to the request for "problem patients to be sent to the clinic." The approach developed in working with these patients utilized some of the principles of brief psychotherapy, psychodynamic formulation, personality diagnosis, and supportive psychotherapy. It was the policy of the clinic that once registered, patients were never discharged and were informed that they could make use of the clinic on an as-needed basis after they were not required to attend any longer.

These patients were high utilizers of medical services, including emergency room and inpatient hospitalization, and were generally not amenable to psychiatric referral. A pilot study (Lipsitt 1964) showed that many of these patients, previously "no-shows" when referred to the department of psychiatry, could accept a setting in the medical outpatient area that did not threaten their need to retain a physical definition of illness. The nondescript name of the clinic reinforced their denial of emotional problems.

A first visit usually began with "tell me about your problems." This almost invariably elicited an "organ recital" of complaints, customarily ending in the expectation that now, finally, someone would fulfill their unrealistic expectation that all would be made well. Such expectations and dependent idealizations of the physician were aborted with a comment like "I don't know why Dr. X thought I would be able to help." Those who questioned this response were informed by the psychiatrist that he needed more time to get to know them, that they had already had a lot of treatment and nothing seemed to help very much. Those who urged the therapist to read their chart were told that it would be more useful to hear their story from themselves than to read what someone else had written about them. The objective was to establish a relationship these patients could tolerate without needing to use barriers of medications and unfulfilled promises as a way of perpetuating their complaints and somatizations. Their histories were punctuated with projections shared with their physicians that "those pills didn't work, we'll try something else," or "maybe something was missed" (often a metaphor for "the doctor didn't listen to me, didn't understand, or wasn't interested").

It was the psychiatrist's intent to have the patient perceive him or her as having no investment in the presence or absence of symptoms but only in what the patient had to say. Only in rare instances were requests for additional appointments granted on the basis of intensification of symptoms, and virtually never was a symptom that was present one month but absent the next inquired about. It was anticipated that patients who were so dependent would need an approach that simultaneously permitted dependency but encouraged independence, a technique that often requires the consultation-liaison psychiatrist to "walk a very fine line." For the most part, these patients needed to be able to trust, to experience an honest relationship, and to be assured that they would not be abandoned. Efforts to provide these reassurances more often took the form of actions than of words, with indications that the patient could make telephone calls that would, at some point, be answered and that they would never be refused access to the clinic. Testing by patients of this kind of intervention usually occurred earlier in treatment but eventually diminished when they assured themselves of the availability of doctors and the clinic.

Improvement was measured by decreased telephone calls, by decreased visits to medical facilities, and ultimately by decreased visits to the integration clinic. If a patient eventually wanted to stop clinic visits "unless something comes up," he or she was given an appointment for a "checkup whether you have symptoms or not" to diminish the connection between visits and symptoms. Other evidence of change appeared in the patient's eventual shift away from the "organ recital" to conversation about family, activities, or interests. This shift usually occurred without prompting by the outpatient consultation-liaison psychiatrist when the relationship was acceptable and tolerable without the presence of physical complaints.

Month-long intervals between appointments diminished the potential for regression while fulfilling patients' need for attachment. Unfortunately, this "attenuated" form of treatment, although requiring small expense of time and money, is not understood or readily accepted by the new approach promoted by insurance companies, managed programs, and health maintenance organizations. This approach clearly has economic and preventive value but requires further controlled research to measure its apparent efficacy on somatizing high utilizers of health care services. It encompasses elements of a variety of approaches, including interpersonal, psychodynamic, cognitive, behavioral, supportive, and reconstructive, and, as such, is a gratifying example of the eclecticism and versatility required of the consultation-liaison psychiatrist in general medical settings.

CONCLUSION

The concept of the consultation-liaison psychiatrist as psychotherapist is relatively recent. It was not until well after World War II that descriptions of actual therapeutic interventions began to appear.

Because of the broad array of patients seen by the consultation-liaison psychiatrist, especially in the inpatient general medical setting, strict adherence to one intervention approach is untenable. A consultation-liaison psychiatrist is a generalist as well as a subspecialist who has familiarity with a spectrum of therapeutic tools. Psychotherapy should be prescribed "cafeteria-style," according to the needs of the patient rather than in an ideologically orthodox manner. The consultation-liaison psychiatrist is thus challenged to synthesize both evaluative

and therapeutic dimensions of the consultative opportunity and to apply, most flexibly, those therapeutic models (or aspects of them) that most usefully fit the time and circumstances as they exist.

The consultation-liaison psychiatrist encounters, in the rich milieu of the general hospital, countless opportunities to be helpful to patients, to educate other caretakers in the biopsychosocial approach, and to be personally and professionally gratified.

REFERENCES

Balint M: The Doctor, His Patient and the Illness. London, Pitman, 1964

Bibring E: Psychoanalysis and the dynamic psychotherapies. J Am Psychoanal Assoc 2:745–770, 1954

Blacher RS: The briefest encounter: psychotherapy for medical and surgical patients. Gen Hosp Psychiatry 6:226–232, 1984

Bloom BL: Focused single-session therapy: initial development and evaluation, in Forms of Brief Therapy. Edited by Budman S. New York, Guilford, 1981, pp 131–175

Budman SH, Stone J: Advances in brief psychotherapy: a review of recent literature. Hosp Community Psychiatry 34:939–946, 1983

Davanloo H: Basic Principles and Techniques in Short-Term Dynamic Psychotherapy. New York, Spectrum, 1978

Deutsch F: The associative anamnesis. Psychoanal Q 8:354–381, 1939

Deutsch F: The Mysterious Leap From the Mind to the Body. New York, International Universities Press, 1959

Deutsch F, Murphy W: The Clinical Interview. New York, International Universities Press, 1955

Fenichel O: Brief psychotherapy, in The Collected Papers of Otto Fenichel, Second Series. New York, WW Norton, 1954, pp 243–259

Frances AJ, Clarkin JF: No treatment as the prescription of choice. Arch Gen Psychiatry 142:922–926, 1981

Gabbard GO: Psychodynamic Psychiatry in Clinical Practice. Washington, DC, American Psychiatric Press, 1990

Gitelson M: On the curative factors in the first phase of analysis, in Psychoanalysis: Science and Profession. Edited by Gitelson M. New York, International Universities Press, 1973, pp 311–341

Green SA: Principles of medical psychotherapy, in Psychiatric Care of the Medical Patient. Edited by Stoudemire A, Fogel BS. New York, Oxford University Press, 1993, pp 1–18

Greenhill MH: Liaison psychiatry, in American Handbook of Psychiatry, Vol 7: Advances and New Directions, 2nd Edition. Edited by Arieti S, Brodie HKH. New York, Basic Books, 1981, pp 672–702

Groves JE, Kurcharski A: Brief psychotherapy, in Massachusetts General Hospital Handbook of General Hospital Psychiatry, 3rd Edition. Edited by Cassem NH. St Louis, MO, CV Mosby, 1991, pp 321–341

Hackett TP, Weisman AD: Psychiatric management of operative syndromes, II: psychodynamic factors in formulation and management. Psychosom Med 22:356–372, 1960

Hamburg D, Adams JE: A perspective on coping behavior. Arch Gen Psychiatry 17:277–284, 1967

Harrison SI, Carek DJ: A Guide to Psychotherapy. Boston, MA, Little, Brown, 1966

Hersen M, Bellack AS: Perspectives in the behavioral treatment of depression. Behav Modif 6:95–106, 1982

Horowitz MJ, Kaltreider NB: Brief therapy for the stress response syndrome. Psychiatr Clin North Am 2:365–377, 1979

Horowitz MJ, Marmar C, Krupnick J, et al: Personality Styles and Brief Psychotherapy. New York, Basic Books, 1984

Jacobs J: Family therapy in the context of chronic medical illness, in Psychiatric Care of the Medical Patient. Edited by Stoudemire A, Fogel BS. New York, Oxford University Press, 1993, pp 19–30

Kahana RJ, Bibring GL: Personality types in medical management, in Psychiatry and Medical Practice in a General Hospital. Edited by Zinberg NE. New York, International Universities Press, 1964, pp 108–123

Klerman GL, Weissman MM, Rounsaville BR, et al: Interpersonal Psychotherapy of Depression. New York, Basic Books, 1984

Liberzon I, Goldman RS, Hendrickson WJ: Very brief psychotherapy in the psychiatric consultation setting. Int J Psychiatry Med 22:65–75, 1992

Lipowski ZJ: Consultation-liaison psychiatry: the first half century. Gen Hosp Psychiatry 8:305–315, 1986

Lipsitt DR: Integration clinic: an approach to the teaching and practice of medical psychology in an outpatient setting, in Psychiatry and Medical Practice in a General Hospital. Edited by Zinberg NE. New York, International Universities Press, 1964, pp 231–249

Lipsitt DR: Some problems in the teaching of psychosomatic medicine, in Psychosomatic Medicine: Current Trends and Clinical Applications. Edited by Lipowski ZJ, Lipsitt DR, Whybrow PC. New York, Oxford University Press, 1977, pp 599–611

Lipsitt DR: Therapeutic alliance in psychiatric consultation, in Psychiatry, Vol 2. Edited by Michels R, Cavenar JO Jr, Brodie HKH, et al. Philadelphia, PA, JB Lippincott, 1985

Luborsky L: Theory and technique in dynamic psychotherapy-curative factors and training therapists to maximize them. Psychother Psychosom 53:50–57, 1990

Malan DH: A Study of Brief Psychotherapy. London, Tavistock, 1963

Mann J: Time-Limited Psychotherapy. Cambridge, MA, Harvard University Press, 1973

Marmor J: The physician as psychotherapist, in Psychiatry in General Medical Practice. Edited by Usdin G, Lewis JM. New York, McGraw-Hill, 1979a

Marmor J: Short-term dynamic psychotherapy. Am J Psychiatry 136:149–155, 1979b

Melges FT: Family approaches to health and disease, in Psychiatry, Vol 2. Edited by Michels R, Cavenar JO Jr, Brodie HKH, et al. Philadelphia, PA, JB Lippincott, 1985

Mohl PC, Burstein AG: The application of Kohutian self-psychology to consultation-liaison psychiatry. Gen Hosp Psychiatry 4:113–119, 1982

Nadelson T: Engagement before alliance. Psychother Psychosom 33:76–86, 1980

Polatin P: A Guide to Treatment in Psychiatry. Philadelphia, PA, JB Lippincott, 1966

Sifneos P: Short-Term Psychotherapy and Emotional Crisis. Cambridge, MA, Harvard University Press, 1972

Sifneos PE: The prevalence of "alexithymic" characteristics in psychosomatic patients. Psychother Psychosom 22:255–262, 1973

Spira JL, Spiegel D: Group psychotherapy of the medically ill, in Psychiatric Care of the Medical Patient. Edited by Stoudemire A, Fogel BS. New York, Oxford University Press, 1993, pp 31–50

Stein A, Weiner S: Group therapy with medically ill patients, in Psychotherapeutic Approaches to Medicine. Edited by Karasu TB, Steinmuller RI. New York, Grune & Stratton, 1978, pp 223–242

Strain JJ, Grossman S: Psychological Care of the Medically Ill. New York, Appleton-Century-Crofts, 1975

Strupp HH, Binder JL: Psychotherapy in a New Key: A Guide to Time-Limited Dynamic Psychotherapy. New York, Basic Books, 1984

Ursano RJ, Hales RE: A review of brief individual psychotherapies. Am J Psychiatry 143:1507–1517, 1986

Viederman M: The active dynamic interview and the supportive relationship. Compr Psychiatry 25:147–157, 1984

Viederman M: Psychotherapeutic approaches in the medically ill, in Psychiatry, Vol 2. Edited by Michels R, Cavenar JO Jr, Brodie HKH, et al. Philadelphia, PA, JB Lippincott, 1985

Waldinger RJ: Psychiatry for Medical Students, 2nd Edition. Washington, DC, American Psychiatric Press, 1990

Yalom ID: Theory and Practice of Group Psychotherapy. New York, Basic Books, 1975

Zeiss AM, Lewinsohn PM, Munoz RF: Nonspecific improvement effects in depression using interpersonal, cognitive and pleasant events focused treatments. J Consult Clin Psychol 47:427–439, 1979

Chapter 34

Behavioral Medicine

Andrew B. Littman, M.D.
Mark W. Ketterer, Ph.D.

Behavioral medicine is a field that was initially inspired by the potential application of classical and operant learning theory to behavioral problems in medical patients (G. E. Schwartz and Weiss 1978). While evolving into a theoretically and therapeutically more eclectic arena, practitioners of behavioral medicine continue to find behavioral techniques (relaxation and hypnosis, environmental modification, biofeedback, cognitive-behavioral therapy) useful and effective. Studies on the underdiagnosis and inadequate treatment of patients with psychiatric disorders in nonpsychiatric medical settings (Katon 1987; Katon et al. 1992) and the primacy of depression in determining disability status (Von Korff et al. 1992; Wells et al. 1989) now complement the observation that patients undergoing psychotherapy evidence a decrease in medical system utilization (Borus et al. 1985; Budman et al. 1984; Rosen and Wiens 1979).

Central to the behavioral medicine approach is a belief that the arousal of emotion fosters disease end points in the psychophysiological disorders—or symptoms, in the case of the somatoform disorders—by way of either psychoneuroendocrine or psychobehavioral pathways. Psychoneuroendocrine pathways encompass the downstream neural and/or endocrine effects of chronic or acute emotional arousal (Chrousos and Gold 1992). Psychopathophysiological arousal may be the result of genetic-constitutional factors, early life experiences that subsequently shape interpersonal beliefs and coping, or environments that are sometimes universally and sometimes idiosyncratically stressful. Intervention can be instituted in an attempt to influence any or all of these modifiable elements.

In an early approach to psychosomatic disorders, several investigators attempted to demonstrate "specificity" of relations between particular personality characteristics and particular medical conditions (Alexander 1950; Dunbar 1947). Behavioral medicine has taken a less theoretically constrained, and more empirically driven, approach to understanding psyche-soma relations. Some of the psychological phenomena that have been the focus of investigation are probably "subclinical" psychiatric disorders, whereas others seem to call for an entirely new way of conceptualizing psychopathology in this arena. For example, it is striking that the DSM system contains large sections on depressive and anxiety disorders but no focused discussion of anger, a central concern in the behavioral treatment of ischemic heart disease (IHD), as discussed below (see "Cardiovascular Diseases"). Other examples of phenomena that are difficult to categorize within the DSM nosology include the impact of high-demand and/or low-control jobs, low social support, and vital exhaustion, each of which is associated with physical disease outcomes. The currently used DSM-IV (American Psychiatric Association 1994) diagnostic entity "316.00—psychological factors affecting a physical condition" is unsatisfying because each of the entities listed above potentially implies a different treatment strategy. A new categorization of these behavioral factors must be developed. We have based the material in this chapter on an empirical, outcome-based approach to evaluating the clinical significance of behavioral treatment in various medical conditions.

■ CARDIOVASCULAR DISEASES[1]

Numerous studies have been performed demonstrating the influence of psychosocial and behavioral risk factors in the etiology of IHD (Blumenthal and Kamarck 1987). The most well-known of these factors is type A behavior, the chronic and habitual response of the individual to perceived demands with time urgency and/or easily provoked annoyance, anger, and aggression (Friedman and Ulmer 1984). The initial enthusiasm for the global type A concept, including elements such as perfectionism, mistrust, competitiveness, arrogance, practicality, and controlling nature or hyperresponsibility, waned in the middle to late 1980s as hostility was found to be the "toxic" element of the syndrome (Dembroski et al. 1989; Shekelle et al. 1985). Whereas global type A behavior is not always predictive of IHD risk, hostility is (Dimsdale 1988).

Depressive symptoms are fairly ubiquitous in patients after a myocardial infarction (MI) and are considered to be reactive in etiology, self-limited, and of minimal importance (Wishnie et al. 1971). Klerman (1989) pointed out that, traditionally, depressive symptoms are minimized in clinical settings as "demoralization," "expectable reactions," and "neurotic" depression. However, 18%–40% of patients with IHD have depressive symptoms that predate the diagnosis of IHD or MI (Cay et al. 1972; Lloyd and Cawley 1978), confirming the impression that depressive symptoms are common among patients with IHD before the onset of symptomatic IHD.

Depressive symptoms significantly affect health outcomes beyond depressive symptoms' considerable influence on functional status and quality of life. For instance, adherence to treatment is lower in patients with IHD who have depressive symptoms (Blumenthal et al. 1982; Finnegan and Suler 1985). Depressive symptoms predict lack of improvement of exercise functioning in patients with IHD who are undergoing cardiac rehabilitation (Downing et al. 1992; A. B. Littman, unpublished data, 1993; Milani et al., in press). In a population-based study of 2,800 American adults (Anda et al. 1993), after controlling for demographic and risk factors, the investigators found that individuals with depressed mood and hopelessness had higher IHD morbidity and mortality.

[1]Portions of this section originally appeared in Littman AB: "Review of Psychosomatic Aspects of Cardiovascular Disease." *Psychotherapy and Psychosomatics* 60:148–167, 1993. Permission for use was obtained from the editor.

No controlled psychopharmacological or psychotherapeutic treatment trials of patients with IHD with depressive symptoms are currently available, but evidence suggests that treatment of the type A behavior pattern by cognitive-behavioral group therapy is associated with significant reductions in both levels of anxiety and depressive symptoms (Fava et al. 1991).

Several studies demonstrate that patients with major depressive disorder have higher mortality from IHD (Murphy et al. 1987; Rubins et al. 1985). Studies also show that, after traditional cardiac risk factors are controlled, untreated major depression predicts major cardiac events, including death, after diagnosis of IHD (Ahern et al. 1990; Carney et al. 1988; Ladwig et al. 1991). In a recent study, 18% of patients hospitalized for MI had major depressive disorder, and depression predicted mortality at 6 months, with a relative risk of 4.3, after other risk factors were controlled (Frasure-Smith et al. 1993). The impact of major depression on cardiovascular mortality is at least equivalent to that of left ventricular dysfunction and history of previous MI, among the most potent known indicators of prognosis (Frasure-Smith et al. 1993).

The term *denial* has at least two presumably correlated meanings as applied to populations of patients with cardiac disease. First, patients sometimes deny their emotions during the initial phases of cardiac illness. Second, patients sometimes deny acute cardiac symptoms themselves. Denial independently predicts better medical outcomes during acute hospitalization for unstable angina (Levenson et al. 1989). During hospitalization for MI or bypass surgery, deniers spend fewer days in the intensive care unit (ICU) (Levine et al. 1987). However, these benefits are short-lived. Over the subsequent year, these same deniers are more noncompliant with medical recommendations and require more days of rehospitalization compared with other patients. Similarly, denying emotional distress during the acute phase

of an MI is associated with increased likelihood of returning to work and being sexually active at 1 year follow-up but also with resumption of smoking (Stern et al. 1976). Thus, it appears that emotional denial during acutely stressful medical events, such as MI or cardiac surgery, is adaptive in the short run but deleterious over the long haul (Suls and Fletcher 1985).

A study examined the relation between emotional and symptomatic denial. A total of 60% of all MIs result in death before hospital admission (American Heart Association 1991). At least 25% of all nonfatal MIs are unrecognized on their occurrence (Bertolet and Hill 1989). Up to 80% of all patients with diagnosed MIs arrive at an emergency facility too late to fully benefit from modern thrombolytic therapy or emergency revascularization. Patient interviews reveal that patients spend most of the time before admission deciding if they are ill, or ill enough, to warrant immediate care. Thus, reality-based cognitive processing of anginal symptoms is the primary determinant of delay of treatment-seeking behavior.

A variety of behavioral and psychological interventions can reduce type A behavior in both healthy individuals (Gill et al. 1985) and patients with IHD (Friedman et al. 1984).

A meta-analysis of type A–reduction treatment studies in patients with IHD demonstrated a 3-year reduction of 50% for combined mortality and recurrent MI (Nunes et al. 1987). A recent comparison of the efficacy of behavioral with medical and surgical interventions to reduce the risk of nonfatal MI and cardiac death showed behavioral therapies to be superior to all methods of treatment, except the use of aspirin in patients with unstable angina and bypass surgery in patients who were classified as "high-risk" (Ketterer 1993). The largest single project to date to evaluate the effects of group treatment of type A behavior is the Recurrent Coronary Prevention Project, involving 862 post-MI patients (Friedman et al. 1987). Four and one-half years after the start of the study, 35% of the treatment group, compared with

10% of the placebo care group, markedly reduced their type A behavior. The rate of recurrence of MI was significantly lower in the type A treatment group than among the placebo care group (13% versus 21%, respectively). The type A treatment group showed a significant reduction in cardiac death (2.7% versus 6.7%) when patients with preexisting severe heart damage were excluded from the analysis.

Ornish et al. (1990) used a multifaceted treatment of comprehensive lifestyle change, including low-fat vegetarian diet (8% of calories as dietary fat), stress management training (yoga, meditation, and group therapy), and moderate exercise, in an attempt to reduce coronary atherosclerosis without the use of lipid-lowering agents. Over a 1-year period, the coronary lesions in the treatment group regressed in 82% of the subjects, whereas the lesions progressed in the usual care group. Overall adherence to the treatment intervention was the best predictor of the extent of atherosclerotic regression (Ornish et al. 1990). Four-year follow-up data showed a highly significant difference in outcomes between the two groups, with continued regression (between 39.7% and 43.6% in average percentage diameter of coronary artery stenosis) in the comprehensive lifestyle change group, and continued progression (41.6%–51.4%) in the usual care group (Ornish et al. 1993).

Pharmacotherapy for Type A Behavior, Hostility, and Anger

The specific effects of pharmacological treatments on type A behaviors and associated clinical outcomes are not well studied in controlled settings. β-Blockers have had inconsistent and modest effects on type A behavior (Schmiedler et al. 1983). Benzodiazepines reduce catecholamines, cortisol, and blood pressure responses to acute mental stress in patients with type A behavior (Williams et al. 1986) and significantly reduce duration of silent ischemia in a small sample ($n = 8$) of patients with coronary disease (Shell and Swan 1986). However, benzodiazepines do not alter type A behavior or hostility. Recently, investigators have hypothesized the presence of lowered central serotonergic function in patients with hostility associated with elevated risk for IHD (Littman et al. 1993). Anger attacks are common (44%) in individuals with major depression, and treatment with fluoxetine, a selective serotonin reuptake inhibitor (SSRI), reduces the presence of these anger outbursts by 70% (Fava et al. 1993). In patients with IHD with hostility and type A behavior but no Axis I psychiatric disorder, a clinical trial demonstrated that buspirone, a central serotonin$_{1A}$ partial agonist, significantly reduced hostility and type A behavior (Littman et al. 1993).

Cholesterol and Behavior

A clear association exists between elevated serum cholesterol and risk for IHD. Lower serum cholesterol reduces IHD events and IHD mortality in both primary and secondary prevention trials yet is not associated with improvement in overall survival (Jacobs et al. 1992). A meta-analysis of these trials showed that counterbalancing the reduction in IHD mortality was an increase in deaths due to accidents, suicide, and violence (Muldoon et al. 1990). The most recent meta-analysis of lipid-lowering trials showed an increased risk of death from violence and suicide only for subjects using medications to lower their cholesterol. This finding is consistent with another study that showed that patients with IHD who were receiving medical treatment for hypercholesterolemia reported significantly more symptoms of depression than those who were not being treated (Ketterer et al. 1993).

Physical Activity

Physical activity appears to have numerous beneficial effects in individuals who are healthy or already have developed IHD. Cardiac rehabilitation programs, primarily exercise programs, reduce mortality by 25% from all causes, including cardiovascular (Oldridge et al. 1988). The Multiple Risk Factor Intervention Trial (MRFIT) (Leon et al. 1987) classified individuals at high risk for IHD in levels of low, moderate, and high tertiles of leisure time physical activity. Moderate levels of leisure time physical activity were associated with 63% fewer cardiovascular deaths and 70% fewer total deaths compared with low leisure time physical activity. Interestingly, mortality rates for the high leisure time physical activity group were similar to those of the moderate leisure time physical activity group. The study showed that 30–60 minutes of predominately light- to moderate-intensity activities on a daily basis is the optimal level to reduce cardiovascular risk (Leon et al. 1987). In addition, the Centers for Disease Control and Prevention reviewed existing observational studies of healthy individuals and found a significant and graded relation between physical inactivity and risk of coronary artery disease (Powell et al. 1987). A study from the Cooper Clinic with more than 13,000 subjects showed a strong, stepwise, and consistent inverse relation between physical fitness and mortality, with the major burden for morbidity and mortality in the lowest quintile of fitness (Blair et al. 1989).

Exercise and dieting appear to have equal efficacy in reducing plasma lipids in overweight sedentary men (Wood et al. 1988). Adherence to a regular exercise routine appears to be difficult, with about half of those enrolled in a well-equipped and staffed program dropping out within the first several months, and many of the remainder within 2 years. Surveys suggest that despite the cultural fascination with fitness, two-thirds of Americans do not exercise on a regular basis, and between 30% and 45% do not exercise at all (Martin and Dubbert 1985).

Obesity and Weight Loss

Weight loss is often urged for patients with cardiac disease because of the adverse effects of being overweight on hypertension, diabetes mellitus, lipid abnormalities, and physical inactivity. This encouragement occurs, unfortunately, despite strong evidence that weight loss is a futile goal for the majority of people. Although about one-third of individuals seem to be able to lose weight and maintain the loss (Schachter 1982), relapse is inevitable for a large majority of people (NIH Technology Assessment Conference Panel 1992; Stunkard 1980). *Consumer Reports* (1993) confirmed these findings in a report titled "Losing Weight: What Works, What Doesn't," an evaluation of the differential effectiveness of the various commercial diet plans available. Because genetic factors play a strong role in obesity (Stunkard et al. 1990), it is possible that urging patients to lose weight as a goal is merely setting them up for frustration, demoralization, and "weight-cycling"—worse outcomes than the initial problem (Garner and Wooley 1991). If a patient is mildly or moderately overweight, not hypertensive or diabetic, or these two conditions are present but controlled, and if the patient exercises, it may be most productive to encourage weight maintenance.

Systemic Arterial Hypertension

Numerous studies have demonstrated that social factors, such as social stress and conflict, and low degrees of social support are associated with elevated blood pressure (Dressler et al. 1986, 1988). The nonpharmacological approaches to the treatment of hypertension are relaxation training, biofeedback, weight loss, exercise, dietary sodium restriction, and nutritional supplementation (calcium, magnesium, potassium, and fish oil) (Chesney et al. 1987). Biofeedback methods are effective in reducing blood pressure, and this effect on blood pressure has been shown to generalize from practice sessions to daily life and sleep periods with some degree of persistence (Chesney et al. 1987).

Only one study (Patel et al. 1985), with 192

hypertensive patients, showed the efficacy of multimodal stress management in reducing blood pressure at 8 weeks and 4 years. A meta-analysis of nine other controlled studies of stress management with 733 subjects found a significant effect (2 mm Hg) only in diastolic blood pressure in nonmedicated patients and no effect in patients who were already taking medication (Kaufman et al. 1988). A study of 2,200 subjects comparing four nonpharmacological interventions (weight reduction, dietary sodium restriction, stress management, and nutritional supplementation) on blood pressure in individuals with high baseline blood pressure demonstrated significant effects on blood pressure only from weight reduction and sodium restriction (Trials of Hypertension Prevention Collaborative Research Group 1992). Despite conventional wisdom and hopes to the contrary, recent studies cast serious doubt on whether relaxation therapies significantly reduce blood pressure (Littman 1993).

Smoking Cessation

Cigarette smoking is the single most avoidable cause of death in society (Shopland 1984). Studies indicate that patients with coronary artery disease who stop smoking have a lower mortality than those who continue to smoke (Vlietstra et al. 1986). In addition, passive cigarette smoking also poses an increased risk to those who are in smoky environments (L'Enfant and Liu 1980).

Public awareness of the health benefits of stopping smoking has motivated many individuals to quit. Despite a dramatic decline over the last 40 years in the United States in the percentage of adults who smoke (J. L. Schwartz 1987), a larger proportion of smokers cannot quit, continue to smoke heavily, and are addicted to nicotine (Shopland 1984).

Historically, most organized treatments designed to assist in smoking cessation have been behaviorally or psychologically based. Long-term quit rates associated with these programs

have averaged 30% (J. L. Schwartz 1987). Pharmacological approaches have been developed more recently to provide adjunctive means to help smokers quit. Randomized trials, including double-blind placebo-controlled studies with nicotine chewing gum—the most widely used pharmacological agent for smoking cessation—indicate that the use of nicotine gum improves long-term quit rates (Hughes and Miller 1984). The efficacy of the chewing gum seems to be attributable to its ability to relieve symptoms of nicotine withdrawal, including irritability, anxiety, difficulty concentrating, and restlessness (Hughes and Hatsukami 1986).

The effectiveness of nicotine gum in smoking cessation depends on several factors. First, when nicotine gum is used to stop smoking independent of specialized smoking cessation services, it appears to have minimal effect (Hughes et al. 1989). Other factors that may adversely affect successful smoking cessation without a formal program include lack of personal support and lack of instructions on the correct use of the nicotine gum. Finally, nicotine gum with specialized smoking cessation treatment appears to significantly increase treatment efficacy. This treatment efficacy with nicotine gum is maximized when combined with specific behavioral skills training rather than a standard didactic approach (Goldstein et al. 1989).

Transdermal nicotine patches are also available for smoking cessation (Abelin et al. 1989). The constant delivery system offers nicotine to an individual without the regular reinforcing behaviors of cigarette smoking and nicotine gum use.

Sexual Functioning

Most patients with IHD experience a decline in quantity and quality of sexual activity. A majority of patients with IHD continue to have reduced frequency of sexual activity, and decreased sexual desire and impotence are commonly seen (Hlatky et al. 1986). A randomized trial of counseling of the wives of men with MI resulted in significantly less anxiety among the wives at 6 months posthospitalization than among control subjects (Thompson and Meddis 1990). It is critical to provide patients with unambiguous information about when it is safe to resume sexual activity. A patient's physiological readiness to resume sexual activity is frequently evaluated by observing his or her capacity to climb two flights of stairs at a brisk pace (McLane et al. 1980). For those patients who experience angina during sex, positioning and prophylactic use of nitro compounds is helpful (Blaustein et al. 1984). Both patient and spousal beliefs and fears about the likelihood of having an MI during sexual activity should be explored and corrected. It is also critical to keep in mind that patients with IHD frequently have vascular, medication-related, or neurogenic causes for impotence or lack of vaginal responsiveness during sex. For example, β-blockers can decrease libido and cause impotence (Kolodny et al. 1979).

Noncardiac Chest Pain

Many patients who are seen in cardiology and general medical practices complain of chest pain or discomfort that is not associated with objectively verifiable cardiac conditions. When no medical condition is found to explain the chest discomfort, these patients have historically received a diagnosis of "cardiac neurosis," "neurocirculatory asthenia," or "hyperventilation syndrome" (Mayou 1989). Among cardiologists, a term that is sometimes heard is *syndrome X* (Cannon et al. 1992). Of all patients who are seen in cardiology clinics who have nonanginal or atypical chest pain, 59% have panic disorder (Beitman et al. 1987). Other studies have shown that a high incidence of psychiatric symptoms, such as anxiety, depression, and hypochondriasis, exists among patients who complain of "nonorganic" chest pain.

GASTROINTESTINAL DISEASES

Whitehead and Bosmajian (1982), after reviewing several studies, concluded that psychological stress exacerbates esophageal motility disorders. However, no clear-cut data to date demonstrate that treatment of psychological stress can reduce symptoms of these esophageal disorders.

Although emotional factors do play a role in the pathogenesis of peptic ulcer disease, the development of highly cost-effective histamine-receptor antagonists as well as new antibiotic treatments places behavioral therapies in a secondary role. Behavioral treatment may improve medication compliance or affect emotional factors that are operative in the initiation or aggravation of peptic ulcer disease (Whitehead and Bosmajian 1982).

As many as 50%–90% of patients suspected of having peptic ulcer disease do not, on examination, have evidence of an ulcer. Functional (nonulcer) dyspepsia is characterized by chronic or recurrent upper abdominal pain or discomfort for at least 3 months without endoscopic evidence of other disease (Drossman et al. 1990). Psychiatric comorbidity among patients with dyspepsia is high—87% of patients with functional (nonulcer) dyspepsia have one or more anxiety disorders as compared with 25% of those with dyspepsia associated with endoscopic evidence of gastrointestinal (GI) disease (Magni et al. 1987). Functional (nonulcer) dyspepsia and irritable bowel syndrome (IBS) overlap a great deal diagnostically. No studies have evaluated the efficacy of behavioral or psychopharmacological interventions in patients with functional (nonulcer) dyspepsia (Whitehead 1992).

IBS is a disturbance characterized by at least 3 months' duration of abdominal discomfort, relieved with defecation or associated with a change in frequency or consistency of stool, along with an irregular pattern of defecation at least 25% of the time that includes two or more of the following: altered stool frequency, altered stool form, passage of mucus, and bloating, without the presence of demonstrable GI pathology (Drossman et al. 1990). In the past 15 years, there have been numerous studies of psychological treatment for IBS, with investigators examining the efficacy of behavioral therapies alone or in combination with standard medical therapies. Brief, insight-oriented psychotherapy in combination with medical therapy has been shown to be superior to medications alone in reducing abdominal pain and diarrhea (Guthrie et al. 1991; Svedlund et al. 1983). Relaxation and stress management (Bennett and Wilkinson 1985) or hypnotherapy alone (Whorell et al. 1984) has been found to reduce abdominal pain and diarrhea. Biofeedback, on the other hand, has been found to have equivocal results in symptom alteration (Radnitz and Blanchard 1988).

There is no objective evidence that emotional stress produces or worsens the symptoms of inflammatory bowel disease (IBD), Crohn's disease, or ulcerative colitis (Whitehead and Bosmajian 1982). Patients with Crohn's disease have more psychological symptoms than do patients with ulcerative colitis, but this difference is not present when controlling for severity of physical symptoms (Drossman et al. 1991).

IMMUNE-RELATED ILLNESSES

Psychoneuroimmunology is a term that is used to identify the field of investigation directed at understanding how behavior and mental states affect immune function (Ader et al. 1991). Although it has long been suspected that host resistance is influenced by emotional well-being, only with the availability of increasingly precise technology for measuring immune cell activity has it become possible to conduct in vitro tests of the potential association between various psychosocial factors and immune activity.

Only randomly assigned, controlled treatment studies can demonstrate experimentally that a true causal relation exists between external events and internal immune function (Kiecolt-Glaser and Glaser 1992). Three studies attempting to utilize this paradigm have been published. The first of these studies involved nursing home residents who were randomly assigned to receive relaxation training. The treatment group had increased in vitro natural killer cell activity and decreased herpes simplex virus antibody titers compared with those who received only social contact or no intervention (Kiecolt-Glaser et al. 1985). The two other studies were performed on young and healthy subjects. In healthy medical students who participated in a stress management program, the percentage of helper T cells was positively related to the amount of practice of relaxation (Kiecolt-Glaser et al. 1986). Healthy undergraduates who wrote essays about traumatic events displayed better mitogen response to phytohemagglutinin than those who wrote about emotionally neutral topics (Pennebaker et al. 1988).

CANCER

A large body of literature has established the existence of a relation between psychosocial events and cancer. Some correlational studies have suggested that cancer onset or survival is partially associated with life stressors (Geyer 1991) or personality (Dean and Surtees 1989; Derogatis et al. 1979; Greer et al. 1979). This relation may also be explained by indirect behavioral-lifestyle factors associated with the psychosocial variables. As discussed above, outcome studies remain the acid test in establishing causality. Such studies can significantly reduce the possibility that the effect is mediated by behavioral-lifestyle factors by concomitantly observing changes in such factors in the treatment and control groups and then controlling for them in analyses.

Inadequate randomization of baseline staging of illness can easily distort the findings of intervention studies that attempt to influence the course of illness in patients with cancer (Morganstern et al. 1984). Spiegel and colleagues (1989) found significantly increased survival in patients with breast cancer who were randomized to participate in an emotional support group in contrast to those receiving standard care alone (Spiegel et al. 1989). This finding provides a compelling case for considering emotional support as a potentially important intervention that influences the course of disease as well as quality of life. Although this result has evinced much skepticism, equivalent results from a drug or surgery trial would be greeted much more enthusiastically. One line of argument that limits the interpretability of these results derives from the observation that the overall survival rate was low, with the treatment group's survival approximating that seen nationally in patients with breast cancer (Fox 1992). Such an argument implies that the randomization procedures failed in Spiegel's study. The staging of illness was the only variable associated with prognosis that marginally favored ($P < .07$) the treatment group, and analysis of treatment efficacy controlled for this finding. To control for the variability of site-specific survival, a study using site-specific, matched comparison data from nationally gathered breast cancer data is under way (B. H. Fox, personal communication, May 1993). Several replication studies are also currently under way (Cunningham and Lockwood 1992; LeShan 1991; Spiegel 1992).

Anticipatory nausea and vomiting are common side effects in patients undergoing chemotherapy. Patients with heightened autonomic reactivity, measured by slower autonomic habituation, appear to be most susceptible to this phenomenon (Andrykowski 1990; Kvale et al. 1991). In severe instances, patients report nausea elicited simply by their driving on the side of town where they receive their treatment. Approximately 25% of patients on chemotherapy discontinue treatment because of the impact of nausea and vomiting on their quality of life. Morrow and Dobkin (1988) reported the first effort at controlling anticipatory nausea and vomiting via relaxation procedures. A significant reduction in nausea and vomiting was observed, a result that has since been replicated several times (Andrykowski 1990).

INFECTIOUS DISEASES

Stress has also been found to co-vary with infectious diseases (Cohen and Williamson 1991). Herpes titers and visible sores, upper respiratory infections, tuberculosis, pyorrhea, and tularemia are more common, or more virulent, in individuals with high stress levels (Antoni et al. 1990). Manipulation of infectious agent exposure in three studies also confirmed an associative relation and supported the notion of a causal role for stress (Cantor 1972; Glaser et al. 1992; Meyer and Haggerty 1962). For example, the clinical expression of deliberate exposure to cold viruses relates to emotional distress in a dose-response relation (Cohen et al. 1991). As with all psychophysiological disorders, both psychoneuroendocrine and psychobehavioral pathways may help to explain some of these results, and only treatment studies provide true experimental evidence for a possible causal role. At least one treatment study in a geriatric population undergoing relaxation training indicated a reduction in herpes simplex virus titers and an increase in natural killer cell activity above their pretreatment baseline (Kiecolt-Glaser et al. 1985).

Although CD4 T-cell counts, per se, are not associated with emotional distress within a population of persons with acquired immunodeficiency syndrome (AIDS) (Rabkin et al. 1991), disease progression is associated with emotional distress (Cecchi 1984; Coates et al. 1984; Donlau et al. 1985; Solomon and Temoshok 1987). It is important to note that studies to date that show this association have not addressed the question of psychological impact of knowledge of disease progression and deteriorating prognosis. Neither have they addressed specific psychiatric predispositions of individuals who were infected by the virus in early years of the epidemic as opposed to later years. Preliminary evidence demonstrates that cognitive-behavioral stress management may be associated with improved CD4 counts, natural killer cell counts, and in vitro lymphocyte response in a randomly assigned, controlled treatment study of patients who had positive tests for infection with the human immunodeficiency virus (HIV) (Antoni et al. 1991). However, another group did not find a similar effect (Coates et al. 1989). No studies using hard clinical end points, such as mortality or length of survival, are yet published (Kelly and Murphy 1992). The degree to which HIV disease progression causes distress and the degree to which distress causes progression remain undefined for HIV disease and other immune-related disorders.

HYPERIMMUNE DISORDERS

The prevalence of hay fever in shy and inhibited children and their parents is approximately double that observed in more socially outgoing children (Bell et al. 1990; Kagan et al. 1991). When present, it is unclear whether these personality traits are fostered by the allergic condition or treatment regimens or are simply manifestations of an underlying biochemical phenomenon. Treatment studies have not yet been undertaken to test the viability of behavioral approaches to managing patients with allergic conditions (Marshall 1993).

Several dermatological conditions are responsive to behavioral treatments. Two different behavioral therapies are successful in treating psychogenic pruritus (Daniels 1973; Dobes 1977). Chronic hyperhidrosis, or excessive sweating, is related to psychological stress in many patients. Biofeedback therapies reduce sweating and associated stress symptoms (Duller and Gentry 1980).

The morbidity and mortality associated with asthma have increased in recent decades, quite possibly because of soaring levels of environmental pollutants and adverse effects of chronic bronchodilator use (Sly 1988). Psychoeducational programs directed at improving self-management of asthma and its therapies increase accuracy of medication and peak flowmeter use, improve the patient's sense of control, and decrease outpatient medical system use (Klingelhofer and Gershwin 1988). The effect of relaxation, particularly facial muscle relaxation, or biofeedback on pulmonary function seems to indicate increased bronchiolar smooth muscle relaxation, decreased frequency of attacks, and decreased medication use (Lehrer et al. 1992).

AUTOIMMUNE DISORDERS

Suspicion that emotional stress may trigger exacerbations of autoimmune conditions is long-standing. In addition, the relatively high prevalence of emotional distress among patients with autoimmune disorders is commonly attributed to reactions to such disorders. Although the "arthritic personality" (passive, conscientious, "catastrophizing," perfectionistic, and emotionally constricted) was initially dismissed as a reaction to the illness rather than a premorbidly existent character style (Anderson et al. 1985), it appears clear that patients with postmorbid coping characterized by these traits have poorer psychosocial functioning (Young 1992). The role of poor coping and emotional distress in determining functional outcome for such patients is strong. For example, anxiety and depression are stronger correlates of increased pain in patients with rheumatoid arthritis (RA) than are physical indices of disease severity such as erythrocyte sedimentation rate and number of swollen joints (Hagglund et al. 1989).

RA is a condition that continues to be widely believed to be aggravated by psychological stress. Most studies to date indicate that acute stressors (life events, marital conflict) may occur more frequently before RA flare-ups than during quiescent periods (Anderson et al. 1985). At least nine controlled treatment studies have been done in patients with RA. Those that were designed to decrease pain or pain behaviors were consistently successful in decreasing reported pain and constriction of activities of daily living (ADLs), whereas those directed at traditional mental health targets alone (depression and anxiety) were not (Young 1992). The utility of stress management in improving pain-related dysfunction and distress seems well established.

There is much speculation, based on cross-sectional or retrospective studies, that psychosocial stress initiates the autoimmune attack of β cells, thus causing diabetes mellitus or further alterations in glucose metabolism in brittle diabetic patients (McClelland et al. 1991; Robinson and Fuller 1986). No prospective studies exist to test this hypothesis. Some studies have demonstrated consistent associations between poor glucose control and anxiety, depression, familial conflict and dysfunction, loss of social contacts, social alienation, and impulsivity (Lustman et al. 1991; Mazze et al. 1984; McClelland et al. 1991; Nagasawa et al. 1990). Such correlational observations may be the result of indirect mechanisms such as noncompliance but also may be neuropsychiatric outcomes of poor control and systemic hyperglycemia (C. S. Holmes et al. 1983). There is clear evidence of the acute and long-term effect of diabetes on diminished cognitive functioning (Cox and Gonder-Frederick 1992). The cognitive dysfunction is generally of "subclinical" intensity—creating interpersonal problems at times because of misconstrual by others.

CHRONIC PAIN CONDITIONS

Most chronic pain conditions exact a heavy toll on patients' levels of psychosocial functioning (Turk and Flor 1987). Patients who have chronic pain conditions may benefit from behavioral therapies regardless of whether the etiology of the pain is clearly the result of known pathophysiologies. Many patients with arthritis, neuropathies, sickle cell disease, Crohn's disease, reflex sympathetic dystrophy, temporomandibular joint syndrome, and cancer-related pain may minimize analgesic use and/or increase ADLs that they are able to engage in if exposed to cognitive-behavioral treatment (Hendler 1981). The increased sense of control and increased sense of usefulness are important in improving mood and quality of life. Even for patients with somatoform pain disorders, it is this loss of control and the development of dependency and helplessness that seem to foster depression. In one national survey, 14% of the general population reported having chronic pain. However, depression occurred in less than one-fourth of those reporting chronic pain (Magni et al. 1990). The depression that is observed in patients with chronic pain usually occurs temporally with pain exacerbations (Atkinson et al. 1988; Brown 1990; Gamsa 1990; Goldberg et al. 1991; Roy et al. 1984; Rudy et al. 1988). Treatment of the chronic pain seems to resolve most cases of depression among patients with chronic pain (Kramlinger et al. 1983; Maruta et al. 1989). It is important to note, however, that patients with chronic pain often have a strong family history of depression (Magni 1987). Although treatment of a patient with depression and chronic pain with antidepressant medication will often improve mood and reported pain, it is also necessary to alter the pain behavior and cognition, with its self-debilitating impact, to achieve a relatively stable long-term outcome (Keefe et al. 1992; Pilowsky and Barrow 1990; Workman 1991; Zitman et al. 1990).

Perhaps the best studied of chronic pain conditions is low back pain. Fordyce et al. (1973) and Turk et al. (1987) recognized that the well-intended solicitousness of the interpersonal environment fosters distress and disability. When combined with the sole use of mood-modulating chronic analgesic and/or psychotropic therapies, there is a risk that this reinforcement fosters "pain behavior" (Table 34–1).

Fordyce used operant principles to extinguish pain behavior in an inpatient program and found that he could increase activity levels, decrease analgesic use, and decrease ruminative preoccupation with pain (Fordyce 1976; Fordyce et al. 1986). These insights have focused clinicians on the primary role of the patient's cognition and interpersonal environment, particularly the spouse, in maintaining pain behavior (Flor et al. 1987a, 1987b; Kerns et al. 1990). For example, increased faith in one's capacity to cope and control are associated with decreased pain intensity, lower degree of disability, and higher endorphin levels (Bandura et al. 1987; Toomey et al. 1991). In addition, attention to, rather than distraction from, chronic pain seems to foster healthy adaptation (J. A. Holmes and Stevenson 1990). Cognitive-behavioral treatment also decreases medical clinic utilization (Caudill et al. 1991).

The role of secondary gain is clearly important, too, with patients actively involved in litigation being less likely to respond to treatment. In clinical settings, premorbid personality dysfunction, the patient's perception that his or her job is emotionally unrewarding, and patients who have several traits suggested by Hackett and Bouckoms's (1987) MADISON scale are prone to prolonged, disabling pain (Table 34–2). Other important aspects of the treatment of chronic pain include monitoring of the patient's propensity for doctor shopping and analgesic and/or psychotropic dependence. Many patients with chronic pain need detoxification before treatment can begin in earnest.

Compared with no treatment, cognitive-behavioral treatment of patients with chronic low back pain decreases physical inactivity, pain, depression, hospitalizations, and analgesic and psychotropic use and increases the likelihood of return to employment (Guck et al. 1985). Compared with control subjects on waiting lists or those who are randomly assigned to control groups, patients in cognitive-behavioral programs exhibit improved mood and decreased pain-related distress, disability,

Table 34–1. Pain behavior

Dependency

Passivity

"Catastrophizing"

Attentional diversion

Avoidance of activity

Nonverbal expressiveness

Belief that the intensity of the pain is entirely uncontrollable by the patient

Anticipatory analgesic use

Table 34–2. MADISON Scale

Multiplicity	The pain occurs in more than one place or is of more than one variety. Successful treatment leads to a new pain.
Authenticity	The patient is at least as interested in your accepting the pain as real as he or she is in a cure.
Denial	The patient denies emotional problems or the impact of emotional state on pain.
Interpersonal relationships	Pain is consistently exacerbated by physical or mental presence of a significant other.
Singularity	The patient insists that his or her pain is unique in some way.
Only you	The patient treats the current physician as omniscient and omnipotent, at least initially.
Nothing helps/ No change	The pain does not vary from hour to hour, day to day, year to year, or only gets worse.

Source.   Adapted from Hackett and Bouckoms 1987.

passivity, and analgesic and psychotropic use and increased exercise tolerance, with maintenance up to 12 months (Basler and Rehfisch 1991; Peters and Large 1990; Phillips 1987).

Most patients with headache do not have life-threatening conditions. Although such patients commonly receive classification of their headaches as vascular or tension in origin, it remains unclear whether the majority of these patients truly follow different courses or merely have clinical variations of a common ailment (Bakal 1982). Cognitive-behavioral techniques represent well-established and well-studied treatment for headaches (Blanchard 1992). When compared with medication therapies (generally amitriptyline, propranolol, diazepam, or ergotamine), behavioral therapies demonstrate a roughly equivalent reduction in headache load along with reduced analgesic use and adverse effects. Even more important is that patients who undergo behavioral therapy maintain these gains for up to 3 years longer than do patients treated with standard medication therapies. The mechanisms that account for these effects are as yet unclear. The most sophisticated examination of various psychophysiological pathways (muscle tension, thermal biofeedback, vascular relaxation and contraction) seems to imply that the effect is at least partly due to attributional processes—patients who believe they are doing well at their relaxation exercises, even if incorrect, also report reduction in their headaches (Holroyd et al. 1984).

Fibromyalgia is a disorder long suspected to be associated with depression. Psychometric profiles of patients with fibromyalgia suggest that psychological abnormality is frequent and not specific to depression (Belfer et al. 1991). However, no controlled studies of psychological or psychopharmacological treatment in fibromyalgia exist.

A history of sexual abuse is common in patients seen with chronic pelvic pain (Toomey et al. 1993). Other psychological characteristics found in patients with chronic pelvic pain include vocational and social dysfunction, medical disability, somatic amplification, and emotional distress (Walker et al. 1992). Combining behavioral and medical treatment decreases pain, anxiety, and depression, and improves psychosocial, occupational, and sexual functioning (Kames et al. 1990).

◼ SUMMARY

Research in behavioral medicine interventions demonstrates that specific behavioral techniques are useful for various chronic, intractable conditions. Treatments are effective in the modification of deleterious behavior patterns, reduction in morbidity and mortality in individuals with comorbid medical conditions, and enhancement of quality of life. The integration of behavioral medicine research with psychiatric diagnostic phenomenology is a recent one. For example, psychiatry has generally ignored the importance of hostility as well as depressive symptoms in the treatment of patients with comorbid medical illnesses. Similarly, behavioral medicine has, until recently, tended to ignore the evaluation of the effect of psychiatric conditions on psychosomatic processes. Research in the area of behavioral medicine practice is needed to assess the potential effect of psychosocial interventions on offsetting the cost of medical care.

◼ REFERENCES

Abelin T, Buehler A, Muller P, et al: Controlled trial of transdermal nicotine patch in tobacco withdrawal. Lancet 1:7–10, 1989

Ader R, Felton DL, Cohen N (eds): Psychoneuroimmunology. New York, Academic Press, 1991

Ahern DK, Gorkin L, Anderson JL, et al: Biobehavioral variables and mortality or cardiac arrest in the Cardiac Arrhythmia Pilot Study (CAPS). Am J Cardiol 66:59–62, 1990

Alexander F: Psychosomatic Medicine. New York, WW Norton, 1950

American Heart Association: Heart and Stroke Facts. Dallas, TX, American Heart Association, 1991

American Psychiatric Association: Diagnostic and Statistical Manual of Mental Disorders, 4th Edition. Washington, DC, American Psychiatric Association, 1994

Anda R, Williamson D, Jones D, et al: Depressed affect, hopelessness, and the risk of ischemic heart disease in a cohort of U.S. adults. Epidemiology 4:285–294, 1993

Anderson KO, Bradley LA, Young LD, et al: Rheumatoid arthritis: review of psychological factors related to etiology, effects and treatment. Psychol Bull 98:358–387, 1985

Andrykowski MA: The role of anxiety in the development of anticipatory nausea in cancer chemotherapy: a review and synthesis. Psychosom Med 52:458–475, 1990

Antoni MH, Schneiderman N, Fletcher MA, et al: Psychoneuroimmunology and HIV-1. J Consult Clin Psychol 58:38–49, 1990

Antoni MH, Bagget L, Ironson G, et al: Cognitive-behavioral stress management intervention buffers distress responses and immunologic changes following notification of HIV-1 seropositivity. J Consult Clin Psychol 59: 906–915, 1991

Atkinson JH, Slater MA, Grant I, et al: Depression and stressful life events in chronic pain. Psychosom Med 50:198–204, 1988

Bakal DA: The Psychobiology of Chronic Headache. New York, Springer, 1982

Bandura A, O'Leary A, Taylor CB, et al: Perceived self-efficacy and pain control: opioid and nonopioid mechanisms. J Pers Soc Psychol 53:563–571, 1987

Basler HD, Rehfisch HP: Cognitive/behavioral therapy in patients with ankylosing spondylitis in a German self-help organization. J Psychosom Res 35:345–354, 1991

Beitman BD, Basha I, Flaker G, et al: Atypical or nonanginal chest pain, panic disorder or coronary artery disease? Arch Intern Med 147: 1548–1552, 1987

Belfer P, Robbins M, Goldenberg D: Fibromyalgia: psychological characteristics of individuals seeking group pain management treatment (abstract). Proceedings of the Society of Behavioral Medicine XII:141, 1991

Bell IR, Jasnoski ML, Kagan J, et al: Is allergic rhinitis more frequent in young adults with extreme shyness? Psychosom Med 52:517–525, 1990

Bennett P, Wilkinson S: A comparison of psychological and medical treatment of the irritable bowel syndrome. Br J Clin Psychol 24: 215–216, 1985

Bertolet BD, Hill JA: Unrecognized myocardial infarction, in Acute Myocardial Infarction. Edited by Pepine CJ. Philadelphia, PA, FA Davis, 1989

Blair SN, Kohl HW, Paffenberger RS, et al: Physical fitness and all-cause mortality: a prospective study. JAMA 262:2395–2401, 1989

Blanchard EB: Psychological treatment of benign headache disorders. J Consult Clin Psychol 60:537–551, 1992

Blaustein AS, Heller GV, Kolman BS: Adjunctive nifedipine therapy in high-risk, medically refractory, unstable angina pectoris. Am J Cardiol 52:950–954, 1984

Blumenthal JA, Kamarck T: Assessment of the type A behavior pattern, in Applications in Behavioral Medicine and Health Psychology: A Clinician's Source Book. Edited by Blumenthal JA, McKee DC. Sarasota, FL, Professional Resource Exchange, 1987, pp 3–39

Blumenthal JA, Williams RS, Wallace AG, et al: Physiological and psychological variables predict compliance to prescribed exercise therapy for inpatients recovering from myocardial infarction. Psychosom Med 44:519–527, 1982

Borus JF, Olendzki MC, Kessler L, et al: The "offset effect" of mental health treatment on ambulatory medical care utilization and charges. Arch Gen Psychiatry 42:573–578, 1985

Brown GK: A causal analysis of chronic pain and depression. J Abnorm Psychol 99:121–137, 1990

Budman SH, Demby A, Feldstein ML: Insight into reduced use of medical services after psychotherapy. Professional Psychology: Research and Practice 15:353–361, 1984

Cannon RO, Camici RG, Epstein SE: Pathophysiological dilemma of syndrome X. Circulation 85:883–892, 1992

Cantor A: Changes in mood during incubation of acute febrile disease and the effects of pre-exposure psychologic status. Psychosom Med 34:424–430, 1972

Carney RM, Rich MW, Friedland KE: Major depressive disorder predicts cardiac events in patients with coronary artery disease. Psychosom Med 50:627–633, 1988

Caudill M, Zuttermeister P, Benson H, et al: Decreased clinic utilization by chronic pain patients after behavioral medicine intervention (abstract). Proceedings of the Society of Behavioral Medicine XII:133, 1991

Cay EL, Vetter N, Philip AE, et al: Psychological status during recovery from an acute heart attack. J Psychosom Res 16:425–435, 1972

Cecchi RL: Stress: prodrome to immune deficiency. Ann N Y Acad Sci 437:286–289, 1984

Chesney MA, Agras WS, Benson H, et al: Nonpharmacologic approaches to the treatment of hypertension. Circulation 76 (suppl I): 104–109, 1987

Chrousos GP, Gold PW: The concepts of stress and stress system disorders. JAMA 267:1244–1252, 1992

Coates TJ, Temoshok L, Mandel J: Psychosocial research is essential to understanding and treating AIDS. Am Psychol 39:1309–1314, 1984

Coates TJ, McKusick L, Kuno R, et al: Stress reduction training changed number of sexual partners but not immune function in men with HIV. Am J Public Health 79:885–887, 1989

Cohen S, Williamson GM: Stress and infectious disease in humans. Psychol Bull 109:5–24, 1991

Cohen S, Tyrrell DAJ, Smith AP: Psychological stress and susceptibility to the common cold. N Engl J Med 325:606–612, 1991

Cox DJ, Gonder-Frederick L: Major developments in behavioral diabetes research. J Consult Clin Psychol 60:628–638, 1992

Cunningham AJ, Lockwood GA: There is simply no valid methodological alternative to randomization of subjects. Adv Cancer Res 8(2):80–82, 1992

Daniels LK: Treatment of urticaria and severe headache by behavior therapy. Psychosomatics 14:347–351, 1973

Dean C, Surtees PG: Do psychological factors predict survival in breast cancer? J Psychosom Res 33:561–569, 1989

Dembroski TM, MacDougall JM, Costa PT, et al: Components of hostility as predictors of sudden death and myocardial infarction in the Multiple Risk Factor Intervention Trial. Psychosom Med 51:514–522, 1989

Derogatis LR, Abeloff MD, Melisaratos N: Psychological coping mechanisms and survival time in metastatic breast cancer. JAMA 242: 1504–1508, 1979

Dimsdale JE: A perspective on type A behavior and coronary artery disease. N Engl J Med 318: 110–112, 1988

Dobes RW: Amelioration of psychosomatic dermatitis by reinforced inhibition of scratching. J Behav Ther Exp Psychiatry 8:185–187, 1977

Donlau JN, Wolcott MS, Gottlieb MS, et al: Psychosocial aspects of AIDS and AIDS-related complex: a pilot study. Journal of Psychosocial Oncology 3:39–55, 1985

Downing J, Littman A, Scheer J, et al: Depressive symptoms in cardiac rehabilitation patients correlates with blunted training effect (abstract). J Am Coll Cardiol 19:257A, 1992

Dressler WW, Mata A, Chavez A, et al: Social support and arterial pressure in a Central Mexican community. Psychosom Med 48:338–349, 1986

Dressler WW, Grell GA, Gallagher PN, et al: Blood pressure and social class in a Jamaican community. Am J Public Health 78:714–716, 1988

Drossman DA, Thompson WG, Talley NJ, et al: Identification of subgroups of functional gastrointestinal disorders. Gastroenterology International 3:159–172, 1990

Drossman DA, Leserman J, Mitchell CM, et al: Health status and health care use in persons with inflammatory bowel disease: a national sample. Dig Dis Sci 36:1746–1755, 1991

Duller P, Gentry WD: Use of biofeedback in treating chronic hyperhydrosis. Br J Dermatol 103:143–146, 1980

Dunbar F: Mind and Body: Psychosomatic Medicine. New York, Random House, 1947

Fava M, Littman A, Halperin P, et al: Psychological and behavioral benefits of a stress/type A reduction program for healthy middle-aged army officers. Psychosomatics 32:337–342, 1991

Fava M, Rosenbaum JF, Pava JA, et al: Anger attacks in unipolar depression, part 1: clinical correlates and response to fluoxetine treatment. Am J Psychiatry 150:1158–1163, 1993

Finnegan DL, Suler JR: Psychological factors with maintenance of improved health behaviors in postcoronary patients. J Psychol 119:81–94, 1985

Flor H, Turk DC, Scholz OB: Impact of chronic pain on the spouse: marital, emotional and physical consequences. J Psychosom Res 31:63–71, 1987a

Flor H, Kerns RD, Turk DC: The role of spouse reinforcement, perceived pain and activity levels of chronic pain patients. J Psychosom Res 31:251–259, 1987b

Fordyce WE: Behavioral Methods for Chronic Pain and Illness. St Louis, MO, CV Mosby, 1976

Fordyce WE, Fowler RS, Lehmann JF, et al: Operant conditioning in the treatment of chronic pain. Arch Phys Med Rehabil 54:399–408, 1973

Fordyce WE, Brockway JA, Bergman JA, et al: Acute back pain: a control-group comparison of behavioral versus traditional management methods. J Behav Med 9:127–140, 1986

Fox BH: LeShan's hypothesis is provocative, but is it plausible? Adv Cancer Res 8(2):82–84, 1992

Frasure-Smith N, Lesperance F, Talajic M: Depression following myocardial infarction: impact on 6-month survival. JAMA 270:1819–1825, 1993

Friedman M, Ulmer D: Treating Type A Behavior and Your Heart. New York, Fawcett-Crest, 1984

Friedman M, Thoreson CE, Gill JJ, et al: Alteration of type A behavior and reduction in cardiac recurrences in postmyocardial infarction patients. Am Heart J 108:237–248, 1984

Friedman M, Thoreson CE, Gill JJ, et al: Alteration of type A behavior and its effect on cardiac recurrences in postmyocardial infarction patients: summary results of the recurrent coronary prevention project. Am Heart J 114:483–490, 1987

Gamsa A: Is emotional disturbance a precipitator or a consequence of chronic pain? Pain 42:183–195, 1990

Garner DM, Wooley SC: Confronting the failure of behavioral and dietary treatments for obesity. Clinical Psychology Review 11:729–780, 1991

Geyer S: Life events prior to manifestation of breast cancer: a limited prospective study covering eight years before diagnosis. J Psychosom Res 35:355–363, 1991

Gill JJ, Price VA, Friedman M, et al: Reduction in type A behavior in healthy middle-aged American military officers. Am Heart J 110:503–514, 1985

Glaser R, Kiecolt-Glaser JK, Bonneau RH, et al: Stress-induced modulation of the immune response to recombinant hepatitis B vaccine. Psychosom Med 54:22–29, 1992

Goldberg GM, Kerns RD, Rosenberg R, et al: Activities, marital support and depression in chronic pain patients (abstract). Proceedings of the Society of Behavioral Medicine XII:130, 1991

Goldstein MG, Niaura R, Follick MJ, et al: Effects of behavioral skills training and schedule of nicotine gum administration on smoking cessation. Am J Psychiatry 146:56–60, 1989

Greer S, Morris T, Pettingale KW: Psychological response to breast cancer: effect on outcome. Lancet 2:785–787, 1979

Guck TP, Skultety FM, Meilman PW, et al: Multidisciplinary pain center followup study: evaluation with a nontreatment control group. Pain 21:295–306, 1985

Guthrie E, Creed F, Dawson D, et al: A controlled trial of psychological treatment for the irritable bowel syndrome. Gastroenterology 100:450–457, 1991

Hackett TP, Bouckoms A: The pain patient: evaluation and treatment, in Massachusetts General Hospital Handbook of General Hospital Psychiatry, 2nd Edition. Edited by Hackett TP, Cassem NH. Littleton, MA, PSG Publishing, 1987, pp 42–68

Hagglund KJ, Haley WE, Reveille JD, et al: Predicting individual differences in pain and functional impairment among patients with rheumatoid arthritis. Arthritis Rheum 32:851–858, 1989

Hendler N: Diagnosis and Nonsurgical Management of Chronic Pain. New York, Raven, 1981

Hlatky MA, Haney T, Barefoot JC, et al: Medical, psychological and social correlates of work disability among men with coronary artery disease. Am J Cardiol 58:911–915, 1986

Holmes CS, Hayford JT, Gonzalez JL, et al: A survey of cognitive functioning at different levels in diabetic persons. Diabetes Care 6(2):180–185, 1983

Holmes JA, Stevenson CAZ: Differential effects of avoidant and attentional coping strategies on adaptation to chronic recent onset pain. Health Psychol 9:577–584, 1990

Holroyd KA, Penzien DB, Hursey KG, et al: Change mechanisms in EMG biofeedback training: cognitive changes underlying improvements in tension headache. J Consult Clin Psychol 52:1039–1053, 1984

Hughes JR, Hatsukami D: Signs and symptoms of tobacco withdrawal. Arch Gen Psychiatry 43:289–294, 1986

Hughes JR, Miller SA: Nicotine gum to help stop smoking. JAMA 252:2855–2858, 1984

Hughes JR, Gust SW, Keenan RM, et al: Nicotine versus placebo gum in general medical practice. JAMA 261:1300–1305, 1989

Jacobs D, Blackburn H, Higgins M, et al: Report of the conference on low cholesterol: mortality associations. Circulation 86:1046–1060, 1992

Kagan J, Snidman N, Julia-Sellers M, et al: Temperament and allergic symptoms. Psychosom Med 53:332–340, 1991

Kames LD, Rapkin AJ, Naliboff BD, et al: Effectiveness of an interdisciplinary pain management program for the treatment of chronic pelvic pain. Pain 41:41–46, 1990

Katon W: The epidemiology of depression in medical care. Int J Psychiatry Med 17:93–112, 1987

Katon W, VonKorff M, Lin E, et al: Adequacy and duration of antidepressant treatment in primary care. Med Care 30:67–76, 1992

Kaufman PG, Jacob RG, Ewart CK: Hypertension intervention pooling project. Health Psychol 7(suppl):209–224, 1988

Keefe FJ, Dunsmore J, Burnett R: Behavioral and cognitive-behavioral approaches to chronic pain: recent advances and future directions. J Consult Clin Psychol 60:528–536, 1992

Kelly JA, Murphy DA: Psychological interventions with AIDS and HIV: prevention and treatment. J Consult Clin Psychol 60:576–585, 1992

Kerns RD, Haythornthwaite J, Southwick S, et al: The role of marital interaction in chronic pain and depressive symptom severity. J Psychosom Res 34:401–408, 1990

Ketterer MW: Secondary prevention of ischemic heart disease: the case for aggressive behavioral monitoring and intervention. Psychosomatics 34:478–484, 1993

Ketterer MW, Brymer J, Rhoads K, et al: Lipid-lowering therapy and violent death: is depression a culprit? Proceedings of the Academy of Psychosomatic Medicine 40:28–29, 1993

Kiecolt-Glaser JK, Glaser R: Psychoneuroimmunology: can psychological interventions moderate immunity? J Consult Clin Psychol 60:569–575, 1992

Kiecolt-Glaser JK, Glaser R, Williger D, et al: Psychosocial enhancement of immunocompetence in a geriatric population. Health Psychol 4:25–41, 1985

Kiecolt-Glaser JK, Glaser R, Strain E, et al: Modulation of cellular immunity in medical students. J Behav Med 9:5–21, 1986

Klerman GL: Depressive disorders: further evidence for increased medical morbidity and impairment of social functioning. Arch Gen Psychiatry 46:856–858, 1989

Klingelhofer EL, Gershwin KD: Asthma self management programs: premises, not promises. J Asthma 25:89–101, 1988

Kolodny RC, Masters WH, Johnson VE: Textbook of Sexual Medicine. Boston, MA, Little, Brown, 1979

Kramlinger KG, Swanson DW, Maruta T: Are patients with chronic pain depressed? Am J Psychiatry 140:747–749, 1983

Kvale G, Hugdahl K, Asbjornsen A: Anticipatory nausea and vomiting in cancer patients. J Consult Clin Psychol 59:894–898, 1991

Ladwig KH, Kieserm M, Konig J, et al: Affective disorder and survival after acute myocardial infarction: results from the post infarction late potential study. Eur Heart J 12:959–964, 1991

Lehrer PM, Sargunaraj D, Hochron S: Psychological approaches to the treatment of asthma. J Consult Clin Psychol 60:639–643, 1992

L'Enfant C, Liu BM: (Passive) smokers versus (voluntary) smokers (editorial). N Engl J Med 302:742–743, 1980

Leon AS, Connett J, Jacobs DR, et al: Leisure-time physical activity levels and risk of coronary heart disease and death: the Multiple Risk Factor Intervention Trial. JAMA 258:2388–2395, 1987

LeShan L: A new question in studying psychosocial interventions and cancer. Adv Cancer Res 7:69–71, 1991

Levenson JL, Mishra A, Hamer RM, et al: Denial and medical outcome in unstable angina. Psychosom Med 51:27–35, 1989

Levine J, Warrenburg S, Kerns R, et al: The role of denial in recovering from coronary heart disease. Psychosom Med 49:109–117, 1987

Littman AB: Prevention of disability due to cardiovascular diseases. Heart Disease and Stroke 2:274–277, 1993

Littman AB, Fava M, McKool K, et al: The use of buspirone in the treatment of stress, hostility and type A behavior in cardiac patients: an open trial. Psychother Psychosom 59:107–110, 1993

Lloyd GG, Cawley RH: Psychiatric morbidity in men one week after first acute myocardial infarction. BMJ 2:1453–1454, 1978

Lustman PJ, Frank BL, McGill JB: Relationship of personality characteristics to glucose regulation in adults with diabetes. Psychosom Med 53:305–312, 1991

Magni G: On the relationship between chronic pain and depression when there is no organic lesion. Pain 31:1–21, 1987

Magni G, di Mario F, Bernasconi G, et al: DSM-III diagnoses associated with dyspepsia of unknown cause. Am J Psychiatry 144:1222–1223, 1987

Magni G, Caldieron C, Rigatti-Luchini S, et al: Chronic musculoskeletal pain and depressive symptoms in the general population: an analysis of the first national health and nutrition examination survey data. Pain 43:299–307, 1990

Marshall PS: Allergy and depression: a neurochemical threshold model of the relation between the illnesses. Psychol Bull 113:23–43, 1993

Martin JE, Dubbert PM: Adherence to exercise, in Exercise and Sport Sciences Reviews, Vol 13. Edited by Terjung RL. New York, Macmillan, 1985, pp 137–167

Maruta T, Vatterott MK, McHardy MJ: Pain management as an antidepressant: long-term resolution of pain-associated depression. Pain 36:335–337, 1989

Mayou R: Atypical chest pain. J Psychosom Res 33:393–406, 1989

Mazze RS, Lucido D, Shamoon H: Psychological and social correlates of glycemic control. Diabetes Care 7:360–366, 1984

McClelland DC, Patel V, Brown D, et al: The role of affiliative loss in the recruitment of helper cells among insulin dependent diabetics. Behav Med 17:5–14, 1991

McLane M, Krop H, Mehta J: Psychosexual adjustment and counseling after myocardial infarction. Ann Intern Med 92:514–519, 1980

Meyer RJ, Haggerty RJ: Streptococcal infections in families. Pediatrics 29:539–549, 1962

Milani R, Littman A, Lavie C: Depressive symptoms predict functional improvement following cardiac rehabilitation and exercise program. Journal of Cardiopulmonary Rehabilitation (in press)

Morganstern H, Gellert GA, Walter SD, et al: The impact of a psychosocial support program on survival with breast cancer: the importance of selection bias in program evaluation. Journal of Chronic Diseases 37:273–276, 1984

Morrow GR, Dobkin PL: Anticipatory nausea and vomiting in cancer patients undergoing chemotherapy treatment: prevalence, etiology and behavioral interventions. Clinical Psychology Review 8:517–556, 1988

Muldoon MF, Manuck SB, Matthews KA: Lowering cholesterol concentrations and mortality: a quantitative review of primary prevention trials. BMJ 301:309–314, 1990

Murphy JM, Monson RR, Oliver DC, et al: Affective disorders and mortality. Arch Gen Psychiatry 44:473–480, 1987

Nagasawa M, Smith MC, Barnes JH, et al: Meta-analysis of correlates of diabetes patients' compliance with prescribed medications. Diabetes Educator 16:192–200, 1990

NIH Technology Assessment Conference Panel: Methods for voluntary weight loss and control. Ann Intern Med 116:942–949, 1992

Nunes EV, Frank KA, Kornfeld DS: Psychologic treatment for the type A behavior pattern and coronary artery disease: a meta-analysis of the literature. Psychosom Med 48:159–173, 1987

Oldridge NB, Guyett GH, Fischer ME, et al: Cardiac rehabilitation after myocardial infarction: combined experience of randomized clinical trials. JAMA 260:945–950, 1988

Ornish D, Brown SE, Scherwitz LW, et al: Can lifestyle changes reverse coronary heart disease? Lancet 336:129–133, 1990

Ornish D, Brown SE, Billings JH, et al: Can lifestyle changes reverse coronary atherosclerosis? Four-year results of the Lifestyle Heart Trial (abstract). Abstracts from the 66th Scientific Sessions of the American Heart Association, November 1993. Circulation 88:1–385, 1993

Patel C, Marmot MG, Terry DJ, et al: Trial of relaxation in reducing coronary risk: four year followup. BMJ 290:1103–1106, 1985

Pennebaker JW, Kiecolt-Glaser JK, Glaser R: Disclosure of traumas and immune function: health implications for psychotherapy. J Consult Clin Psychol 56:239–245, 1988

Peters JL, Large RG: A randomized control trial evaluating in and outpatient pain management programmes. Pain 41:283–293, 1990

Phillips HC: The effects of behavioral treatment on chronic pain. Behav Res Ther 25:365–377, 1987

Pilowsky I, Barrow CG: A controlled study of psychotherapy and amitriptyline used individually and in combination in the treatment of chronic intractable, "psychogenic" pain. Pain 40:3–19, 1990

Powell KE, Thompson PD, Casperson CJ, et al: Physical activity and the incidence of coronary artery disease. Annu Rev Public Health 8:253–287, 1987

Rabkin JG, Williams JBW, Remien RH: Depression, distress, lymphocyte subsets and human immunodeficiency virus symptoms on two occasions in HIV-positive homosexual men. Arch Gen Psychiatry 48:111–119, 1991

Radnitz CL, Blanchard EB: Bowel sound biofeedback as a treatment for irritable bowel syndrome. Biofeedback Self Regul 13:169–179, 1988

Robinson N, Fuller JH: Severe life events and their relationship to the etiology of insulin-dependent (type I) diabetes mellitus. Pediatric Adolescent Endocrinology 15:129–133, 1986

Rosen JC, Wiens AN: Changes in medical problems and use of medical services following psychological intervention. Am Psychol 34:420–431, 1979

Roy R, Thomas M, Matas M: Chronic pain and depression: a review. Compr Psychiatry 25:96–103, 1984

Rubins PV, Harris K, Koven S: High fatality rates of late life depression associated with cardiovascular disease. J Affect Disord 9:165–167, 1985

Rudy TE, Kerns RD, Turk DC: Chronic pain and depression: toward a cognitive-behavioral mediation model. Pain 34:53–60, 1988

Schachter S: Recidivism and self-cure of smoking and obesity. Am Psychol 37:436–444, 1982

Schmiedler R, Freidrich G, Neus H, et al: The influence of beta blockers on cardiovascular reactivity and type A behavior pattern in hypertensives. Psychosom Med 45:417–423, 1983

Schwartz GE, Weiss SM: Behavioral medicine revisited: an amended definition. J Behav Med 1:249–251, 1978

Schwartz JL: Review and evaluation of smoking cessation methods: the United States and Canada, 1978–1985. U.S. DHHS Public Health Service, NIH Publication No 87–2940, U.S. Government Printing Office, Washington, DC, 1987

Shekelle RB, Hulley SB, Neaton JD, et al and the MRFIT Research Group: The MRFIT behavior pattern study. Am J Epidemiol 122:559–570, 1985

Shell WE, Swan HJC: Treatment of silent myocardial ischemia with transdermal nitroglycerine added to beta-blockers and alprazolam. Cardiol Clin 4:697–704, 1986

Shopland D: The Health Consequences of Smoking: Chronic Obstructive Lung Disease: A Report of the Surgeon General. USDHEW Publication PHS-84-50205. Washington, DC, U.S. Government Printing Office, 1984

Sly RM: Mortality from asthma: 1979–1984. J Allergy Clin Immunol 82:705–717, 1988

Solomon GF, Temoshok L: A psychoneuroimmunologic perspective on AIDS research: questions, preliminary findings and suggestions. Journal of Applied Social Psychology 17:286–308, 1987

Spiegel D: Our goal is to see to it that every cancer patient who wants it has access to supportive/expressive therapy. Adv Cancer Res 8:85–86, 1992

Spiegel D, Bloom JR, Kraemer HC, et al: Effect of psychosocial treatment on survival of patients with metastatic breast cancer. Lancet 2:888–891, 1989

Stern M, Pascale L, McLoone J: Psychosocial adaptation following an acute myocardial infarction. Journal of Chronic Diseases 29:513–526, 1976

Stunkard AJ (ed): Obesity. Philadelphia, PA, WB Saunders, 1980

Stunkard AJ, Harris JR, Pederson NL, et al: The body mass index of twins who have been reared apart. N Engl J Med 322:1483–1487, 1990

Suls J, Fletcher B: The relative efficacy of avoidant and nonavoidant coping strategies: a meta-analysis. Health Psychol 4:249–288, 1985

Svedlund J, Sjodin I, Ottosson JO, et al: Controlled study of psychotherapy in irritable bowel syndrome. Lancet 2:589–592, 1983

Thompson DR, Meddis R: Wives' responses to counseling early after myocardial infarction. J Psychosom Res 34:249–258, 1990

Toomey TC, Mann JD, Abashian S, et al: Relationship between perceived self-control of pain, pain description and functioning. Pain 45:129–133, 1991

Toomey TC, Hernandez JT, Gittelman DF, et al: Relationship of sexual and physical abuse to pain and psychological assessment variables in chronic pelvic pain patients. Pain 53:105–109, 1993 [comment in Pain 56:361, 1994]

Trials of Hypertension Prevention Collaborative Research Group. The effects of nonpharmacologic interventions on blood pressure of persons with high normal levels. JAMA 267:1213–1220, 1992

Turk DC, Flor H: Pain and pain behaviors: the utility and limitations of the pain behavior construct. Pain 31:277–295, 1987

Turk DC, Flor H, Rudy TE: Pain and families, I: etiology, maintenance and psychosocial impact. Pain 30:3–27, 1987

Vlietstra RE, Kronmal RA, Oberman A, et al: Effect of cigarette smoking on survival of patients with angiographically documented coronary artery disease. JAMA 255:1023–1027, 1986

Von Korff M, Ormel J, Katon W, et al: Disability and depression among distressed high utilizers of healthcare. Arch Gen Psychiatry 49:91–100, 1992

Walker EA, Katon WJ, Neraas K, et al: Dissociation in women with chronic pelvic pain. Am J Psychiatry 149:534–537, 1992

Wells KB, Stewart A, Hays RD, et al: The functioning and well-being of depressed patients: results from the Medical Outcome Study. JAMA 262:914–919, 1989

Whitehead WE: Behavioral medicine approaches to gastrointestinal disorders. J Consult Clin Psychol 60:605–612, 1992

Whitehead WE, Bosmajian LS: Behavioral medicine approaches to gastrointestinal disorders. J Consult Clin Psychol 50:672–683, 1982

Whorell PJ, Prior A, Faragher EB: Controlled trial of hypnotherapy in the treatment of severe refractory irritable bowel syndrome. Lancet 2:1232–1234, 1984

Williams RB, Schanberg SM, Kuhn CM, et al: Influence of alprazolam on neuroendocrine and cardiovascular response to stress in type A men. Paper presented at the annual meeting of the American College of Neuropsychopharmacology, Washington, DC, September 1986

Wishnie HA, Hackett TP, Cassem NH: Psychological hazards of convalescence following myocardial infarction. JAMA 215:1292–1296, 1971

Wood PD, Stefanick ML, Dreon DM, et al: Changes in plasma lipids and lipoproteins in overweight men during weight loss through dieting as compared with exercise. N Engl J Med 319:1173–1179, 1988

Workman EA: Multimodal treatment of chronic pain: combining medical and behavioral interventions (abstract). Proceedings of the Society of Behavioral Medicine XII:132, 1991

Young LD: Psychological factors in rheumatoid arthritis. J Consult Clin Psychol 60:619–627, 1992

Zitman FG, Linssen ACG, Edelbroek PM, et al: Low dose amitriptyline in chronic pain: the gain is modest. Pain 42:35–42, 1990

Index

Page numbers printed in **boldface** type refer to tables or figures.